PROGRESS IN BRAIN RESEARCH

VOLUME 58

MOLECULAR AND CELLULAR INTERACTIONS
UNDERLYING HIGHER BRAIN FUNCTIONS

Recent volumes in PROGRESS IN BRAIN RESEARCH

PROGRESS IN BRAIN RESEARCH

VOLUME 58

MOLECULAR AND CELLULAR INTERACTIONS UNDERLYING HIGHER BRAIN FUNCTIONS

Proceedings of the 9th Meeting of the International Neurobiology Society, held at the Abbaye Royale de Fontevraud (France), on September 1–4, 1981

EDITED BY

J.-P. CHANGEUX

Collège de France and Institut Pasteur, 75724 Paris Cédex 15 (France)

J. GLOWINSKI

Collège de France, 75231 Paris Cédex 05 (France)

M. IMBERT

Collège de France, 75231 Paris Cédex 05 (France)

and

F.E. BLOOM

The Salk Institute, San Diego, CA 92138 (U.S.A.)

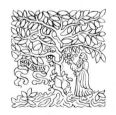

ELSEVIER SCIENCE PUBLISHERS B.V.
AMSTERDAM — NEW YORK
1983

PUBLISHED BY:
ELSEVIER BIOMEDICAL PRESS
1 MOLENWERF, P.O. BOX 211
AMSTERDAM, THE NETHERLANDS

SOLE DISTRIBUTOR FOR THE U.S.A. AND CANADA:
ELSEVIER SCIENCE PUBLISHING CO. INC.
52 VANDERBILT AVENUE
NEW YORK, NY 10017, U.S.A.

ISBN FOR THE SERIES 0-444-80104-9
ISBN FOR THE VOLUME 0-444-80432-3

Library of Congress Cataloging in Publication Data

International Neurobiology Society.   Meeting (9th :
    1981 : Abbaye de Fontevrault)
    Molecular and cellular interactions underlying higher
brain functions.

    (Progress in brain research ; v. 58)
    Includes index.
    1. Higher nervous activity--Congresses.   2. Neural
transmission--Congresses.   3. Cytoarchitectonics--
Congresses.   4. Developmental neurology--Congresses.
I. Changeux, Jean-Pierre. II. Title. III. Series.
[DNLM: 1. Higher nervous activity--Congresses.   2. Cell
communication--Congresses.   3. Central nervous system--
Anatomy and histology--Congresses.   4. Central nervous
system--Growth and development--Congresses.   W1 PR667J

v. 58 / WL 102 I6196 1981m]
QP376.P7 vol. 58 [QP395]   599'.0188   83-5521
ISBN 0-444-80432-3

WITH 182 ILLUSTRATIONS AND 16 TABLES

PRINTED IN THE NETHERLANDS

List of Contributors

W.B. Adams, Friedrich Miescher-Institut, P.O. Box 273, CH-4002 Basel, Switzerland

P. Andersen, Institute of Neurophysiology, University of Oslo, Norway

D.J. Anderson, Laboratory of Cell Biology, The Rockefeller University, New York, NY 10021, U.S.A.

D. Aunis, Unité INSERM U-44, Centre de Neurochimie, 5 rue Blaise Pascal, F-67084 Strasbourg Cédex, France

M.-F. Bader, Unité INSERM U-44, Centre de Neurochimie, 5 rue Blaise Pascal, F-67084 Strasbourg Cédex, France

C.A. Barnes, Institute of Neurophysiology, University of Oslo, Norway

B. Berger, INSERM U. 134, Laboratoire de Neuropathologie Charles Foix, Hôpital Salpétrière, 75651 Paris Cédex 13, France

P. Bernd, Department of Pharmacology, NYU School of Medicine, 550 First Avenue, New York, NY 10016, U.S.A.

D.M. Berson, Division of Biology and Medicine, Brown University, Providence, RI 02912, U.S.A.

M.M. Black, Department of Pharmacology, NYU School of Medicine, 550 First Avenue, New York, NY 10016, U.S.A.

G. Blobel, Laboratory of Cell Biology, The Rockefeller University, New York, NY 10021, U.S.A.

F.E. Bloom, Arthur V. Davis Center for Behavioral Neurobiology, The Salk Institute, P.O. Box 85800, San Diego, CA 92138, U.S.A.

B.B. Boycott, Medical Research Council Cell Biophysics Unit, King's College, 26–29 Drury Lane, London WC2B 5RL, U.K.

Y. Burnod, INSERM U3, CNRS, Hôpital Salpétrière, 47 Bd. Hôpital, Paris, France

D.E. Burnstein, Department of Pathology, NYU School of Medicine, 550 First Avenue, New York, NY 10016, U.S.A.

J. Calvet, INSERM U3, CNRS, Hôpital Salpétrière, 47 Bd. Hôpital, Paris, France

S. Chang, Department of Biological Sciences, Stanford University, Stanford, CA 94305, U.S.A.

J.-P. Changeux, Collège de France and Neurobiologie Moléculaire, Laboratoire associé au Centre National de la Recherche Scientifique, Interactions Moléculaires et Cellulaires, Institut Pasteur, 25, rue du Docteur Roux, 75015 Paris, France

G. Chevalier, Laboratoire de Physiologie des Centres Nerveux, Université Pierre et Marie Curie, 4, place Jussieu, 75230 Paris Cédex 5, France

J. Ciesielski-Treska, Unité INSERM U-44, Centre de Neurochimie, 5 rue Blaise Pascal, F-67084 Strasbourg Cédex, France

J.L. Connolly, Department of Pathology, Harvard Medical School, Boston, MA 02215, U.S.A.

M.-C. Daguet, INSERM U 114, Collège de France, 11, place Marcelin Berthelot, 75231 Paris Cédex 05, France

J.M. Deniau, Laboratoire de Physiologie des Centres Nerveux, Université Pierre et Marie Curie, 4, place Jussieu, 75230 Paris Cédex 5, France

U. Di Porzio, Laboratorio Embriologia Molecolare, Via Toiano 2, Arco Felice, Napoli, Italy

D.S. Faber, Division of Neurobiology, Department of Physiology, SUNY at Buffalo, Buffalo, NY, U.S.A.

B. Fass, Department of Physiology, University of Virginia School of Medicine, Charlottesville, VA 22098, U.S.A.

E. Fenwick, Max-Planck-Institut für biophysikalische Chemie, Postfach 968, D-3400 Göttingen, F.R.G.

A. Ferron, Groupe NB INSERM U 114, Collège de France, 11, place Marcelin Berthelot, 75231 Paris Cédex 05, France

R. Fischer-Colbrie, Department of Pharmacology, Univ. of Innsbruck, A-6020, Innsbruck, Austria

Y. Fregnac, Laboratoire de Neurobiologie du Développement, Bâtiment 440, Université de Paris-Sud, 91405 Orsay Cédex, France

A.G. Garcia, Department of Pharmacology and Experimental Therapeutics, Medicine Faculty, Autonomous University, Arzobispo Morcillo 1, Madrid 32, Spain

S. Ghandour, Centre de Neurochimie du CNRS, F-67084 Strasbourg Cédex, France

A. Ghysen, Laboratoire de Génétique, Université Libre de Bruxelles, 67, rue des Chevaux, 1640 Rhode-St-Genèse, Belgium

C.D. Gilbert, Department of Neurobiology, Harvard Medical School, Boston, MA 02115, U.S.A.

J. Glowinski, Groupe NB INSERM U 114, Collège de France, 11, place Marcelin Berthelot, 75231 Paris Cédex 05, France

P.S. Goldman-Rakic, Section of Neuroanatomy, Yale University School of Medicine, 333 Cedar Street, New Haven, CT 06510, U.S.A.

G. Gombos, Centre de Neurochimie du CNRS, F-67084 Strasbourg Cédex, France

C.S. Goodman, Department of Biological Sciences, Stanford University, Stanford, CA 94305, U.S.A.

C. Goridis, Centre d'Immunologie INSERM-CNRS de Marseille-Luminy, Case 906, F-13288 Marseille Cédex 9, France

M. Gray, INSERM U. 134, Laboratoire de Neuropathologie Charles Foix, Hôpital Salpétrière, 75651 Paris Cédex 13, France

A.M. Graybiel, Department of Psychology and Brain Science, Massachusetts Institute of Technology, Cambridge, MA 02139, U.S.A.

L.A. Greene, Department of Pharmacology, NYU School of Medicine, 550 First Avenue, New York, NY 10016, U.S.A.

C.E. Henderson, Institut Pasteur, Neurobiologie Moléculaire, 25 rue du Docteur Roux, 75015 Paris, France

A. Herbet, INSERM U 114, Collège de France, 11, place Marcelin Berthelot, 75231 Paris Cédex 05, France

M. Hirn, Centre d'Immunologie INSERM-CNRS de Marseille-Luminy, Case 906, F-13288 Marseille Cédex 9, France

R. Ho, Department of Biological Sciences, Stanford University, Stanford, CA 94305, U.S.A.

C.E. Holt, MRC Biophysics Unit, King's College, London University, 26–29 Drury Lane, London WC2B 5RL, U.K.

O. Hornykiewicz, Institute of Biochemical Pharmacology, University of Vienna, A-1090 Vienna, Austria

H. Hörtnagl, Institute of Biochemical Pharmacology, University of Vienna, A-1090 Vienna, Austria

E. Hösli, Department of Physiology, University of Basel, Vesalgasse 1, CH-4051 Basel, Switzerland

L. Hösli, Department of Physiology, University of Basel, Vesalgasse 1, CH-4051 Basel, Switzerland

M. Imbert, Laboratoire de Neurobiologie du Développement, Bâtiment 440, Université de Paris-Sud, 91405 Orsay Cédex, France

L.Y. Jan, Department of Physiology, School of Medicine, University of California, San Francisco, CA 94143, U.S.A.

Y.N. Jan, Department of Physiology, School of Medicine, University of California, San Francisco, CA 94143, U.S.A.

H. Korn, INSERM U3, CHU Pitié Salpétrière, 91 Blvd. de l'Hôpital, Paris B, France

O.K. Langley, Centre de Neurochimie du CNRS, F-67084 Strasbourg Cédex, France

I.A. Langmoen, Institute of Neurophysiology, University of Oslo, Karl Johansgt. 47, Oslo, Norway

J.R. Lemos, Friedrich Miescher-Institut, P.O. Box 273, CH-4002 Basel, Switzerland

I.B. Levitan, Friedrich Miescher-Institut, P.O. Box 273, CH-4002 Basel, Switzerland

A. Limat, Friedrich Miescher-Institut, P.O. Box 2534, CH-4002 Basel, Switzerland

C. Llorens Cortes, Unité 109 de Neurobiologie, Centre Paul Broca de l'INSERM, 2ter, rue d'Alésia, 75014 Paris, France

J. Mariani, Département de Biologie Moléculaire, Institut Pasteur, Paris Cédex 15, France

A. Marty, Max-Planck-Institut für biophysikalische Chemie, Postfach 968, D-3400 Göttingen, F.R.G.

K.A.C. Martin, Department of Experimental Psychology, South Parks Road, Oxford, OX1 3UD, U.K.

B. Maton, INSERM U3, CNRS, Hôpital Salpétrière, 47 Bd. Hôpital, Paris, France

W.D. Matthew, Department of Physiology, University of California, San Francisco, CA 94143, U.S.A.

B.L. McNaughton, Department of Anatomy, University College London, Gower Street, London WC1E 6BT, U.K.

D. Monard, Friedrich Miescher-Institut, P.O. Box 2534, CH-4002 Basel, Switzerland

N. Morel, Département de Neurochimie, Neurobiologie Cellulaire, CNRS, 91190 Gif-sur-Yvette, France

I.G. Morgan, Department of Behavioural Biology, Research School of Biological Sciences, Australian National University, P.O. Box 475, Canberra City, ACT 2601, Australia

E. Neher, Max-Planck-Institut für biophysikalische Chemie, Postfach 968, D-3400 Göttingen, F.R.G.

J. Nicolet, INSERM U3, CHU Pitié-Salpétrière, 91 Bd. de l'Hôpital, 75634 Paris Cédex 13, France

E. Niday, Friedrich Miescher-Institut, P.O. Box 2534, CH-4002 Basel, Switzerland

I. Novak-Hofer, Friedrich Miescher-Institut, P.O. Box 273, CH-4002 Basel, Switzerland

J. O'Keefe, Cerebral Functions Group, Department of Anatomy, University College London, Gower Street, London WC1E 6BT, U.K.

C.R. Olson, Department of Psychology and Brain Science, Massachusetts Institute of Technology, Cambridge, MA 02139, U.S.A.

R. Parvari, Department of Neurobiology, The Weizmann Institute of Science, Rehovot, Israel

L. Peichl, Max-Planck-Institut für Hirnforschung, Deutschordenstr. 46, D-6000 Frankfurt 71, F.R.G.

V.H. Perry, Department of Experimental Psychology, South Parks Road, Oxford OX1 3UD, U.K.

H. Pollard, Unité 109 de Neurobiologie, Centre Paul Broca de l'INSERM, 2ter, rue d'Alésia, 75014 Paris, France

A. Prochiantz, INSERM U 114, Collège de France, 11, place Marcelin Berthelot, 75231 Paris Cédex 05, France

T.T. Quach, Unité 109 de Neurobiologie, Centre Paul Broca de l'INSERM, 2ter, rue d'Alésia, 75014 Paris, France

G. Rager, Institut für Anatomie und spezielle Embryologie I, rue Gockel, CH-1700 Fribourg, Switzerland

P. Rakic, Section of Neuroanatomy, Yale University School of Medicine, 333 Cedar Street, New Haven, CT 06510, U.S.A.

J.A. Raper, Department of Biological Sciences, Stanford University, Stanford, CA 94305, U.S.A.

L.F. Reichardt, Department of Physiology, University of California, San Francisco, CA 94143, U.S.A.

C. Rose, Unité 109 de Neurobiologie, Centre Paul Broca de l'INSERM, 2ter, rue d'Alésia, 75014 Paris, France

A. Rukenstein, Department of Pharmacology, NYU School of Medicine, 550 First Avenue, New York, NY 10016, U.S.A.

E. Schlögl, Institute of Biochemical Pharmacology, University of Vienna, A-1090 Vienna, Austria

W. Schmidt, Department of Pharmacology, University of Innsbruck, A-6020, Innsbruck, Austria

J.-C. Schwartz, Unité 109 de Neurobiologie, Centre Paul Broca de l'INSERM, 2ter, rue d'Alésia, 75014 Paris, France

P.J. Seeley, Department of Pharmacology, NYU School of Medicine, 550 First Avenue, New York, NY 10016, U.S.A.

M.M. Segal, Center for Neurobiology and Behavior, Physiology Department, College of Physicians and Surgeons, Columbia University, 722 W. 168th Street, New York, NY 10032, U.S.A.

I. Silman, Department of Neurobiology, The Weizmann Institute of Science, Rehovot, Israel

F. Solomon, Department of Biology and Center for Cancer Research, MIT, Cambridge, MA 02139, U.S.A.

H. Soreq, Department of Neurobiology, The Weizmann Institute of Science, Rehovot, Israel

G. Sperk, Institute of Biochemical Pharmacology, University of Vienna, A-1090 Vienna, Austria

G.S. Stent, Department of Molecular Biology, University of California, Berkeley, CA 94720, U.S.A.

O. Steward, Department of Neurosurgery, University of Virginia School of Medicine, Charlottesville, VA 22098, U.S.A.

E. Teugels, Laboratoire de Génétique, Université Libre de Bruxelles, 67, rue des Chevaux, 1640 Rhode-St-Genèse, Belgium

A.M. Thierry, Groupe NB INSERM U 114, Collège de France, 11, place Marcelin Berthelot, 75231 Paris Cédex 05, France

D. Thierse, Unité INSERM U-44, Centre de Neurochimie, 5 rue Blaise Pascal, F-67084 Strasbourg Cédex, France

A. Triller, INSERM U3, CHU Pitié-Salpétrière, 91 Bd. de l'Hôpital, 75634 Paris Cédex 13, France

C. Verney, INSERM U. 154, Hôpital Saint Vincent de Paul, 74 avenue Denfert-Rochereau, 75674 Paris Cédex 14, France

A. Vigny, Institut de Biologie physico-chimique, 12 rue Pierre Curie, 75005 Paris, France

H. Wässle, Max-Planck-Institut für Hirnforschung, Deutschordenstr, 46, D-6000 Frankfurt 91, F.R.G.

A. Weber, Department of Pharmacology, Univ. of Innsbruck, A-6020, Innsbruck, Austria

D.A. Weisblat, Department of Molecular Biology, University of California, Berkeley, CA 94720, U.S.A.

T.N. Wiesel, Department of Neurobiology, Harvard Medical School, Boston, MA 02115, U.S.A.

H. Winkler, Department of Pharmacology, University of Innsbruck, A-6020 Innsbruck, Austria

S. Zeki, Department of Anatomy, University College London, Gower Street, London WC1E 6BT, U.K.

Preface

This volume constitutes the proceedings of the 9th Meeting of the International Neurobiology Society on ''Molecular and Cellular Interactions Underlying Higher Brain Functions'', held at the Abbaye Royale de Fontevraud (France) from September 1 to 4, 1981.

The organizing committee consisted of Drs. Jean-Pierre Changeux, Jacques Glowinski, Michel Imbert (all France) and Floyd Bloom (San Diego, CA, U.S.A.). About 110 participants from 13 countries attended the meeting.

The meeting could not have been held without the generous support of several organizations. It is a pleasure to acknowledge, with gratitude, the financial assistance given by the following:

Centre National de la Recherche Scientifique,
Fondation Hugot du Collège de France,
Laboratoire SPECIA.

Jean-Pierre Changeux
Jacques Glowinski
Michel Imbert
Floyd Bloom

**Dedicated
to the memory of
Stephen Kuffler**

Contents

Section III — Rules of Development of the Central Nervous System

xvi

SECTION I

Molecular Mechanisms of
Information Transfer

Chemical Communication in the CNS: Neurotransmitters and Their Function

FLOYD E. BLOOM

Arthur V. Davis Center for Behavioral Neurobiology, The Salk Institute, P.O. Box 85800, San Diego, CA 92138 (U.S.A.)

INTRODUCTION

In considering current work on neurotransmitters at least four major categories of information merit our attention. First, there is the process of transmitter discovery, and the likelihood that future application of molecular genetics methods may accelerate and broaden the search for those neurotransmitters which await discovery (see Bloom, 1981; Baxter this volume). Second, there are the cellular strategies by which already discovered transmitters are localized, and their mechanisms of cell–cell communication expressed. From these sorts of studies the spatial and functional domains over which specific transmitters operate can be characterized and contrasted (see Bloom, 1979; Siggins and Bloom, 1981). Third, are parallel molecular level studies which for some transmitters permit biochemical assessment of functions other than direct electrophysiological regulation of target cells and which may represent other facets of a set of holistic actions. Finally, a fourth body of work attempts to relate cellular and molecular actions of transmitters to regulation of behaviors. In this essay I will briefly comment on the metabolic properties of the presumed cortical transmitter vasoactive intestinal polypeptide (VIP), and on the mechanisms possibly underlying the behavioral effects of arginine-vasopressin (AVP) a hypothalamic peptide presumed to operate as a neurotransmitter as well as in a more classical endocrine hormone role.

METABOLIC ACTIONS OF PRESUMPTIVE TRANSMITTERS: VIP

VIP is a 28 amino acid polypeptide first isolated from porcine intestine by Said and Mutt (1970). It shares structural homologies with other gastrointestinal peptides such as glucagon, secretin and gastric inhibitory peptide. Biological effects range from systemic vasodilatation, increased cardiac output and hyperglycemia, to smooth muscle relaxation, regulation of secretory processes in the gastrointestinal tract and stimulation of glycogenolysis in liver slices (see Said, 1980). VIP-immunoreactive material occurs in highest concentration in cerebral cortex; here neurons with VIP-like immunoreactivity release the peptide in vitro. Furthermore, brain membranes specifically bind radiolabeled VIP (Taylor and Pert, 1979) and a VIP-stimulated adenylate cyclase has been identified in various areas of the central

[3]

nervous system (Quik et al., 1978; Deschodt-Lanckman et al., 1977). We have employed the method of Quach et al. (1978) to determine whether cortical actions of VIP include evidence of metabolic control functions such as glycogenolysis (Magistretti et al., 1981).

Effects of VIP on [³H]glycogen levels

On incubations in vitro, mouse brain slices incorporate glucose; the [³H]glycogen content increases linearly during 30 min of incubation. VIP 10^{-7} M, added after 30 min of incubation, induces a rapid fall in the [³H]glycogen content. This glycogenolytic action of VIP was concentration-dependent. The Eadie–Hofstee plot of the dose–response curve yields an EC_{50} of 26 nM and a maximal glycogenolytic effect of 77% of basal levels (correlation coefficient of regression line: 0.992).

Effects of other substances on [³H]glycogen levels

Norepinephrine (NE) also displays glycogenolytic action as shown by Quach et al. (1978) and confirmed by us (Magistretti et al., 1981). An Eadie–Hofstee plot of the dose–response curve gives an EC_{50} of 500 nM and a maximal glycogenolytic effect of 70.5% of basal levels (correlation coefficient of regression line: 0.972). Secretin at a 5×10^{-7} M concentration also decreased the [³H]glycogen content of the slices to 40.6% of basal levels (Table I). Glucagon had no glycogenolytic effect. Other putative cortical neurotransmitters, such as γ-aminobutyric acid (GABA), glutamic acid, aspartic acid and somatostatin did not decrease the [³H]glycogen levels in the slices (Table I). Carbamylcholine, a cholinergic agonist, was similarly inactive (Table I). Preliminary results indicate that somatostatin does not antagonize the glycogenolytic effect induced by VIP.

Interactions between VIP and NE

The decrease in [³H]glycogen levels induced by 10^{-6} M NE was effectively blocked ($P < 0.01$) by D, L-propranolol, 10^{-5} M, a β-adrenergic antagonist (Table I).

TABLE I

P = statistical significance assessed by one way analysis of variance, followed by paired comparisons with a Newman–Keul test. Tests here based on quadruplicate results from one series; similar results obtained in 2–4 replicate series. (Data from Magistretti et al., 1981.)

Drug tested (M)	% Glycogenolysis	P
VIP (5×10^{-7} M)	66.5	<0.01
NE (10^{-6} M)	60.9	<0.01
NE + VIP	64.4	<0.01
NE + propranolol (10^{-5} M)	12.9	n.s.
VIP + propranolol	64.4	<0.01
Propranolol (10^{-5} M)	−1.2	n.s.
Secretin (5×10^{-7} M)	40.6	<0.01
No effects at 10^{-5} M		
GABA, Glu, Asp, carbamylcholine		
Somatostatin, glucagon		

In contrast to this result, D,L-propranolol did not antagonize the glycogenolytic action of VIP, 10^{-7} M. The β-adrenergic blocker did not affect the [^{3}H]glycogen levels when tested alone.

No significant difference in the glycogenolytic effect of 10^{-7} M VIP was apparent between mice in which an 85% depletion in cortical NE was induced by intracisternal 6-hydroxydopamine (6-OHDA) injection and control mice. Finally, VIP and NE tested together at supramaximal concentrations showed no additive effects (Table I).

Thus, among the various putative neurotransmitters tested, only VIP and NE had an effect on [^{3}H]glycogen levels: they induced a concentration-dependent hydrolysis of the newly synthesized [^{3}H]polysaccharide. The EC_{50} for this effect was 26 nM for VIP and 500 nM for NE. The maximal [^{3}H]glycogen hydrolysis induced by both neurotransmitters was 75–80% of basal levels. A common feature which distinguishes NE and VIP from other cortical neurotransmitters is their ability to stimulate the membrane-bound enzyme adenylate cyclase. This action suggests a possible molecular mechanism responsible for the glycogenolytic action of the two substances. Quach et al. (1978) have demonstrated that the effect of NE on [^{3}H]glycogen levels was potentiated by the phosphodiesterase inhibitor isobutyl-methylxanthine (IBMX) and mimicked by dibutyryl-cyclic-AMP. In our studies, the effect of VIP also was potentiated by IBMX (see Magistretti et al., 1981), suggesting that the glycogenolytic action of the peptide was mediated by cyclic AMP. Glycogen hydrolysis induced by the two cortical neurotransmitters, will result in an increased glucose availability for the generation of phosphate-bound energy in those cellular elements receiving terminals from VIP and NE neurons. This similar action of the two neurotransmitters at the cellular level is particularly interesting, given the neuronal organization of the cortical noradrenergic and VIP systems. Recently we have obtained a detailed immunohistochemical characterization of the cortical VIP neurons; our observations indicate that individual VIP neurons extend across the entire vertical thickness of the cerebral cortex, but arborize in a narrow radial column with minimal branching in the horizontal plane. This orthogonal pattern of spatial organization, confers upon the VIP neuron the capacity to regulate energy metabolism locally, within individual columnar modules. This anatomical profile for VIP contrasts with the mainly tangential organization of the coeruleo-cortical noradrenergic projection, which thus has spatial capacity to exert similar metabolic actions more globally, throughout a vast expanse of cortex. More detailed electrophysiological observations are needed to determine whether NE and VIP share other functional effects on target cell activity (see Bloom, 1979). However, VIP and NE do display similar glycogenolytic actions in peripheral tissues. This shared action may indicate that certain substances, with specific hormonal roles in several cell systems, may also exert the same homeostatic functions at the cellular level within the central nervous system, where their effects are constrained by the spatio-temporal function precision inherent to neural transmission.

VASOPRESSIN AND BEHAVIORAL REGULATION IN THE RAT

Substantial evidence exists to support the hypothesis that neurohypophyseal hormones, in addition to integrating fluid volume, blood pressure, and temperature, may also be involved in adaptive behavior, perhaps even "memory". In early work,

TABLE II

Effects of arginine-vasopressin and a peptide antagonist of arginine-vasopressin and a peptide antagonist on the rate of extinction of active avoidance responding

(Results from Koob et al., 1981.)

Experimental condition	*Mean number avoidance responses (±S.E.M.)*
First extinction trial	7.98 ± 0.15 (27)
Second extinction trial (2 h)	
Saline + saline	5.65 ± 0.65
Saline + 6 μg AVP	6.25 ± 0.75
dPTyr-(Me)AVP + AVP	5.65 ± 0.65
Third extinction trial (4 h)	
Saline + saline	2.80 ± 0.7
Saline + 6 μg AVP	6.05 ± 0.5*
dPTyr-(Me)AVP + AVP	2.65 ± 0.4
Fourth extinction trial (6 h)	
Saline + saline	1.75 ± 0.7
Saline + 6 μg AVP	6.20 ± 0.7*
dPTyr-(Me)AVP + AVP	1.55 ± 0.7

* Results significantly different from control (saline) or AVP + dPTyr-(Me)AVP injected rats.

hypophysectomized rats were found deficient in a number of behavioral situations, especially the acquisition and extinction of aversively motivated tasks (see De Wied, 1980 for review). These deficiencies were reversible by administration of a crude pituitary extract, Pitressin, and in later work by arginine-vasopressin (AVP) in microgram amounts injected subcutaneously. Furthermore, lysine-vasopressin delayed extinction in an active avoidance task in intact animals and improved retention of a passive avoidance task. In more recent work, intraventricular injection of nanogram quantities of AVP significantly delayed extinction of the active avoidance response (De Wied, 1976), while anti-vasopressin serum inhibited the retention in the passive avoidance test (Van Wimersma Greidanus et al., 1975).

We have sought to reproduce and extend some of the findings of De Wied and his colleagues regarding the effects of vasopressin on learned behavior. More specifically, we sought to examine the effects of both subcutaneous and intraventricular injection of vasopressin and a new vasopressin antagonist on the extinction of an active avoidance response (see Table II). Our methods and detailed results are reported elsewhere (Le Moal et al., 1981; Koob et al., 1981).

BEHAVIORAL EFFECTS OF ARGININE VASOPRESSIN AND THE VASOPRESSIN ANTAGONIST PEPTIDE dPTyr-(Me)AVP

Injection of 1 μg AVP subcutaneously after the first 10 extinction trials significantly prolonged the extinction of the avoidance response. Similar effects were seen with intraventricular injections of AVP. At a dose of 1 ng, AVP again significantly prolonged extinction of the avoidance response. However, higher doses of AVP failed to produce this effect and the highest dose (50 ng/rat) actually produced a more rapid extinction.

To test for actions of the AVP antagonist peptide (Bankoski et al., 1978) shock levels were augmented to produce greater resistance to extinction in the control (saline injected) rats. Subcutaneous injection of [1-deaminopenicillamine-2-(O-methyl)-tyrosine]arginine-vasopressin (dPTyr-(Me)AVP) produced a dose-dependent facilitation (more rapid) of extinction of the avoidance response; this effect reached significance at 100 μg/rat. However, in contrast to the results seen with intraventricular injection of AVP itself, dPTyr-(Me)AVP failed to significantly alter extinction after intraventricular injection except at the highest dose, 10 μg/rat (see Koob et al., 1981).

Despite these data suggesting a vasopressin action on behavior of extraordinarily long duration presumably elicited wholly within the CNS, the precise site and mechanism of this AVP action is not at all clear. In addition, peripheral administration of a new vasopressin antagonist peptide revealed the opposite effect, a facilitation of extinction, while intraventricular injection of the antagonist had little effect except at doses close to those found to antagonize blood pressure and behavioral effects of AVP after peripheral injection (Le Moal et al., 1981). This suggests a site of action for AVP that is not easily accessible via the intraventricular route.

De Wied and colleagues have emphasized that peptide fragments and analogs of AVP which exhibit little or no peripheral "endocrine-like" actions also exhibit behavioral effects similar to AVP. They interpret this lack of correspondence between endocrine and behavioral actions to indicate specialized central receptive processes operating directly on memory and learning mechanisms. Our current view is somewhat different. We view the ability of dPTyr-(ME)AVP to antagonize both the vascular and behavioral effects of AVP as strongly suggestive evidence that the sites mediating the two effects have – at the minimum – quite similar molecular recognition properties. Furthermore, we reason that the brain must possess mechanisms by which to monitor the status of visceral functions (such as blood pressure, blood glucose, body temperature, etc.), as well as a means to monitor the execution of those commands necessary to make appropriate adaptive responses (e.g. to secrete hormones). Therefore, we propose that the ability of AVP or non-endocrine subfragments to alter behavior may not reflect actions on a "memory" process per se, but rather indicates the detection by the brain of a logical mismatch between the current visceral needs of the body and the just executed secretory commands for hormones dealing with these needs. When peptides are injected intracerebroventricularly in the absence of either a peripheral signal or a brain command to secrete, the mismatch – detected as an unrequested visceral response (i.e. blood pressure elevation) or as an unrequested occupancy of a central monitor's receptors (such as those presumed to exist in the circumventricular organ system) – may evoke alerting signals to which the animal responds by either prolonging or altering previously effective behaviors. Under this view, it is not surprising that many AVP effects on behavior are disrupted by lesions of the dorsal noradrenergic bundle, since many alerting signals in the external environment would appear to be manifest upon forebrain cortical targets through this monoaminergic system (Iversen, 1981; Aston-Jones and Bloom, 1981; Swanson and Mogenson, 1981).

CONCLUSIONS

Although it is unlikely that the majority of transmitters remain to be discovered, existing data support the view that the behavioral effects of a transmitter substance must be viewed within the context of the spatial organization of the neurons utilizing a given transmitter, the cellular mechanisms by which it produces these effects and the general range of molecular events which characterize the transmitter's effects. Thus, while common actions on membrane ion or energy fluxes may underlie most responses to transmitters at the molecular level, the overall behavioral effect depends on the relationships between the cell circuits in which these actions occur, and the external and internal contingencies which then exist.

ACKNOWLEDGEMENTS

Supported by USPHS Grants AA 03504 and DA 01785. I thank my colleagues Drs. Magistretti, Morrison, Shoemaker, Le Moal, Koda and Koob for our many helpful discussions, and Mrs. Nancy Callahan for manuscript preparation.

REFERENCES

Aston-Jones, G. and Bloom, F.E. (1981) Norepinephrine-containing locus coeruleus neurons in behaving rats exhibit pronounced responses to non-noxious environmental stimuli. *J. Neurosci.*, 1: 887–900.

Bankoski, K., Manning, M., Haldar, J. and Sawyer, W.H. (1978) Design of potent antagonists of the vasopressor response to arginine-vasopressin. *J. med. Chem.*, 21: 850–853.

Bloom, F.E. (1979) Chemical Integrative Processes in the Central Nervous System. In F.O. Schmitt and F.G. Worden (Eds.), *The Neurosciences, Fourth Study Program*, MIT Press, Cambridge, MA, pp. 51-58.

Bloom, F.E. (1981) Recombinant DNA strategies of neurotransmitter research. In *Proc. Eighth International Congress on Pharmacology*, Tokyo, Japan, Vol. 2, pp. 189–200.

Borghi, C., Nicosia, S., Giachetti, A. and Said, S.I. (1979) Vasoactive intestinal polypeptide (VIP) stimulates adenylate cyclase in selected areas of rat brain. *Life Sci.*, 24: 65–70.

De Wied, D. (1976) Behavioral effects of intraventricularly administered vasopressin and vasopressin fragments. *Life Sci.*, 19: 685–690.

De Wied, D. (1980) Behavioural actions of neurohypophysial peptides. *Proc. roy. Soc. B*, 210: 183–195.

Deschodt-Lanckman, M., Robberect, P. and Christopher, J. (1977) Characterization of VIP-sensitive adenylate cyclase in guinea pig brain. *FEBS Lett.*, 83: 76–80.

Fuxe, K., Hökfelt, T., Said, S.I. and Mutt, V. (1977) Vasoactive intestinal polypeptide (VIP) and the nervous system: immunohistochemical evidence for localization in central and peripheral neurons, particularly intracortical neurons of the cerebral cortex. *Neurosci. Lett.*, 5: 241–246.

Iversen, S.D. (1981) Neuropeptides: do they integrate body and brain? *Nature (Lond.)*, 291: 452.

Koob, G.F., Le Moal, M., Gaffori, O., Manning, M., Sawyer, W.H., Rivier, J. and Bloom, F.E. (1981) Effects of arginine vasopressin and a vasopressin antagonist, dPTyr-(Me)-AVP, on extinction of active avoidance behavior in rats. *Regulatory Peptides*, 2: 153–164.

Le Moal, M., Koob, G.F., Koda, L.Y., Bloom, F.E., Manning, M., Sawyer, W.H. and Rivier, J. (1981) Vasopressor receptor antagonist prevents behavioural effects of vasopressin. *Nature (Lond.)*, 291: 491–493.

Magistretti, P., Morrison, J.H. Shoemaker, W.J., Sapin, V. and Bloom, F.E. (1981) Vasoactive intestinal polypeptide induces glycogenolysis in mouse cortical slices: a possible regulatory mechanism for the local control of energy metabolism. *Proc. nat. Acad. Sci. U.S.A.*, 78: 6535–6539.

Phillis, J.W., Kirkpatrick, J.R. and Said, S.I. (1978) Vasoactive intestinal polypeptide excitation of central neurons. *Canad. J. Physiol. Pharmacol.*, 56: 337–340.

Quach, T.T., Rose, C. and Schwartz, J.C. (1978) [^{3}H]Glycogen hydrolysis in brain slices: responses to neurotransmitters and modulation of noradrenaline receptors. *J. Neurochem.*, 30: 1335–1341.

Quik, M., Iversen L.L. and Bloom, S.R. (1978) Effect of vasoactive intestinal peptide (VIP) and other peptides on cAMP accumulation in rat brain. *Biochem. Pharmacol.*, 27: 2209–2213.

Said, S.I. (1980) Vasoactive intestinal peptide (VIP): isolation, distribution, biological actions, structure–function relationships, and possible functions. In G.J.B. Glass (Ed.), *Gastrointestinal Hormones*, Raven Press, New York, pp. 245–273.

Said, S.I. and Mutt, V. (1970) Polypeptide with broad biological activity: isolation from small intestine. *Science*, 169: 1217–1218.

Siggins, G.R. and Bloom, F.E. (1981) Modulation of unit activity by chemically coded neurons, In O. Pompeiano and C. Ajmone-Marsan (Eds.), *Brain Mechanisms and Perceptual Awareness*, Raven Press, New York, pp. 431–448.

Swanson, L.W. and Mogenson, G.J. (1981) Neural mechanisms for the functional coupling of autonomic, endocrine and somatomotor responses in adaptive behavior. *Brain Res. Rev.*, 3: 1–35.

Taylor, D.P. and Pert, C.B. (1979) Vasoactive intestinal polypeptide: specific binding rat brain membranes. *Proc. nat. Acad. Sci. U.S.A.*, 76: 660–664.

Van Wimersma Greidanus, T.J.B., Dogterom, J., and De Wied, D. (1975) Intraventricular administration of anti-vasopressin serum inhibits memory consolidation in rats. *Life Sci.*, 16: 637–644.

Molecular Mechanisms of Neurotransmitter Storage and Release: A Comparison of the Adrenergic and Cholinergic Systems

H. WINKLER, W. SCHMIDT, R. FISCHER-COLBRIE and A. WEBER

Department of Pharmacology, University of Innsbruck, A-6020 Innsbruck (Austria)

INTRODUCTION

Amongst the transmitter-containing organelles, those storing catecholamines and acetylcholine are the best characterized ones. This is due to the fact that pure preparations of these vesicles can be isolated from adrenal medulla and sympathetic nerve (see Winkler, 1976; Lagercrantz, 1976; Winkler and Westhead, 1980) or from the electric organ of *Torpedo* fish (see Zimmermann, 1979; Morris, 1980). In this limited review we would like to compare these adrenergic and cholinergic vesicles with each other and by doing so arrive at some common properties in terms of molecular function. We have, of course, to be aware of the fact (see Fig. 1) that in the adrenergic system most data are available for the chromaffin granules and the

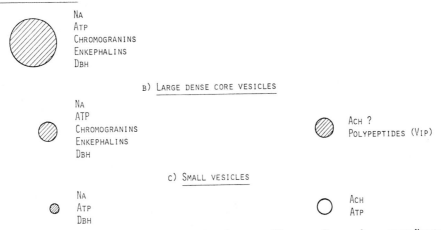

Fig. 1. Storage organelles in the adrenergic and cholinergic system. The organelles are drawn according to their approximate size (chromaffin granules, 280 nm; large dense core vesicles, 100 nm; small adrenergic vesicles, 50 nm; small cholinergic vesicles of *Torpedo marmorata*, 80 nm). The most important constituents are given, further details are discussed in the text. DBH, dopamine-β-hydroxylase; NA, noradrenaline; ACH, acetylcholine.

[11]

12

large dense core vesicles, which appear, as far as biochemical criteria are concerned, very similar to each other (see Winkler, 1976; Lagercrantz, 1976). The small dense core vesicles are much less characterized; however, recent studies indicate (De Potter and Chubb, 1977; Fried et al., 1978; Fried, 1978) that at least their membrane may be quite similar to that of the other two adrenergic organelles. In the cholinergic system the small vesicles have been studied in great detail (see Morris, 1980; Zimmermann, 1979) and we will compare these with the adrenergic organelles. For the large cholinergic vesicles it is interesting to note that they contain a specific polypeptide, i.e. the vasoactive intestinal polypeptide (VIP; Johansson and Lundberg 1981), which finds its parallel in the enkephalin content of the adrenergic vesicles (see, e.g., Viveros et al., 1979).

STORAGE PROPERTIES OF TRANSMITTER-CONTAINING ORGANELLES

Figure 2 gives the number of small molecules present in the two types of organelles. The common feature of cholinergic and adrenergic vesicles is the high concentration of the respective transmitter, of nucleotides (mainly ATP) and of calcium. Their concentrations in chromaffin granules add up to an osmolarity which is significantly higher than that of the cytoplasm, whereas in cholinergic vesicles this difference is less significant. Obviously, at least in the adrenergic system, mechanisms must exist to reduce this osmolarity inside the organelles to avoid lysis by water which can permeate the membrane. Furthermore, the possible contribution of a stable storage complex to the maintenance of the transmitter store has to be considered. Since, for chromaffin granules, these problems have recently been reviewed in great detail (Winkler and Westhead, 1980), it suffices here to restate some conclusions mainly derived from nuclear magnetic resonance studies (Daniels

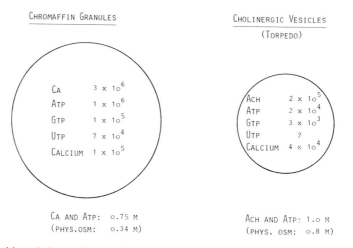

Fig. 2. Composition of chromaffin granules and cholinergic vesicles. The data for a single chromaffin granule are taken from the review by Winkler and Westhead (1980) and most of those for the cholinergic vesicle of the electric organ (*Torpedo marmorata*) from Morris (1980). The value of calcium for the cholinergic vesicles was calculated from Israel et al. (1980). The concentration of GTP was obtained from the study of Wagner et al. (1978) on the cholinergic vesicles from the electric organ of *Narcine*.

et al., 1978; Sen et al., 1979). (a) Chromaffin granules do not contain a stable storage complex involving catecholamines and nucleotides. These molecules are present in solution within the granule. However, a certain degree of interaction with each other and with the soluble proteins, the acidic chromogranins, is likely to reduce the "free" concentration of these molecules which can leak from the organelles by diffusion. This leakage is also reduced by a membrane, which is practically impermeable to these molecules at 0 °C, but is less so at 37 °C. (b) The interaction of these molecules just mentioned is able to reduce the osmolarity within these organelles sufficiently to prevent their lysis within the cytoplasm.

For cholinergic vesicles much less is known about the state of the molecules in the vesicle content. However, a recent nuclear magnetic resonance study indicates a similarity to the adrenergic system (Stadler and Füldner, 1980). The acetylcholine within the vesicles is present in solution and not in any stable storage complex. Whether it interacts with the molecules of ATP or the acidic groups of the glycosaminoglycans present in these organelles (Stadler and Whittaker, 1978) deserves further attention.

UPTAKE OF SMALL MOLECULES BY TRANSMITTER-CONTAINING ORGANELLES

In the absence of any stable storage complex, mechanisms must exist in these organelles which allow the accumulation and maintenance of the high concentrations of small molecules.

In the adrenergic system a carrier-mediated uptake of catecholamines has been characterized in great detail (see Winkler, 1977). A significant breakthrough of our understanding of this process occurred when Radda and collaborators (see Njus and Radda, 1978) established that the driving force is an electrochemical proton gradient maintained by the ATPase of the granule membrane. According to Johnson and Scarpa (1979), both the electrical and the chemical part of this gradient are responsible for amine uptake. Nucleotides are also taken up into chromaffin granules through a carrier-mediated process (Kostron et al., 1977; Aberer et al., 1978; Phillips and Morton, 1978; Carmichael et al., 1980; Weber and Winkler, 1981) which is competitively inhibited by atractyloside (Aberer et al., 1978). Recent studies indicate that the nucleotide carrier has a relatively broad specificity. Besides ATP and ADP also GTP and UTP (see Table I) are transported with similar affinities (Weber and Winkler, 1981). This lack of specificity goes even further since phosphoenolpyruvate, phosphate and even sulfate (see Table I) can bind to, or are transported by, this carrier (Grueninger et al., 1980; Weber and Winkler, 1983). The fact that sulfate is a substrate for this carrier has to be considered for uptake studies with chromaffin granules. Many investigators use $MgSO_4$ in mM concentrations for the activation of the ATPase. This sulfate will be transported into the granules and interfere with nucleotide uptake. Thus under these conditions catecholamine uptake is accompanied by some sulfate accumulation, whereas in the absence of this anion only nucleotides will be transported by the nucleotide carrier (see below).

For both nucleotide and catecholamine uptake the proton pumping ATPase is an essential partner since it provides the driving force. Apps and Schatz (1979) have recently shown that the ATP-splitting component of this enzyme is closely similar to

14

TABLE I

*The specificity of the nucleotide carrier in chromaffin
granules and Torpedo vesicles*

The apparent K_m of the uptake of the various
nucleotides and SO_4^{2-} are given in mM. The results
for chromaffin granules are taken from Weber and
Winkler (1981, 1983) and those for the *Torpedo*
vesicles from Luqmani (1981).

	Chromaffin granules $K_m (mM)$	Torpedo vesicles $K_m (mM)$
ATP	0.9	1.3
GTP	0.3	1.2
UTP	0.7	2.0
SO_4^{2-}	0.4	?

the F_1-complex present in mitochondria. The morphological equivalent for this
mitochondrial enzyme are the stalked particles seen on the inner membrane of these
organelles (see Racker, 1975). As proposed in a recent review (Winkler and
Westhead, 1980), it seemed likely therefore that chromaffin granules should possess
similar particles on their surface. In fact such particles of 8 nm diameter have now
been discovered in negatively stained or freeze-etched preparations of chromaffin
granules (Schmidt et al., 1982). As shown schematically in Fig. 3 a single chromaffin
granule possesses on average 22 of these typical particles on its surface – a number
quite close to the value of 10 which was predicted (see Winkler and Westhead, 1980)
from biochemical data.

Thus we can conclude for the adrenergic system that we have already quite a
coherent picture of the molecular mechanisms by which these organelles accumulate
catecholamines and nucleotides. For cholinergic vesicles any progress in this question was impossible for a long time since isolated vesicles apparently did not take up
any acetylcholine. However, recent studies (Giompres and Luqmani, 1980; Michaelson and Angel, 1981; Koenigsberger and Parsons, 1980) have finally succeeded in

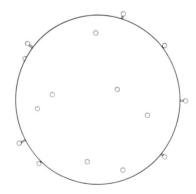

Fig. 3. Schematic drawing of the surface particles on chromaffin granules. When chromaffin granules are
subjected to negative staining, stalked particles can be seen on their membranes (Schmidt et al., 1982). In
this study it could be calculated that a single granule possesses 22 of these particles. The size, number and
distribution of these particles is presented schematically for one chromaffin granule.

demonstrating such an uptake. This process is saturable and therefore different from the passive permeation of acetylcholine (Carpenter et al., 1980). A direct relationship of this uptake to the activity of an ATPase has not yet been established in these vesicle preparations. However, a study on acetylcholine uptake in intact tissue (PC12 clonal line of rat pheochromocytoma) indicated that the uptake into the vesicles was dependent on ATP and possibly on a proton gradient present in them (Toll and Howard, 1980). Thus these most recent results reveal similarities to the adrenergic system. These parallels become even more striking if we consider the nucleotide uptake into cholinergic vesicles (Luqmani, 1981). The transport is saturable and inhibited by atractyloside. The specificity of the carrier resembles that of chromaffin granules very closely (see Table I). Inhibition of the uptake by SCN^- (Luqmani and Giompres, 1981), which as a lipid permeant anion abolishes membrane potentials, is consistent with the involvement of such a potential as the driving force just as it is in chromaffin granules (for acetylcholine uptake see the recent paper by Anderson et al., 1982).

Finally, cholinergic vesicles do possess a Mg^{2+}-activated ATPase (Breer et al., 1977; Michaelson and Ophir, 1980). That this enzyme is part of a proton pumping system seems quite possible considering the foregoing discussion. It will be interesting to study the cholinergic vesicles by negative staining in order to find a morphological equivalent of such an enzyme. Since these vesicles are small (50–80 nm diameter versus 280 nm for chromaffin granules, giving the cholinergic vesicles less than 10% of the surface of chromaffin granules), one has of course to search for an even smaller number of molecules than the 22 reported for a single chromaffin granule.

Let us now return to the chromaffin granules for a few comments on the molecular mechanisms of membrane transport of catecholamines and nucleotides. Johnson and Scarpa (1979) proposed a model in which catecholamines are taken up as uncharged molecules. However, Knoth et al. (1981) have recently presented evidence that actually the charged form is carried. Furthermore, the possibility of a cotransport of anions, e.g. nucleotides, was not considered in the model by Johnson and Scarpa (1979). Since atractyloside, which inhibits nucleotide transport, does not interfere with the initial rate of catecholamine accumulation (Kostron et al., 1977) this seemed justified. However, when the total amount of catecholamines taken up during longer incubations is measured in the presence of atractyloside a reduction becomes obvious (Scherman and Henry, 1980). This indicates some coupling between catecholamine and nucleotide uptake. In fact under physiological conditions (mM concentration of ATP in cytoplasm) catecholamine transport will always be accompanied by nucleotide accumulation. In Fig. 4 we are presenting a scheme which considers these points (see also Phillips and Apps, 1980; Njus et al., 1981). Catecholamines are taken up as charged molecules with a rate 8 times faster than that of nucleotides (Weber and Winkler, 1981). Since amines, especially in uncharged form, are likely to leak from the granule more than nucleotides do, the final catecholamine/ATP ratio in the granules will still be around 4. Since catecholamines and nucleotides are accumulated together the charged catecholamines will not contribute to the membrane potential and therefore continuous uptake of catecholamines can occur. If, however, nucleotide transport is inhibited, catecholamine uptake will finally increase the membrane potential to such a degree that further proton transport, and consequently catecholamine uptake, will be blocked. This

16

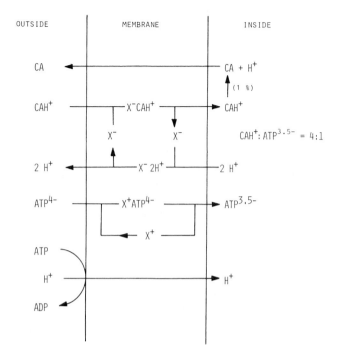

Fig. 4. A model of catecholamine and nucleotide uptake into chromaffin granules. The charged catecholamine (CA) molecule binds to a carrier (X) which "transports" the amine through the membrane. After dissociation of the catecholamines inside the granules (pH 5.6) the carrier takes up $2H^+$, releases them to the exterior and becomes available for a further cycle. Nucleotides bind to a positively charged carrier. $\Delta\psi$ "drives" this complex which has now an overall negative charge. After nucleotide release into the granule interior the now positively charged carrier returns to its original position (or conformation). Catecholamine uptake occurs at 8 times the rate of nucleotide transport. In order to account for the 4:1 catecholamine/ATP ratio in intact granules a preferential leakage of uncharged catecholamine is assumed.

concept would explain the above mentioned effect of atractyloside (Scherman and Henry, 1980) on catecholamine transport.

MOLECULAR MECHANISM OF SECRETION

It seems well established that secretion from both the adrenergic (see Smith and Winkler, 1972) and cholinergic (see Zimmermann, 1979) systems occurs by a process of exocytosis. Since in this process the membrane of the storage organelle is an essential partner, knowledge of the molecular organization of this structure is crucial for defining the molecular events during exocytosis. The molecular topography of the membranes of chromaffin granules has recently been reviewed in great detail (see Winkler and Westhead, 1980) and therefore only the main features will be restated here (for references see review). The granule membrane contains quite a number of proteins (>20), although some of the minor components may be contaminants (adsorbed from the cytosol or contaminating membranes). Functionally defined components are dopamine-β-hydroxylase (molecular weight of subunits 75,000), F_1-ATPase (51,000, 50,000 and 28,000), actin (42,000) and cytochrome b-561 (=chromomembrin B: 21,000). Most of these proteins (Abbs and

Phillips, 1980) are present on the outer surface of these chromaffin granules with dopamine-β-hydroxylase and the other glycoproteins as the notable exceptions (Huber et al., 1979). Two of these glycoproteins (GP II and GP III: see Huber et al., 1979) have recently been isolated, analyzed and used for immunization (Fischer-Colbrie et al., 1981). An immunological analysis of subcellular fractions of bovine adrenal medulla revealed that these two proteins are specifically confined to the membranes of chromaffin granules.

Let us now compare these data with the protein composition of pure cholinergic vesicles isolated from the electric organ which has been characterized in two independent studies (Stadler and Tashiro, 1979; Wagner and Kelly, 1979). Both groups agree that major protein bands of molecular weights of about 20,000, 35,000 and 42,000 are present. Additional proteins of 70,000 (Wagner and Kelly, 1979) and about 150,000 (Stadler and Tashiro, 1979) have been described. The topographical arrangement of the proteins in the cholinergic system is similar to that of chromaffin granules, with the majority of the proteins accessible on their outer surface (Wagner and Kelly, 1979). There is as yet only one protein, i.e. actin, which appears to be common to cholinergic and adrenergic vesicles. One of the "cholinergic" proteins (band 11 of molecular weight 34,000: Stadler and Tashiro, 1979) has been considered (see Luqmani, 1981) to represent the nucleotide carrier. If this is the case it should also be present in chromaffin granules. On the other hand, the cholinergic vesicles might contain the F_1-ATPase subunits found in chromaffin granules as minor components. Thus we might gain useful knowledge from a thorough comparison of the membrane proteins of these two organelles. A specific search for defined components might be rewarding even if these proteins are minor constituents in the respective organelles. At present one can only predict that two major components of the adrenergic membranes, i.e. dopamine-β-hydroxylase and probably also the cytochrome (see Winkler and Westhead, 1980) which are essential for catecholamine synthesis, will be absent from the cholinergic vesicles.

Despite the considerable knowledge of the organization of the storage vesicle membranes we are still not in a position to present an established molecular model for exocytosis, although numerous hypotheses have been put forward (see, e.g., the recent review by Plattner, 1981). One of the main reasons for this slow progress was the lack of adequate models for an in vitro study of this phenomenon. This, however, may have been overcome by two recent developments: (a) Konings and De Potter (1981) demonstrated that release of catecholamines can be elicited in an in vitro system consisting of isolated chromaffin granules and plasma membranes. If this system does indeed represent exocytosis in vitro the influence of various agents and antibodies can now be studied easily (see also Lelkes et al., 1980); (b) Baker and Knight (1979) are investigating isolated cells which are made "leaky" by electric currents. Since the membrane of these cells is permeable to small molecules their influence on exocytosis can be studied directly without any of the usual problems of permeation through the plasma membrane. Essential requirements of amine release in this system are low concentrations of calcium (10^{-6} M), Mg^{2+} and ATP. Up till now results on these cells seem to disprove at least two hypotheses: (i) the osmotic exocytosis hypothesis (see, e.g., Zinder and Pollard, 1980) – in this model the positive membrane potential of chromaffin granules is supposed to lead to an uptake of anions when the granule becomes attached to the plasma membrane during secretion. This anion uptake finally causes osmotic fission. If this were the case inhibitors of the proton pump providing the membrane potential necessary for anion uptake and uncouplers which abolish this potential should block exocytosis. However, this was not observed (Knight and Baker, 1982); (ii) participation of contractile proteins – Compounds interfering with these proteins do not influence exocytosis in leaky cells (Knight and Baker, 1982) and therefore participation of these proteins in exocytosis seems unlikely. At present one can only speculate that during exocytosis ATP is split by a Mg^{2+}-activated enzyme. This enzyme might be localized in the plasma membrane or on the granules. Whether this ATPase drives some ionic pump or changes the membrane properties, or whether the inorganic phosphate formed plays some role, is not known. One might of course recall that amorphous calcium phosphate leads to the release of catecholamines from isolated granules (Lishajko, 1970). However, this system in the absence of plasma membranes is hardly a suitable model for exocytosis. Therefore, it seems futile to speculate further. The new methical developments in this field should soon provide answers on the mechanism of exocytosis.

CONCLUSIONS

By comparing adrenergic and cholinergic vesicles we have come to the conclusion that significant similarities exist in the molecular organization and function of these organelles. We probably have stressed the similarities in a biased way; however, we present this approach as a challenge to others to attempt to disprove this concept.

ACKNOWLEDGEMENTS

The original work of the authors quoted in this review was supported by the Fonds zur Förderung der wissenschaftlichen Forschung (Austria) and by the Dr. Legerlotz-Stiftung.

REFERENCES

Abbs, M.T. and Phillips, J.H. (1980) Organization of the proteins of the chromaffin granule membrane. *Biochim. biophys. Acta*, 595: 200–221.

Aberer, W., Kostron, H., Huber, E. and Winkler, H. (1978) A characterization of the nucleotide uptake by chromaffin granules of bovine adrenal medulla. *Biochem. J.*, 172: 353–360.

Anderson, D.C., King, S.C. and Parsons, S.M. (1982) Proton gradient linkage to active uptake of [^{3}H]acetylcholine by *Torpedo* electric organ synaptic vesicles. *Biochemistry*, 21: 3037–3043.

Apps, D.K. and Schatz, G. (1979) An adenosine triphosphatase isolated from chromaffin granule membranes is closely similar to F_1-adenosine triphosphatase of mitochondria. *Europ. J. Biochem.*, 100: 411–419.

Baker, P.F. and Knight, D.E. (1979) The "leaky" adrenal medullary cell. A new preparation for investigating the mechanism of neurosecretion by exocytosis. *Trends, NeuroSci.*, 2: 288–291.

Breer, H., Morris, S.J. and Whittaker, V.P. (1977) Adenosine triphosphatase activity associated with purified cholinergic synaptic vesicles of *Torpedo marmorata*. *Europ. J. Biochem.*, 80: 313–318.

Carmichael, S.W., Weber, A. and Winkler, H. (1980) Uptake of nucleotides and catecholamines by chromaffin granules from pig and horse adrenal medulla. *J. Neurochem.*, 35: 270–272.

Carpenter, R.S., Koenigsberger, R. and Parsons, S.M. (1980) Passive uptake of acetylcholine and other organic cations by synaptic vesicles from *Torpedo* electric organ. *Biochemistry*, 19: 4373–4379.

Daniels, A.J., Williams, R.J.P. and Wright, P.E. (1978) The character of the stored molecules in chromaffin granules of the adrenal medulla: a nuclear magnetic resonance study. *Neuroscience*, 3: 573–585.

De Potter, W.P. and Chubb, I.W. (1977) Biochemical observations on the formation of small noradrenergic vesicles in the splenic nerve of the dog. *Neuroscience*, 2: 167–174.

Fischer-Colbrie, R., Schachinger, M., Zangerle, R. and Winkler, H. (1982) Dopamine β-hydroxylase and other glycoproteins from the soluble content and the membranes of adrenal chromaffin granules: isolation and carbohydrate analysis. *J. Neurochem.*, 38: 725–732.

Fried, G. (1978) Cytochrome b-561 in sympathetic nerve terminal vesicles from rat vas deferens. *Biochim. biophys. Acta*, 507: 175–177.

Fried, G., Lagercrantz, H. and Hökfelt, T. (1978) Improved isolation of small noradrenergic vesicles from rat seminal ducts following castration. A density gradient and morphological study. *Neuroscience*, 3, 1271–1291.

Giompres, P. and Luqmani, Y.A. (1980) Cholinergic synaptic vesicles isolated from *Torpedo marmorata*: demonstration of acetylcholine and choline uptake in an in vitro system. *Neuroscience*, 5: 1041–1052.

Grueninger, H., Weber, A., Apps, D., Phillips, J., Westhead, E. and Winkler, H. (1980) Effects of phosphoenolpyruvate on ATP transport in chromaffin granules. *Hoppe-Seylers Z. Physiol. Chem.*, 361: 1290.

Huber, E., König, P., Schuler, G., Aberer, W., Plattner, H. and Winkler, H. (1979) Characterization and topography of the glycoproteins of adrenal chromaffin granules. *J. Neurochem.*, 32: 35–47.

Israel, M., Manaranche, R., Marsal, J., Meunier, F.M., Morel, N., Frachon, P. and Lesbats, B. (1980) ATP-dependent calcium uptake by cholinergic synaptic vesicles isolated from *Torpedo* electric organ. *J. Membrane Biol.*, 54: 115–126.

Johansson, O. and Lundberg, J.M. (1981) Ultrastructural localization of VIP-like immunoreactivity in large dense-core vesicles of cholinergic-type, nerve terminals in cat exocrine glands. *Neuroscience*, 6: 847–862.

Johnson, R.G. and Scarpa, A. (1979) Proton-motive force and catecholamine transport in isolated chromaffin granules. *J. biol. Chem.*, 254: 3750–3760.

Knight, D.E. and Baker, P.F. (1982) Calcium-dependence of catecholamine release from bovine adrenal medullary cells after exposure to intense electric fields. *J. Membrane Biol.*, 68: 107–190.

Knoth, J., Isaacs, J.M. and Njus, D. (1981) Amine transport in chromaffin granule ghosts: pH-dependence implies cationic form is translocated. *J. biol. Chem.*, 256: 6541–6543.

Koenigsberger, R. and Parsons, S.M. (1980) Bicarbonate and magnesium ion-ATP dependent stimulation of acetylcholine uptake by *Torpedo* electric organ synaptic vesicles. *Biochem. biophys. Res. Commun.*, 94: 305–312.

Konings, F. and De Potter, W. (1981) Calcium-dependent in vitro interaction between bovine adrenal medullary cell membranes and chromaffin granules as a model for exocytosis. *FEBS Lett.*, 126: 103–106.

Kostron, H., Winkler, H., Peer, L.J. and König, P. (1977) Uptake of adenosine triphosphate by isolated adrenal chromaffin granules. A carrier-mediated transport. *Neuroscience*, 2: 159–166.

Lagercrantz, H. (1976) On the composition and function of large dense cored vesicles in sympathetic nerves. *Neuroscience*, 1: 81–92.

Lelkes, P.I., Lavie, E., Naquira, D., Schneeweiss, F., Schneider, A.S. and Rosenheck, K. (1980) Acetylcholine-induced in vitro fusion between cell membrane vesicles and chromaffin granules from the bovine adrenal medulla. *FEBS Lett.*, 115: 129–133.

Lishajko, F. (1970) Releasing effect of calcium and phosphate on catecholamines, ATP and protein from chromaffin cell granules. *Acta physiol. scand.*, 79: 575–584.

Luqmani, Y.A. (1981) Nucleotide uptake by isolated cholinergic synaptic vesicles: evidence for a carrier of adenosine 5'-triphosphate. *Neuroscience*, 6: 1011–1021.

Luqmani, Y.A. and Giompres, P. (1981) On the specificity of uptake by isolated *Torpedo* synaptic vesicles. *Neurosci. Lett.*, 23: 81–85.

Michaelson, D.M. and Angel, I. (1981) Saturable acetylcholine transport into purified cholinergic synaptic vesicles. *Proc. nat. Acad. Sci. U.S.A.*, 78: 2048–2052.

Michaelson, D.M. and Ophir, I. (1980) Sidedness of (calcium, magnesium) adenosine triphosphatase of purified *Torpedo* synaptic vesicles. *J. Neurochem.*, 34: 1483–1490.

Morris, S.J. (1980) The structure and stoichiometry of electric ray synaptic vesicles. *Neuroscience*, 5: 1509–1516.

Njus, D. and Radda, G.K. (1978) Bioenergetic processes in chromaffin granules. A new perspective on some old problems. *Biochim. biophys. Acta*, 463: 219–244.

Njus, D., Knoth, J. and Zallakian, M. (1981) Proton-linked transport in chromaffin granules. *Curr. Topics Bioenergetics*, 11: 107–147.

Phillips, J.H. and Apps, D.K. (1980) Stoichiometry of catecholamine/proton exchange across the chromaffin granule membranes. *Biochem. J.*, 192: 273–278.

Phillips, J.H. and Morton, A.G. (1978) Adenosine triphosphate in the bovine chromaffin granule. *J. Physiol. (Paris)*, 74: 503–508.

Plattner, H. (1981) Membrane behaviour during exocytosis. *Cell Biol. Int. Rep.*, 5: 435–459.

Racker, E. (1975) Inner mitochondrial membranes: basic and applied aspects. In G. Weissmann and R. Clairborne (Eds.), *Cell Membranes, Biochemistry, Cell Biology and Pathology*, HP Publishing Co., New York, pp. 135–141.

Scherman, D. and Henry, J.P. (1980) Role of the proton electrochemical gradient in monoamine transport by bovine chromaffin granules. *Biochim. biophys. Acta*, 601: 664–677.

Schmidt, W., Winkler, H. and Plattner, H. (1982) Adrenal chromaffin granules: evidence for an ultrastructural equivalent of the proton-pumping ATPase. *Europ. J. Cell Biol.*, 27: 96–104.

Sen, R., Sharp, R.R., Domino, L.E. and Domino, E.F. (1979) Composition of the aqueous phase of chromaffin granules. *Biochim. biophys. Acta*, 587: 75–88.

Smith, A.D. and Winkler, H. (1972) Fundamental mechanisms in the release of catecholamines. In H. Blaschko and E. Muscholl (Eds.), *Handbook of Experimental Pharmacology, Vol. 33*, Springer-Verlag, Berlin, pp. 538–617.

Stadler, H. and Füldner, H.H. (1980) Proton NMR detection of acetylcholine status in synaptic vesicles. *Nature (Lond.)*, 286: 293–294.

Stadler, H. and Tashiro, T. (1979) Isolation of synaptosomal plasma membranes from cholinergic nerve terminals and a comparison of their proteins with those of synaptic vesicles. *Europ. J. Biochem.*, 101: 171–178.

Stadler, H. and Whittaker, V.P. (1978) Identification of vesiculin as a glycosaminoglycan. *Brain Res.*, 153: 408–413.

Toll, L. and Howard, B.D. (1980) Evidence that an ATPase and a proton motive force function in the transport of acetylcholine into storage vesicles. *J. biol. Chem.*, 255: 1787–1789.

Viveros, O.H., Diliberto, E.J., Hazum, E.J. and Chang, K.J. (1979) Opiate-like materials in the adrenal medulla: evidence for storage and secretion with catecholamines. *Molec. Pharmacol.*, 16: 1101–1108.

Wagner, J.A. and Kelly, R.B. (1979) Topological organization of proteins in an intracellular secretory organelle: the synaptic vesicle. *Proc. nat. Acad. Sci. U.S.A.*, 76: 4126–4130.

Wagner, J.A., Carlson, S.S. and Kelly, R.B. (1978) Chemical and physical characterization of cholinergic synaptic vesicles. *Biochemistry*, 17: 1199–1206.

Weber, A. and Winkler, H. (1981) Specificity of nucleotide transport in chromaffin granules. *Neuroscience*, 6: 2269–2276.

Weber, A. and Winkler, H. (1983) Specificity and properties of the nucleotide carrier in the chromaffin granules from bovine adrenal medulla. *Biochem. J.*, in press.

Winkler, H. (1976) The composition of adrenal chromaffin granules: an assessment of controversial results. *Neuroscience*, 1: 65–80.

Winkler, H. (1977) The biogenesis of adrenal chromaffin granules. *Neuroscience*, 2: 657–683.

Winkler, H. and Westhead, E. (1980) The molecular organization of adrenal chromaffin granules. *Neuroscience*, 5: 1803–1823.

Zimmermann, H. (1979) Vesicle recycling and transmitter release. *Neuroscience*, 4: 1773–1803.

Zinder, O. and Pollard, H.B. (1980) The chromaffin granule: Recent studies leading to a functional model for exocytosis. In M.B.H. Youdim, W. Lovenberg, D.F. Sharman and J.R. Lagnado (Eds.), *Essays in Neurochemistry and Neuropharmacology, Vol. 4*, John Wiley, pp. 125–162.

Contractile Proteins in Chromaffin Cells

MARIE-FRANCE BADER, ANTONIO G. GARCIA*, JAROSLAVA CIESIELSKI-TRESKA,
DANIÈLE THIERSE and DOMINIQUE AUNIS**

*Unité INSERM U-44, Centre de Neurochimie, 5 rue Blaise Pascal, F-67084 Strasbourg Cedex (France)
and *Department of Pharmacology and Experimental Therapeutics, Medicine Faculty, Autonomous
University, Arzobispo Morcillo 1, Madrid 34 (Spain)*

INTRODUCTION

Neurons and chromaffin cells share a common embryological origin, the neural crest. The adrenal chromaffin cell is a modified post-ganglionic sympathetic ganglion cell and releases its noradrenergic and adrenergic neurotransmitters into the blood stream, where they act as hormones. On a cell biology basis, the chromaffin cells should be regarded as the relatives of the neurons on the basis of their structure, function, metabolism and origin. According to criteria proposed by Fujita (1977), the chromaffin cell is a typical paraneuron. Due to experimental ease, and because of the homogenous population of adrenal paraneurons, the morphology, biochemistry, physiology, pharmacology and pathology of these neural elements have been extensively studied; many important biological concepts have been developed from studies on the adrenal medulla, and extended and extrapolated to peripheric and central neurons.

The catecholamines of the adrenal medulla are stored in chromaffin granules and, upon stimulation by acetylcholine liberated from endings of splanchnic nerve derivations, the content of the granule is released to the exterior of the cell. The secretion mechanism occurs by exocytosis in which the secretory stimulus first causes the storage granule to fuse with the surface cell membrane, the fused membrane then opens to the cell exterior and through this opening the granule content is extruded from the cell. The similarities between stimulus–secretion coupling and stimulus–contraction coupling in muscle (Douglas, 1975; Trifaro, 1977) suggest that contractile proteins could play a role in release mechanism.

Recent studies have shown the presence of contractile proteins in the bovine adrenal medulla. A myosin-like (Trifaro and Ulpian, 1976; Creutz, 1977; Hesketh et al., 1977, 1978; Johnson et al., 1977) and an actin-like (Phillips and Slater, 1975; Lee et al., 1979) proteins have been isolated from bovine adrenal medullary tissue and characterized. Using immunofluorescent techniques, it has been shown that adrenal vessels were heavily fluorescent when stained with anti-myosin antibody while chromaffin cells were poorly but definitely labeled (Creutz, 1977; Aunis et al., 1980a, b).

In order to investigate more directly the role of contractile proteins in the mechanism of release, experiments were performed on isolated chromaffin cells.

** To whom correspondence should be addressed.

IS CATECHOLAMINE SECRETION FROM ISOLATED CHROMAFFIN CELLS MEDIATED BY CONTRACTILE PROTEINS?

Chromaffin cells were isolated essentially as described by Fenwick et al. (1978) using sequential digestion of bovine adrenal medullary tissue with collagenase (Aunis and Garcia, 1981). The number of isolated cells varied in every experiment between 1.5 and 4×10^6 cells/adrenal medulla. Under the light microscope the cell suspension contained spherical intact chromaffin cells (phase-bright, granular aspect, smooth contour, 20 μm in diameter, approx. 100% viability from exclusion of trypan blue) with few erythrocytes. Figure 1 shows that isolated chromaffin cells are functional since acetylcholine evoked the catecholamine release which was dependent on extracellular Ca^{2+}. The peak secretory response was 5.0 times the basal release. Increasing doses of hexamethonium progressively inhibited catecholamine release evoked by acetylcholine, indicating that nicotinic receptors are important in mediating the release from isolated cells. Immunochemical staining of isolated cells with specific anti-myosin, anti-actin and anti-α-actinin antibodies gave an intense fluorescence (Fig. 2) indicating the presence of contractile proteins within chromaffin cells. Cytochalasin B and phalloidin are known to act on actin filaments (Lin and Lin, 1979; Lin et al., 1979, 1980; Brenner and Korn, 1979; Brown and Spudich, 1979; Wehland et al., 1977) and colchicine on microtubules (see Dustin, 1978). It was interesting to test their effects on the catecholamine secretory response from isolated chromaffin cells, since diffusion barriers were removed. Results are depicted in Fig. 3. At a concentration of 10^{-5} M, cytochalasin B blocked release by 50% while colchicine at a concentration of 10^{-4} M inhibited release by 40%. Phalloidin did not seem to have any effect on the release, in contrast with what has been described using synaptosomes (Babitch et al., 1979).

Cytochalasin B has also been shown to block neurotransmitter release from sympathetic nerves (Thoa et al., 1972) and from synaptosomal preparations (Nicklas

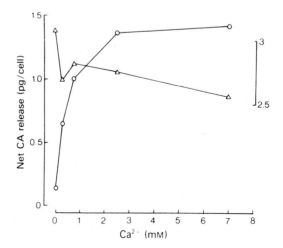

Fig. 1. Dependence of catecholamine (CA) secretion from isolated bovine chromaffin cells on Ca^{2+} concentration. Cells (suspended in Krebs medium; 28 °C, 2×10^5) were stimulated for 10 min with 10^{-4} M acetylcholine in the presence of 10^{-5} M physostigmine. Left ordinate scale (open circle) is the net CA release; right ordinate scale (open triangle) shows the CA cell content at the end of each experiment.

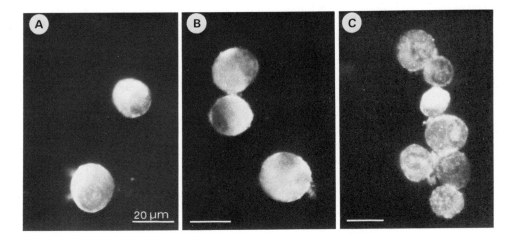

Fig. 2. Indirect immunofluorescence staining of isolated bovine adrenal chromaffin cells by anti-actin antibody (A), anti-myosin antibody (B) and anti-α-actinin antibody (C). Chromaffin cell suspensions were smeared on glass slides and air-dried. Fixation and staining by the standard immunofluorescence test were as described by Trifaro et al. (1978). Controls with pre-immune sera or with adsorbed antisera were negative.

and Berl, 1974). From these data, if one considers that the movement of granules to the cell periphery, the attachment of the granules to the cell membrane, or the expulsion of the granular contents during exocytosis are the results of the actin-myosin interaction with secretory granules, it is crucial to know the subcellular distribution of contractile elements in the chromaffin cell and whether contractile proteins are conspicuous components of the secretory granule.

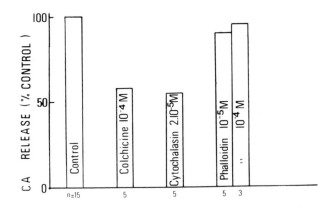

Fig. 3. Effect of colchicine, cytochalasin B and phalloidin on catecholamine secretion from isolated bovine adrenal chromaffin cells. Drugs at the indicated concentration were added 15 min before stimulation with acetylcholine (10^{-4} M, 28 °C, 10 min). Release in control experiments was 2.05 pg/cell.

LOCALIZATION OF CONTRACTILE PROTEINS IN THE CHROMAFFIN CELL

Subcellular fractionation of cellular organelles on sucrose gradients allows us to determine the distribution of contractile proteins, particularly in the purified granule fraction. However, redistribution and artefactual binding to membrane structures during the homogenization procedure of adrenal medullary tissue must not be excluded. A complementary approach would be to localize protein in cultured chromaffin cells using immunocytochemical techniques, although culturing cells might introduce some reorganization of contractile elements because process out-growth, exaggerated granule transport and morphological changes have been repor-ted (see Aunis et al., 1980b; Unsicker et al., 1980; Kilpatrick et al., 1980; Kenigsberg and Trifaro, 1980).

Hesketh et al. (1977) studied the subcellular distribution of myosin using the $(K^+,EDTA)$-ATPase activity associated with the myosin molecule. Myosin is asso-ciated with the plasma membrane of chromaffin cells, and very little activity is found with the purified chromaffin granule fraction. Electrophoretic analysis confirmed the absence of myosin heavy chains in the vesicle fraction. In contrast, several reports demonstrated the presence of actin associated on the granule membrane (Phillips and Slater, 1975; Meyer and Burger, 1979; Jockusch et al., 1977; Aunis et al., 1980b), although actin is highly concentrated in the cytosol of the adrenal medulla (Phillips and Slater, 1975; Lee et al., 1979). Actin has also been localized in the plasma membrane-enriched fraction (Zinder et al., 1978).

α-Actinin appears as a very interesting element of the contractile machinery. α-Actinin is localized in the Z-disc of skeletal muscle myofibrils (Schollmeyer et al., 1973, 1974) and is also present in cardiac and smooth muscles (Robson and Zeece, 1973; Schollmeyer et al., 1973) and non-muscle systems (Lazarides and Burridge, 1975; Lazarides, 1976). On the basis of biochemical properties of α-actinin (Suzuki et al., 1976; Podlubnaya et al., 1975), this molecule could serve as an attachment site or organizing template for actin filaments, controlling the orientation of actin filaments. A recent study showed that α-actinin is associated with the chromaffin granule membrane (Jockusch et al., 1977) and Aunis et al. (1980b) extended this observation by solubilizing and purifying α-actinin from the limiting vesicle mem-brane. In addition, a cross-reactivity with the antibody raised against muscle α-actinin was found.

Using two-dimensional gel electrophoresis (isoelectrofocusing in the first dimen-sion and separation according to molecular weight in the second dimension) as an analytical tool, α-actinin has been identified as a conspicuous component of the chromaffin granule membrane (Fig. 4). α-Actinin is not a major component, and the recovery is variable from one granule preparation to another because the molecule is progressively lost when the granules are isolated by conventional sucrose gradients at low ionic strength. α-Actinin from chromaffin granule membrane has a molecular weight of 97,000 and a pH_i of 6.4. How α-actinin is associated or integrated in the limiting vesicle membrane is not yet answered. One major question is the orientation of α-actinin, facing the outside or the inside of the granule. Intact granules were radiolabeled with $Na^{125}I$/lactoperoxidase and few components were subsequently found to be radioactive; actin and α-actinin were poorly radioactive. Following digestion with pronase of the crude chromaffin granule fraction, intact granules were

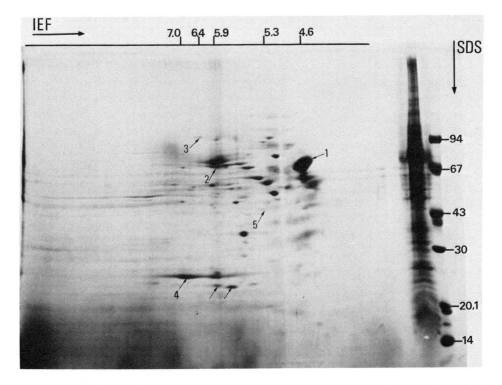

Fig. 4. Two-dimensional electrophoretogram of chromaffin granule membrane proteins. Two-dimensional gel electrophoresis was performed as described by O'Farrell (1975). Many components are separated; some of them have been identified: 1, chromogranin A; 2, dopamine-β-hydroxylase; 3, α-actinin; 4, chromomembrin B or cytochrome b_{561}; 5, actin. Actual pHs are indicated (IEF, isoelectrofocussing, 1st dimension) and molecular weight standards are indicated on the right (SDS, 2nd dimension).

separated by centrifugation and membrane proteins analyzed by two-dimensional gel electrophoresis. The polypeptide profile was completely altered: many spots disappeared and α-actinin was completely digested. These experiments strongly suggest that α-actinin is facing the cytoplasmic side of the chromaffin granule. An in vitro interaction between rabbit actin, chicken myosin and bovine chromaffin granules has been previously described by Burridge and Phillips (1975). Is α-actinin playing a potential role in the attachment of actin filaments to granule membrane?

To answer this crucial question, we used chemically tritiated (Cohen et al., 1978) actin. As shown in Fig. 5, [^{3}H]actin binds to granule membrane (1.5 nmol actin monomer per mg membrane protein), and there was a linear relationship between actin binding and actin concentration (at least in the concentration range tested in this study). However, when membranes were pre-incubated with specific anti-α-actinin antibody, a dramatic decrease of the actin binding was observed (Fig. 5), which was dependent on the antibody concentration (Fig. 6). These results show that α-actinin binds actin and that the attachment can be prevented by anti-α-actinin antibody. A recent study has shown that binding of [^{3}H]actin to chromaffin granule membranes can be partially inhibited by cytochalasin B (Wilkins and Lin, 1981). Actin nuclei are present in the chromaffin granule membrane; there is an interaction between these nuclei and α-actinin, the nature of which remains to be elucidated.

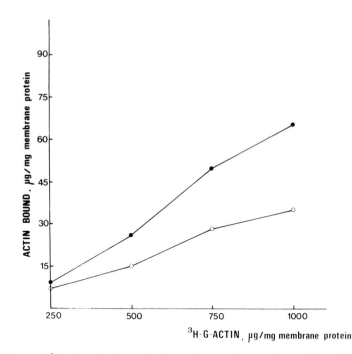

Fig. 5. Inhibition of [³H]actin attachment to chromaffin granule membrane. Chromaffin granule membranes (250 μg) were pre-incubated in phosphate buffer containing 0.25 mg pre-immune rabbit immunoglobulin (control; closed symbol) or 0.25 mg anti-α-actinin immunoglobulins (open symbol) at 4 °C for 18 h. Membranes were then collected by centrifugation, washed and assayed for [³H]actin binding. Membranes were incubated at a concentration of 1 mg protein/ml with increasing concentration of actin for 120 min at 20 °C in the actin binding buffer (5 mM NaH_2PO_4, 1 mM ATP, 0.75 mM β-mercaptoethanol, 1 mM $MgCl_2$, pH 6.5, 0.25 ml). Membrane suspension was then layered onto sucrose gradient, centrifuged at 32,800 g_{max} for 30 min. Radioactivity was measured in the membrane fraction and actin bound calculated as μg per mg membrane protein.

Using immunofluorescence techniques with specific antibodies to myosin, actin and α-actinin, each of these contractile elements were localized in chromaffin cells in culture (Aunis et al., 1980b; Hesketh et al., 1981). When maintained in culture, bovine adult chromaffin cells started to grow expansions with typical bulbous tips. The number and length of processes varied considerably, but most of the processes displayed varicosities, lateral branches and growth cone-like structures (Bader et al., 1981). In these cultured cells, α-actinin was localized in a punctate pattern in cytoplasm and neuritic-like expansions, suggesting α-actinin to be associated with chromaffin granules (Aunis et al., 1980b). Chromaffin cells stained strongly with anti-actin antibody (Aunis et al., 1980b; Hesketh et al., 1981). Fine filament bundles were seen, and also diffuse staining in cytoplasm, some punctate labeling and staining of the plasma membrane of sub-membranous cytoplasm. Colchicine caused retraction of neuritic extensions and formation of lateral growth cones. Cytochalasin B caused ballooning of terminal tips and phalloidin stimulated microspike formation. These observations show that contractile proteins are also related to cell functions as process outgrowth and morphological changes in addition to the neurosecretory function.

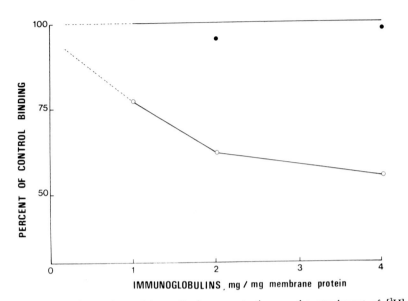

Fig. 6. Effect of increasing anti-α-actinin antibody concentration on the attachment of [³H]actin to chromaffin granule membrane. Chromaffin granule membranes were incubated with increasing immunoglobulin concentration as indicated (pre-immune, closed symbols; anti-α-actinin, open symbols).

CONCLUSIONS

Interactions of contractile proteins with synaptic vesicles (Puszkin and Kochwa, 1974), with the secretory granules of neurohypophysis (Ostlund et al., 1977) and with chromaffin granules from adrenal medulla (Burridge and Phillips, 1975; present data) have been described. At the ultrastructural level, Le Beux and Willemot (1975a, b) have shown evidence of a microfilament lattice in the neuron, which has anchorage points in the synaptic membrane and sends projections forming contacts with the synaptic vesicles. A similar observation has been recently made by Alonso et al. (1981) concerning neurohypophysis and neurohormone-containing granules. The frequent binding of actin filaments to fusing vesicles (Alonso et al., 1981) suggests that the contractile machinery participates in the fusion of vesicles and axonal membranes leading to neurotransmitter release.

During the last decade, contractile proteins have been actively studied in a variety of cell systems, including nerve cells and paraneurons. These proteins may participate in many cellular functions, such as axonal transport, transmitter release, receptor modulation and membrane retrieval (see Trifaro, 1978), and many hypotheses have been proposed. Chromaffin cells appear as a very promising and interesting working model and should help in future in the understanding of the role of contractile proteins in the mechanism of neurohormone and neurotransmitter liberation. Obviously further work is necessary and attention must now be paid to the role of regulatory proteins, on the interaction of contractile elements with cellular organelles and cell membrane by the development of biochemical and ultrastructural techniques.

ACKNOWLEDGEMENTS

Original studies in our laboratory were supported by grants from French DGRST (79-7-1058) and INSERM (CRL 806017).

REFERENCES

Alonso, G., Gabrion, J., Travers, E. and Assenmacher, I. (1981) Ultrastructural organization of actin filaments in neurosecretory axons of the rat. *Cell Tiss. Res.*, 214: 323–341.

Aunis, D. and Garcia, A.G. (1981) Correlation between catecholamine secretion from bovine isolated chromaffin cells and (^{3}H)-ouabain binding to plasma membranes. *Brit. J. Pharmacol.*, 72: 31–40.

Aunis, D., Hesketh, J.E. and Devilliers, G. (1980a) Immunohistochemical and immunocytochemical localization of myosin, chromogranin A and dopamine-β-hydroxylase in nerve cells in culture and adrenal glands. *J. Neurocytol.*, 9: 255–274.

Aunis, D., Guerold, B., Bader, M.F. and Ciesielski-Treska, J. (1980b) Immunocytochemical and biochemical demonstration of contractile proteins in chromaffin cells in culture. *Neuroscience*, 5: 2261–2277.

Babitch, J.A., Gage, F.H. and Valdes, J.J. (1979) Effects of phalloidin on K$^+$-dependent, Ca^{2+}-independent neurotransmitter efflux and Ca^{2+}-dependent neurotransmitter release, *Life Sci.*, 24: 117–124.

Bader, M.F., Ciesielski-Treska, J., Thierse, D., Hesketh, J. and Aunis, D. (1981) Immunocytochemical study of microtubules in chromaffin cells in culture and evidence that tubulin is not an integral protein of the chromaffin granule membrane. *J. Neurochem.*, 37: 917–933.

Brenner, S.L. and Korn, E.D. (1979) The effects of cytochalasin on actin polymerization and actin ATPase provide insights into the mechanism of polymerization. *J. biol. Chem.*, 255: 841–844.

Brown, S.S. and Spudich, J.A. (1979) Nucleation of polar actin filament assembly by a positively charged surface, *J. Cell Biol.*, 80: 499–504.

Burridge, K. and Phillips, J.H. (1975) Association of actin and myosin with secretory granule membranes. *Nature (Lond.)*, 254: 526–529.

Cohen, C.M., Jackson, P.L. and Branton, D. (1978) Actin–membrane interactions: association of G-actin with the red cell membrane. *J. Supramol. Struct.*, 9: 113–124.

Creutz, C.E. (1977) Isolation, characterization and localization of bovine adrenal medullary myosin. *Cell Tiss. Res.*, 178: 17–38.

Douglas, W.W. (1975) Secretomotor control of adrenal medullary reaction: synaptic, membrane and ionic events in stimulus-secretion coupling. In H. Blaschko, G. Sayers and A.D. Smith (Eds.), *Handbook of Physiology, Vol. 6*, Amer. Physiol. Soc., Washington, DC, pp. 367–388.

Dustin, P. (1978) *Microtubules*. Springer Verlag, Berlin.

Fenwick, E.M., Fajdiga, P.B., Howe, V.B.S. and Livett, B.G. (1978) Functional and morphological characterization of isolated bovine adrenal medullary cells. *J. Cell Biol.*, 76: 12–30.

Fujita, T. (1977) Concept of paraneurons. *Arch. Histol. Jap.*, 40: 1–12.

Hesketh, J.E., Aunis, D., Pescheloche, M. and Mandel, P. (1977) Subcellular distribution of myosin (K$^+$,EDTA)-ATPase in bovine adrenal medulla. *FEBS Lett.*, 80; 324–328.

Hesketh, J.E., Aunis, D., Mandel, P. and Devilliers, G. (1978) Biochemical and morphological studies of bovine adrenal medullary myosin. *Biol. Cell.*, 33: 199–208.

Hesketh, J.E., Ciesielski-Treska, J. and Aunis, D. (1981) A phase-contrast and immunofluorescence study of adrenal medullary chromaffin cells in culture: neurite formation, actin and chromaffin granule distribution. *Cell Tiss. Res.*, 218: 331–343.

Jockusch, B.M., Burger, M.M., Da Prada, M., Richards, J.G., Chaponnier, C. and Gabbiani, G. (1977) α-Actinin attached to membranes of secretory vesicles. *Nature (Lond.)*, 270: 628–629.

Johnson, D.H., McCubbin, W.D. and Kay, C.M. (1977) Isolation and characterization of a myosin-like protein from bovine adrenal medulla. *FEBS Lett.*, 77: 69–74.

Kenigsberg, R.L. and Trifaro, J.M. (1980) Presence of high affinity uptake system for catecholamines in cultured bovine adrenal chromaffin cells. *Neuroscience*, 5: 1547–1556.

Kilpatrick, D.L., Ledbetter, F.H., Carson, K.A., Kirshner, A.G., Slepetis, R. and Kirschner, N. (1980) Stability of bovine adrenal medulla cells in culture. *J. Neurochem.*, 35: 679–682.

Lazarides, E. (1976) Actin, α-actinin and tropomyosin interaction in the structural organization of actin filaments in non-muscle cells. *J. Cell Biol.*, 68: 202–219.

Lazarides, E. and Burridge, K. (1975) α-Actinin: immunofluorescent localization of a muscle structural protein in non-muscle cells. *Cell*, 6: 289–298.

Le Beux, Y.J. and Willemot, J. (1975a) An ultrastructural study of the microfilaments in rat brain by means of heavy meromyosin labeling, I. The perikaryon, the dendrites and the axon. *Cell Tiss. Res.*, 160: 1–36.

Le Beux, Y.J. and Willemot, J. (1975b) An ultrastructural study of the microfilaments in rat by means of E-PTA staining and heavy meromyosin labeling. II. The synapses. *Cell Tiss. Res.*, 160: 37–68.

Lee, R.W.H., Mushinski, W.E. and Trifaro, J.M. (1979) Two forms of cytoplasmic actin in adrenal chromaffin cells. *Neuroscience*, 4: 843–852.

Lin, D.C. and Lin, S. (1979) Actin polymerization induced by a motility-related high affinity cytochalasin binding complex from human erythrocyte membranes. *Proc. nat. Acad. Sci. U.S.A.*, 76: 2345–2349.

Lin, D.C., Tobin, K.D., Grumet, M. and Lin, S. (1980) Cytochalasin inhibits nuclei-induced actin polymerization by blocking filament elongation. *J. Cell. Biol.*, 84: 455–460.

Lin, S., Lin, D.C., Flanagan, M.D. and Grumet, M. (1979) Control of actin polymerization by high-affinity cytochalasin binding complexes. *J. Cell. Biol.*, 83: 317a.

Meyer, D.I. and Burger, M.M. (1979) The chromaffin granule surface: the presence of actin and the nature of its interaction with the membrane. *FEBS Lett.*, 101: 129–133.

Nicklas, W.J. and Berl, S. (1974) Effects of cytochalasin B on uptake and release of putative neurotransmitters by synaptosomes and on brain actomyosin-like protein. *Nature (Lond.)*, 247: 471–473.

O'Farrell, P.H. (1975) High-resolution two-dimensional electrophoresis of proteins, *J. biol. Chem.*, 250: 4007–4021.

Ostlund, R.E., Leung, J.T. and Kipnis, D.M. (1977) Muscle actin filaments bind pituitary secretory granules in vitro. *J. Cell. Biol.*, 73: 78–87.

Phillips, J.H. and Slater, A. (1975) Actin in the adrenal medulla. *FEBS Lett.*, 101: 129–133.

Podlubnaya, Z.A., Tskhovrebova, L.A., Zaalishvili, M.M. and Stefanenko, G.A. (1975) Electron microscopic study of α-actinin. *J. Molec. Biol.*, 92: 357–359.

Puszkin, S. and Kochwa, S. (1974) Regulation of neurotransmitter release by a complex of actin in the relaxing protein isolated from rat brain synaptosomes. *J. biol. Chem.*, 249: 7711–7714.

Robson, R.M. and Zeece, M.G. (1973) Comparative studies of α-actinin from porcine cardiac and skeletal muscle. *Biochim. biophys. Acta*, 295: 208–224.

Schollmeyer, J.E., Goll, D.E., Robson, R.M. and Stromer, H.M. (1973) Localization of α-actinin and tropomyosin in different muscles, *J. Cell. Biol.*, 59: 306a.

Schollmeyer, J.V., Goll, D.E., Stromer, M.H., Dayton, W., Singh, I. and Robson, R.M. (1974) Studies on the composition of the Z-disk. *J. Cell. Biol.*, 63: 303a.

Suzuki, A., Goll, D.E., Singh, I., Allen, R.E., Robson, R.M. and Stromer, M.H. (1976) Some properties of purified skeletal muscle α-actinin. *J. biol. Chem.*, 251: 6860–6870.

Thoa, N.B., Wooten, G.F., Axelrod, J. and Kopin, I.J. (1972) Inhibition of release of dopamine-β-hydroxylase and norepinephrine from sympathetic nerves by colchicine, vinblastine or cytochalasin B. *Proc. nat. Acad. Sci. U.S.A.*, 69: 520–522.

Trifaro, J.M. (1977) Common mechanisms of hormone secretion. *Ann. Rev. Pharmacol. Toxicol.*, 17: 27–47.

Trifaro, J.M. (1978) Contractile proteins in tissues originating in the neural crest. *Neuroscience*, 3: 1–24.

Trifaro, J.M. and Ulpian, C. (1976) Isolation and characterization of myosin from the adrenal medulla. *Neuroscience*, 1: 483–488.

Trifaro, J.M., Ulpian, C. and Preiksaitis, H. (1978) Anti-myosin stains chromaffin cells. *Experientia*, 34: 1568–1571.

Unsicker, K., Griesser, G.H., Lindmar, R., Loffelholz, K. and Wolf, V. (1980) Establishment, characterization and fiber outgrowth of isolated bovine adrenal medullary cells in long-term culture. *Neuroscience*, 5: 1445–1460.

Wehland, J., Osborn, M. and Weber, K. (1977) Phalloidin-induced actin polymerization in the cytoplasm of cultured cells interferes with cell locomotion and growth. *Proc. nat. Acad. Sci. U.S.A.*, 74: 5613–5617.

Wilkins, J.A. and Lin, S. (1981) Association of actin with chromaffin granule membranes and the effect of cytochalasin B on the polarity of actin filament elongation. *Biochim. biophys. Acta*, 642: 55–66.

Zinder, O., Hoffman, P.G., Bonner, W.H. and Pollard, H.B. (1978) Comparison of chemical properties of purified plasma membranes and secretory vesicle membranes from the bovine adrenal medulla. *Cell Tiss. Res.*, 188: 153–170.

Plasma Membrane of *Torpedo* Synaptosomes: Morphological Changes During Acetylcholine Release and Evidence for a Specific Protein*

NICOLAS MOREL

Département Neurochimie, Neurobiologie Cellulaire, CNRS, 91190 Gif sur Yvette (France)

INTRODUCTION

Torpedo electric organs have an abundant and purely cholinergic innervation (Feldberg et al., 1940) and are therefore very convenient for biochemical studies of neurotransmission at peripheral synapses. As is the case for brain (Gray and Whittaker, 1960; De Robertis et al., 1961), nerve terminals pinched off during tissue subfractionation can be isolated as sealed particles = synaptosomes (Israël et al., 1976; Morel et al., 1977; Michaelson and Sokolovsky, 1978). The main advantage of *Torpedo* synaptosomal fractions is that all the synaptosomes are cholinergic. This permits the study of their physiological properties without interference from non-cholinergic materials. The large field electron micrograph (Fig. 1) illustrates the homogeneity and purity of the synaptosomal fraction.

EFFECT OF STIMULATION: ACETYLCHOLINE RELEASE

It is possible to label synaptosomal acetylcholine (ACh) by incubating the synaptosomes in the presence of a radioactive precursor, choline or acetate (Morel et al., 1977). The use of acetate appeared very convenient since, for low external concentrations (less than 40 μM), all the synaptosomal radioactivity was found as labeled ACh (Morel et al., 1979, 1980). It is then possible to consider that the released radioactivity provides a good measurement of transmitter release. It has been shown (Morel et al., 1979, 1980) that K^+ depolarization (50 or 100 μM) triggers a calcium-dependent ACh release. This release is transient and subsides in a minute, though K^+ is still present and only a small fraction of synaptosomal ACh (about 5%) has been released. If KCl is further increased after the first depolarization, a further ACh release can be obtained (Morel and Meunier, 1981).

ACh release can also be triggered by application of a venom (GV) extracted from

*This work was performed in collaboration with M. Israel, R. Manaranche, and B. Lesbats, *Neurobiologie Cellulaire, CNRS, 91190 Gif sur Yvette* and T. Gulik-Krzywicki, *Centre de Génétique Moléculaire, CNRS, 91190 Gif sur Yvette.*

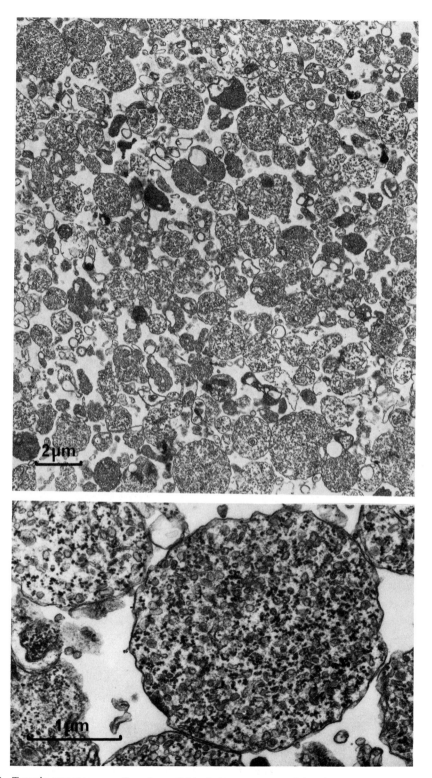

Fig. 1. *Torpedo* synaptosomes. Top: large field of the synaptosomal fraction prepared from *Torpedo* electric organ. Bottom: a typical *Torpedo* synaptosome. Note the absence of postsynaptic membrane attachment and the large size of the synaptosome. Intraterminal mitochondria are rarely observed.

Glycera convoluta (Manaranche et al., 1980). Figure 2 compares the ACh releases induced, on the same synaptosomal fraction, either by KCl depolarization or by GV application. In the latter case, ACh release is much more prolonged and larger amounts of ACh are released. GV action is not dependent upon the external calcium concentration since GV can induce ACh release from *Torpedo* synaptosomes even in the absence of external calcium and in the presence of EGTA (Israël et al., 1981).

Recently Israël and Lesbats (1980) developed a chemiluminescent method for measuring ACh. They were able to follow quantitatively and continuously the release of ACh from synaptosomes, and to determine immediately the changes in their internal ACh compartmentalization (Israël and Lesbats, 1981). As is the case for various cholinergic tissues or other neurotransmitters (for review, see Israël et al., 1980), it is possible to distinguish two different neurotransmitter compartments within *Torpedo* synaptosomes. After freezing and thawing the synaptosomes, a so-called "free" compartment is lost (Morel et al., 1977) or released in the external medium (Israël and Lesbats, 1981). This compartment is labeled with a higher specific radioactivity than the other (bound) compartment, which is rather insensitive to the freezing-thawing procedure (Morel et al., 1977). On the basis of sub-fractionation arguments, "bound" ACh is assumed to be located within synaptic vesicles. Israël and Lesbats (1981) have measured successively on the same samples, in conditions where ACh resynthesis is absent, the amounts of released, "free" and bound ACh. After GV application, released ACh amounted to the size of the "free" pool which was exhausted, whereas the "bound" (vesicular) pool was not modified. After KCl depolarization, "free" ACh was diminished whereas bound ACh was unchanged. Therefore ACh appears to be released from the "free" ACh compartment in *Torpedo* synaptosomes, as has been shown in *Torpedo* electric organ (see

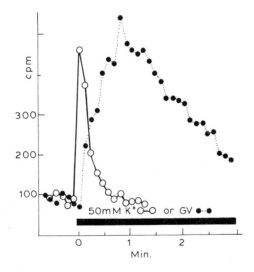

Fig. 2. ACh release. Synaptosomal ACh was labeled using [1-^{14}C]acetate (40 μM) for 2 h at 20 °C. Synaptosomes were concentrated by centrifugation and 100–200 μl aliquots were introduced into a perfusion chamber (see Morel et al., 1979, 1980). Radioactivity was determined in each drop of the effluent. After a washing period, a constant background activity was obtained. Stimulation was started by perfusion in a medium containing either 50 mM K$^+$ or a venom (GV, 0.05 gland/ml final concentration) extracted from *Glycera convoluta* (see Manaranche et al., 1980).

Israël et al., 1980, for a review). The "free" pool of ACh, which is clearly different from the pool bound to synaptic vesicles, is at least partly cytoplasmic since choline acetyltransferase is a soluble enzyme (Fonnum, 1967). The existence of a sub-compartment of "free" ACh, loosely bound to some unknown intraterminal structure, cannot be excluded.

EFFECT OF STIMULATION: ULTRASTRUCTURAL CHANGES

Freeze-fracture methods have been used to follow morphological modifications accompanying neurotransmitter release, since a large surface of the presynaptic membrane can be analyzed (Pfenninger et al., 1972; Heuser et al., 1974; Ceccarelli et al., 1979). Ultrarapid freezing procedures permit the avoidance of any chemical fixation and are, therefore, very suitable to catch transient membrane modifications (Heuser et al., 1979; Morel et al., 1980). Using the "sandwich freezing" procedure (Gulik-Krzywicki and Costello, 1978) for the ultrarapid freezing of *Torpedo* synaptosomes in suspension, large surface areas of the synaptosomal membrane were analyzed in conditions causing ACh release. An increase of the number of pits in the P and E faces of the synaptosomal membrane was noticed after KCl depolarization (Fig. 3). This increase, like ACh release, was dependent on the presence of extracellular calcium and was transient (Morel et al., 1980). These pits are probably related to the endo–exocytotic cycle of synaptic vesicles, which has been demonstrated by the internalization of extracellular markers (Ceccarelli et al., 1973; Heuser and Reese, 1973; Fried and Blaustein, 1978). Surprisingly, the number of pits in the presynaptic membrane was not increased after 40 s of GV action, whereas ACh release was already important (Israël et al., 1981). It is therefore possible to dissociate ACh release and the endo–exocytotic cycle of synaptic vesicles.

A second type of modification of the presynaptic membrane was observed, which concerned the density of intramembrane particles (Israël et al., 1981). The major result is the observation of an important decrease of the small (5–8 nm) P face particles after KCl depolarization or GV action. This decrease was calcium-dependent after KCl depolarization but not after GV action (like ACh release). This result is in good agreement with previous works (Fesce et al., 1980; Tokunaga et al., 1979) and suggests redistributions or reassociations of intramembrane proteins during synaptic activity.

Besides these ultrastructural modifications of the synaptosomal membrane, ACh release is also accompanied by a presynaptic ATP release which has the same time course (Morel and Meunier, 1981). The stoichiometry of ACh to ATP release is about 50 after KCl depolarization and 10 after GV action and, therefore, higher than the ACh/ATP ratio within isolated synaptic vesicles (about 5).

The study of ACh release suffers from the impossibility of controlling the intracellular composition of synaptosomes. The isolation of presynaptic membrane sacs would perhaps permit one to perform the type of experiments described above on particles less complex than synaptosomes and to study the relationships between ACh release and metabolic or membrane processes triggered by stimulation.

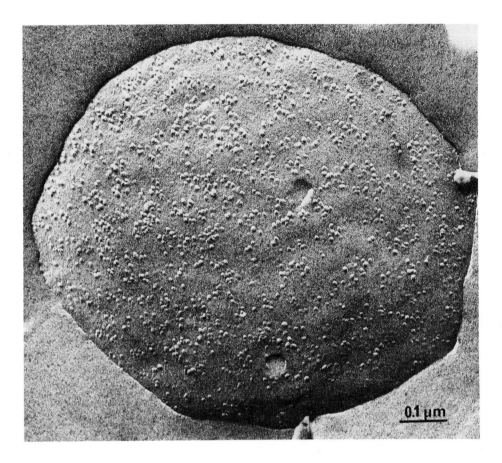

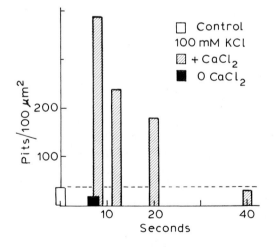

Fig. 3. Pits in KCl-depolarized synaptosomes. The micrograph shows a *Torpedo* synaptosome depolarized in 100 mM KCl for 20 s. Two pits are visible in the smooth surface of the presynaptic membrane (P face). The density of pits is maximal after 7 s of KCl depolarization (100 mM) and returns to control levels in less than 40 s. No increase was found in the absence of calcium (for details, see Morel et al., 1980).

ISOLATION OF THE SYNAPTOSOMAL PLASMA MEMBRANE

With *Torpedo* synaptosomes one overcomes a major difficulty usually encountered in the isolation of presynaptic membranes, i.e. the absence of a specific biochemical or immunological marker. We have taken advantage of the high purity of the synaptosomal fraction (see Fig. 1) to assume that most of the plasma membrane we isolate after lysis of the synaptosomes and equilibrium centrifugation on sucrose density gradients must correspond to the synaptosomal plasma membrane. Such an assumption has already been made in the previous work of Stadler and Tashiro (1979). The most likely contaminants are postsynaptic plasma membrane fragments, easily recognized by their high nicotinic ACh receptor content. We were able to clearly separate two related plasma membrane fractions (F_3 and F_4) from postsynaptic plasma membranes on the basis of their equilibrium density (Morel et al., 1982). Morphological analysis of F_3 and F_4 demonstrated the absence of synaptic vesicles or myelin fragments. These membrane fragments have the same intramembrane particle density as the freeze-fractured synaptosomal membrane. They are rich in acetylcholinesterase. Their polypeptide pattern was analyzed by polyacrylamide gel electrophoresis in SDS (see Fig. 4; Morel et al., 1982).

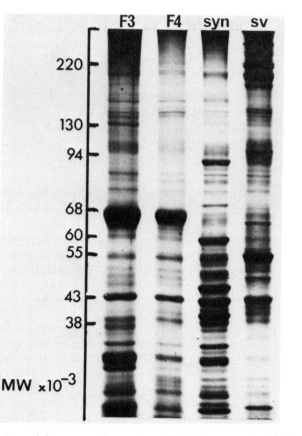

Fig. 4. The protein pattern of the presynaptic membrane (F_3, F_4) is compared with that of synaptosomes (syn) and of crude synaptic vesicles (sv) isolated as described by Israël et al. (1980). Each sample contains about 40–50 μg protein.

It appeared complex with numerous bands, great similarities being evident between F_3 and F_4. A major band (67,000 daltons molecular weight) appears specific for the presynaptic membrane since it was not found in F_5, which contains the postsynaptic membranes, or in a crude fraction of synaptic vesicles. Furthermore, there is a great enrichment of this band in presynaptic membranes when compared to synaptosomes.

This work raises the possibility of an immunochemical characterization of the plasma membrane of cholinergic nerve terminals. An immunological marker would also permit a large scale purification of this membrane, necessary to envisage experiments concerning the functional properties of these proteins.

REFERENCES

Ceccarelli, B., Hurlbut, W.P. and Mauro, A. (1973) Turnover of transmitter and synaptic vesicles at the frog neuromuscular junction. *J. Cell Biol.*, 57: 499–524.

Ceccarelli, B., Grohovaz, F. and Hurlbut, W.P. (1979) Freeze-fracture studies of frog neuromuscular junctions during intense release of neurotransmitter. II. Effects of electrical stimulation and high potassium. *J. Cell Biol.*, 81: 178–192.

De Robertis, E., Pellegrino de Iraldi, A., Rodriguez de Lores Arnaiz, G. and Salganicoff, L. (1961) Electron microscope observations on nerve endings isolated from rat brain. *Anat. Rec.*, 139: 220.

Feldberg, W., Fessard, A. and Nachmansohn, D. (1940) The cholinergic nature of the nervous supply to the electrical organ of the torpedo (*Torpedo marmorata*). *J. Physiol. (Lond.)*, 97: 3P.

Fesce, R., Grohovaz, F., Hurlbut, W.P. and Ceccarelli, B. (1980) Freeze-fracture studies of frog neuromuscular junctions during intense release of neurotransmitters. III A morphometric analysis of the number and diameter of intramembrane particles. *J. Cell Biol.*, 85: 337–345.

Fonnum, F. (1967) The compartmentation of choline acetyltransferase within the synaptosome. *Biochem. J.*, 103: 262–270.

Fried, R.C. and Blaustein, M.P. (1978) Retrieval and recycling of synaptic vesicle membrane in pinched-off nerve terminals (synaptosomes). *J. Cell Biol.*, 78: 685–700.

Gray, E.G. and Whittaker, V.P. (1960) The isolation of synaptic vesicles from the central nervous system. *J. Physiol. (Lond.)*, 153: 35P–37P.

Gulik-Krzywicki, T. and Costello, M.J. (1978) The use of low temperature X-ray diffraction to evaluate freezing methods used in freeze-fracture electron microscopy. *J. Microsc.*, 112: 103–113.

Heuser, J.E. and Reese, T.S. (1973) Evidence for recycling of synaptic vesicle membrane during transmitter release at the frog neuromuscular junction. *J. Cell Biol.*, 57: 315–344.

Heuser, J.E., Reese T.S. and Landis, D.M.D. (1974) Functional changes in frog neuromuscular junctions studied with freeze-fracture. *J. Neurocytol.*, 3: 109–131.

Heuser, J.E., Reese, T.S., Dennis, M.J., Jan, Y., Jan, L. and Evans, L. (1979) Synaptic vesicle exocytosis captured by quick freezing and correlated with quantal transmitter release. *J. Cell Biol.*, 81: 275–300.

Israël, M. and Lesbats, B. (1980) Détection continue de la libération d'acétylcholine de l'organe électrique de la Torpille à l'aide d'une réaction de chimiluminescence. *C.R. Acad. Sci. (Paris)*, 291: 713–715.

Israël, M. and Lesbats, B. (1981) Continuous determination of transmitter release and compartmentation in *Torpedo* electric organ synaptosomes, studied with a chemiluminescent method detecting acetylcholine. *J. Neurochem.*, in press.

Israël, M., Manaranche, R., Mastour, P. and Morel, N. (1976) Isolation of pure cholinergic nerve endings from the electric organ of *Torpedo marmorata*. *Biochem. J.*, 160: 113–115.

Israël, M., Dunant, Y. and Manaranche, R. (1979) The present status of the vesicular hypothesis. *Progr. Neurobiol.*, 13: 237–275.

Israël, M., Manaranche, R., Marsal, J., Meunier, F.M., Morel, N., Frachon, P. and Lesbats, B. (1980) ATP dependent calcium uptake by cholinergic synaptic vesicles isolated from *Torpedo* electric organ, *J. Membrane Biol.*, 54: 115–126.

Israël, M., Manaranche, R., Morel, N., Dedieu, J.C., Gulik-Krzywicki, T. and Lesbats, B. (1981) Redistribution of intramembrane particles related to acetylcholine release by cholinergic synaptosomes. *J. Ultrastruct. Res.* in press.

38

Manaranche, R., Thieffry, M. and Israël, M. (1980) Effect of the venom of *Glycera convoluta* on the spontaneous quantal release of transmitter. *J. Cell Biol.*, 85: 446–458.

Michaelson, D.M. and Sokolovsky, M. (1978) Induced acetylcholine release from active purely cholinergic *Torpedo* synaptosomes. *J. Neurochem.*, 30: 217–230.

Morel, N. and Meunier, F.M. (1981) Simultaneous release of ACh and ATP from stimulated cholinergic synaptosomes. *J. Neurochem.*, 36: 1766–1773.

Morel, N., Israël, M., Manaranche, R. and Mastour, P. (1977) Isolation of pure cholinergic nerve endings from *Torpedo* electric organ. Evaluation of their metabolic properties. *J. Cell Biol.*, 75: 43–55.

Morel, N., Israël, M., Manaranche, R. and Lesbats, B. (1979) Stimulation of cholinergic synaptosomes isolated from *Torpedo* electric organ. In S. Tuček (Ed.), *The Cholinergic Synapse, Progress in Brain Research, Vol. 49*, Elsevier/North-Holland, Amsterdam, pp. 191–202.

Morel, N., Manaranche, R., Gulik-Krzywicki, T. and Israël, M. (1980) Ultrastructural changes and transmitter release induced by depolarization of cholinergic synaptosomes. *J. Ultrastruct. Res.*, 70: 347–362.

Morel, N., Manaranche, R., Israël, M. and Gulik-Krzywicki, T. (1982) Isolation of a presynaptic plasma membrane fraction from *Torpedo* cholinergic synaptosomes: evidence for a specific protein. *J. Cell Biol.*, 93: 349–356.

Pfenninger, K., Akert, K., Moor, H. and Sandri, C. (1972) The fine structure of freeze-fractured presynaptic membranes. *J. Neurocytol.*, 1: 129–149.

Stadler, H. and Tashiro, T. (1979) Isolation of synaptosomal plasma membranes from cholinergic nerve terminals and a comparison of their proteins with those of synaptic vesicles. *Europ. J. Biochem.*, 101: 171–178.

Tokunaga, A., Sandri, C. and Akert, K. (1979) Increase of large intramembranous particles in the presynaptic active zone after administration of 4-aminopyridine. *Brain Res.*, 174: 207–219.

Ionic Channels for Signal Transmission and Propagation

ERWIN NEHER, ALAIN MARTY and ELIZABETH FENWICK*

*Max-Planck-Institut für biophysikalische Chemie (*Abt. Neurochemie), Postfach 968, D-3400 Göttingen (F.R.G.)*

INTRODUCTION

The ability to propagate and transmit signals is conferred to neurons by proteins embedded in the lipid membrane. A knowledge of the molecular properties of these macromolecules would therefore provide a sound basis for the understanding of neuronal functions. A great deal of information on such molecular functions has been provided by two recently developed electrophysiological techniques: noise analysis and single channel recording. Both these techniques allow the study of integral proteins which are assumed to function as so-called ionic channels or membrane pores regulating the flow of ions across the membrane. As such, these proteins must span the whole membrane thickness, and provide a hydrophilic pathway across the membrane. In addition, they must be able to undergo conformational changes between states of different ionic permeabilities in order to switch the membrane current on and off. Both noise analysis and single channel recording aim at answering questions such as: how much current does a single ionic channel carry in its high or low permeability state? What is the number of such entities per unit area of membrane? For how much time does a channel stay in one or the other state? What are the physical or chemical stimuli which induce transitions between the states?

Single channel recording answers these questions by resolving microscopic current contributions from individual ionic channels in experimental situations where channel opening is a rare event, and where background noise of the recording can be sufficiently reduced. Thereby, some of the above questions are answered by mere inspection of the current records.

Noise analysis works on the macroscopic fluctuations in membrane current, which result from the statistical superposition of many microscopic unit responses. Exploiting some fundamental laws of statistics it deduces from the macroscopic fluctuations the properties of the elementary units which constitute them (see also Fig. 1). Noise analysis is applicable to a wider range of preparations and experimental conditions; however, it depends on certain assumptions, the validity of which, in turn, has to be proven by single channel recording.

This article gives a summary of some of the molecular features of ionic channels encountered in nerve and nerve-like cells. It will focus on results obtained by single channel recording. Where necessary, it will also include noise results.

[39]

40

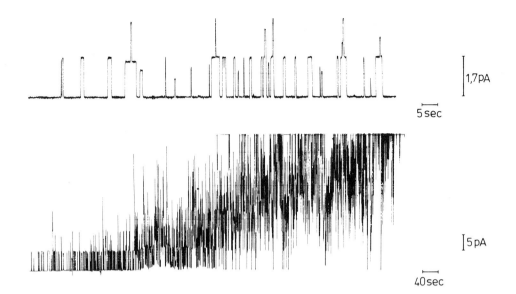

1,7pA

5 sec

5 pA

40 sec

Fig. 1. The relationship between membrane current fluctuations and single channel events. The two traces of the figure show recordings of membrane current flowing through artificial bimolecular lipid membranes treated with the channel-forming polypeptide gramicidin A. In the upper trace, a steady-state situation had been reached with a low number of channels incorporated into the membrane. Experimental conditions were chosen such that single channel responses of approximately 2 pA and 1 s mean duration appeared at a constant low frequency. In the lower trace, a larger amount of gramicidin was added to the experimental chamber shortly before the start of the record. Some well-separated single channel responses appeared in the first few seconds of the records. Then, while more and more gramicidin was incorporated into the membrane, channel responses became more frequent, and overlapped, to produce large fluctuations in current. Single steps cannot be resolved at the end of the record due to excessive overlap. Still, the pulse parameters can be estimated by the method of noise analysis. For instance, the information on the size of the unit step is contained in the relation between the size of the fluctuations and the mean current (see Neher and Stevens, 1977, for review).

A NEURON NEEDS AT LEAST THREE SETS OF IONIC CHANNELS

Nerve impulses are propagated along axons by a mechanism involving voltage and time dependent membrane permeability changes. Hodgkin and Huxley (1952) were able to separate the complex current pattern into two components: an early transient inward current, carried by Na, which depolarizes the nerve fiber during an action potential; and a delayed, maintained outward current, carried by K ions which repolarizes the fiber. The ionic channels underlying these currents have been studied on the single channel level in a number of preparations: in squid giant axon (Conti and Neher, 1980), in rat embryonic muscle cells (Sigworth and Neher, 1980), and in bovine chromaffin cells (Fenwick et al., 1981).

Besides propagating impulses a neuron must be able to integrate incoming information along its dendritic surface, and it must have a means of transmitting its activity to follower cells. Both tasks are largely fulfilled by chemical synapses, where the neuron plays the role of the postsynaptic or presynaptic part, respectively (Katz, 1966). In its presynaptic function the neuron must be able to release transmitter substance in response to an action potential. Release, by vesicle exocytosis, is stimulated by an increase in internal Ca concentration (see article by H. Winkler et al., this volume) which, in turn, results from an increase in Ca permeability. This Ca permeability is voltage dependent and resembles the nerve Na permeability in its activation properties; however it does not inactivate in many preparations (Llinas et al., 1981). Single channel properties of Ca channels were studied in snail neurons (Lux and Nagy, 1982) and in bovine chromaffin cells (Fenwick et al., 1981). The latter cells, in many respects, are model cells for nerve terminals.

Besides Ca channels, neurosecretory cells seem to require extra voltage-dependent K channels which are controlled by intracellular, or membrane-bound Ca (for review see Thompson and Aldrich, 1981). These channels act to hyperpolarize cells after periods of activity. They may constitute a feedback element or may serve a safety function which is required due to the fact that Ca currents do not inactivate. Different types of Ca-dependent K single channels have been studied in bovine chromaffin cells (Marty, 1981) and in snail neurons (Lux et al., 1981).

The third set of channels is connected to the neuron's postsynaptic function. Transmitter substances either depolarize or hyperpolarize neurons or muscle cells mostly by activating ionic channels which are either permeable for Na *and* K (for excitatory transmitters) or for Cl *or* K (for inhibitory transmitters). Acetylcholine (ACh) and its action as an excitatory transmitter has been best studied so far. This transmitter and the ionic channel activated by it have also stimulated the development of both noise analysis (Katz and Miledi, 1972; Anderson and Stevens, 1973) and single channel recording techniques (Neher and Sakmann, 1976). Next to ACh the action of glutamate as an excitatory transmitter at crustacean neuromuscular junctions (Usherwood, 1980) and the action of GABA and glycine at spinal cord neurons (Mathers et al., 1981; Borman et al., 1982) has been studied by single channel techniques.

THE PATCH TECHNIQUE OFFERS FOUR RECORDING CONFIGURATIONS FOR STUDYING IONIC CHANNELS IN MEMBRANE PATCHES AND IN SMALL CELLS

In order to resolve current signals from individual ionic channels two conditions must be met: first, the background noise must be small; secondly, the overall activity must be low, such that individual events can be separated. Both requirements are met if the total membrane area on which the recording is done is sufficiently small. For noise considerations a membrane area of $1000 \, \mu m^2$, corresponding to a spherical cell $18 \, \mu m$ in diameter, would be small enough (Neher, 1982). For the second requirement an even smaller area might be better. Since it is general experience that electrophysiological recording from such small cells is difficult, if not impossible, we tried to meet the requirements by electrically isolating for the purpose of the measurement small patches of membrane from larger structures. We achieved this by placing a heat-polished glass pipette of small dimensions onto the surface of an enzymatically cleaned muscle fiber (Neher and Sakmann, 1976). The success of such a measurement depends critically on the quality of the contact between glass pipette and membrane. This contact establishes the seal separating the membrane patch on which the measurement is performed from the rest of the cell. Upon plain contact this seal is in the range 10–50 MΩ (resistance measured between pipette interior and bath). Under favorable circumstances this seal can be irreversibly increased to 1–100 GΩ (Neher, 1982). The improved seal (giga-seal), then, together with simple mechanical manipulations, allows four different types of measurement to be performed (Hamill et al., 1981).

(a) *Cell attached patch recording*: recording of current flowing through a pipette which is sealed to a relatively large cell. This is essentially an extracellular recording. Extracellular type action potentials (biphasic) can be observed if the cell is spontaneously active. The membrane potential of the patch can be changed with respect to the rest of the cell by changing the potential in the pipette. Voltage-clamp-type currents originating from the microscopic patch are measured if the rest of the cell is large enough to "clamp" the intracellular potential to the normal resting value. This is usually the case if the cell is larger than approximately 30 μm in diameter. The membrane patch can be stimulated locally both electrically (see above) and chemically (by adding a low concentration of transmitter substance to the pipette filling solution).

(b) *Whole cell recording employing a patch pipette*: once a giga-seal has formed the membrane adheres to the glass pipette so tightly that the membrane patch can be broken without the seal being affected. Then there is a low-resistance connection between the pipette interior and the cell. The whole assembly has a "leakage" against bath solution better than 10 GΩ. In this situation current-clamp- or voltage-clamp-type recording from the whole cell can be performed. If the patch pipette opening is made relatively wide (≥1 μm inner diameter) the cell interior is being efficiently dialyzed against the pipette solution. This is similar to the internal perfusion techniques developed for larger cells (Kristhal and Pidoplichko, 1975; Lee et al., 1978). Voltage-clamp conditions are met for cells smaller than 15 μm in diameter (see Fig. 2).

If the pipette is slowly withdrawn from the cell in any of the above two configurations the membrane does not separate from the pipette, nor does it tear a large hole into the cell. Rather, a cone- or cylinder-shaped bridge is pulled out of the cell by the recording pipette, which becomes longer and thinner as the separation increases. Finally, the bridge ties off. Afterwards, there is an intact cell left behind, and a pipette which is tightly closed off by microscopic pieces of membrane. This leads to two more recording configurations (Hamill et al., 1981).

(c) *The outside-out patch*: if the pipette is withdrawn starting from a "whole-cell recording" configuration, it is being closed off by a patch of membrane which has its previously extracellular surface exposed to the bath fluid. Its previously cytoplasmic face is exposed to the pipette solution. This configuration is very well suited for studying single channels activated by outwardly directed receptors (e.g. ACh-activated channels), since the concentration of the agonist can be changed at ease. The patches are very stable, since their integrity no longer depends on a mechanically stable micromanipulator.

(d) *The inside-out patch*: if the pipette is withdrawn starting from a "cell-attached" configuration, a closed, vesicle-like structure forms in the pipette. Withdrawal, so to speak, folds a new membrane over the already existing one. The second membrane can be destroyed by air exposure (Hamill and Sakmann, 1981), or else it can be made leaky if the procedure is performed in Ca-free media with fluoride as the major anion (Horn and Patlak, 1980). In both cases, effectively, a single bilayer remains as the main barrier for ion flow. It has its previously cytoplasmic face

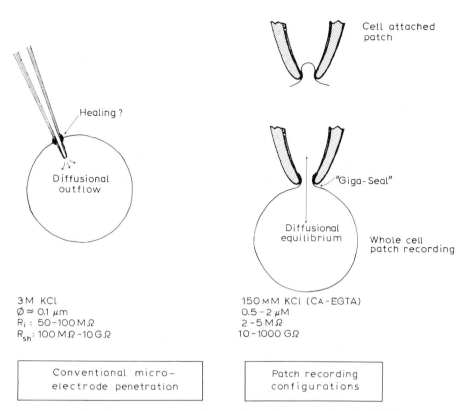

Fig. 2. A comparison between conventional recording techniques and patch pipette measurements. Schematic diagrams which compare the different ways of recording from small cells with respect to the following parameters: filling solution, inner diameter of pipette opening, typical internal resistance R_i, and the shunt resistance R_{sh} between pipette interior and bath fluid.

exposed to the bath solution. This configuration allows single ionic channels to be studied under accurate control of the "inside" ionic milieu. It has a vast potential for studying effects of internal Ca (Marty, 1981) or other substances thought to function as intracellular second messengers.

THE CHROMAFFIN CELL: A MODEL "NEURON"

Chromaffin cells from adrenal medulla are derived ontogenetically from the neuronal crest and have many similarities to sympathetic neurons. They possess the complete sets of ionic channels mentioned above (Fenwick et al., 1981), and in this sense can serve the function of model "neurons".

Bovine chromaffin cells are obtained as dispersed cells in large quantities (Fenwick et al., 1978) and can be kept in short-term tissue culture. They fire action potentials, which either occur spontaneously, or can be elicited by current stimulation or by stimulation with ACh. This is illustrated in Fig. 3 which shows a whole cell recording under current-clamp conditions. Voltage-clamp records normally display Hodgkin–Huxley-type Na and K currents (Fig. 4). In medium lacking Na, a non-

44

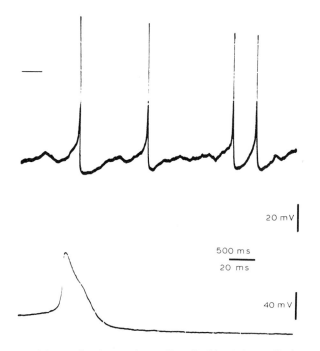

Fig. 3. Intracellular potential recording from a chromaffin cell with a "giga-seal" pipette. The upper trace shows spontaneous action potentials (APs) of 80–100 mV amplitude starting from a resting potential fluctuating around −60 mV. The lower trace gives one of these APs at better time resolution. The parallel combination of seal resistance and cell membrane resistance was >10 GΩ in this cell. Room temperature; filter bandwidth was 1 kHz.

inactivating Ca current can be observed. This current component is very similar to the Ca current of squid giant synapse (Llinas et al., 1981).

ACh at concentrations between 10 and 100 μM induces inward currents of up to 200 pA (at −80 mV).

On the single channel level (in "cell-attached" or outside-out patch recording configuration), discrete current pulses corresponding to all four current components mentioned so far can be observed. In addition, a fifth type of unit event appears. This extra current is a K current of large unit size which depends on intracellular Ca (Marty, 1981).

Single Na channels are most prominent when the cell is maintained at a hyper-polarized level of −80 to −90 mV and then intermittently stimulated by 30–50 mV depolarizing pulses. They are inwardly directed current pulses of 1–2 pA amplitude and of approximately 1 ms duration (Fig. 5). At larger depolarizations small outward unit events also occur, which probably represent the delayed K-rectifier.

Unit currents of the Ca-type can be observed if Ba is the main cation in the extracellular medium (Fenwick et al., 1981). Stimulation by ACh induces single channels of 45 pS unit conductance and ≈30 ms mean open time. Individual channels sometimes trigger an action potential. This illustrates an interesting feature of small cells regarding the relationship between unit channel size and whole cell conductance properties.

In large cells which are, for technical reasons, usually preferred for elec-

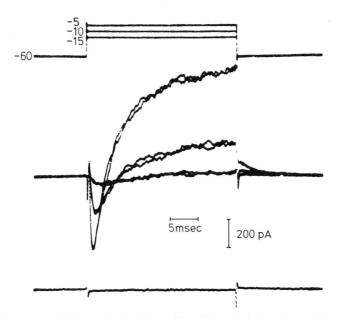

Fig. 4. Voltage-clamp records from a bovine chromaffin cell in a "whole cell recording" configuration. Depolarizing command voltage steps of 35, 45 and 55 mV amplitude are given starting from a resting potential of −60 mV. Room temperature. Two traces are superimposed for each value of the command signal. The bath fluid was normal mammalian Ringer; the pipette was filled with a solution containing 140 mM KCl, 1.05 mM EGTA, 1 mM $CaCl_2$, 2 mM $MgCl_2$ and 10 mM HEPES, pH 7.6. The currents display Hodgkin–Huxley-type Na and K currents. They differ from standard voltage-clamp records (e.g. from squid) in two respects: (1) current scale, currents are smaller than 1 nA due to the small size of the cells (<20 μm); and (2) the currents show relatively large random fluctuations due to the small numbers of ionic channels involved. The background noise of the recording can be estimated from the lowermost current trace, which shows a single response to a 55 mV hyperpolarizing voltage pulse. This record also demonstrates the low leakage conductance and fast settling time of the clamp. No leakage subtraction, but capacitance transient cancellation (Hamill et al., 1981) was applied.

trophysiological measurements, unit channel conductance is a vanishing quantity. The quantum nature of the channel hardly reflects itself in the cell's behavior. This is very different in cells of 10–20 μm in diameter, which sizewise are probably more representative for cells in the animal kingdom. Consider a chromaffin cell of 15 μm diameter. It has an input resistance in the range 10 GΩ (Hamill et al., 1981). A single ACh channel (25 GΩ internal resistance) can depolarize it by 10–20 mV if it happens to open for a time longer than the cell's time constant. Thus, statistics of single channels can dominate the cell's resting behavior. This fact reflects itself in the noisy baseline of voltage recordings in Fig. 3. During an action potential, however, many channels are active. Maximum Na currents under optimal stimulation are in the range 1 nA which represents the superposition of at least 500–1000 channels. Even if only 10% of these channels were active during an action potential, the number would still be large enough to average out the statistical nature of the unit channel. Also, the total number of ACh channels on a chromaffin cell is well above 100 (fast application of 100 μM ACh elicits up to 200 pA of current at −80 mV). Since a single channel can fire an action potential it can be expected that there is efficient transduction.

46

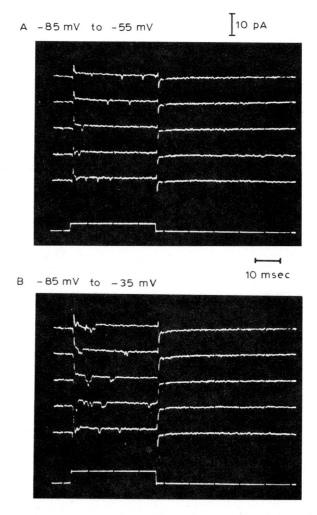

Fig. 5. Single Na currents in response to depolarizing voltage stimuli. This is an "outside-out" patch recording at room temperature and with a holding potential of −85 mV. Depolarizing voltage commands to either −55 mV (A) or −35 mV (B) are given repeatedly. Single Na channel currents appear during the stimulation period. At the smaller depolarization they are short in duration and spread out over the whole stimulation interval. At the larger depolarization they are longer in duration and appear predominantly early during the stimulation interval.

CONCLUSIONS

Most of the well-known electrophysiological ionic processes have been shown to be made up of unit current contributions occurring statistically. The amplitude range of these single channel conductances is 5–50 pS. Their time-course has the shape of rectangular square pulses or of groups ("bursts") of these pulses. These parameters are such that a single event may dominate the resting behavior in cells of 10–20 μm diameter – a size range probably most common in animal tissue. During action potentials, however, a large number of channels has to act in concert, such that the statistical nature of the unit signals is averaged out.

Comparison of single channel currents with macroscopic voltage-clamp currents can be very helpful for separating individual current components in cells with complex electrophysiology. Analysis of single channel waveforms gives kinetic information more detailed than that of the macroscopic currents.

ACKNOWLEDGEMENTS

A. Marty and E. Neher were partially supported by the Deutsche Forschungsgemeinschaft. E. Fenwick was supported by a von Humboldt fellowship.

REFERENCES

Anderson, C.R. and Stevens, C.F. (1973) Voltage clamp analysis of acetylcholine produced end-plate current fluctuations at frog neuromuscular junction. *J. Physiol. (Lond.)*, 235: 655–691.

Borman, J., Hamill, O.P. and Sakmann, B. (1982) Voltage and chemically activated channels in spinal cord neurons, in preparation.

Conti, F. and Neher, E. (1980) Single channel recordings of K^+ currents in squid axons. *Nature (Lond.)*, 285: 140–143.

Fenwick, E.M., Fajdiga, P.B., Howe, N.B.S. and Livett, B.G. (1978) Functional and morphological characterization of isolated bovine adrenal medullary cells. *J. Cell Biol.*, 76: 12–30.

Fenwick, E.M., Marty, A. and Neher, E. (1981) Voltage clamp and single channel recording from bovine chromaffin cells. *J. Physiol. (Lond.)*, abstract, in press.

Hamill, O.P. and Sakmann, B. (1981) A cell-free method for recording single channel currents from biological membranes. *J. Physiol. (Lond.)*, 312: 41–42P.

Hamill, O.P., Marty, A., Neher, E., Sakmann, B. and Sigworth, F.J. (1981) Improved patch-clamp techniques for high-resolution current recording from cells and cell-free membrane patches. *Pflügers Arch.*, in press.

Hodgkin, A.L. and Huxley, A.F. (1952) A quantitative description of membrane current and its application to conduction and excitation in nerve. *J. Physiol. (Lond.)*, 117: 500–544.

Horn, R. and Patlak, J.B. (1980) Single channel currents from excised patches of muscle membrane. *Proc. nat. Acad. Sci. U.S.A.*, 77: 6930–6934.

Jackson, M.B. and Lecar, H. (1979) Single postsynaptic channel currents in tissue cultured muscle. *Nature (Lond.)*, 282: 863–864.

Katz, B. (1966) *Nerve, Muscle, and Synapse*, McGraw-Hill, New York.

Katz, B. and Miledi, R. (1972) The statistical nature of the acetylcholine potential and its molecular components. *J. Physiol. (Lond.)*, 224: 665–699.

Kristhal, O.A. and Pidoplichko, V.I. (1975) Intracellular perfusion of Helix neurons. *Neirofiziol. (Kiev)*, 7: 258–259.

Lee, K.S., Akaike, N. and Brown, A.M. (1978) Properties of internally perfused, voltage clamped, isolated nerve cell bodies. *J. gen. Physiol.*, 71: 489–508.

Llinas, R., Steinberg, I. Z. and Walton, K. (1981) Presynaptic Ca currents in squid giant synapse. *Biophys. J.*, 33: 289–322.

Lux, H.D. and Nagy, K. (1982) Single channel Ca currents in *Helix pomatia* neurons. *Pflüger's Arch.*, in press.

Lux, H.D., Neher, E. and Marty, A. (1981) Single channel activity associated with the calcium dependent outward current in *Helix pomatia*, *Pflügers. Arch.*, 389: 293–295.

Marty, A. (1981) Ca-dependent K channels with large unitary conductance in chromaffin cell membrane. *Nature (Lond.)*, 291: 497.

Mathers, D.A., Jackson, M.B., Lecar, H. and Barker, J.L. (1981) Single channel currents activated by GABA, muscimol, and pentobarbitol in cultured mouse spinal neurons. *Biophys. J.*, 33: 14a.

Neher, E. (1982) Unit conductance studies in biological membranes. In P.F. Baker (Ed.), *Techniques in Cellular Physiology*, Elsevier/North-Holland, Amsterdam.

48

Neher, E. and Sakmann, B. (1976) Single-channel currents recorded from membrane of denervated frog muscle fibres. *Nature* (*Lond.*), 260: 799–802.

Neher, E. and Stevens, C.F. (1977) Conductance fluctuations and ionic pores in membranes. *Ann. Rev. Biophys. Bioengng*, 6: 345–381.

Nelson, D.J. and Sachs, F. (1979) Single ionic channel observed in tissue-cultured muscle. *Nature* (*Lond.*), 282: 861–863.

Sigworth, F.J. and Neher, E. (1980) Single Na^+ channel currents observed in cultured rat muscle cells. *Nature* (*Lond.*), 287: 447–449.

Thompson, S.H. and Aldrich, R.W. (1981) Membrane potassium channels. In C.W. Cotman, G. Poste and G.L. Nicolson (Eds.), *The Cell Surface and Neuronal Function*, Elsevier/North-Holland, Amsterdam.

Usherwood, P.N.R. (1980) Neuromuscular transmitter receptors of insect muscle. In D.B. Satelle (Ed.), *Receptors for Neurotransmitters, Hormones and Pheromones in Insects*, Elsevier/North-Holland, Amsterdam.

Some Features of Peptidergic Transmission

Y.N. JAN and L.Y. JAN

Department of Physiology, School of Medicine, University of California, San Francisco, CA 94143 (U.S.A.)

INTRODUCTION

In the nervous system, neurons communicate with each other mainly through the use of chemical transmitters. From a simplistic point of view, one could imagine that one excitatory and one inhibitory transmitter would be sufficient for a nervous system to function. However, this does not seem to be true in view of the recent discovery of many peptides in the nervous system. At present, about two dozen peptides are regarded as putative transmitters (for review, see Snyder, 1980). Considering that many of these neuropeptides were discovered serendipitously, it seems likely that many more will be discovered. This raises a question: why are there so many transmitters? Finding an explanation for this "diversity of transmitters" may provide much insight to our understanding of the nervous system. To approach this problem, first, one would like to know whether peptides indeed function as neurotransmitters, then one may ask whether the actions of peptides are qualitatively different from those of the classical transmitters such as acetylcholine and monoamines. The possibility that peptides act as neurotransmitters has been investigated extensively in recent years (for review, see Snyder, 1980; Nicoll et al., 1980). In the central nervous system, the best documented case for a peptide transmitter is that of substance P. Substance P is present in small cells of dorsal root ganglia and is released upon stimulation of the dorsal roots. Exogenous application of substance P depolarizes some of the dorsal horn neurons which are known to receive sensory input. Whether substance P mimics all the effects of the natural sensory transmitter remains to be established. Taken together the evidence for substance P to be a sensory transmitter in the spinal cord is strong, but not compelling. The evidence is far less complete for most other peptides. This is mainly due to the intrinsic difficulty of studying the effects of peptides or those of the natural transmitter in the central nervous system. The use of a simple model system could circumvent much of this difficulty. Simple model systems have proven very useful in the past; for instance, the knowledge of synaptic transmission gained from studies of the frog neuromuscular junction seems to apply to fast chemical transmission in general.

The study of peptidergic transmission may benefit from a similar strategy. A sufficiently simple preparation may permit a rigorous and detailed characterization of peptidergic transmission. Promising model systems are provided by the autonomic nervous system. Autonomic ganglia are relatively simple in structure and receive a number of peptidergic inputs. Nishi and Koketsu (1968) first discovered a slow, non-cholinergic synaptic potential in the frog and named it the late slow excitatory postsynaptic potential (EPSP). Similar slow, non-cholinergic potentials have since been found in several autonomic ganglia including superior cervical ganglia of rabbit (Ashe and Libet, 1981), myenteric plexus and interior mesenteric ganglia of guinea pigs (Katayama and North, 1978; Neild, 1978; Konishi et al., 1979). Recent experiments indicate that those slow synaptic potentials may be mediated by peptides.

PEPTIDERGIC TRANSMISSION IN SYMPATHETIC GANGLIA OF THE FROG

We chose to work on sympathetic ganglia of the bullfrog because the preparations are simple and accessible to a variety of experimental manipulations. In addition, much background knowledge was available from the work of many investigators (for review, see Skok, 1973; Nishi, 1974; Kuba and Koketsu, 1978; Libet, 1970).

Variety of synaptic responses

We usually used the 9th and 10th ganglia, the two most caudal ganglia of the paravertebral sympathetic chain, for our experiments. Neurons in these ganglia (the principal cells) can be divided into two groups according to their size and innervation. The large cells (with diameters of 30–70 μm) are called B cells. Their axons conduct at about 2 m/s. C cells are generally smaller (with diameters of 10–45 μm and their axons conduct at about 0.2 m/s. For us, the greatest attraction of this preparation is that the ganglionic neurons exhibit four different types of synaptic potentials with vastly different time courses ranging from milliseconds to minutes (Fig. 1).

(1) The nicotinic fast EPSP (lasting for 30–50 ms). This cholinergic response is found in both B and C cells. The receptors mediating this synaptic potential are nicotinic cholinergic receptors which are blocked by dihydro-β-erythroidine.

(2) The muscarinic slow EPSP (lasting 30–60 s). This response is usually found in B cells. The receptors mediating this synaptic potential are muscarinic cholinergic receptors which are blocked by atropine.

(3) The slow IPSP (lasting 1–2 s). This response is found in C cells and is also blocked by muscarinic blockers (Horn and Dudd, 1981).

(4) The late slow EPSP (lasting for several minutes). This slow response is recorded in both B and C cells. It is not blocked by nicotinic or muscarinic cholinergic blockers (Nishi and Koketsu, 1968).

The late slow EPSP is mediated by a luteinizing hormone-releasing hormone (LH-RH)-like peptide

The most striking feature of the late slow EPSP is its long duration. Typically, the time course of a late slow EPSP is several minutes, about 10^4 times longer than that of the fast EPSP. Intuitively, one might expect the underlying mechanism of the late slow EPSP to be much different from that of the fast synaptic potentials. To study the function and underlying mechanisms of this slow synaptic potential, we first attempted to identify its transmitter. The results obtained so far suggest strongly that the transmitter is an LH-RH-like peptide (Jan et al., 1979, 1980a, b).

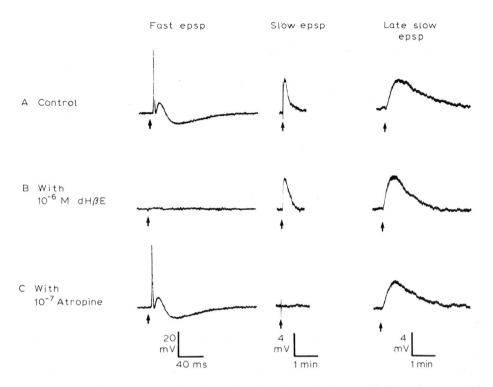

Fig. 1. Effects of a nicotinic cholinergic blocker, dihydro-β-erythroidine (dHβE), and a muscarinic cholinergic blocker, atropine, on the fast EPSP, slow EPSP, and late slow EPSP recorded from the same B cell. Arrows indicate time of nerve stimulation. The fast EPSP was initiated by a single stimulus of the sympathetic chain above the seventh ganglion. The slow EPSP was induced by stimulating the chain at 30 Hz for 0.7 s. Two separate nerves, the 7th and 8th spinal nerves, were stimulated at 5 Hz for 20 s to induce the late slow EPSP. (From Jan and Jan, 1982, with permission.)

In the following, we review the criteria used to qualify the LH-RH-like peptide as the transmitter for the late slow EPSP.

(1) *The LH-RH-like peptide is present in the presynaptic terminals*
This conclusion is based on two lines of evidence.

(a) Radioimmunoassays (RIA). By using an antiserum highly specific for LH-RH (Nett et al., 1973) in radioimmunoassays, we found that each sympathetic chain contained 100–800 pg of an LH-RH-like substance. This LH-RH-like substance was resistant to heating in a boiling water bath but totally destroyed by α-chymotrypsin. By using gel filtration chromatography, we estimated that the substance has a molecular weight of about 1000. Therefore, the LH-RH-like substance is probably a peptide (Jan et al., 1979). Its exact sequence has not been identified. High pressure liquid chromatography indicates that it is not identical to LH-RH. However, RIAs and bioassays indicate that it closely resembles the structure of mammalian LH-RH (Eiden and Eskay, 1980; Rivier et al., 1981). To localize the LH-RH-like peptide in the ganglia, we studied the effect of denervation. It was known previously that cutting preganglionic nerves caused failure of synaptic transmission and degenera-

52

tion of terminals within 5 days. Such operation caused no sign of degeneration of the ganglionic neurons. With RIA, we found that 5 days after ipsilateral preganglionic axons were cut, 95% of the LH-RH-like peptide disappeared from the ganglia, while the amount of LH-RH-like peptide tripled in the 7th and 8th spinal nerves proximal to the cut region, suggesting that the LH-RH-like peptide is contained in preganglionic fibers.

(b) *Immunohistochemical localization.* To determine directly the distribution of LH-RH-like peptide within the ganglia, we did immunocytochemical experiments using either immunofluorescence or the peroxidase–antiperoxidase technique of Sternberger and coworkers (1970), and rabbit antisera to LH-RH as the primary antisera. Synaptic boutons on the ganglia cell soma were stained (Fig. 2). Preadsorption of the primary rabbit antisera with LH-RH completely eliminated the staining (Jan et al., 1980b). Thus, the LH-RH-like peptide is contained in presynaptic terminals.

(2) *Calcium-dependent release of the LH-RH-like peptide*

If the LH-RH-like peptide in the presynaptic nerve terminals is the transmitter

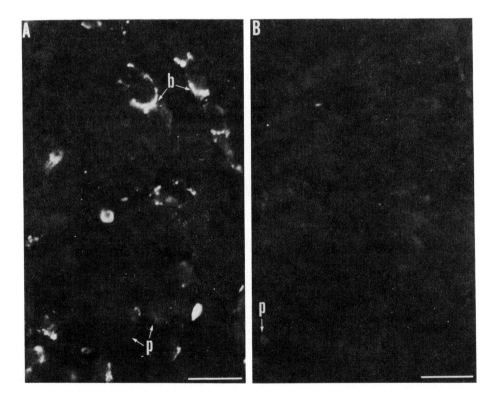

Fig. 2. A; immunofluorescent staining of LH-RH-positive terminals on sympathetic neurons. B: preadsorption control in which the rabbit anti-LH-RH sera (1:200 dilution) were adsorbed with synthetic LH-RH (60 μg/ml) overnight before the staining procedure. b represents boutons that are red due to the rhodamine-labeled second antibodies; p represents pigment granules that are autofluorescent (yellow). Calibration bar represents 70 μm. (From Jan and Jan, 1982, with permission.)

for the late slow EPSP, it should be released either by stimulation of the pre-ganglionic fibers or by raising the external potassium concentration. Indeed, both methods were effective in causing release of the LH-RH-like peptide. This release requires Ca^{2+}. Little LH-RH-like immunoreactivity is detected in the bathing solution when the external Ca^{2+} was replaced with Mg^{2+}.

(3) *The LH-RH-induced depolarization of sympathetic neurons mimics the late slow EPSP*

If the transmitter for the late slow EPSP is an LH-RH-like peptide, application of LH-RH to the ganglionic neuron should mimic the effects of natural transmitter. By passing brief pulses of pressure through a micropipette containing LH-RH, we could deliver small amounts of the peptide near a ganglion cell. This caused a slow depolarization of the neurons (Fig. 3). To decide whether the slow depolarization was due to a postsynaptic action of the peptide, we replaced Ca^{2+} in the Ringer's solution with Mg^{2+} to block release of transmitters. Under such conditions, nerve stimulation became ineffective, while direct application of LH-RH still depolarized the ganglionic neurons to approximately the same extent (Jan et al., 1980a). This experiment shows that the effect of LH-RH on ganglionic neurons is due predominantly to a direct, postganglionic action.

The LH-RH-induced response and the nerve evoked late slow EPSP are similar in many aspects (Jan et al., 1980a; Jan and Jan, 1982).

(a) They are associated with similar conductance changes. In the majority of the cells tested, both caused a marked increase in membrane resistance.

(b) Their amplitudes vary in parallel as the membrane potential is shifted over a wide range, suggesting that similar ionic mechanisms are involved.

(c) Both responses increase the excitability of the neurons.

(d) The responses interact with the cholinergic PSPs in a parallel manner.

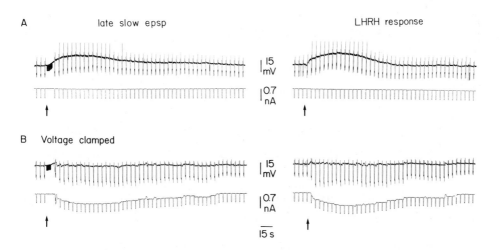

Fig. 3. A: increase in input resistance during a late slow EPSP (left) and an LH-RH-induced response (right) in the same ganglion cell. The voltage change produced by the current pulse increased during the depolarization. B: same stimulation but with the membrane potential manually clamped at its resting level (about -50 mV). (From Jan and Jan, 1982, with permission.)

54

(4) *LH-RH antagonists block both the LH-RH response and late slow EPSP*

Among the hundreds of LH-RH analogs synthesized, several were found to be effective antagonists in mammals (Rivier and Vale, 1978). Drs. W. Vale and J. Rivier of the Salk Institute kindly provided us with several antagonists of LH-RH. These LH-RH analogs blocked both the late slow EPSP and the LH-RH response in frog sympathetic ganglia. An example is shown in Fig. 4. This antagonist appeared to be specific for the peptidergic responses. It did not alter the membrane potential, membrane conductance, or any of the cholinergic responses.

Taken together, the existing evidence strongly supports that an LH-RH-like peptide is the transmitter for the late slow EPSP.

Features of peptidergic transmission

With this relatively well-defined peptidergic synapse, we recently began to analyze this peptidergic transmission in detail. Interesting features have started to emerge.

(1) *Peptides diffuse and act on neurons many microns away from the release site*

A surprising observation made in the immunocytochemical experiments is that the peptidergic synaptic boutons are localized only on C cells (Jan et al., 1980b). As described before, the sympathetic ganglia contain two types of neurons: B cells and C cells. These two types of neurons are interspersed in the 9th and 10th ganglia. All the neurons have both cholinergic and peptidergic synaptic potentials. The preganglionic cholinergic synaptic boutons on B cells arise from preganglionic fibers contained in the 3rd, 4th and 5th spinal nerves, while synaptic boutons on C cells

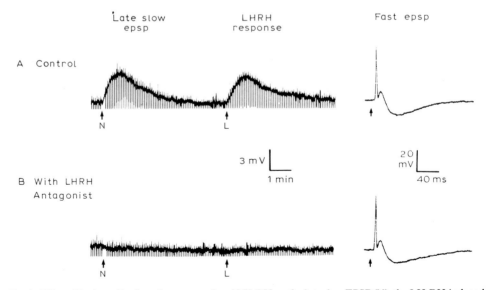

Fig. 4. Effect of bath application of an antagonist of LH-RH on the late slow EPSP (N), the LH-RH-induced response (L), and the cholinergic fast EPSP. Applying an antagonist, [D-pGlu^1, D-Phe^2, D-Trp^{3,6}]-LH-RH, to the bathing medium at a final concentration of 10^{-5} M had no effect on the membrane potential, the membrane resistance or the cholinergic fast EPSP, but completely blocked both the late slow EPSP and the LH-RH-induced response. (From Jan and Jan, 1982, with permission.)

arise from preganglionic fibers contained in the 7th and 8th spinal nerves. Cutting the sympathetic chain rostral to the 7th ganglion removed all nerve terminals on B cells, but did not eliminate the late slow EPSP in B cells. To verify this, we have recorded from B cells 5 days after the sympathetic chain was cut, and demonstrated that they show only the late slow EPSP but not any cholinergic responses; we then serial sectioned the same cells for electron microscopy. No terminals were found on these B cells (Jan et al., 1980b). Therefore, the B cells must be able to respond to LH-RH-like peptide released from peptidergic terminals on C cells, which are microns away. This conclusion is supported by physiological experiments (Jan and Jan, 1982) (Fig. 5). Applying antagonist of LH-RH onto a B cell during a late slow EPSP caused the slow potential to be truncated, indicating that for many seconds the peptide transmitters are still in the vicinity of the receptor (they may be in the extracellular space or bound to the receptors). The long range and long lasting action of the peptidergic transmitters may turn out to be a general feature of peptidergic transmission (see below).

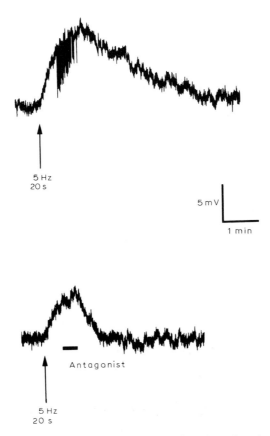

Fig. 5. Effect of an antagonist of LH-RH on the late slow EPSP. After a late slow EPSP was initiated by stimulating the 7th and 8th spinal nerves at 5 Hz for 20 s, pressure application of [Ac-Δ^3-Pro^1, pF-D-Phe^2, D-Trp^{3,6}]-LH-RH, an antagonist of LH-RH (1 psi, 25 s), reduced both the amplitude and the duration of the late slow EPSP. The antagonist by itself has no effect on the membrane potential of this cell. Notice that the spontaneously occurring action potentials during the late slow EPSP were also eliminated. (From Jan and Jan, 1982, with permission.)

(2) *Coexistence and corelease of acetylcholine and the LH-RH-like peptide from the same preganglionic fibers*

The question as to whether a neuron can produce and release more than one transmitter has attracted considerable interest. One difficulty in settling this question is that so far the classical criteria for transmitters have not been fulfilled for two substances within any given neuron (for review, see Hökfelt et al., 1980). In frog sympathetic ganglia, both acetylcholine (ACh) and LH-RH-like peptides are almost certain to be neurotransmitters. Thus, this preparation could lend itself to a rigorous test of the idea of coexistence and corelease of transmitters.

Our preliminary results indicate that ACh and the LH-RH-like peptide are indeed contained within and released from the same preganglionic C fibers.

(a) Intracellular recording demonstrated that a cell usually receives 3–5 different cholinergic inputs which have different thresholds. By stimulating the preganglionic nerves at different strengths, we found that each time a cholinergic fiber was recruited, initiating an additional fast EPSP, there was a corresponding increment in the peptidergic response. Thus, the threshold of cholinergic fibers correlate well with the threshold of peptidergic fibers, suggesting that the same preganglionic fibers for C cells supply both cholinergic and peptidergic inputs.

(b) We marked all terminals on C cells either by filling preganglionic fibers with horseradish peroxidase or by using a monoclonal antibody specific for synaptic vesicles (Matthew et al., 1981), and then stained the same sections using antibodies specific for LH-RH. At least 90% of all preganglionic terminals on C cells contained the LH-RH-like immunoreactivity, suggesting that at least some terminals contain both the LH-RH-like peptide and ACh. Therefore, it appears that most, if not all, preganglionic fibers for C cells contain and release both ACh and the LH-RH-like peptide.

(3) *Some speculations about peptidergic synaptic transmission*

Figure 6 summarizes the actions of ACh and the LH-RH-like peptide in the sympathetic ganglia of the frog. When preganglionic C fibers are activated, both ACh and the LH-RH-like peptide are released (probably from the same nerve terminals in close contact with C cells). Of the two transmitters, ACh acts focally on C cells and has no obvious effect on B cells, while the LH-RH-like peptide apparently diffuses for microns and exerts its effects on both B and C cells. This example led to the following postulation:

Perhaps peptide transmitters generally act upon neurons within many microns from the release site.

If this postulation is true, one expects the peptidergic transmitters to have the following properties:

(a) The responses mediated by peptides should be considerably slower than those caused by the focal action of transmitters such as ACh.

If we assume the average distance a peptide molecule travels is of the order of one or a few cell diameters, say 50 μm, then assuming free diffusion, the time, t, it takes for a molecule to reach its receptor can be roughly estimated with $\bar{X}^2 = 2\,Dt$, where $\bar{X}$ is the mean distance travelled by a peptide molecule, and D is the diffusion constant. A value of $10^{-6}\,\text{cm}^2/\text{s}$ for D should be a reasonable estimate. Then, t would

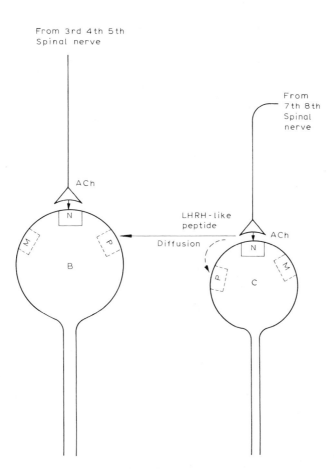

Fig. 6. Scheme of innervation of neurons in 9th or 10th ganglia. Cholinergic axons for B neurons arise from the 3rd, 4th and 5th spinal nerves, whereas preganglionic fibers for C cells come through the 7th and 8th spinal nerves. LH-RH-positive nerve terminals are present only on C cells. Most likely both the LH-RH-like peptide and acetylcholine are contained and released from the same preganglionic fibers for C cells. N, nicotinic cholinergic receptors; M, muscarinic cholinergic receptors; P, peptidergic receptors. Of the three types of receptors the nicotinic cholinergic receptors have been localized. They are situated right in opposition to the synaptic boutons (see Marshall, 1981).

be several seconds. This implies that a peptidergic response should take at least several seconds to reach its peak value. In a number of preparations (mostly autonomic ganglia) where peptides are suspected of mediating some of the synaptic potentials, almost without exception those responses are slow in onset (hundreds of ms) and take seconds to reach their peak value (Ashe and Libet, 1981; Katayama and North, 1978; Neild, 1978; Konishi et al., 1979).

(b) The peptide receptors should have high affinity for the ligands. At a synapse such as the skeletal neuromuscular junction, where the sites of transmitter release are in close opposition to the receptors, the peak concentration of the transmitter during a synaptic response could be as high as 10^{-3} M in the vicinity of the receptors. In this case, the receptors need not have a very high affinity for the transmitter molecules. In contrast, for peptides to act on receptors microns away from the release sites, their concentration will be greatly reduced before they reach the receptors. Thus, one would expect peptide receptors to have a considerably higher affinity so that they can detect low levels of peptides. Results of receptor binding studies are consistent with this speculation. Peptide receptors studied thus far appear to have high affinity for peptides. The dissociation constants were found to be in the range of 10^{-10} to 10^{-9} M, which is $10–10^4$ times lower than that of classical transmitters such as ACh and amino acids (e.g. Moody et al., 1978; Taylor and Pert, 1979; Hanley et al., 1980).

The action of peptidergic transmitters may be intermediate between the focal action of classical transmitters such as ACh and the global action of hormones. One usually thinks of precise circuitry of synaptic contacts as the only means by which selective communications between neurons are achieved, especially in regions of the nervous system where several different types of neurons are interspersed. However, in situations where the speed of action is not crucial or perhaps a slower and prolonged influence is more desirable, conceivably the "presynaptic" neurons may terminate in the vicinity of the "postsynaptic" neurons without making synaptic contacts. Such an arrangement would work if the transmitter released can diffuse for a distance of several cell diameters before acting on receptors. Selective communication is possible if different neurons in a given region express different subsets of receptors on their surface, so that a transmitter released from the "presynaptic" cell influences only those neurons in the vicinity which have receptors for that transmitter. Intuitively this arrangement seems more economical and conceivably plasticity might invoke merely an alteration in the type of receptors expressed on the surface of the "postsynaptic" cell. For this type of interneuronal communication to be used extensively in the nervous system without cross-talks between parallel pathways, a necessary requirement is that many different molecules are used as transmitters.

REFERENCES

Ashe, J.H. and Libet, B. (1981) Orthodromic production of noncholinergic slow depolarizing response in superior cervical ganglion of rabbit. *J. Physiol. (Lond.)*, 320: 333–346.
Eiden, L.E. and Eskay, R.L. (1980) Characterization of LRF-like immunoreactivity in the frog sympathetic ganglia: non identity with LRF decapeptide. *Neuropeptides*, 1: 29–37.
Hanley, M.R., Sandberg, B.E.B., Lee, C.M., Iversen, L.L., Brundish, D.E. and Wade, R. (1980) Specific binding of [^{3}H] substance P to rat brain membrane. *Nature (Lond.)*, 286: 810–812.
Hökfelt, T., Johannson, O., Ljungdahl, Å., Lundberg, J.M. and Schultzberg, M. (1980) Peptidergic neurones. *Nature (Lond.)*, 284: 515–521.
Horn, J.P. and Dodd, J. (1981) Monosynaptic muscarinic activation of K^+ conductance underlies the slow inhibitory postsynaptic potential in sympathetic ganglia. *Nature (Lond.)*, 292: 625–627.
Jan, L.Y. and Jan, Y.N. (1982) Peptidergic transmission in sympathetic ganglia of the frog. *J. Physiol. (Lond.)*, 327: 219–246.
Jan, Y.N., Jan, L.Y. and Kuffler, S.W. (1979) A peptide as a possible transmitter in sympathetic ganglia of the frog. *Proc. nat. Acad. Sci. U.S.A.*, 76: 1501–1505.
Jan, Y.N., Jan, L.Y. and Kuffler, S.W. (1980a) Further evidence for peptidergic transmission in sympathetic ganglia. *Proc. nat. Acad. Sci. U.S.A.*, 77: 5008–5012.
Jan, L.Y., Jan, Y.N. and Brownfield, M.S. (1980b) Peptidergic transmitters in synaptic boutons of sympathetic ganglia. *Nature (Lond.)*, 288: 380–382.
Katayama, Y. and North, R.A. (1978) Does substance P mediate slow synaptic excitation within the myenteric plexus? *Nature (Lond.)*, 274: 387–388.
Konishi, S., Tsunoo, A. and Otsuka, M. (1979) Substance P and noncholinergic excitatory synaptic transmission in guinea pig sympathetic ganglia. *Proc. Jap. Acad.*, 55, Ser. B: 525–530.

Kuba, K. and Koketsu, K. (1978) Synaptic events in sympathetic ganglia. *Progr. Neurobiol.*, 11: 77–169.

Libet, B. (1970) Generation of slow inhibitory and excitatory postsynaptic potentials. *Fed. Proc.*, 29: 1945–1956.

Marshall, L.M. (1981) Synaptic localization of α-bungarotoxin binding which blocks nicotinic transmission at frog sympathetic neurons. *Proc. nat. Acad. Sci. U.S.A.*, 78: 1948–1952.

Matthew, W.D., Tsavaler, L. and Reichardt, L.F. (1981) Monoclonal antibodies to synaptic membranes and vesicles. In *Monoclonal Antibodies to Neural Antigens*, Cold Spring Harbor, pp. 163–191.

Moody, T.W., Pert, C.B., Rivier, J. and Brown, M. (1978) Bombesin: Specific binding of to rat brain membranes. *Proc. nat. Acad. Sci. U.S.A.*, 75: 5372–5376.

Nicoll, R.A., Shenker, C. and Leeman, S.E. (1980) Substance P as a transmitter candidate. *Ann. Rev. Neurosci.*, 3: 227–268.

Nield, T.O. (1978) Slowly-developing depolarization of neurons in the guinea pig inferior mesenteric ganglion following repetitive stimulation of the preganglionic nerves. *Brain Res.*, 140: 231–239.

Nett, T.M., Akbar, A.M., Niswender, G.D., Hedlund, M.T. and White, W.F. (1973) A radioimmunoassay for gonadotropin-releasing hormone in serum. *J. clin. Endocr. Metab.*, 36: 880–885.

Nishi, S. (1974) Ganglionic transmission. In J.I. Hubbard (Ed.), *The Peripheral Nervous System*, Plenum Press, New York, pp. 225–255.

Nishi, S. and Koketsu, K. (1968) Early and late after-discharges of amphibian sympathetic ganglion cells. *J. Neurophysiol.*, 31: 109–121.

Rivier, J.E. and Vale, W.W. (1978) [D-pGlu^1, D-Phe^2, D-trp^{3,6}]-LRF. A potent LRF antagonist *in vitro* and inhibitor of ovulation in the rat. *Life Sci.*, 23: 869–876.

Rivier, J.E., Spiess, J., Rivier, C., Branton, D., Miller, R. and Vale, W. (1981) HPLC purification of rat extrahypothalamic somatostatin, frog brain LRF and ovian CRF. In *Proc 7th American Peptide Symposium*.

Skok, V.I. (1973) Physiology of Autonomic Ganglia, Igaka Shoin, Tokyo.

Snyder, S.H. (1980) Brain peptide as neurotransmitters? *Science*, 209: 976–983.

Sternberger, L.A., Hardy, P.H., Cuculus, J.J. and Meyer, H.G. (1970) The unlabeled antibody–enzyme method of immunohistochemistry. Preparation and properties of soluble antigen–antibody complex (HRP and anti-HRP) and its use in identification of spirochetes. *J. Histochem. Cytochem.*, 18: 315–333.

Taylor, D.P. and Pert, C.B. (1979) Vasoactive intestinal polypeptide: Specific binding to rat brain membranes. *Proc. nat. Acad. Sci. U.S.A.*, 76: 660–664.

Some Mechanisms Controlling Hippocampal Pyramidal Cells

IVER ARNE LANGMOEN*

Institute of Neurophysiology, University of Oslo, Karl Johansgt. 47, Oslo (Norway)

INTRODUCTION

Early studies of the neuromuscular junction and on motoneurons formed certain classical concepts about mechanisms controlling excitable cells (reviewed by Eccles, 1964; Katz, 1966). Excitation was shown to be caused by a relatively non-specific permeability increase of the synaptic membrane ("short-circuit"), while inhibition was shown to be due to a specific permeability increase, letting only ions carrying an outward current pass the membrane. Following these early studies, synaptic transmission has been subjected to intensive investigations, not least in lower animals (for reviews see Krnjević, 1974, 1976; Bennett, 1974; Gerschenfeld, 1973; Takeuchi, 1977). However, relatively little is known about the detailed mechanisms of control in mammalian cortical cells. This refers to the mechanisms producing excitatory postsynaptic potentials (EPSPs), the mechanism of action of most neurotransmitters as well as postsynaptic interaction between synaptic potentials.

In the present paper some studies on mechanisms involved in the control of the CA1 hippocampal pyramidal cell (HPC) are reviewed. Technical details may be found in Langmoen and Andersen (1981) and in the original papers.

THE MECHANISM GENERATING THE EPSP

In the motoneuron and in the peripheral nervous system it has been shown that excitation is due to a short-circuiting of the membrane that produces a postsynaptic depolarization (Eccles, 1964). In agreement with this Hablitz and Langmoen (1982) found that the EPSP in HPCs increased with hyperpolarization and decreased with depolarization. When the membrane potential was moved above 0 mV, the EPSP was reversed, and appeared as a negative potential deflection. In Fig. 1, the size of the EPSP is plotted against the membrane potential. The reversal potential found by fitting a linear regression line to these points was -9.0 mV. In cells with a pure EPSP the mean E_{EPSP} was -2.8 mV ± 9.6 (S.D.).

The EPSPs were, however, generated in the dendritic tree $50–150\ \mu$m from the soma. It must therefore have been some attenuation of the potentials between the site of the synapses and the soma. The true reversal potential is therefore somewhat

---

*Present address: Dept. of Neurosurgery, Ullevål Hospital, Oslo, Norway.

62

more negative than reported above. Anyway, the results indicate that the EPSP is produced by an increased permeability to ions carrying an inward current.

GLUTAMATE AS AN EXCITATORY TRANSMITTER

Several studies have suggested glutamate and/or aspartate as excitatory transmitters in the hippocampus (Biscoe and Straughan, 1966; Schwarzkroin and Andersen, 1975; Segal, 1976; Spencer et al., 1976; Storm-Mathisen and Iversen, 1979). Recently a more specific study has supported the role of glutamate in the fibers from the ipsilateral CA3 (Malthe-Sørensen et al., 1979).

Iontophoretically applied L-glutamate reliably depolarizes HPCs (Hablitz and Langmoen, 1982). The depolarization is highly localized and obtained with low ejection currents (1–10 nA). The effect is exerted directly on the pyramidal cell and not via interneurons, since it persists after blockade of the synaptic transmission by adding 4 mM manganese chloride.

The amplitude of the glutamate potential is dependent on the membrane potential and decreases with depolarization (Hablitz and Langmoen, 1982). By injecting Cs^+ into the cells the fall in input resistance observed during large depolarizations is abolished and it is possible to depolarize the cells to between +20 and +50 mV. The Glu-response/MP relationship was reliably linear and crossed the abscissa near 0 mV. The mean E_{Glu} in 11 cells was -1.5 ± 6.7 mV (S.D.). Control studies indicated that Cs^+ did not affect E_{Glu}. A comparison between E_{Glu} and E_{EPSP} in the same cell is shown in Fig. 1. Linear regression lines indicate $E_{Glu} = -6.2$ mV and $E_{EPSP} = -9.0$ mV. The close fit between E_{Glu} (-1.5 ± 6.7) and E_{EPSP} (-2.8 ± 9.6) supports the proposed function of glutamate as a neurotransmitter in HPCs.

Replacing NaCl in the incubation fluid with TRIS-HCl caused a considerable reduction of the amplitude of the glutamate potential (Hablitz and Langmoen, 1982).

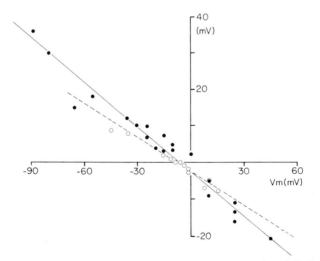

Fig. 1. Comparison between E_{Glu} and E_{EPSP}. The EPSP (open circles, dotted line) and the glutamate response (closed circles, continuous line) have been plotted against the membrane potential (abscissa). The continuous and the dotted lines are linear regression lines fitted to the values of the glutamate potential and EPSP respectively. They indicate a reversal potential of -9.0 mV for the EPSP and -6.4 mV for the glutamate response. (Hablitz and Langmoen, unpublished observations.)

When Na$^+$ was reduced to 25%, the reversal potential was shifted 30 mV in a negative direction. It thus appears likely that Na$^+$ is a major carrier of the synaptic current evoked by glutamate.

Chloride injections did not affect E_{Glu} in one cell and did not change the amplitude of the glutamate depolarization in several other cells tested. In view of the fact that E_{Glu} is situated between E_K and E_{Na}, it is suggested that the synaptic current consists of potassium in addition to sodium. Possible participation of divalent cations can at present, however, not be excluded.

SUMMATION OF SEPARATE EPSPs

Possible postsynaptic interaction between separate excitatory systems has been tested by using two afferent inputs to the HPC, one ending proximally and one distally in the dendritic tree (Langmoen and Andersen, 1983).

Two examples are shown in Fig. 2. In both parts of the figure the upper trace represents the EPSP due to stimulation of fibers ending proximally on the dendritic tree and the second trace the EPSP evoked by distal fibers. The lower trace shows the algebraic sum of the two separate EPSPs superimposed upon the EPSP due to simultaneous activation of the two inputs (observed sum). Summation is evidently non-linear in the cell shown in Fig. 2A as the amplitude of the EPSP due to double activation was smaller than the algebraic sum of the separate EPSPs. In the cell shown in Fig. 2B, however, summation is linear. Out of a total of 47 cells, 38 (81%) showed non-linear summation when tested at or close to the resting potential, whereas the EPSPs in the remaining 9 cells (19%) added linearly at the resting potential. The non-linear summation illustrated can be explained by interaction between the two synaptic populations. Another possibility exists, however. Simultaneous activation activated a larger number of the surrounding pyramidal cells (the population spike increased), this must in turn have activated more basket cells and thus a more powerful IPSP in the pyramidal cell recorded from. Since the recurrent

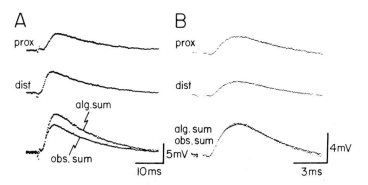

Fig. 2. Summation of distal and a proximal EPSP. The figure shows results obtained from two different cells. In both parts the upper trace shows averaged EPSPs due to activation of fibers synapsing in the proximal dendritic tree. The middle traces represent EPSPs due to activation of distally terminating fibers. The lower parts of A and B show superimposed traces of: (1) the algebraic sum of the proximal and the distal EPSP, and (2) the EPSP produced by activating the proximal and distal fibers simultaneously (observed sum). The summation was linear in the cell shown in B, whereas it was non-linear in the cell in A. (Langmoen and Andersen, unpublished observations.)

64

IPSP normally interacts with the EPSP (Dingledine and Gjerstad, 1980) the non-linear summation seen in Fig. 2A can be due to reinforcement of the IPSP.

In order to test this hypothesis the mode of summation was tested at different membrane potentials. Hyperpolarization regularly decreased the non-linearity. Of the 38 cells where the EPSPs added non-linearly an increase in the membrane potential gave linear summation in 35. Linear summation took place when the cell was hyperpolarized to an extent which made the peak of the EPSP due to simultaneous input appear at $-11\,mV \pm 5$ (S.D.) negative to the resting potential. This is similar to the reversal potential for the IPSP and the hyperpolarizing GABA effect (Andersen et al., 1980). A direct comparison between the reversal potential of the IPSP and the membrane potential at which linear summation took place, confirmed this.

In addition, the mode of summation was tested before and after application of penicillin which blocks the IPSPs (Dingledine and Gjerstad, 1980). After IPSP blockade, summation was linear (two cells).

The non-linear summation of EPSPs, therefore, seems to be chiefly due to IPSP interaction. Direct interaction between different populations of excitatory synapses, however, is most likely small or negligible.

THE MECHANISM GENERATING THE IPSP

The terminals of the basket cell axons give rise to a plexus of terminals around the somata of pyramidal cells (Ramón y Cajal, 1893; Lorente de Nó, 1934). The synapses are of Gray's type II (Blackstad and Flood, 1963). IPSPs were demonstrated in the hippocampus by Kandel et al. (1961) and Andersen et al. (1964a). From several lines of evidence Andersen et al. (1964b) concluded that the IPSP was of the recurrent type and was mediated by the basket cells. The same authors reported that the IPSP was highly potential sensitive and probably was caused by an outward current at the soma. Later studies have confirmed this (Dingledine and Langmoen, 1980) and shown that the postsynaptic membrane is permeable to small anions (Eccles et al., 1977; Allen et al., 1977).

GABA AS AN INHIBITORY TRANSMITTER

There is considerable evidence that GABA is the transmitter of the basket cell synapse (Biscoe and Straughan, 1966; Curtis et al., 1970, 1971; Storm-Mathisen and Fonnum, 1971; Storm-Mathisen, 1972, 1975; Barber and Saito, 1976; Ozawa and Okada, 1976; Nadler et al., 1977; Ribak et al., 1978; Dingledine and Gjerstad, 1980). HPCs show two responses to GABA (Langmoen et al., 1978). Application of GABA to the cell body hyperpolarizes the cells. When applied to the dendrites, however, GABA depolarizes the cells. The hyperpolarization is associated with decreased input resistance and is reversed by hyperpolarizing the cell membrane (Andersen et al., 1980). Following reduced Cl⁻ concentration in the incubation fluid, the response is decreased. Cl⁻ ions are thus likely carriers of the GABA-induced current. The reversal potentials for GABA and the IPSP are similar.

The depolarizing GABA effect is also associated with decreased input resistance (Andersen et al., 1980). The response decreases with depolarization and extrapola-

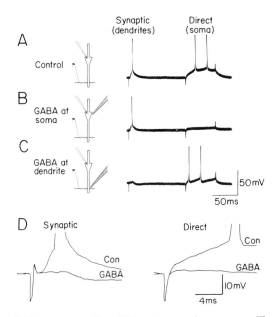

Fig. 3. Discriminative inhibitory effect of GABA. A: control responses. The cell first received an orthodromic volley which evoked an EPSP with a superimposed action potential. After 120 ms it was directly activated by a current pulse through the recording electrode in the soma, which evoked two action potentials. B: GABA application to the soma abolished the discharge due to the depolarizing pulse, whereas the orthodromic response due to the synaptic input in the dendrites was unchanged. C: GABA application to the site of synaptic input in the apical dendrite abolished the synaptic response evoked at this site. The response to direct stimulation at the soma was, however, facilitated. D: on the left, the cell was orthodromically activated. The control response consisted of an EPSP with a superimposed action potential. GABA applied to the site of afferent input in the dendrite 'clamped' the EPSP and thereby abolished the spike discharge. On the right, the cell was given a depolarizing pulse through the intracellular electrode, the control response consisting of a membrane depolarization triggering an action potential. GABA applied near to the soma 'clamped' the depolarization and thereby abolished spike discharges. (Langmoen, Gjerstad and Andersen, unpublished observations.)

tion indicated a reversal potential close to -40 mV as "seen" from the soma. Both responses to GABA persist after blocking synaptic transmission, showing that GABA acts directly on the cell membrane and not via interneurons. Bicuculline and picrotoxin reduce both types of GABA responses and also suppress the IPSP (Langmoen, Gjerstad and Andersen, unpublished results).

Both somatic and dendritic GABA applications shunt local depolarizations (Fig. 3). Interestingly, however, the dendritic application simultanously facilitates proximal inputs (Fig. 3). The term *discriminative inhibition* has been proposed for this phenomenon (Andersen et al., 1980).

NOREPINEPHRINE AS AN INHIBITORY TRANSMITTER

The hippocampus receives an inhibitory projection from the pontine nucleus locus coeruleus which probably uses norepinephrine (NE) as transmitter (Blackstad et al., 1967; Ungerstedt, 1971; Pickel et al., 1974; Segal and Bloom, 1974a, b; Storm-Mathisen and Guldberg, 1974).

Intracellular recordings have shown that NE hyperpolarizes HPCs (Langmoen et al., 1981). The hyperpolarization is associated with decreased input resistance (mean 22%) suggesting that the hyperpolarization is produced by increased permeability to ions carrying an outward current. The I/V plot in Fig. 4 suggests a reversal potential of −7.8 mV relative to the resting membrane potential in this cell.

The response to depolarizing current pulses is reduced more than the response to hyperpolarizing pulses (Fig. 5A and B). In addition, the depolarizing potentials are reduced with a faster time course. This stronger effect on depolarizations can be explained by a NE-induced reduction of anomalous rectification. Fig. 5 shows the input resistance at different membrane potentials. The control (Fig. 5C, open circles) shows an apparent increase in input resistance starting just below the discharge threshold, i.e. anomalous rectification (Fig. 5C, open circles). After NE application (Fig. 5C, closed circles), there is an overall decrease in resistance, which would equally affect hyperpolarizations and depolarizations. In addition, however, the increase in input resistance at depolarized levels (anomalous rectification) is abolished. The latter must profoundly reduce the response to depolarizing current pulses and is the most likely explanation for the selective reduction of slow depolarization seen during NE action.

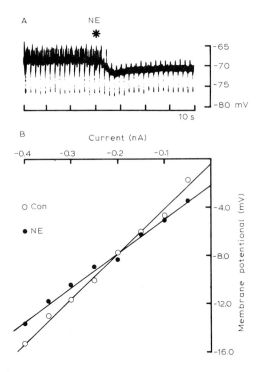

Fig. 4. Response to norepinephrine. A: continuous recording of the membrane potential during application of norepinephrine (NE) which hyperpolarized the cell. The downward vertical deflections are responses to constant hyperpolarizing current pulses, indicating the input resistance. The shorter pulses after NE application indicate an increased ionic permeability. B: an example of an I/V plot before (open circles) and after (closed circles) NE application. The slope is less steep after NE, indicating a decreased input resistance. Linear regression lines fitted to the observations suggest a reversal potential of 7.8 mV negative to the resting potential. (Part A modified from Langmoen et al., 1981.)

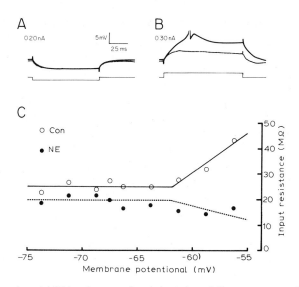

Fig. 5. Voltage-dependent inhibition by norepinephrine. A and B: responses to hyperpolarizing and depolarizing current pulses, respectively. Continuous line before, and dotted line after, NE application. NE hyperpolarized the cell and the response to the hyperpolarizing pulse was slightly decreased. In contrast, there was a substantial reduction of the depolarizing response following NE application. The reason is shown in C, where the input resistance has been tested at different membrane potentials. Before NE (open circles) the input resistance increases considerably just subthreshold to cellular firing (−55 mV). After NE this rise in input resistance is abolished. The bend in the plot usually observed is lacking in the post-NE plot for this cell, but has been illustrated with the dotted line. (From Langmoen, 1981.)

REFERENCES

Allen, G.I., Eccles, J., Nicoll, R.A., Oshima, T. and Rubia, F.J. (1977) The ionic mechanisms concerned in generating the i.p.s.ps. of hippocampal pyramidal cells. *Proc. roy. Soc. B*, 198: 363–384.

Andersen, P., Dingledine, R., Gjerstad, L., Langmoen, I.A. and Mosfeldt Laursen, A. (1980) Two different responses of hippocampal pyramidal cells to application of gamma-amino butyric acid. *J. Physiol. (Lond.)*, 305: 279–296.

Andersen, P., Eccles, J.C. and Løyning, Y. (1964a) Location of post-synaptic inhibitory synapses on hippocampal pyramids. *J. Neurophysiol.*, 27: 592–607.

Andersen, P., Eccles, J.C. and Løyning, Y. (1964b) Pathway of post-synaptic inhibition in the hippocampus. *J. Neurophysiol.*, 27: 608–619.

Barber, R. and Saito, K. (1976). Light microscopic visualization of GAD and GABA-T in immunocytochemical preparations of rodent CNS. In E. Roberts, T.N. Chase and D.B. Tower (Eds.), *GABA in Nervous System Function*, Raven Press, New York, pp. 113–132.

Bennett, M.V.L. (1974) *Synaptic Transmission and Neuronal Interaction, Society of General Physiologists Series, Vol. 28*, Raven Press, New York.

Biscoe, T.J. and Straughan, D.W. (1966). Micro-electrophoretic studies of neurones in the cat hippocampus. *J. Physiol. (Lond.)*, 183: 341–359.

Blackstad, T.W. (1967) Cortical gray matter. A correlation of light and electron microscopic data. In H. Hydén (Ed.), *The Neuron*, Elsevier, Amsterdam, pp. 49–118.

Blackstad, T.W. and Flood, P.R. (1963) Ultrastructure of hippocampal axo-somatic synapses. *Nature (Lond.)*, 198: 542–543.

Blackstad, T.W., Fuxe, K. and Hökfelt, T. (1967) Noradrenaline nerve terminals in the hippocampal region of the rat and the guinea pig. *Z. Zellforsch.*, 78: 463–473.

Curtis, D.R., Duggan, A.W., Felix, D., Johnston, G.A.R. and McLennan, H. (1971) Antagonism between bicuculline and GABA in the cat brain. *Brain Res.*, 33: 57–73.

Curtis, D.R., Felix, D. and McLennan, H. (1970) GABA and hippocampal inhibition. *Brit. J. Pharmacol.*, 40: 881–883.

Dingledine, R. and Gjerstad, L. (1980) Reduced inhibition during epileptiform activity in the in vitro hippocampal slice. *J. Physiol. (Lond.)*, 305: 297–313.

Dingledine, R. and Langmoen, I.A. (1980) Conductance changes and inhibitory actions of hippocampal recurrent IPSPs. *Brain Res.*, 185: 277–287.

Eccles, J.C. (1964) *The Physiology of Synapses*, Springer-Verlag, Heidelberg, 316 pp.

Eccles, J., Nicoll, R.A., Oshima, T. and Rubia, F.J. (1977) The anionic permeability of the inhibitory postsynaptic membrane of hippocampal pyramidal cells. *Proc. roy. Soc. B*, 198: 345–361.

Gerschenfeld, H.M. (1973) Chemical transmission in invertebrate central nervous systems and neuromuscular junctions, *Physiol. Rev.*, 53: 1–119.

Hablitz, J.J. and Langmoen, I.A. (1982) Excitation of hippocampal pyramidal cells by glutamate. *J. Physiol. (Lond.)*, 325: 317–331.

Kandel, E.R., Spencer, W.A. and Brinley, F.J., Jr. (1961) Electrophsiology of hippocampal neurons. I. Sequential invasion and synaptic organization. *J. Neurophysiol.*, 24: 225–242.

Katz, B. (1966) *Nerve, Muscle and Synapse*, McGraw-Hill, New York, 193 pp.

Krnjević, K. (1974) Chemical nature of synaptic transmission in vertebrates. *Physiol. Rev.*, 54: 418–540.

Krnjević, K. (1976) Inhibitory action of GABA and GABA-mimetics on vertebrate neurons. In E. Roberts, T.N. Chase and D.B. Tower (Eds.), *GABA in Nervous System Function*, Raven Press, New York, pp. 269–281.

Langmoen, I.A. (1981) *Synaptic Mechanisms in Hippocampal Pyramidal Cells*, Thesis, Oslo, 1981.

Langmoen, I.A. and Andersen, P. (1981) The hippocampal slice in vitro. A description of the technique and some examples of the opportunities it offers. In G.A. Kerkut and H. Wheal (Eds.), *Electrophysiology of Isolated Mammalian CNS Preparations*, Academic Press, London, pp. 51–105.

Langmoen, I.A. and Andersen, P. (1983) Summation of excitatory postsynaptic potentials in hippocampal pyramidal cells. *J. Neurophysiol.*, submitted.

Langmoen, I.A., Andersen, P., Gjerstad, L., Mosfeldt Laursen, A. and Ganes, T. (1978) Two separate effects of GABA on hippocampal pyramidal cells in vitro. *Acta physiol. scand.*, 102: 28–29A.

Langmoen, I.A., Segal, M. and Andersen, P. (1981) Mechanisms of norepinephrine actions on hippocampal pyramidal cells in vitro. *Brain Res.*, 208: 349–362.

Lorente de Nó, R. (1934) Studies on the structure of the cerebral cortex. II. Continuation of the study of the ammonic system. *J. Psychol. Neurol.*, 46: 113–177.

Malthe-Sørensen, D., Skrede, K.K. and Fonnum, F. (1979) Calcium-dependent release of D-[^{3}H]aspartate evoked by selective electrical stimulation of excitatory afferent fibres to the hippocampal pyramidal cells in vitro. *Neuroscience*, 4: 1255–1263.

Nadler, J.V., White, W.F., Vaca, K.W. and Cotman, C.W. (1977) Calcium-dependent γ-aminobutyrate release by interneurones of rat hippocampal regions: lesion-induced plasticity. *Brain Res.*, 131: 241–258.

Ozawa, S. and Okada, Y. (1976) Decrease of GABA levels and the appearance of a depolarizing shift in thin hippocampal slice in vitro. In E. Roberts, T.N. Chase and D.B. Tower (Eds.), *GABA in Nervous System Function*, Raven Press, New York, pp. 449–454.

Pickel, V.M., Segal, M. and Bloom, F.E. (1974) A radioautographic study of the efferent pathways of the nucleus locus coeruleus. *J. comp. Neurol.*, 155: 15–42.

Ramón y Cajal, S. (1893) Beiträge zur feineren Anatomie des grossen Hirns. I. Über die feinere Struktur des Ammonhornes. *Z. wiss. Zool.* 56: 615–663.

Ribak, C.E., Vaughn, J.E. and Saito, K. (1978) Immunocytochemical localization of glutamic acid decarboxylase in neuronal somata following colchicine inhibition of axonal transport. *Brain Res.*, 140: 315–332.

Schwartzkroin, P.A. and Andersen, P. (1975) Glutamic acid sensitivity of dendrites in hippocampal slices in vitro. *Advanc. Neurol.*, 12: 45–51.

Segal, M. (1976) Glutamate antagonists in rat hippocampus. *Brit. J. Pharmacol.*, 58: 341–345.

Segal, M. and Bloom, F.E. (1974a) The action of norepinephrine in the rat hippocampus. I. Iontophoretic studies. *Brain Res.*, 72: 79–97.

Segal, M. and Bloom, F.E. (1974b) The action of norepinephrine in the rat hippocampus. II. Activation of the input pathway. *Brain Res.*, 72: 99–114.

Spencer, H.J., Gribkoff, V.K., Cotman, C.W. and Lynch, G.S. (1976) GDEE antagonism of iontophoretic amino acid excitation in the intact hippocampus and in the hippocampal slice preparation. *Brain Res.*, 105: 471–481.

Storm-Mathisen, J. (1972) Glutamate decarboxylase in the rat hippocampal region after lesions of the afferent fibre systems. Evidence that the enzyme is localized in intrinsic neurones. *Brain Res.*, 40: 215–235.

Storm-Mathisen, J. (1975) High affinity uptake of GABA in presumed GABA-ergic nerve endings in rat brain. *Brain Res.*, 84: 409–427.

Storm-Mathisen, J. and Fonnum, F. (1971) Quantitative histochemistry of glutamate decarboxylase in the rat hippocampal region. *J. Neurochem.*, 18: 1105–1111.

Storm-Mathisen, J. and Guldberg, H.C. (1974) 5-Hydroxytryptamine and noradrenaline in the hippocampal region: effect of transection of afferent pathways on endogenous levels, high affinity uptake and some transmitter related enzymes. *J. Neurochem.*, 22: 793–803.

Storm-Mathisen, J. and Iversen, L.L. (1979) Uptake of [³H]glutamic acid in excitatory nerve endings: light and electronmicroscopic observations in the hippocampal formation of the rat. *Neuroscience*, 4: 1237–1253.

Takeuchi, A. (1977) Junctional transmission. I. Postsynaptic mechanisms. In J.M. Brookhart and V.B. Mountcastle, (Eds.), *Handbook of Physiology, Section 1: The Nervous System, Volume I* (E.R. Kandel, Ed.) *Cellular Biology of Neurons*, American Physiological Society, Bethesda, MD, pp. 295–327.

Ungerstedt, U. (1971) Stereotaxic mapping of the monoamine pathways in the brain. *Acta physiol. scand.*, Suppl. 367: 1–48.

A Role for Protein Phosphorylation in the Regulation of Electrical Activity of an Identified Nerve Cell

IRWIN B. LEVITAN, WILLIAM B. ADAMS, JOSÉ R. LEMOS and ILSE NOVAK-HOFER

Friedrich Miescher-Institut, P.O. Box 273, CH-4002 Basel (Switzerland)

INTRODUCTION

The large size and ready identifiability of many molluscan neurons makes them particularly convenient for combined biochemical and electrophysiological studies on individual nerve cells. Recently, a number of laboratories have taken advantage of these favorable properties to investigate the role of intracellular second messengers in neurotransmitter actions and have implicated cyclic AMP (cAMP) in the effects of serotonin (5-HT) on several different molluscan neurons (Kaczmarek et al., 1978; Klein and Kandel, 1978; Drummond et al., 1980; Levitan and Drummond, 1980; Deterre et al., 1981). Our studies have focused on the identified neuron R15, in the abdominal ganglion of the marine mollusc *Aplysia californica*. R15 is an endogenous "bursting" neuron; it exhibits a pattern of spontaneous activity comprising bursts of action potentials separated by interburst hyperpolarizations (Fig. 1). We have found that 5-HT causes R15 to hyperpolarize and stop bursting (Fig. 1). This hyperpolarization results from an increase in K^+ conductance and is mediated by cAMP (Drummond et al., 1980; Levitan and Drummond, 1980). In this report we present biochemical and electrophysiological evidence that protein phosphorylation is involved in the regulation of K^+ conductance in neuron R15.

STEADY-STATE I–V CURVES

To investigate the ionic mechanisms of the 5-HT response in R15 we have used a voltage-clamp to generate "steady-state" current–voltage (I–V) curves, the slopes of which are a measure of the total ionic conductance of the cell's membrane. 5-HT causes an increase in the slope of the steady-state I–V curve (Fig. 2A), indicative of an increase in membrane conductance to K^+ (Drummond et al., 1980). This is the basic paradigm which has been used to study the role of protein phosphorylation in R15's response to 5-HT.

[71]

72

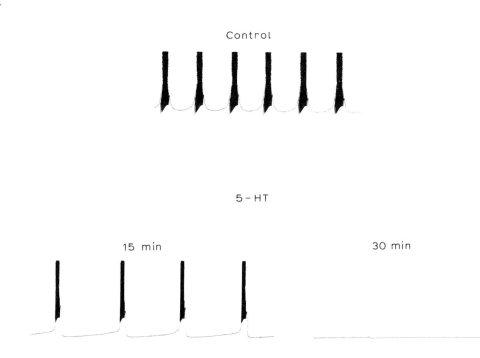

Control

5 - HT

15 min 30 min

Wash 35 min

40 mV

20 sec

Fig. 1. 5-HT causes neuron R15 to hyperpolarize. Intracellular voltage recording from neuron R15, in the absence and presence of 1 μM 5-HT. Note that 5-HT selectively enhances the interburst hyper-polarization, and in some cells bursting is completely abolished. The pattern returns to normal following a prolonged wash with normal medium. (Modified from Drummond et al., 1980.)

PROTEIN KINASE INHIBITOR

Protein kinase inhibitor (PKI) is a 10,000 dalton protein which binds with high affinity to the active catalytic subunit of cAMP-dependent protein kinase and inhibits its activity (Walsh et al., 1971). We have found that PKI purified to homogeneity from rabbit skeletal muscle (Demaille et al., 1977) is a potent inhibitor of cAMP-dependent protein kinase from *Aplysia* (Adams and Levitan, 1981). Accordingly, we injected PKI via a microelectrode directly into neuron R15, and found that the increase in K^+ conductance normally elicited by 5-HT (Fig. 2A) was completely blocked several hours after PKI injection (Fig. 2B). To test the selectivity of this

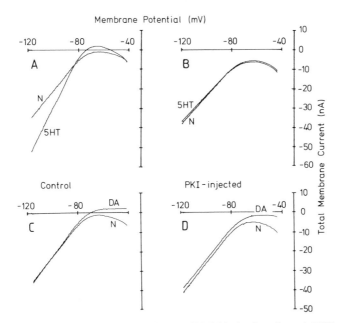

Fig. 2. Intracellular injection of protein kinase inhibitor (PKI) blocks the effect of 5-HT on neuron R15. Steady-state I–V curves generated using a conventional two-electrode voltage clamp. The increase in K$^+$ conductance (seen as the increase in slope of the I–V curve) normally elicited by 5-HT is shown in A. There is no effect of 5-HT 2 h after intracellular injection of PKI (B). In contrast, the decrease in inward (negative) current normally elicited by DA (C) is unchanged 3 h after PKI injection (D). (Modified from Adams and Levitan, 1981.)

inhibition by PKI, we examined R15's response to dopamine (DA). DA also causes R15 to hyperpolarize (Ascher, 1972), but the ionic response is different from that produced by 5-HT (Wilson and Wachtel, 1978) and the DA response does *not* appear to be mediated by cAMP (Levitan and Drummond, 1980). As shown in Fig. 2C, DA causes a decrease in voltage-dependent inward current, thought to be due to a decrease in Na$^+$ conductance (Wilson and Wachtel, 1978). A comparison of Figs. 2C and D demonstrates that PKI injection does not affect this DA response. Furthermore, we have found that the 5-HT response is normal following the injection of other proteins into R15, indicating that the PKI inhibition cannot be attributed simply to injection of protein per se (Adams and Levitan, 1981). Thus, the blockage of the neurotransmitter effect appears to be produced *specifically* by PKI, and is *selective* for the 5-HT-induced, cAMP-mediated increase in K$^+$ conductance. We conclude from these experiments employing a highly specific molecular probe, that cAMP-dependent protein phosphorylation is involved in the regulation of electrical activity in neuron R15.

PROTEIN PHOSPHORYLATION INSIDE A SINGLE LIVING NERVE CELL

Having implicated protein phosphorylation in the control of K$^+$ conductance in R15, we are now attempting to identify phosphoproteins which may be involved in

74

this regulation. Previous attempts to measure protein phosphorylation in individual nerve cells have involved incubating ganglia with ^{32}P-labeled inorganic phosphate, followed by isolation of individual nerve cell bodies and analysis of radioactive phosphoproteins (Levitan and Barondes, 1974; Levitan et al., 1974; Jennings et al., 1979; Paris et al., 1980). Although this approach has provided useful information, it suffers from several disadvantages: (1) the cell body can never be isolated totally free of glia and even portions of neighboring neuronal cell bodies, which will contribute to the labeling pattern; (2) perhaps more importantly, the neuropil axonal and dendritic processes of the cell, which are the sites at which all synaptic contacts occur, are not sampled by this procedure. To circumvent these problems we have developed methods to inject [γ-^{32}P]ATP directly into R15, in amounts sufficient to

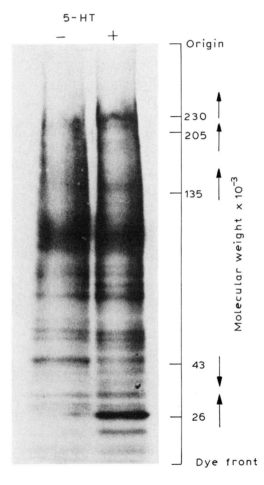

Fig. 3. 5-HT alters the phosphorylation of specific proteins within living neuron R15. Autoradiograms of SDS-polyacrylamide gels containing phosphoproteins from abdominal ganglia, incubated either in the absence or presence of 5-HT. In each ganglion neuron R15 had been injected with [γ-^{32}P]ATP, so the bands on the autoradiograms represent phosphoproteins labeled within R15. The neuron R15 in the 5-HT-treated ganglion showed a large increase in K$^+$ conductance (comparable to that in Fig. 2A). The arrows are adjacent to bands whose phosphorylation state (measured by quantitative densitometry of the autoradiograms) appears to be specifically altered by 5-HT. (Modified from Lemos et al., 1982.)

label phosphoproteins. We have confirmed, by autoradiography of sections of the abdominal ganglion, that all the radioactivity remains within neuron R15 following such injections (Lemos, Novak-Hofer and Levitan, unpublished). Thus, we can process the entire abdominal ganglion, including the neuropil region, for gel electrophoresis and be confident that any radioactive phosphoproteins we observe originate within R15. It is also important to note that we monitor the physiological properties of the cell with intracellular microelectrodes throughout the labeling period, so changes in the phosphoprotein labeling pattern may be related to changes in membrane conductance. As shown in Fig. 3, at least 15 phosphoproteins are labeled in R15 following the injection of $[\gamma\text{-}^{32}P]$ATP. The extent of labeling of three high-molecular weight phosphoprotein bands (molecular weights 230,000, 205,000 and 135,000 daltons), as well as of a 26,000 dalton band, is significantly increased in cells in which K^+ conductance has been increased by treatment with 5-HT (Fig. 3; Lemos et al., 1982). 5-HT also decreases the labeling of a 43,000 dalton band (Fig. 3). It is tempting to speculate that one or more of these phosphoproteins may constitute a regulatory component of a specific K^+ channel in the R15 membrane. Kinetic and pharmacological experiments designed to test this possibility are under way.

SUMMARY

The favorable properties of molluscan neurons have made it possible to investigate the hypothesis (Greengard, 1979) that cAMP-dependent protein phosphorylation may mediate certain actions of neurotransmitters. Results from other laboratories, demonstrating that intracellular injection of the catalytic subunit of protein kinase alters neuronal electrical activity (Kaczmarek et al., 1980; Castellucci et al., 1980; De Peyer et al., 1982) are complemented by our finding that protein phosphorylation may mediate the regulation of a specific ion channel by a neurotransmitter. The development of techniques to measure protein phosphorylation within individual living neurons opens up the possibility of identifying specific phosphoproteins which play a role in ion channel regulation.

ACKNOWLEDGEMENT

We are grateful to Dr. E. Fischer, University of Washington (Seattle), for his generous gift of purified protein kinase inhibitor.

REFERENCES

Adams, W.B. and Levitan, I. (1982) Intraceullar injection of protein kinase inhibitor blocks the serotonin-induced increase in K^+ conductance in *Aplysia* neurone R15. *Proc. nat. Acad. Sci. U.S.A.*, 79: 3877–3880.

Ascher, P. (1972) Inhibitory and excitatory effects of dopamine on *Aplysia* neurons. *J. Physiol. (Lond.),* 225: 173–209.

Castellucci, V., Kandel, E.R., Schwartz, J.H., Wilson, F.D., Nairn, A.C. and Greengard, P. (1980) Intracellular injection of the catalytic subunit of protein kinase simulates facilitation of transmitter release underlying behavioral sensitization in *Aplysia. Proc. nat. Acad. Sci. U.S.A.*, 77: 7492–7496.

De Peyer, J.E., Cachelin, A.B., Levitan, I.B. and Reuter, H. (1982) Ca^{++}-activated K^+ conductance in internally perfused snail neurons is enhanced by protein phosphorylation. *Proc. nat. Acad. Sci. U.S.A.*, 79: 4207–4211.

Demaille, J.G., Peters, K. and Fischer, E.H. (1977) Isolation and properties of the rabbit skeletal muscle protein inhibitor of cAMP-dependent protein kinases. *Biochemistry*, 16: 3080–3086.

Deterre, P., Paupardin-Tritsch, D., Bockaert, J. and Gerschenfeld, H.M. (1981) Role of cAMP in a serotonin-evoked slow inward current in snail neurons. *Nature (Lond.)*, 290: 783–785.

Drummond, A.H., Benson, J.A. and Levitan, I.B. (1980) Serotonin-induced hyperpolarization of an identified *Aplysia* neuron is mediated by cyclic AMP. *Proc. nat. Acad. Sci. U.S.A.*, 77: 5013–5017.

Greengard, P. (1979) Cyclic nucleotides, phosphorylated proteins and the nervous system. *Fed. Proc.*, 38: 2208–2217.

Jennings, K., Kaczmarek, L. and Strumwasser, F. (1979) Protein phosphorylation during afterdischarge of the neuroendocrine bag cells in *Aplysia*. *Neurosci. Abstr.*, 5: 249.

Kaczmarek, L.K., Jennings, K. and Strumwasser, F. (1978) Neurotransmitter modulation, phosphodiesterase inhibitor effects and cAMP correlates of afterdischarge in peptidergic neurons. *Proc. nat. Acad. Sci. U.S.A.*, 75: 5200–5204.

Kaczmarek, L.K., Jennings, K., Strumwasser, F., Nairn, A.C., Walter, U., Wilson, F.D. and Greengard, P. (1980) Microinjection of catalytic subunit of cAMP-dependent protein kinase enhances calcium action potentials of bag cell neurons in cell culture. *Proc. nat. Acad. Sci. U.S.A.*, 77: 7487–7491.

Klein, M. and Kandel, E.R. (1978) Presynaptic modulation of voltage-dependent Ca^{++} current: mechanism for behavioral sensitization in *Aplysia*. *Proc. nat. Acad. Sci. U.S.A.*, 75; 3512–3516.

Lemos, J.R., Novak-Hofer, I. and Levitan, I.B. (1982) Serotonin alters the phosphorylation of specific proteins inside a single living nerve cell. *Nature (Lond.)*, 298: 64–65.

Levitan, I.B. and Barondes, S.H. (1974) Octopamine- and serotonin-stimulated phosphorylation of specific protein in the abdominal ganglion of *Aplysia californica*. *Proc. nat. Acad. Sci. U.S.A.*, 71: 1145–1148.

Levitan, I.B. and Drummond, A.H. (1980) Neuronal serotonin receptors and cAMP: biochemical, pharmacological and electrophysiological analysis. In U. Littauer et al. (Eds.), *Neurotransmitters and Their Receptors*, John Wiley and Sons, London, pp. 163–176.

Levitan, I.B., Madsen, C.J. and Barondes, S.H. (1974) Cyclic AMP and amine effects on phosphorylation of specific protein in abdominal ganglion of *Aplysia*: localization and kinetic analysis. *J. Neurobiol.*, 5: 511–525.

Paris, C.G., Kandel, E.R. and Schwartz, J.H. (1980) Serotonin stimulates phosphorylation of a 137,000 dalton membrane protein in the abdominal ganglion of *Aplysia*. *Neurosci. Abstr.*, 6: 844.

Walsh, D.A., Ashby, C.D., Gonzales, C., Calkins, D., Fischer, E.H. and Krebs, E.G. (1971) Purification and characterization of a protein inhibitor of cAMP-dependent kinases. *J. biol. Chem.*, 246: 1977–1985.

Wilson, W. and Wachtel, H. (1978) Prolonged inhibition in burst firing neurons: synaptic inactivation of the slow regenerative inward current. *Science*, 202: 772–775.

Regulation of Intracellular Protein Traffic

GÜNTER BLOBEL

Laboratory of Cell Biology, The Rockefeller University, New York, NY 10021 (U.S.A.)

INTRODUCTION

A cell contains millions of protein molecules. These are steadily being synthesized and degraded. At homeostasis, a given species of protein is represented by a characteristic number of molecues that is kept constant within a narrow range. Very little is known about the cell's accounting procedures, i.e. how it balances and controls biosynthesis and biodegradation.

An important aspect of biosynthesis (Blobel, 1980), as well as biodegradation (Blobel, 1979), is the intracellular topology of proteins. Many protein species spend their entire life in the same compartment in which they are synthesized, others have to be translocated across the hydrophobic barrier of one, or in some cases, two distinct cellular membranes in order to reach the intracellular compartment or extracellular site where they exert their function. Numerous protein species have to be integrated asymmetrically into distinct cellular membranes. For many proteins this requires partial translocation, i.e. selective transfer of one or several *distinct hydrophilic* or *charged segments* of the polypeptide chain across the hydrophobic barrier of one or two intracellular membranes. Following complete or partial translocation across a translocation-competent membrane(s), subpopulations may undergo further "post-translocational" traffic (Palade, 1975). Soluble or membrane proteins may be shipped in bulk or by receptor-mediated processes from a translocation-competent donor compartment to a translocation-incompetent receiver compartment. This post-translocational traffic may be unidirectional (in which case the protein ends up as a permanent resident of a particular cellular membrane) or may follow a cyclic pattern between distinct cellular membranes (e.g. recycling of receptors).

The collective term "topogenesis" has been introduced (Blobel, 1980) to encompass protein translocation (partial or complete) across membranes as well as subsequent post-translocational protein traffic. Not included in these processes that define topogenesis are distinct traffic patterns that may be required for protein degradation. Theoretical considerations on the topology of protein degradation have been presented elsewhere (Blobel, 1979) and will not be dealt with here: in essence, these considerations argue for the existence of three (animal cells) or even four (plant cells) distinct and separate compartments for protein degradation, each containing a distinct set of proteases. Detailed proposals have also been made for protein topogenesis (Blobel, 1980). The essence of these proposals is that the information for intracellular protein topogenesis resides in *discrete* "topogenic" sequences that constitute a permanent or transient part of the polypeptide chain. The repertoire of distinct topogenic sequences was predicted to be relatively small

[77]

because many different proteins would be topologically equivalent, i.e. targeted to the same intracellular address. Four types of topogenic sequences were distinguished (Blobel, 1980): (i) *Signal* sequences, they initiate translocation of proteins across specific membranes and are decoded by protein translocators that, by virtue of their signal sequence-specific domain and their location in distinct cellular membranes, effect unidirectional translocation of proteins across specific cellular membranes; (ii) *Stop-transfer* sequences, they interrupt the translocation process that was previously initiated by a signal sequence and, by excluding a distinct segment of the polypeptide chain from translocation, yield asymmetric integration of proteins into translocation-competent membranes; (iii) *Sorting* sequences, they act as determinants for post-translocational traffic of subpopulations of proteins, originating in translocation-competent donor membranes (and compartments) and leading to translocation-incompetent receiver membranes (and compartments); and (iv) *Insertion* sequences interact with the lipid bilayer directly and thereby anchor a protein to the hydrophobic core of the lipid bilayer.

An attempt is made here to amplify some of these previous proposals and to discuss some of the recent experimental data that are relevant to these proposals.

TRANSLOCATION OF PROTEINS ACROSS MEMBRANES

Translocation is understood here as transport of an entire polypeptide chain across one (or two) membrane(s), proceeding undirectionally from the protein biosynthetic compartment. Not considered here will be ectopically synthesized proteins (e.g. toxins such as the colicins or diphtheria toxins) although their entry into cells may also require complete or partial translocation of polypeptide chains across a membrane, either the plasma membrane directly or an intracellular membrane, following uptake by endocytosis.

Hypothetical models for intracellular protein translocation must deal with two essential tenets which appear to underly the observed phenomenology of this process. First, the permeability barrier of the membrane appears to be reversibly modified for the passage of each translocated polypeptide chain while being maintained for other solutes. Second, the species of protein to be translocated, as well as the type of membrane across which a given protein is translocated, are highly specific. Both of these tenets can be readily satisfied by postulating that protein translocation is a receptor-mediated process (Blobel, 1980) in which specificity is achieved by "signal" sequences in the proteins to be translocated and by signal-sequence-specific translocation systems that are restricted in their location to distinct cellular membranes.

BIOLOGICAL MEMBRANES ENDOWED WITH
PROTEIN TRANSLOCATION SYSTEMS

Several signal-sequence specific translocation systems have been postulated to exist (Blobel, 1980). Table I lists the biological membranes or membrane pairs that have been proposed to be endowed each with *one* signal sequence-specific translocation system (in multiple copies) that is able to decode the information of *one* type

TABLE I

Cellular membranes proposed to be endowed with a transport system (translocator)
for the unidirectional translocation of nascent or newly synthesized proteins

Each of the translocation-competent membranes listed here (a–i) is proposed to contain only *one* distinct "translocator" (in multiple copies). Each translocator responds to *one* type of signal sequence. Translocation can proceed across a *single* membrane (a–g), or *two* membranes (h–i), cotranslationally (a–d), or post-translationally (e–i). Suggested abbreviations for these translocation-competent membranes might serve as useful codes. For example, a signal sequence (Si) addressed to the rough endoplasmic reticulum (RER), to the chloroplast envelope (CEN), etc., might be designated Si(RER), Si(RER), Si(CEN), etc. Likewise, a particular signal receptor (SiR), or signal peptidase (SiP) could be classified as SiR(RER), SiR(CEN), or SiP(RER), SiP(CEN), etc. (From Blobel, 1980, with permission.)

Mode of translocation	Membrane	Code
Cotranslational	a. prokaryotic plasma membrane	PPM
	b. inner mitochondrial membrane	IMM
	c thylakoid membrane	TKM
	d. rough endoplasmic reticulum	RER
Post-translational	e. outer mitochrondrial membrane	OMM
(across *one* membrane)	f. outer chloroplast membrane	OCM
	g. peroxisomal membrane	PXM
Post-translational	h. mitochondrial envelope	MEN
(across *two* membranes)	i. chloroplast envelope	CEN

of signal sequence. Two modes of translocation have been distinguished, a cotranslational and a post-translational mode. In cotranslational translocation (Redman and Sabatini, 1966; Blobel, 1980) the passage of the polypeptide chain across the membrane appears to be strictly coupled to translation, whereas in post-translational translocation (Dobberstein et al., 1977; Blobel, 1980) the polypeptide can traverse the membrane post-translationally uncoupled from its synthesis.

The conjecture was made (Blobel, 1980), based on possible evolutionary relationships between various cellular membranes (see below, Fig. 4) that the contemporary cotranslational translocation systems (Table Ia–d) were derived from a common ancestral system and that they might be highly conserved. A high degree of conservation has indeed been demonstrated for the rough endoplasmic reticulum (RER) translocation system within the animal and plant kingdoms (Dobberstein and Blobel, 1977). Moreover, it has been demonstrated that a signal sequence of a eukaryotic protein addressed to the RER translocation system can be decoded by its putative analogue in the prokaryotic plasma membrane (Talmadge et al., 1980a, b). The existence of two other cotranslational translocation systems, namely those in the inner mitochondrial membrane and in the thylakoid membrane, has been postulated (Blobel, 1980) because of the presence of membrane-bound polysomes in thylakoid membranes (Chua et al., 1973) and in the inner mitochondrial membrane (Kuriyama and Luck, 1973). These cotranslational translocation systems are most likely involved in partial translocation, i.e. translocation only of a distinct segment of the nascent chain (and not of the entire polypeptide) and therefore function in the integration of membrane proteins (see below).

Post-translational translocation systems have been postulated (Blobel, 1980) for translocation of cytoplasmically synthesized proteins across a *single* membrane (peroxisomal-, outer mitochrondrial-, outer chloroplast membrane) or across *two* membranes (outer and inner membranes of mitochrondria and chloroplasts).

Evidence for the existence of a post-translational translocation system in the peroxisomal membrane rests on the demonstration that liver catalase and uricase (two enzymes located in the peroxisome) are synthesized by free ribosomes and not by membrane-bound ribosomes (Goldman and Blobel, 1978). Conclusive evidence for the existence of post-translational translocation systems in the outer mitochondrial membrane (Maccecchini et al. 1979b) and across both outer and inner membranes of chloroplasts (Dobberstein et al., 1977; Highfield and Ellis, 1978; Chua and Schmidt, 1978), and mitochrondria (Maccecchini et al., 1979a) was first derived from data of in vitro translation and translocation experiments which were subsequently confirmed by numerous laboratories. The existence of a post-translational translocation system in the outer chloroplast membrane analogous to that in the outer mitochrondrial membrane has not yet been demonstrated.

SIGNAL SEQUENCES

The existence of a "signal sequence" for translocation across the RER was first postulated on theoretical grounds (Blobel and Sabatini, 1971). Subsequently, cell-free synthesis of secretory proteins showed them to be synthesized as larger precursors (Milstein et al., 1972; Swan et al., 1972; Schechter et al., 1974; Devillers-Thiery et al., 1975) and in vitro translocation experiments provided evidence that the sequence extension present in these precursors functions as a "signal sequence" in translocation (Blobel and Dobberstein, 1975a, b; Szczesna and Boime, 1976). Thereafter, signal sequences were discovered, by similar in vitro approaches, for translocation across the prokaryotic plasma membrane (Inouye et al., 1977; Inouye and Beckwith, 1977), the chloroplast envelope (Dobberstein et al., 1977; Highfield and Ellis, 1978), the two mitochondrial membranes (Maccecchini et al., 1979a) and the outer mitochrondrial membrane (Maccecchini et al., 1979b).

Translocation is not always accompanied by cleavage of the signal sequence and there are now numerous examples for uncleaved signal sequences. Further, the signal sequence is not always located at the NH_2-terminus (Lingappa et al., 1979; Garoff et al., 1980) and there may be more than one signal sequence in a polypeptide (Blobel, 1980; Garoff et al., 1980).

The complete primary structure is known for the signal sequence addressed to: (a) the RER (numerous examples, see compilation by Steiner et al., 1980); (b) the prokaryotic plasma membrane (numerous examples, see compilation by Emr et al., 1980), and (c) the chloroplast envelope (so far one one example, Schmidt et al., 1979).

As expected on evolutionary grounds (Blobel, 1980), and as demonstrated experimentally (Talmadge et al., 1980a, b), the signal sequence addressed to the RER plasma membrane is similar to that addressed to the prokaryotic plasma membrane. At present it is not obvious, at least not from the primary structure of the numerous examples, what features of the signal sequence constitutes a consensus structure for the receptor (see below). Elegant experiments with mutants (see review by Emr et al., 1980) and with amino acids analogues (Hortin and Boime, 1980) have shown that replacement in the signal sequence of hydrophobic residues by charged or hydrophilic residues interfere with translocation.

As expected, the primary structure of the signal sequence addressed to the chloroplast envelope (Schmidt et al., 1979) differs dramatically from that addressed to the RER or to the prokaryotic plasma membrane. However, the primary structure of more examples needs to be elucidated before one could recognize features of a consensus structure for the corresponding receptor(s) of the chloroplast envelope translocation system.

It should be emphasized that a signal sequence was postulated only to be involved in the initiation of chain translocation (Blobel and Dobberstein, 1975a). Implicit in this postulate was that the rest of the polypeptide chain must be compatible with the translocation machinery (see "stop-transfer" sequences below); for example, a polyleucine or a non-secretory protein (Moreno et al., 1980) linked to a signal sequence may be non-permissive for translocation.

MECHANISMS OF TRANSLOCATION

Until recently, the postulated translocation machinery (Blobel and Sabatini, 1971; Blobel and Dobberstein, 1975a; Blobel, 1980) remained largely undefined, so much so that it was deemed unnecessary (von Heijne and Blomberg, 1979; Wickner, 1979; Garnier et al., 1980; Engelman and Steitz, 1981). Only after the development of an in vitro translocation system (Blobel and Dobberstein, 1975b) that was able to reproduce translocation across the ER membrane (isolated in form of closed microsomal vesicles) with apparent fidelity, did it become possible to assay and to characterize the ER's translocation activity *in vitro*. Two approaches were taken to dissect the membrane translocation activity: salt extraction (Warren and Dobberstein, 1978; Walter and Blobel, 1980) and limited proteolysis (Walter et al., 1979; Meyer and Dobberstein, 1980a). Both approaches yielded membrane vesicles that were largely translocation-inactive; translocation activity, however, could be restored by readdition of the salt- or tryptic-extract. These findings provided an assay for the purification of the active components of the salt extract (Walter and Blobel, 1980) and of the proteolytic extract (Meyer and Dobberstein, 1980b). The purified active component of the proteolytic extract consisted of an apparently single polypeptide chain (Meyer and Dobberstein, 1980b) whereas the purified active component of the salt extract was shown to be an 11S protein of $\approx$250,000 daltons that consisted of six polypeptide chains which could not be separated from each other by a variety of non-denaturing procedures (Walter and Blobel, 1980). The precise relationship between the purified proteins from the proteolytic- and the salt-extract remains to be investigated (see below).

Studies on the role of the 11S protein in the translocation process revealed that it is involved in the recognition of the signal sequence and therefore it was termed "Signal Recognition Protein" (SRP) (Walter et al., 1981). When SRP is present in the cell-free translation system in the absence of salt-extracted microsomal membranes it was found to inhibit selectively only the translation of mRNA for secretory protein (bovine prolactin) but not of mRNA for cytosolic proteins (α and β chain of rabbit globin; Walter et al., 1981). Moreover, SRP was found to bind with a relatively low affinity (apparent K_d 5×10^{-5} M) to ribosomes, but was shown to bind with a 6000-fold higher affinity (apparent K_d 8×10^{-9} M) when ribosomes are engaged in the translation of mRNA for secretory proteins (Walter et al., 1981). Most interestingly, this high affinity binding of SRP causes a site-specific and signal sequence-induced arrest of chain elongation (Walter and Blobel, 1981b). The elongation-arrested peptide of nascent preprolactin was shown to be $\approx$70 amino acid residues long (Walter and Blobel, 1981b). Because the signal sequence of nascent bovine preprolactin comprises 30 residues (Jackson and Blobel, 1980), and because about 40 residues of the nascent chain are buried (protected from proteases) in the large ribosomal subunit (Malkin and Rich, 1967; Blobel and Sabatini, 1970), it was concluded (Walter and Blobel, 1981b) that it is the signal sequence of the nascent chain (fully emerged on the outside of the large ribosomal subunit) that causes high affinity binding of SRP which, in turn, modulates translation and causes arrest in chain elongation.

Most strikingly, elongation arrest is released upon binding of the elongation-arrested ribosome to salt-extracted microsomal membranes (K-RM) resulting in chain elongation and translocation into the microsomal vesicle (Walter and Blobel, 1981a). Binding of the translating ribosome to K-RM occurs only in the presence of SRP. Further, treatment of K-RM with low concentrations of trypsin abolishes SRP-mediated binding of the translating ribosome to K-RM (Walter and Blobel, 1981a). This latter finding suggests that besides SRP (which could be considered a peripheral membrane protein) integral membrane proteins are required for translocation to proceed. It is likely, but remains to be proven, that it is the hydrophilic cytoplasmic domains of these integral membrane proteins (severed by proteolytic enzymes in such a manner that they retain reconstitutability to their parent molecules; (Walter and Blobel, 1979; Meyer and Dobberstein, 1980a) that have recently been purified (Meyer and Dobberstein, 1980b).

Taken together, these data provide the strongest support to date for the most pivotal (and most contested) postulate of the signal hypothesis (Blobel and Dobberstein, 1975a; Blobel 1980), namely that protein translocation across the ER is a receptor-mediated process. These data thus definitively rule out alternative hypotheses that have postulated that chain translocation across the ER occurs spontaneously, without the mediation by proteins, (Bretscher, 1973; Wickner, 1979; Garnier et al., 1980; Engelman and Steitz, 1981). They also rule out translocation models that, although relying on the participation of specific proteins, have postulated a primary interaction of the signal sequence (because of its hydrophobic nature) with the lipid bilayer (DiRienzo et al., 1978; von Heijne and Blomberg, 1979; Steiner, 1980). Thus, the initial events that lead to translocation and provide for its specificity are protein–protein (signal sequence plus ribosome–SRP) and *not* protein–lipid (signal sequence–lipid bilayer) interactions.

The ability of SRP to arrest chain elongation and the finding that microsomal membranes release this arrest is of teleological interest. If this mechanism also operates in vitro it would provide the cell with a means to stop the synthesis of secretory proteins (some of which might be harmful if completed in the cytosol) unless sites on the ER are available so that translocation and segregation into the intracisternal space are insured. These sites in the microsomal membranes could consist of several integral membrane proteins which might form an ensemble undergoing cyclic disassembly and reassembly for each chain translocation event

(Blobel and Dobberstein, 1975a). Signal peptidase and core sugar transferase might, as integral membrane proteins, participate in the formation of this ensemble or might be transiently associated with it. Other components of this ensemble might be the so-called ribophorins (Kreibich et al., 1978a, b), although their involvement in protein translocation has not yet been demonstrated.

Because of evolutionary considerations (see below) and because of the documented mechanistic similarity of protein translocation across the prokaryotic plasma membrane (Smith et al., 1977; Randall et al., 1978; Chang et al., 1978, 1979; Emr et al., 1980; Talmadge et al., 1980a) to that across the ER, our conjecture (Blobel, 1980) is that there is only *one, cotranslational* translocation system in the bacterial plasma membrane and, moreover, that this system will be essentially similar if not identical to that in the ER. However, it should be noted that this view has been challenged and that a post-translational mode of translocation across the bacterial plasma membrane has been postulated (Wickner, 1979; Koshland and Botstein, 1980).

The discovery of SRP has permitted us to add more detail to and to expand the previously proposed translocation models. The postulated ribosome receptor and signal sequence receptor for the cotranslational translocation system were envisioned to be integral membrane proteins (Blobel, 1980). Because SRP (presumably a peripheral membrane protein) is, at least in part, endowed with these postulated receptor properties, and because additional, integral membrane proteins are required for translocation (translocation activity of trypsinized K-RM cannot be restored by SRP), our present cotranslational translocation model (Walter and Blobel, 1981b) is in detail, not in principle, more complex than previously envisioned (Blobel, 1980).

The discovery of SRP likewise suggests modifications of our models for post-translational translocation. The latter has been envisioned to be in principle similar to cotranslational translocation except that the existence of only signal sequence receptors (again as integral membrane proteins) but not of ribosome receptors was envisioned (Blobel, 1980). If signal sequence-specific SRP analogues would exist also for the various post-translational translocation systems and if, in turn, SRP-specific receptors in various organelle membranes were to control import into organelles, one could envision a cytoplasmic pool of translocation-competent complexes consisting of an SRP analogue plus a protein to be imported. The search of these SRP analogues is now under way in our laboratory.

INTEGRATION INTO MEMBRANES

Many integral membrane proteins (IMPs) require selective translocation of one or more hydrophilic segment(s) of the polypeptide chain in order to acquire their characteristic asymmetric orientation. How could a selective translocation of discrete segment(s) of the polypeptide chain be accomplished?

In considering theoretical solutions to this problem, an arbitrary definition of possible modes of orientation of the polypeptide chain of IMPs with respect to the hydrophobic core and the hydrophilic environment of the lipid bilayer was proposed (Blobel, 1980). IMPs were classified as monotopic, bitopic and polytopic (see Fig. 1). The polypeptide chain of monotopic IMPs exhibits unilateral topology – i.e. each

84

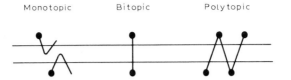

Fig. 1. Classification of integral membrane proteins (IMPs) as monotopic, bitopic and polytopic. The hydrophobic boundary of the lipid bilayer is indicated by two parallel lines. Solid circles on polypeptide chains indicate major hydrophilic domains. The hydrophilic domain of an individual monotopic IMP is exposed only on one side of the lipid bilayer. A hydrophobic domain is indicated to anchor the polypeptide chain to the hydrophobic core of the lipid bilayer. A monotopic IMP may contain several hydrophilic and hydrophobic segments alternating with each other (not indicated here). However, all hydrophilic domains are unilaterally exposed. The polypeptide chain of bitopic IMPs spans the lipid bilayer once and contains a hydrophilic domain on each side of the membrane. In variants of bitopic IMPs (not indicated), the bilateral hydrophilic domains could be further subsegmented by interspersed hydrophobic domains that are capable of monotopic integration. The polypeptide chain of polytopic IMPs spans the membrane more than once and contains multiple hydrophilic domains on both sides of the membrane. The existence of polytopic IMPs remains to be demonstrated. Two structurally monotopic IMPs located on opposite sides of the membrane could interact via their hydrophobic anchorage domains and form a functionally bilateral ensemble.

molecule possesses hydrophilic domain(s) exposed to the hydrophilic environment on only one side of the membrane. The polypeptide chain of bitopic and polytopic IMPs is bilateral in nature, containing two or multiple hydrophilic domains, respectively, exposed on opposite sides of the membrane.

It was proposed (Blobel, 1980) that all of these orientations could be accomplished by invoking, in addition to the signal sequence, only two additional types of topogenic sequences, termed "stop-transfer sequences" and "insertion sequences". The *stop-transfer sequence* was proposed to contain the information to interrupt the chain translocation process that was initiated by a signal sequence – e.g. by effecting premature disassembly of the translocation system (Blobel, 1980).

Because translocation of the polypeptide chain could be expected to proceed sequentially and asymmetrically in both contranslational and post-translational translocation, stop-transfer sequences would be effective means for asymmetric integration of certain IMPs by either modes of translocation (see Table I). There could be as many translocator-specific stop-transfer sequences as there are translocator-specific signal sequences. On the other hand, there could be only one stop-transfer sequence addressed to one component common to all translocators.

The sequence features that constitute a stop-transfer sequence remain to be defined. The stop-transfer sequence may not simply be that stretch of ≈ 25 primarily hydrophobic residues which is found as the transmembrane segment of bitopic IMPs and which might be envisioned to act as a stop-transfer sequence by virtue of being non-permissive with the translocation process. There are, for example, viral bitopic IMPs which possess stretches of at least 28 hydrophobic residues in their ectoplasmic domain (Scheid et al., 1978; Gething et al., 1978). Since this domain is translocated it is clear that a long stretch of hydrophobic residue per se is not sufficient to stop the translocation process.

The *insertion sequence* functions to anchor a protein monotopically to the hydrophobic core of the lipid bilayer. Insertion would be spontaneous and not mediated by specific proteins. It would not be accompanied by the translocation across the membrane's lipid bilayer of large charged segments of the polypeptide chain. The latter can be achieved only by a signal sequence in a receptor-mediated process.

As is the case for the stop-transfer sequence, the structural features of an insertion sequence remain to be defined. It is conceivable that there are several unique insertion sequences that can distinguish lipid composition and therefore insert only into specific membranes. On the other hand, the specificity of insertion into a distinct membrane may be largely dictated by protein–protein interaction (i.e. by an affinity of a protein to be inserted to another IMP).

Although the precise orientation of the polypeptide backbone with respect to the lipid bilayer is unknown for most species of IMPs, the proposed (Blobel, 1980) hypothetical schemes of multiple topogenic sequences (Fig. 2) can explain any one orientation by what essentially are a limited number of highly redundant mechanisms. It is clear from these examples (Fig. 2) that the integration of most proteins into the membrane requires a signal sequence and a translocator, except for one subgroup of monotopic IMPs (see Fig. 2, upper left example). Thus, most IMPs can be integrated directly only into translocation-competent membranes. Because the translocators themselves are likely to consist of IMPs (see above) that require translocation for their integration into the membrane, it follows that Virchow's

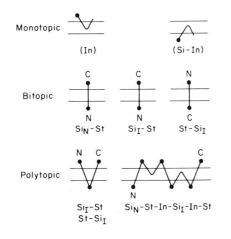

Fig. 2. Program of topogenic sequences for the asymmetric integration into membranes of some representative examples of monotopic, bitopic and polytopic IMPs. (From Blobel, 1980, with permission.) Hydrophobic boundary of lipid bilayer is indicated by two parallel lines, with upper line facing the protein biosynthetic compartment. Solid circles represent major hydrophilic domains which, when indicated, contain amino (N) or carboxy (C) terminus of the polypeptide chain. Topogenic sequences are: insertion sequence (In), signal sequence (Si), and stop-transfer sequences (St). Si_N and Si_I indicate amino-terminal and internal signal sequences, respectively. Examples given here (except for monotopic IMP at upper left) are for cotranslational integration into RER. Similar programs are conceivable also for cotranslational integration into PPM, IMM, and TKM as well as for post-translational integration into PXM, OMM, OCM, IMM [using Si(MEN)], and ICM/TKM [using Si(CEN)] (see Table I). An attempt has been made to list topogenic sequences in order of their location along the polypeptide chain starting from the amino terminus. The problems encountered in predicting the order relate to uncertainties as to the order of chain translocation. In particular, in the case of an internal signal sequence (Si_I) there are several possibilities depending on the order of translocation (Lingappa et al., 1979). The orientation of a polytopic IMP such as indicated at the lower right is entirely hypothetical and is illustrated here only to indicate how such a polypeptide chain could be integrated into the membrane by a program of multiple topogenic sequences.

paradigm on the ontogeny of cells could be extended to membranes and paraphrased to "omnis membrana e membrana".

Information about the mechanism of integration can be derived from assays which mimic the in vivo situation as closely as possible. Isolation of an IMP with detergents and its subsequent reconstitution into lipid vesicles (Kagawa and Racker, 1971), while important for functional studies, cannot yield such information because it is improbable that detergents (either free or bound to proteins) are used by the cell to integrate its IMPs into membranes.

The first example of IMP integration into membranes (RER) under physiological conditions, in an in vitro translocation system (developed for in vitro translocation of secretory proteins; Blobel and Dobberstein, 1975b) was that of a bitopic viral IMP, the glycoprotein G of vesicular stomatitis virus (VSV). It was shown (Lingappa et al., 1978) that this protein is synthesized with a signal sequence, that is addressed to the ER translocation system and which is functionally identical to that of a secretory protein (shown by competition experiments). This in vitro translocation system also reproduced the bitopic asymmetric orientation of G with fidelity; the amino terminal portion of newly synthesized G was translocated into the microsomal vesicles (protected by added proteolytic enzymes) whereas its carboxy-terminal portion remained untranslocated and therefore accessible to proteolytic enzymes (Lingappa et al., 1978). Recently, we have shown (D. Anderson, P. Walter and G. Blobel, in preparation) that integration of IMPs into the RER also requires SRP, as was expected, based on results of the earlier competition experiments (Lingappa et al., 1978).

The finding that SRP causes a signal sequence-induced arrest in chain elongation (Walter and Blobel, 1981b) should be useful for mapping the location (NH_2-terminal or internal; Lingappa et al., 1979) of a signal sequence in those IMPs that contain an uncleaved signal sequence (Bonatti and Blobel, 1979; Schechter et al., 1979). The same approach should also be useful for mapping the location of multiple signal sequences (Garoff et al., 1980).

Together with the rapidly accumulating information on the primary structure of a variety of IMPs and on their precise topology in the membrane, SRP and the in vitro translocation system can also be expected to yield detailed information on the mechanism of integration of those IMPs with other than a simple bitopic orientation.

PHYLOGENY OF MEMBRANES, PROTEIN TRANSLOCATION AND COMPARTMENTS

How then could biological membranes with their characteristic asymmetry of proteins have evolved if their assembly depended on the development of a protein translocation system which, because it was made up in part of IMPs, was itself dependent for its assembly on a protein translocation system?

In an attempt to retrace the "phylogeny" of membranes one could distinguish between precellular and cellular stages of evolution. Starting with lipid vesicles (Fig. 3) the first step in the precellular evolution of biological membranes may have been monotopic integration of proteins into the outer leaflet of lipid vesicles via insertion sequences. Such vesicles could have functioned as capturing devices to collect, on

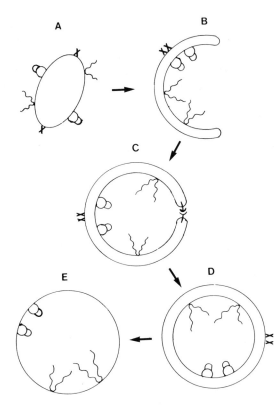

Fig. 3. Schematic illustration of various theoretical stages of precellular evolution on the surface of vesicles culminating in the formation of a primordial cell. (From Blobel, 1980 with permission.) A: vesicles containing monotopic IMPs (not indicated) are able to bind various macromolecules (X) and macromolecular complexes, among them chromatin and ribosomes. B: non-random distribution of bound components on the vesicle surface and beginning invagination. C: formation of a "gastruloid" vesicle, perhaps able to open and to close via protein-protein interaction of bitopic IMPs at the orifice. D. fusion at the orifice, resulting in a primordial cell delimited by two membranes. E: loss of the outer membrane. D could have evolved into Gram-negative bacteria and E into Gram-positive bacteria and eukaryotic cells (see Fig. 4).

their outer surface, components involved in replication, transcription, and translation as well as metabolic enzymes present in the surrounding medium (Fig. 3A). In this way, much of the precellular evolution and assembly of macromolecular complexes (such as the ribosome) may have proceeded on the surface of these vesicles rather than within vesicles. By vesicle fusion, larger vesicles containing a synergistic assortment of functions could have evolved, resulting essentially in the formation of "inside-out cells" (Fig. 3A and B) (Blobel, 1980). Concurrent with the evolution of such inside-out cells could have been the development of mechanisms for the translocation of proteins, thus providing the opportunity to segregate proteins, to colonize (with monotopic IMPs) the interior leaflet of the vesicle's lipid bilayer, and to integrate bitopic IMPs. Toward this end, the ribosome–membrane junction could have been remodeled and the insertion sequence could have evolved into a signal sequence so as to achieve first a cotranslational mode of translocation. The development of the stop-transfer sequence (perhaps as a variant of the signal

88

sequence) to integrate bitopic IMPs may have concluded the precellular evolution of the cotranslational mechanism for the assembly of membranes. The post-translational mode of translocation may have evolved from the cotranslational mode by transposing the information that might be contained in ribosomal protein and adding it to the signal sequence for cotranslational translocation. The integration of bitopic IMPs into the lipid bilayer permitted the development of transport systems and signaling systems. This set the stage for evolution to continue within a closed system (the primordial cell) effectively sealed from some of the hazards of the surrounding medium by the lipid bilayer but able to communicate with the outside via the lipid bilayer-integrated transport and signaling systems. The primordial cell (Fig. 3D) may have possessed two membranes, a plasma membrane delimiting the newly generated

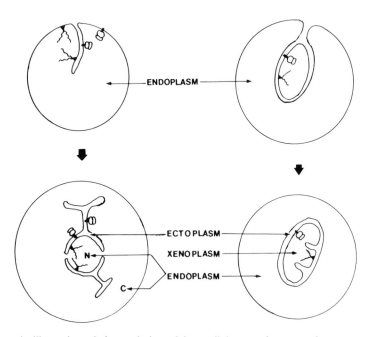

Fig. 4. Schematic illustration of the evolution of intracellular membranes and compartments. (From Blobel, 1980, with permission). Left: aggregation of certain membrane functions in the plane of the pluripotent plasma membrane. Non-random removal of these functions from the plasma membrane by invagination and fission results in the formation of a nuclear envelope (pore complexes omitted) continuous with the endoplasmic reticulum (rough and smooth) and generates an ectoplasmic compartment. The endoplasmic compartment is thereby subdivided into nucleoplasm (N) and cytoplasm (C). Note, however, that N and C remain connected via nuclear pores that do not have a membranous barrier. Other intracellular membranes that are distinct from the endoplasmic reticulum, such as lysosomal, peroxisomal, and Golgi complex membranes, also could have developed by invagination from the plasma membrane or could be outgrowths of the endoplasmic reticulum. Right: symbiotic capture of another cell, generating an additional xenoplasmic compartment. Green plant cells have two such xenoplasmic compartments (mitochondrial matrix and chloroplast stroma). Only the inner mitochondrial membrane and the inner chloroplast membrane (including derived thylakoid membrane) would be of xenoplasmic origin, whereas the outer mitochondrial and chloroplast membranes would be of orthoplasmic origin, like all other cellular membranes. The proposed terminology may be useful for describing the precise topology of IMPs (see Fig. 1). For example, monotopic IMPs of the thylakoid membrane may be exposed ectoplasmically (i.e. toward the intradisc space) or xenoplasmically (i.e. toward the stroma); bitopic IMPs of the outer mitochondrial membrane have an ectoplasmic and an endoplasmic domain. etc.

endoplasmic compartment, and an outer membrane enclosing a periplasmic space that represents the remnant of the intravesicular space of the inside-out cell. Subsequent elimination of the outer membrane would have yielded a cell with only one membrane (Fig. 3E), the plasma membrane, and one compartment, the endoplasmic compartment. All other biological membranes could have originated either directly or indirectly from this primordial plasma membrane.

The membranes of eukaryotic cells could be traced to two distinct sources (Fig. 4). One would be the cell's own primordial plasma membrane, generating by invagination various "orthoplasmic" membranes which delimit a new intracellular compartment, the ectoplasmic compartment (Fig. 4). The other source (based on the theory of endosymbiosis; see Margulis, 1970) would be the plasma membrane of a foreign symbiotic cell (at a "prenuclear" stage of evolution) which after being interiorized would give rise to "xenoplasmic" membranes delimiting a xenoplasmic subcompartment within the ectoplasmic compartment (Fig. 4).

POST-TRANSLOCATIONAL PATHWAYS

The non-random removal of distinct membrane functions from a pluripotent primordial plasma membrane during evolution would generate a number of highly differentiated intracellular membranes that lack a translocator and that are physically not continuous (at least not permanently) with translocation-competent membranes. These translocation-incompetent membranes (or the subcompartments they enclose) therefore must receive their translocation-dependent, constitutive IMPs (or segregated proteins) from translocation-competent membranes (or subcompartments).

The most significant donor membrane (subcompartment) is the RER which probably supplies translocation-dependent proteins to essentially all orthoplasmic membranes and ectoplasmic subcompartments (Palade, 1975). Each of the receiving membranes presumably contains a set of IMPs that are permanent residents (either constitutive to a particular receiving membrane or shared by several other orthoplasmic membranes) and a set of proteins in transit (either on their way to their permanent residence or cycling between orthoplasmic membranes – e.g. carrier proteins, see below).

The information for post-translocational traffic could reside in one (or several) discrete segment(s) of the polypeptide chain. Proteins with an identical travel objective could share this information. These sequences, termed "sorting sequences", would therefore constitute another group of topogenic sequences. Sorting sequences may be required not only for proteins that leave the RER but also for those that need to be anchored there.

It is possible, however, that individual proteins may be able to reach their target without a sorting sequence(s). They could do this merely by association with another protein (piggybacking) that is endowed with a sorting sequence(s). Likewise, sorting sequences (as defined here) may not be needed for the non-random distribution of proteins within physically continuous membranes. Protein–protein interactions to form large ensembles with a decreased rate of diffusion in the plane of the membrane and possibly anchored by cytoskeletal elements could be responsible for the regional differences that are characteristic of continuous membranes.

Decoding of the information contained in the sorting sequences should be effected by specific proteins. For sorting sequences of bilateral IMPs, the effector may be represented by a few distinct peripheral membrane proteins. For sorting sequences of soluble proteins, such as lysosomal enzymes, the effector may be represented by a bilateral IMP that functions as a carrier protein shuttling back and forth between the donor and a receiver compartment. Its ectoplasmic domain may be able to bind reversibly to the sorting sequence(s) of lysosomal enzymes and its endoplasmic domain may contain a sorting sequence for a cyclic traffic pattern between the donor (RER) and receiver compartments (the latter could be represented by a distinct portion of the Golgi apparatus from which primary lysosomes develop; Novikoff, 1976). A defect in the carrier could result in secretion of all lysosomal enzymes.

The need for sorting arose from the use of only one translocator for topologically different proteins. The reverse – namely, the potential to use more than one translocator for topologically equivalent proteins – may have arisen when certain membranes (see Table I) acquired a post-translational translocator. For example, there could be two programs of topogenic sequences for peroxisomal proteins (Table II), both for the "content" proteins of the peroxisome and for those constitutive of the peroxisomal membrane (exemplified by bitopic IMPs). In reality, however, only one

TABLE II

Alternate-choice programs of topogenic sequences for topologically equivalent proteins

Abbreviations as in Table I; St, stop-transfer sequence; So, sorting sequence. Listed are programs only for bitopic IMPs and content proteins that are not integral membrane proteins. Alternate programs analogous to those shown for the peroxisomal membrane are theoretically possible also for the outer membrane of mitochondria and chloroplasts, whereby the "content" proteins would correspond to proteins that are located in the ectoplasmic compartment (intermembrane space) of mitochondria and chloroplasts (see Fig. 4). Likewise, a program analogous to that shown for the inner mitochondrial membrane is conceivable also for the inner membrane of chloroplasts. For the corresponding "content" proteins in the xenoplasmic compartment there most likely is no alternate program of topogenic sequences: proteins are synthesized either within the xenoplasmic compartment or imported via Si(MEN) or Si(CEN). The alternate programs for bitopic IMPs in the thylakoid membrane are similar to those in the inner chloroplast membrane, except that sorting sequences may be required for the program Si(CEN)-St to distinguish between those bitopic IMPs that remain in the inner membrane and those that continue (by invagination) to become residents of TKM. By the same token, one of the programs [Si(OCM)-So] for the corresponding "content" proteins in the intradisc space is based on the possibility that this space communicates transiently with the ectoplasmic space of chloroplasts. (From Blobel, 1980, with permission.)

Membrane	Bitopic IMPs	Content Proteins
Peroxisomal	Si(PXM)-St	Si(PXM)
	Si(RER)-St-So	Si(RER)-So
Inner mitochondrial	Si(IMM)-St	Si(MEN)
	Si(MEN)-St	
Thylakoid	Si(TKM)-St	Si(TKM)
	Si(CEN)-St-So	Si(OCM)-So

program for each group may exist, such as Si(PXM) for peroxisomal content proteins and Si(RER)-St-So for peroxisomal bitopic IMPs, with the alternate program either never developed or eliminated in evolution.

On the other hand, both programs indicated in Table II for the integration of bitopic IMPs into the inner mitochondrial membrane (or the inner membrane of chloroplasts) and into the thylakoid membrane, are likely to exist.

Finally, if topogenic sequences behaved in evolution like "transposable" elements one could conceive of "pleiotopic" proteins that are similar in structure and function but different in topology. Pleiotopic proteins could have arisen by the loss or acquisition of a topogenic sequence(s). Such processes may be important: (a) for achieving dichotomy in the post-translocational pathway of proteins (e.g. secretory and lysosomal proteins); or (b) for achieving either export or retention via binding to membranes (e.g. secreted or membrane-bound form of IgM heavy chains; Rogers et al., 1980); or (c) for diversifying the organellar distribution of proteins (e.g. some proteins that may occur both within peroxisomes and the mitochondrial matrix); or (d) for anchoring polymeric structures in the membrane (e.g. free and membrane-bound forms of cytoskeletal proteins).

REFERENCES

Blobel, G. (1979) Extralysosomal compartments for the turnover of intracellular macromolecules. In G.N. Cohen and H. Holzer (Eds.), *Limited Proteolysis in Microorganisms*, U.S. Department of Health, Education, and Welfare, p. 167.
Blobel, G. (1980) Intracellular protein topogenesis. *Proc. nat. Acad. Sci. U.S.A.*, 77: 1496.
Blobel, G. and Dobberstein, B. (1975a) Transfer of proteins across membranes. I. Presence of proteolytically processed and unprocessed nascent immunoglobulin light chains on membrane-bound ribosomes of murine myeloma. *J. Cell Biol.*, 67: 835.
Blobel, G. and Dobberstein, B. (1975b) Transfer of proteins across membranes. II. Reconstruction of functional rough microsomes from heterologous components. *J. Cell Biol.*, 67: 852.
Blobel, G. and Sabatini, D.D. (1970) Controlled proteolysis in rat liver cell fractions: I. Location of the polypeptides within ribosomes. *J. Cell Biol.*, 45: 130.
Blobel, G. and Sabatini, D. (1971) Ribosome-membrane interaction in eukaryotic cells. In L.A. Manson (Ed.), *Biomembranes* Vol. 2, Plenum Press, New York, p. 193.
Bonatti, S. and Blobel, G. (1979) Absence of a cleavable signal sequence in Sindbis virus glycoproteins PE_2. *J. biol. Chem.*, 254: 12261.
Bretscher, M.S. (1973) Membrane structure: some general principles. *Science*, 181: 622.
Chang, C.N., Blobel, G. and Model, P. (1978) Detection of prokaryotic signal peptidase in an *Escherichia coli* membrane fraction: endoproteolytic cleavage of nascent f_1 pre-coat protein. *Proc. nat. Acad. Sci. U.S.A.*, 75: 361.
Chang, C.N., Model, P. and Blobel, G. (1979) Membrane biogenesis: Cotranslational integration of the bacteriophage f_1 coat protein into an *Escherichia coli* membrane fraction. *Proc. nat. Acad. Sci. U.S.A.*, 76: 1251.
Chua, N.-H. and Schmidt, G.W. (1978) Post-translational transport into intact chloroplasts of a precursor to the small subunit of ribulose-1,5-bisphosphosphate carboxylase. *Proc. nat. Acad. Sci. U.S.A.*, 75: 6110.
Chua, N.-H., Blobel, G., Siekevitz, P. and Palade, G.E. (1973) Attachment of chloroplast polysomes to thylakoid membranes in *Chlamydomonas reinhardtii*. *Proc. nat. Acad. Sci. U.S.A.*, 70: 1554.
Devillers-Thiery, A., Kindt, T., Scheele, G. and Blobel, G. (1975) Homology in amino-terminal sequence of precursors to pancreatic secretory proteins. *Proc. nat. Acad. Sci. U.S.A.*, 72: 5016.
Di Rienzo, J.M., Nakamura, K. and Inouye, M. (1978) The outer membrane proteins of gram negative bacteria: biosynthesis, assembly and functions. *Ann. Rev. Biochem.*, 47: 481.
Dobberstein, B. and Blobel, G. (1977) Functional interaction of plant ribosomes with animal microscomal membranes. *Biochem. biophys. Res. Commun.*, 74: 1675.

Dobberstein, B., Blobel, G. and Chua, N.-H. (1977) In vitro synthesis and processing of a putative precursor for the small subunit of ribulose-1,5-bisphosphate carboxylase of *Chlamydomonas reinhardtii. Proc. nat. Acad. Sci. U.S.A.,* 74: 1082.

Emr, S.D., Hall, M.N. and Silhavy, T.J. (1980) A mechanism of protein localization: the signal hypothesis and bacteria. *J. Cell Biol.,* 86: 701.

Engelman, D.M. and Steitz, T.A. (1981) The spontaneous insertion of proteins into and across membranes: the helical hairpin hypothesis. *Cell,* 23: 411.

Garnier, J., Gaye, P., Mercier, J.C. and Robson, B. (1980) Structural properties of signal peptides and their membrane insertion. *Biochimie,* 62: 231.

Garoff, H., Frischauf, A.M., Simons, K., Lehrach, H. and Delius, H. (1980) Nucleotide sequence of cDNA coding for Semliki Forest virus membrane glycoproteins. *Nature (Lond.),* 288: 236.

Gething, M.J., White, J.M. and Waterfield, M.D. (1978) Purification of the fusion protein of Sindbis virus. Analysis of the NH_2-terminal sequence generated during precursor activation. *Proc. nat. Acad. Sci. U.S.A.,* 75: 2737.

Goldman, B.M. and Blobel, G. (1978) Biogenesis of peroxisomes: intracellular site of synthesis of catalase and uricase. *Proc. nat. Acad. Sci. U.S.A.,* 75: 5066.

Highfield, P.E. and Ellis, R.J. (1978) Synthesis and transport of the small subunit of chloroplast ribulose-bisphosphate carboxylase. *Nature (Lond.),* 271: 420.

Hortin, G. and Boime, I. (1980) Inhibition of preprotein processing in ascites tumor lysates by incorporation of a leucine analogue. *Proc. nat. Acad. Sci. U.S.A.,* 77: 1356.

Inouye, H. and Beckwith, J. (1977) Synthesis and processing of an *E. coli* alkaline phosphatase precursor in vitro. *Proc. nat. Acad. Sci. U.S.A.,* 74: 1440.

Inouye, S., Wang, S., Sekizawa, J., Halegoua, S. and Inouye, M. (1977) Amino acid sequence for the peptide extension on the prolipoprotein of the *Escherichia coli* outer membrane. *Proc. nat. Acad. Sci. U.S.A.,* 74: 1004.

Jackson, R.C. and Blobel, G. (1980) Post-translational processing of full-length presecretory proteins with canine signal peptidase. *Ann. N.Y. Acad. Sci.,* 343: 391.

Kagawa, Y. and Racker, E. (1971) Partial resolution of the enzymes catalyzing oxidative phosphorylation. *J. biol. Chem.,* 246: 5474.

Koshland, D. and Botstein, D. (1980) Secretion of beta-lactamase requires the carboxy end of the protein. *Cell,* 20: 749.

Kreibich, G., Ulrich, B.C. and Sabatini, D.D. (1978a) Proteins of rough microsomal membranes related to ribosome binding. I. Identification of ribophorins I and II, membrane proteins characteristic of rough microsomes. *J. Cell Biol.,* 77: 464.

Kreibich, G., Freienstein, C.M., Pereyra, P.N., Ulrich, B.C. and Sabatini, D.D. (1978b) Proteins of rough microsomal membranes related to ribosome binding. II. Crosslinking of bound ribosomes to specific membrane proteins exposed at the binding sites. *J. Cell Biol.,* 77: 488.

Kuriyama, R. and Luck, D. (1973) Membrane-associated ribosomes in mitochrondria of *Neurospora crassa. J. Cell Biol.,* 59: 776.

Lingappa, V.R., Katz, F.N., Lodish, H.F. and Blobel, G. (1978) A signal sequence for the insertion of a transmembrane glycoprotein. Similarities to the signals of secretory proteins in primary structure and function. *J. biol. Chem.,* 253: 8667.

Lingappa, V.R., Lingappa, J.R. and Blobel, G. (1979) Chicken ovalbumin contains an internal signal sequence. *Nature (Lond.),* 281: 117.

Maccecchini, M.L., Rudin, Y. Blobel, G. and Schatz, G. (1979a) Import of proteins into mitochrondria: precursor forms of the extramitochondrially made F_1-ATPase subunits in yeast. *Proc. nat. Acad. Sci. U.S.A.,* 76: 343.

Maccecchini, M.L., Rudin, Y. and Schatz, G. (1979b) Transport of proteins across the mitochondrial outer membrane. *J. biol. Chem.,* 254: 7468.

Malkin, L.I. and Rich, A. (1967) Partial resistance of nascent polypeptide chains to proteolytic digestion due to ribosomal shielding. *J. molec. Biol.,* 26: 329.

Margulis, L. (1970) *Origin of Eukaryotic Cells,* Yale Univ. Press, New Haven, Ct.

Meyer, D. and Dobberstein, B. (1980a) A membrane component esstential for vectorial translocation of nascent proteins across the endoplasmic reticulum: requirements for its extraction and reassociation with the membrane. *J. Cell Biol.,* 87: 498.

Meyer, D. and Dobberstein, B. (1980b) Identification and characterization of a membrane component essential for the translocation of nascent proteins across the membrane of the endoplasmic reticulum. *J. Cell Biol.,* 87: 503.

Milstein, C., Brownlee, G.G., Harrison, T.M. and Mathews, M.B. (1972) A possible precursor of immunoglobulin light chain. *Nature New Biol.*, 293: 117.

Moreno, F., Fowler, A.V., Hall, M. Silhavy, T.J., Zabin, I. and Schwartz, M. (1980) A signal sequence is not sufficient to lead beta-galactosidase out of the cytoplasm. *Nature (Lond.)*, 286: 356.

Novikoff, A.B. (1976) The endoplasmic reticulum: a cytochemist's view (a Review). *Proc. nat. Acad. Sci. U.S.A.*, 73: 2781.

Palade, G. (1975) Intracellular aspects of the process of protein secretion. *Science*, 189: 347.

Randall, L.L., Hardy, S.J.S. and Josefson, L.G. (1978) Precursors of three exported proteins in *Escherichia coli. Proc. nat. Acad. Sci. U.S.A.*, 75: 1209.

Redman, C.M. and Sabatini, D.D. (1966) Vectorial discharge of peptides released by puromycin from attached ribosomes. *Proc. nat. Acad. Sci. U.S.A.*, 56: 608.

Rogers, J., Early, P., Carter, C., Calame, K., Bond, M., Hood, L. and Wall, R. (1980) Two mRNAs with different 3′ ends encode membrane-bound and secreted forms of immunoglobulin μ chains. *Cell*, 20: 303.

Schechter, I., McKean, D.J., Guyer, R. and Terry, W. (1974) Partial amino acid sequence of the precursor of immunoglobulin light chain programmed by mRNA in vitro. *Science*, 188: 160.

Schechter, I., Burstein, Y., Zemell, R., Ziv, E., Kantor, F. and Papermaster, D.S. (1979) Messenger RNA of opsin from bovine retina: isolation and partial sequence of the in vitro translation product. *Proc. nat. Acad. Sci. U.S.A.*, 76: 2654.

Scheid, A., Graves, M.C., Silver, S.M. and Choppin, P.W. (1978) Studies on the structure and function of paramyxovirus glycoproteins. In B.W.J. Mahy and R.D. Barry (Eds.), *Negative Strand Viruses and the Host Cell*, Academic Press, London, p. 181.

Schmidt, G.W., Devillers-Thiery, A., Desruisseaux, H., Blobel, G. and Chua, N.-H. (1979) NH_2-terminal amino acid sequences of precursors and mature forms of the ribulose-1,5-bisphosphate carboxylase small subunit from *Chlamydomonas reinhardtii. J. Cell Biol.*, 83: 615.

Smith, W.P., Tai, P.C., Thompson, R.C. and Davis, B.D. (1977) Extracellular labeling of nascent polypeptides traversing the membrane of *Escherichia coli. Proc. nat. Acad. Sci. U.S.A.*, 74: 2830.

Steiner, D.F., Quinn, P.S., Chan, S.J., Marsh, J. and Tager, H.S. (1980) Processing mechanisms in the biosynthesis of proteins. *Ann. N.Y. Acad. Sci.*, 343: 1.

Swan, D., Aviv, H. and Leder, P. (1972) Purification and properties of biologically active messenger RNA for a myeloma light chain. *Proc. nat. Acad. Sci. U.S.A.*, 69: 1967.

Szczesna, E. and Boime, I. (1976) mRNA-dependent synthesis of authentic precursor to human placental lactogen: conversion to its mature hormone form in ascites cell-free extracts. *Proc. nat. Acad. Sci. U.S.A.*, 73: 1179.

Talmadge, K., Stahl, S. and Gilbert, W. (1980a) Eukaryotic signal sequence transports insulin antigen in *Escherichia coli. Proc. nat. Acad. Sci. U.S.A.*, 77: 3369.

Talmadge, K., Kaufman, J. and Gilbert, W. (1980b) Bacteria mature preproinsulin to proinsulin. *Proc. nat. Acad. Sci. U.S.A.*, 77: 3988.

Von Heijne, G. and Blomberg, C. (1979) Transmembrane translocation of protein. *Europ. J. Biochem.*, 97: 175.

Walter, P. and Blobel, G. (1980) Purification of a membrane-associated protein complex required for protein translocation across the endoplasmic reticulum. *Proc. nat. Acad. Sci. U.S.A.*, 77: 7112.

Walter, P. and Blobel, G. (1981a) Translocation of proteins across the endoplasmic reticulum. II. Signal Recognition Protein (SRP) mediates the selective binding to microsomal membranes of in vitro assembled polysomes synthesizing secretory protein. *J. Cell Biol.*, 91: 551.

Walter, P. and Blobel, G. (1981b) Translocation of proteins across the endoplasmic reticulum. III. Signal Recognition Protein (SRP) causes signal sequence-dependent and site-specific arrest of chain elongation that is released by microsomal membranes. *J. Cell Biol.*, 91: 557.

Walter, P., Jackson, R.C., Marcus, M.M., Lingappa, V.R. and Blobel, G. (1979) Tryptic dissection and reconstitution of translocation activity for nascent presecretory proteins across microsomal membranes. *Proc. nat. Acad. Sci. U.S.A.*, 76: 1795.

Walter, P., Ibrahimi, I. and Blobel, G. (1981) Translocation of proteins across the endoplasmic reticulum. I. Signal Recognition Protein (SRP) binds to in vitro assembled polysomes synthesizing secretory proteins. *J. Cell Biol.*, 91: 545.

Warren, G. and Dobberstein, B. (1978) Protein transfer across microsomal membranes reassembled from separated membrane components. *Nature (Lond.)*, 273: 569.

Wickner, W. (1979) Assembly of proteins into membranes: the membrane trigger hypothesis. *Ann. Rev. Biochem.*, 48: 23.

In Vitro Biosynthesis of the Subunits
of Acetylcholine Receptor

DAVID J. ANDERSON and GÜNTER BLOBEL

Laboratory of Cell Biology, The Rockefeller University, New York, NY 10021 (U.S.A.)

The acetylcholine receptor (AChR) of electric ray and eel is one of the few neurotransmitter receptors to be isolated and extensively characterized. Furthermore, it occupies a unique position in the catalogue of membrane proteins thus far purified, in that it is the only such protein which exhibits both a receptor and an ionophore activity. Located in the post-synaptic plasma membranes of *Torpedo* electric organ, the AChR is an oligomer of four non-identical subunits, of molecular weights 40,000 (α), 50,000 (β), 60,000 (γ) and 65,000 (δ), which appear to form a cation conductance channel in response to the neurotransmitter acetylcholine (for review, see Heidmann and Changeux, 1978.) The actual organization of these four polypeptides in the lipid bilayer, and their mechanism of functional interaction, however, are still unknown.

The biosynthetic pathway of this molecular complex is an important aspect of the formation and maintenance of neuromuscular junctions. It is, furthermore, a potential paradigm for the manner in which other multi-subunit integral membrane proteins are assembled and transported to the plasmalemma. The biosynthesis of AChRs has been studied primarily in skeletal muscle (Devreotes et al., 1977), where small quantities of material have thus far precluded the preparation of AChR subunit-specific antibodies. As a result, these studies have depended upon the use of the nicotinic antagonist α-bungarotoxin as a specific, irreversible label for the AChR complex. While the affinity of this reagent for mature AChRs is high, its interaction with the receptor probably depends upon quaternary protein associations which do not necessarily exist in the earliest stages of AChR synthesis.

We have approached the problem of biosynthesis of the biochemically well-defined *Torpedo* AChR, by using subunit-specific antibodies to directly examine the primary translation products of AChR mRNA in a cell-free system. When supplemented with rough microsomal vesicles, these in vitro systems have been shown for several representative examples to accurately reproduce the synthesis, glycosylation and asymmetric membrane insertion of single-subunit transmembrane glycoproteins (Katz et al., 1977.)

Previously, Mendez et al. (1980) reported that *Torpedo californica* electroplax mRNA directs the cell-free synthesis of a set of polypeptides immunologically related to AChR. Here we have extended their result to define the primary translation product for each individual subunit, and to demonstrate unequivocally that each polypeptide is the translation product of a separate mRNA. Furthermore, we have shown that in the microsome-supplemented system, the four subunits are independently integrated into the membrane in a co-translational manner (Blobel and Dobberstein, 1975), which results in a trans-bilayer orientation for each poly-peptide. Specific membrane-protected domains are obtained for each subunit after proteolysis with trypsin, and in the cases of the α and δ subunits, their molecular weights are compatible with those reported by Wennogle and Changeux (1980) for mature AChR in plasma membrane vesicles. However, in the in vitro system, the subunits are not associated with one another in the pentameric complex charac-teristic of mature "holoreceptor", and do not bind measureably to α-bungarotoxin. We have therefore apparently reconstructed a stage in the assembly of this multi-subunit membrane protein which is an intermediate, between the asymmetric insertion of the constituent polypeptides into the lipid bilayer, and their subsequent aggregation into a functional oligomeric complex.

To study the biosynthesis of a membrane protein in vitro, one needs an ap-propriate messenger RNA preparation that directs the synthesis of the protein, and an antibody with which to purify the translation products from the reaction mixtures by immunoprecipitation. In the case of the AChR, the electric organs of electric rays have long been known to contain copious quantities of nicotinic receptors, and were therefore apparently the tissue of choice for extracting AChR mRNA. Un-expectedly, this tissue in fact contains very small amounts of RNA. Apparently, the high steady-state levels of AChR in electric organ result from slow turnover of the protein. Despite the fact that the tissue yields only small amounts of mRNA, the receptor polypeptide mRNAs comprise a fairly substantial fraction of them, amounting to almost 2% of the total translation products (Table I). When translated in a wheat germ cell-free system, this mRNA directs the synthesis of a broad spectrum of polypeptides including those with molecular weights over 100,000 daltons, indicating that the RNA is largely intact (Fig. 1). Figure 2, lane 1 shows the

TABLE I

Quantitation of AChR subunit synthesis in vitro

For total cpm values, 25 μl translations were immunoprecipitated with the appropriate antiserum as described in the text. After elution of proteins from the immunoadsorbent (see Experimental Procedures section), TCA-precipitable radioactivity in the supernatant fluid was determined as described in the legend to Fig. 1. "Total Products" radioactivity was determined for a 5 μl aliquot of the translation before immunoprecipitation. Specific radioactivity = total cpm − background. "Background" is the "−mRNA" sample for Total Products, and the "Non-Immune" serum immunoprecipitate for the individual subunits. Relative Met content data are from Vandlen et al. (1979).

Sample	Total cpm per 25 μl	Specific cpm	% Total counts in subunit	Relative Met content	Relative % synthesis adjusted for # of Mets
Total products, −mRNA	176,930	−			
Total products, +mRNA	5,222,250	5,045,320			
α Immunoppt.	37,432	32,964	0.65	1.0	0.65
β Immunoppt.	18,132	13,664	0.27	0.7	0.38
γ Immunoppt.	18,020	13,552	0.27	0.7	0.38
δ Immunoppt.	30,620	26,152	0.52	1.0	0.52
Non-Immune	4,468	−			
					Total: 1.93%

[RNA], A$_{260}$/ml: 0   1   2   4   5   6   12   18

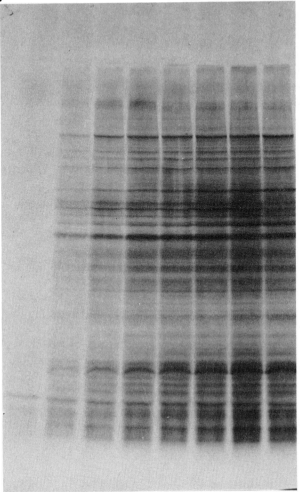

Fig. 1. Analysis of the total translation products of *Torpedo* mRNA by SDS polyacrylamide gel electrophoresis. Total cellular RNA was extracted from frozen electroplax tissue using SDS/phenol/proteinase K. The first precipitation of nucleic acids was performed by adding NaCl to 0.18 M and then 0.6 volumes of isopropanol, followed by an overnight incubation at $-20\,°C$. Prior to this step, the aqueous phase from the phenol extractions were freed of contaminating glycogen by centrifugation at 100,000 *g* for 30 min. Total cellular RNA (separated from contaminating DNA by LiCl precipitation) was translated in a wheat germ cell-free system at the final concentrations indicated. After incubation at 29 °C for 90 min, 10 μl of reaction mixture were diluted with SDS sample buffer and subjected to electrophoresis in 0.1% SDS on a 10–15% linear gradient polyacrylamide gel. Shown is an autoradiograph of the dried gel.

electrophoretic profile of an AChR preparation purified by affinity chromatography on cobratoxin-Sepharose (Froehner and Rafto, 1979). The subunits were separated by preparative electrophoresis in SDS, and eluted as individual polypeptides. The homogeneity of these preparations is shown in lanes 2–5. Using methods established by Jon Lindstrom and his co-workers (1978), these subunits were injected into rats

98

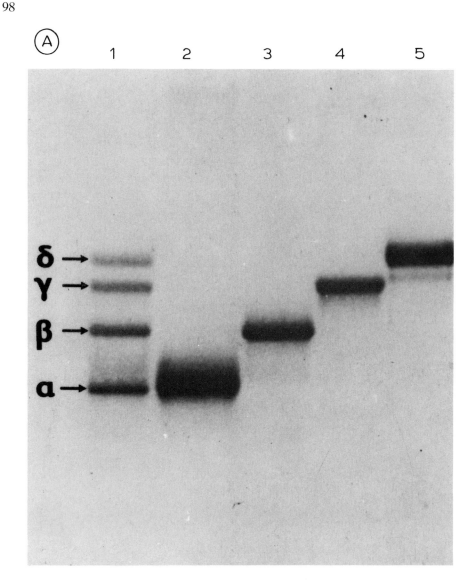

Fig. 2. Purification of *Torpedo* AChR subunits. Shown is a linear gradient 7.5–15% SDS polyacrylamide gel electrophoretogram. Protein was visualized by Coomassie blue staining. Lane 1, AChR eluted from a cobratoxin-Sepharose affinity column. α, β, γ and δ indicate the 40, 50, 60 and 65 kdalton subunits, respectively. Lanes 2–5, the α, β, γ and δ subunits re-run in the same gel system after preparative electrophoresis in SDS. Note the absence of significant cross-contamination in the subunit preparations. (After Anderson and Blobel, 1981, with permission.)

and antisera were produced against each of the subunits. The specificities of these reagents for particular subunits are shown in Fig. 3.

To characterize these antisera, receptor protein was purified and iodinated under non-denaturing conditions. This material is shown in the lane marked "AChR." The subunits were dissociated with SDS and different antisera were tested for their ability to immunoprecipitate these polypeptides.

It is clear that each serum reacts primarily with the subunit to which it was

AChR Triton Immpts.   SDS Immppts

1   2   3   4   5 | 1   2   3   4   5

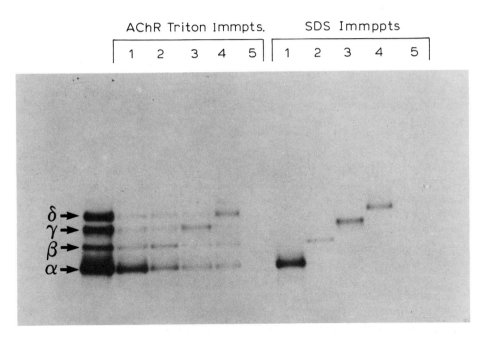

Fig. 3. Characterization of subunit specificities of anti-AChR antisera. AChR purified under non-denaturing conditions (10 ml Tris-HCl, pH 7.4, 0.01% sodium cholate) was radioiodinated using the Iodogen reagent (New England Nuclear, Inc.). "SDS Immppts", parallel samples of [^{125}I]AChR were heated to 100 °C in 1% SDS, 10 mM dithiothreitol (DTT) for 3 min, and then diluted with 4 volumes of buffer containing 1.25% Triton X-100, prior to addition of antisera. "Triton Immppts", samples were diluted with Triton X-100 containing buffer without prior solubilization in SDS. After an overnight incubation with the antibody, immunoprecipitates were adsorbed to protein A-Sepharose, washed and subjected to electrophoresis in the same system described for Fig. 2. Shown is an autoradiograph of the dried gel. Antisera used were: lanes 1–4, anti-α, -β, -γ and -δ, respectively; lane 5, non-immune serum. Lane "AChR" shows the radioiodinated purified receptor. (From Anderson and Blobel, 1981, with permission.)

originally raised ("SDS Immppts.", lanes 1–5). Interestingly, if this same assay is performed using AChR not dissociated in SDS, each serum precipitates all four subunits ("Triton Immppts"). This result reflects the association of the subunits in the oligomeric complex. Hence this latter assay provides an easy way to determine whether multisubunit assembly has occurred in vitro.

Having prepared and characterized these reagents, they were used to isolate the primary translation products corresponding to each of the four AChR subunits. Messenger RNA from the electric organ was translated in a wheat germ cell-free protein synthesizing system in the absence of rough microsomal membranes. Translation products were denatured in SDS, immunoprecipitated with the subunit-specific sera and displayed by electrophoresis on polyacrylamide gels. Figure 4 shows the results obtained for the γ and δ subunits.

The results of this experiment are shown in lanes 2 of both panels. There is a separate band for each of the two subunits, and in both cases the primary translation product is smaller in molecular weight than its mature counterpart. This is to be expected, since all of the AChR subunits are known to be glycosylated (Vandlen et al., 1979), and the primary translation products do not contain carbohydrate. The identity of these translation products was confirmed by the ability of the corresponding unlabeled in vivo-synthesized subunits to compete out the immunoprecipitation of their in vitro-synthesized counterparts (lanes 7). The molecular weights of the primary translation products obtained for the four chains correlate well with those published by Baxter and co-workers (Mendez et al., 1980) using a reticulocyte lysate system and an antiserum that reacted with all four subunits. The primary translation products for the α and β subunits are shown in lanes 2 of Fig. 5. Interestingly, the product corresponding to the β chain co-migrates with its authentic counterpart in this gel system. The reasons for this will be discussed subsequently. As mentioned earlier, one reason for carrying out this study was to determine whether there is a separate mRNA for each subunit, or whether all are derived from a common polyprotein precursor. Such polyproteins are in fact synthesized in the case of viral membrane glycoproteins. The fact that we observed distinct translation products corresponding to each subunit, rather than a common 250,000 dalton species, strongly argues against a polyprotein precursor. However, because cell-free systems contain proteases which might rapidly cleave such a precursor, rigorous evidence was provided with the use of radioactive [^{35}S]formylated methionyl (fMet) tRNA to label the primary translation product (Mihara and Blobel, 1980).

The basis for the experiment is the fact that the first amino acid of a protein sequence, the translation initiation site, and only that site, codes for fMet in eukaryotic mRNAs. A polyprotein precursor would yield, therefore, only one subunit labeled by the initiator methionine. The fact that all four subunits were labeled under these conditions shows that there is a separate mRNA for each chain (Anderson and Blobel, 1981.)

Given this analysis of the primary translation products, the next step was to examine the forms of the subunits that were synthesized when the translation system was supplemented with dog pancreas rough microsomal membranes. (Microsomes from this source are widely used because they function in a variety of cell-free systems without inhibiting protein synthesis (Shields and Blobel, 1978). Microsomal membranes from other tissues such as hen oviduct (Thibodeau and Walsh, 1980), bovine adrenal medulla (Boime et al., 1976) and Ehrlich ascites cells (Szczesna and Boime, 1976) have also been shown to effect proper processing of nascent presecretory proteins synthesized in vitro.)

The results of this experiment are shown for the γ and δ chains in lanes 3 of Fig. 4. A new major form of each chain which, in this gel system, migrates close to the position of the corresponding authentic subunit, is obtained under these conditions. Some minor intermediate species are also seen. All of these new forms can be competed out of the immunoprecipitation by adding an excess of the corresponding unlabeled authentic subunit (lanes 8), indicating that they are immunologically indistinguishable from material synthesized in the absence of membranes (lane 2).

The increase in molecular weight upon addition of microsomal membranes suggests that core glycosylation of the newly synthesized subunits may be occurring in this system. That this is indeed the case will be shown shortly. First, however, we shall describe experiments designed to determine the transmembrane orientation of these AChR subunits synthesized in vitro.

In the case of mature AChR in *Torpedo* plasma membrane vesicles, Wennogle and Changeux (1980) showed that the α and δ subunits are insensitive to proteolytic attack at the extracytoplasmic surface of the membrane, but are readily cleaved once

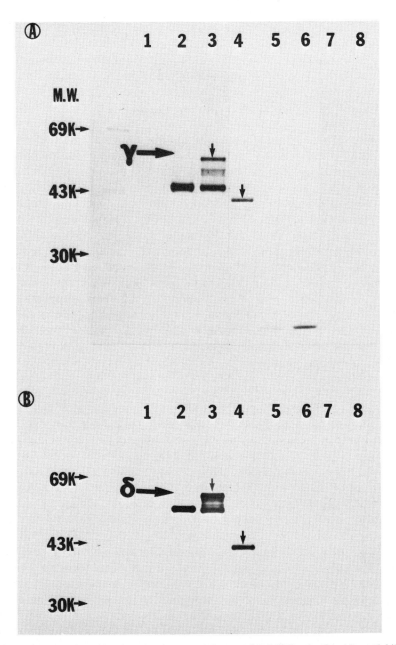

Fig. 4. In vitro synthesis and membrane integration of the γ and δ AChR subunits. After solubilization in 1% SDS and dilution with buffer containing a 5-fold excess of Triton X-100, translation were immunoprecipitated with either anti-γ (panel A) or anti-δ (panel B) antisera. Shown is a fluorograph of a 7.5–15% SDS polyacrylamide gel. M.W., molecular weight markers in kdaltons. Lane 1, purified unlabeled γ subunit (A) or δ subunit (B) was run on the same gel and its position marked by aligning the autoradiographic film with the original gel. Lanes 2–8 contain in vitro translation products labeled with [35S]methionine. Translations were carried out in either the absence (lanes 2, 6, 7) or presence (lanes 3, 4, 5, 8) of 2 A_{280}/ml rough microsomes, and after translation was complete the samples in lanes 2, 6 and 7 received 2 A_{280}/ml of microsomes, and were further incubated for 90 min at 26 °C. In lanes 4, 5 and 6, samples were immunoprecipitated after proteolysis with 300 μg/ml trypsin at 20 °C for 30 min. In lane 5 the trypsinization was performed in the presence of 0.1% Nikkol, a non-ionic detergent. In lanes 7 and 8, immunoprecipitation was performed in the presence of an excess of unlabeled, competing γ(A) or δ(B) subunit. Samples were reduced with 100 mM dithiothreitol (DTT) and alkylated with 500 mM iodoacetamide prior to electrophoresis. (From Anderson and Blobel, 1981, with permission.)

the vesicles are disrupted by sonication or alkaline extraction. This result suggested that both of these subunits had protease-sensitive sites at the cytoplasmic surface of the membrane. No evidence was available for the other two chains, however. The cell-free system used in the present study has the advantage that the rough microsomal membranes containing in vitro-synthesized AChR subunits are topologically inside-out with respect to AChR-rich *Torpedo* vesicles.

The results of this experiment are shown in lane 4 of Fig. 4. Treatment with high concentrations of trypsin caused both γ and δ to be reduced to a smaller fragment. In the case of the δ subunit, this fragment is almost 20 kdalton smaller than the uncleaved polypeptide. In contrast, lanes 6 show that the precursor synthesized in the absence of membranes is completely degraded by this procedure or is reduced to very small fragments. Thus the bands in lane 4 are not due to intrinsic insensitivity of the protein to proteolysis. Finally, if the trypsinization was performed on material synthesized with membranes, but with non-ionic detergent present to disrupt the lipid bilayer, the subunits are again completely degraded, as seen in lane 5. This result shows that the incomplete degradation of subunits in the presence of microsomes is due to protection of part of the chain by the protease-impermeable lipid bilayer. Thus, some part of each subunit has been translocated across or integrated into the membrane. However, the fact that substantial portions of each chain can be cleaved off by this procedure indicates that in fact all four subunits have regions exposed on the cytoplasmic surface of the membrane.

To demonstrate core-glycosylation of the membrane-integrated forms of the AChR subunits, we performed an affinity chromatography of the in vitro translation products using concanavalin A (Con A)-Sepharose. The principle of the fractionation is that glycosylated polypeptides containing the mannose-rich core oligosaccharide will bind to the lectin-agarose, whereas non-glycosylated material is not retained. A representative result is shown for the δ subunit in Fig. 6.

The 60 kdalton "precursor" to δ synthesized in the absence of membranes is not glycosylated, and appears in the fraction not retained by the Con A (group A, lane 3). In contrast, material synthesized in the presence of microsomes (group B, lane 1) can be fractionated into a 65 kdalton form of δ which is adsorbed by the lectin (lane 2), and residual unprocessed "pre-δ" which is not retained (lane 3). To prove that the binding of the 65 kdalton form to the Con A was due to the presence of a specific carbohydrate on the protein, we demonstrated that this binding could be abolished by adding excess α-methylmannoside as a "competitive inhibitor" of the lectin–glycoprotein interaction. In this case, none of the species was adsorbed (lane 4) and all appeared in the flow-through fraction (lane 5).

Additionally, it was shown that the glycosylated residues of δ are contained in that part of the protein which is protected by the membrane from exogenously added protease. Thus, the 44 kdalton trypsin-resistant fragment of δ (group C, lane 1, arrow), when subjected to fractionation on Con A-Sepharose, was specifically adsorbed to the lectin (lane 2, arrow), indicating the presence of mannose residues. The presence of core oligosaccharide on the membrane-integrated forms of the AChR subunits has recently been confirmed by an independent method, using the enzyme endo-β-N-acetylglucosaminidase-H (endo H).

In the cases of the α and β subunits, translation in the presence of rough microsomes yielded more *rapidly* migrating forms of these chains (Fig. 5, lanes 3, upward arrows). The results of Endo H digestion experiments suggest that these are

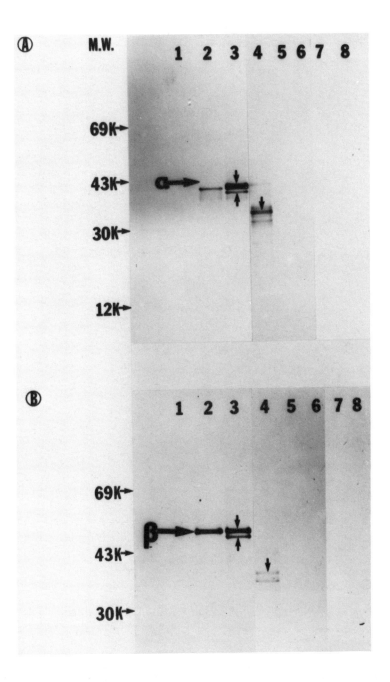

Fig. 5. In vitro synthesis, and membrane integration of the α and β subunits of AChR. Panel A: anti-α antiserum was used for immunoprecipitation. Panel B: anti-β antiserum. The legend is the same as that described for Fig. 4, except that samples were not alkylated prior to electrophoresis, and the α sample was not heated but rather solubilized at room temperature.

104

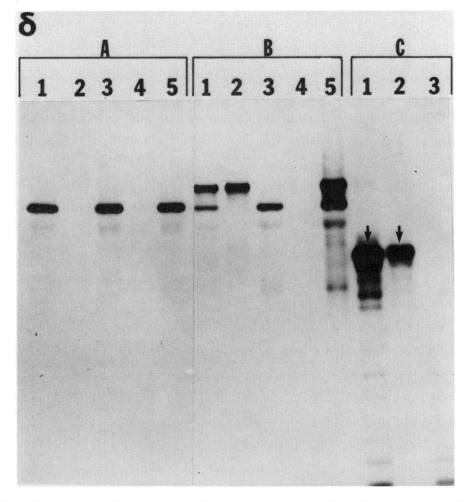

Fig. 6. Demonstration of in vitro glycosylation of the δ subunit by affinity chromatography on Con A-Sepharose. Group A, products synthesized without membranes; groups B and C, products synthesized with membranes. For group C the products were trypsinized immediately after translation (sse Fig. 4, lane 4). Lanes 1, an aliquot immunoprecipitated without further fractionation. Lanes 2, material which was adsorbed to the Con A-Sepharose. Lanes 3, material not retained by the lectin. Groups A and B, lanes 4 and 5 are as lanes 2 and 3 but incubation with the Con A-Sepharose was in the presence of 0.4 M α-methylmannoside. Samples were eluted from the Con A by boiling in 1% SDS, and immunoprecipitated with anti-δ antiserum. The lower bands in lane C1 are contaminants which do not appear in lanes C2 or 3 due to loss of material incurred during the affinity chromatography procedure.
(From Anderson and Blobel, 1981, with permission.)

the signal sequence-cleaved, non-glycosylated forms of these subunits (data not shown.) In the case of the α subunit, there is also a more slowly-migrating glycosylated form (Fig. 5A, lane 3, downward arrow), but in the case of the β subunit, this form co-migrates with the precursor (Fig. 5B, lane 3, downward arrow.) However, this glycosylated form of β can be resolved from the precursor by affinity chromatography on Con A-Sepharose (data not shown.) The α and β subunits also exhibit trypsin-resistant, glycosylated domains protected by the membrane from proteolysis (Fig. 5, lanes 4, downward arrows.) However, minor bands are also seen, which probably arise from the population of molecules which have been integrated into the membrane and had their signal sequences removed, but which have not been glycosylated. In the case of the β chain, this form appears in equal proportion to the glycosylated fragment (lane 4.)

Figure 7 depicts some of the possible topological orientations of the AChR subunits in the membrane. The simplest one, on the left, shows the chain spanning the membrane only once. This is consistent with the fact that the subunits exhibit a single protease-resistant domain which is glycosylated. It is also in keeping with the precedent established for VSV G (Katz et al., 1977) and the HLA antigens (Ploegh et al., 1979). However, the present study is limited by the necessity of im-munoprecipitation, and it is possible that there are some additional membrane-integrated and protease-protected segments that do not react with the antibody used. The more complex orientation implied by this possibility is suggested in the middle diagram. Finally, although by analogy to VSV G one might expect that the amino terminus of the polypeptide is on the inside of the vesicle, one can equally envision the orientation shown in the diagram on the right. Sequencing studies are currently being performed to investigate this issue.

As previously discussed, mature AChR is a pentameric complex of composition $\alpha_2\beta\gamma\delta$ which binds the cholinergic antagonist α-bungarotoxin with extremely high affinity ($K_d = 10^{-11}$ M). When the in vitro-synthesized, membrane-integrated AChR subunits were assayed for toxin binding and oligomeric assembly by several in-dependent methods, neither property could be demonstrated (data not shown.) Trivial explanations for these negative results have been ruled out. Thus, the cell-free system does not contain an inhibitor of α-bungarotoxin binding, since exogenously added mature AChR binds the ligand in a normal manner after incubation in a mock translation. For what reasons might oligomeric assembly and functional maturation not occur in vitro?

If the mechanism of assembly is simply lateral diffusion of the subunits and aggregation in the plane of the membrane, it is unlikely that such an assembly would occur with this system. In the cell, the rough endoplasmic reticulum is an extensive reticulum of membrane sheets. What is added to the cell-free system is a suspension of membranous vesicles, obtained from homogenized tissue. Since electron micro-scopy reveals that each vesicle can accommodate between 4 and 10 polysomes, given that each AChR subunit comprises 0.5% of total protein synthesis – and assuming this

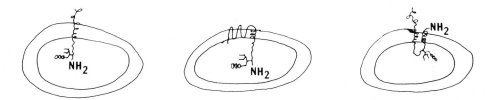

Fig. 7. Possible transmembrane orientations of the δ subunit in the rough endoplasmic reticulum membrane. The inside of the vesicles is topologically equivalent to the outside of the cell. "NH$_2$" indicates the amino terminus of the polypeptide chain. The branched structure represents a core oligosaccharide group, but does not imply that there is only one of these groups per chain, nor that its position in the protein is precisely as indicated.

reflects mRNA abundance – it can be calculated that the probability of getting one polysome for each of the four subunits on a single vesicle is, on the average, about 1 in a million. Another possible reason for the lack of functional assembly of AChR in this system is that under these conditions only those events that normally occur in the rough endoplasmic reticulum are reconstructed, whereas the AChR may require transport to another intracellular organelle, such as the Golgi apparatus, before the toxin binding-site can form.

REFERENCES

Anderson, D.J. and Blobel, G. (1981) In vitro synthesis, glycosylation, and membrane insertion of the four subunits of *Torpedo* acetylcholine receptor. *Proc. natl. Acad. Sci. U.S.A.*, 78: 5598–5602.

Blobel, G. and Dobberstein, B. (1975) Transfer of proteins across membranes. II. Reconstitution of functional rough microsomes from heterologous components. *J. Cell Biol.*, 67: 835–851.

Boime, I., Bielinska, M., Rogers, G. and Ruckinsky, T. (1980) In vitro processing of placental peptide hormones by smooth microsomes. *Ann. N.Y. Acad Sci.*, 343: 69–78.

Devreotes, P.N., Gardner, J.M. and Fambrough, D.M. (1977) Kinetics of biosynthesis of acetylcholine receptor and subsequent incorporation into plasma membranes of cultured chick skeletal muscle. *Cell*, 10: 365–373.

Froehner, S.C. and Rafto, S. (1979) Comparison of the subunits of *Torpedo californica* acetylcholine receptor by peptide mapping. *Biochemistry*, 18: 301–307.

Heidmann, T. and Changeux, J.-P. (1978) Structural and functional properties of the acetylcholine receptor protein in its purified and membrane-bound states. *Ann. Rev. Biochem.*, 47: 317–357.

Katz, F.M., Rothman, J.E., Lingappa, V.R., Blobel, G. and Lodish, H.F. (1977) Membrane assembly in vitro: synthesis, glycosylation and asymmetric insertion of a transmembrane protein. *Proc. nat. Acad. Sci. U.S.A.*, 74: 3278–3282.

Lindstrom, J., Einarson, B. and Merlie, J. (1978) Immunization of rats with polypeptide chains from *Torpedo* acetylcholine receptors causes an autoimmune response to receptors in rat muscle. *Proc. nat. Acad. Sci. U.S.A.*, 75: 769–773.

Mendez, B., Valenzuela, P., Martial, J.A. and Baxter, J.D. (1980) Cell-free synthesis of acetylcholine receptor polypeptides. *Science*, 209: 695–697.

Mihara, K. and Blobel, G. (1980) The four cytoplasmically made subunits of yeast mitochondrial cytochrome c oxidase are synthesized individually and not as a polyprotein. *Proc. nat. Acad. Sci. U.S.A.*, 77: 4160–4164.

Ploegh, H.L., Cannon, L.E. and Strominger, J.L. (1979) Cell-free translation of the mRNAs for the heavy and light chains of HLA-A and HLA-B antigens. *Proc. nat. Acad. Sci. U.S.A.*, 76: 2273–2277.

Shields, D. and Blobel, G. (1978) Efficient cleavage and segregation of nascent presecretory proteins in a reticulocyte lysate supplemented with microsomal membranes. *J. biol. Chem.*, 253: 3753–3756.

Sobel, A., Weber, M. and Changeux, J.-P. (1977) Large scale purification of the acetylcholine receptor protein in its membrane-bound and detergent extracted forms from *Torpedo marmorata* electric organ. *Europ. J. Biochem.*, 80: 215–224.

Szczesna, E. and Boime, I. (1976) mRNA dependent synthesis of authentic precursor to human placental lactogen: conversion to its mature form in ascites cell-free extracts. *Proc. nat. Acad. Sci. U.S.A.*, 73: 1179–1183.

Thibodeau, S.N. and Walsh, K.A. (1980) Processing of precursor proteins by preparations of oviduct microsomes. *Ann N.Y. Acad. Sci.*, 343: 180–191.

Vandlen, F.L., Wu, W.C.-S., Eisenach, J.C. and Raftery, M.A. (1979) Studies of the composition of purified *Torpedo californica* acetylcholine receptor and of its subunits. *Biochemistry*, 18: 1845–1854.

Wennogle, L.P. and Changeux, J.-P. (1980) Transmembrane orientation of proteins present in acetylcholine receptor-rich membranes from *Torpedo marmorata* studied by selective proteolysis. *Europ. J. Biochem.*, 106: 381–393.

Biosynthesis of Acetylcholinesterase in Rat Brain and *Torpedo* Electric Organ is Directed by Scarce mRNA Species

HERMONA SOREQ, RUTI PARVARI and ISRAEL SILMAN

Department of Neurobiology, The Weizmann Institute of Science, Rehovot (Israel)

INTRODUCTION

The principal role of acetylcholinesterase (AChE) is believed to be termination of impulse transmission by hydrolysis of the neurotransmitter acetylcholine, and development of cholinergic synapses is indeed accompanied by accumulation of this enzyme. The biosynthesis of AChE is of interest for a number of reasons: it is a synaptic enzyme whose regulation and assembly may involve both pre- and post-synaptic control (see, for example, Koenig and Vigny, 1978; Silman et al., 1979; Lømo and Slater, 1980; Rubin et al., 1980), and it exists in multiple molecular forms differing in their localization, mode of association with the surface membrane, regulation and, presumably, physiological functions (see, for example, Hall, 1973; Silman et al., 1979; Massoulié, 1980; Jedrzejczyk et al., 1981). Moreover, it may be expected that certain of these molecular forms may undergo novel modes of post-translational processing and modification in the course of their integration into the functional synapse.

A number of groups have studied the appearance and regulation of AChE in cultures of nerve and muscle. Thus it has been shown that after irreversible inhibition of existing enzyme with organophosphate anticholinesterase agents, protein synthesis inhibitors arrest reappearance of activity, providing proof that de novo synthesis is involved (Lanks et al., 1974; Walker and Wilson, 1976; Rieger et al., 1976; Rotundo and Fambrough, 1980).

Meedel and Whittaker (1979) have shown that increases in AChE activity during the early stages of embryogenesis of the ascidian, *Ciona intestinalis*, are inhibited by actinomycin D, and have suggested a possible role for mRNA production in the ontogeny of this enzyme.

In vitro studies of AChE biosynthesis as directed by mRNA are difficult to carry out, since the enzyme comprises only a minor fraction of the total tissue protein. The high turnover number of the enzyme (Vigny et al., 1978), however, permits the detection of minute amounts of active AChE (Johnson and Russell, 1975). This raised the possibility that a bioassay could be developed for the production of active AChE as directed by mRNA. Since in vitro systems are of limited duration, and deficient in their ability to perform post-translational processing and to produce biologically active products (Blobel and Dobberstein, 1975), we chose to develop such a bioassay in microinjected *Xenopus* oocytes.

[107]

The *Xenopus* oocyte system (Gurdon et al., 1971) offers an attractive experimental approach to this issue for a number of reasons: it has been extensively used as a translation system for a variety of microinjected mRNAs, correctly performing translation (Gurdon et al., 1971), processing (Ghysdael et al., 1977) and various post-translational modifications (Lane and Knowland, 1975); in the case of mRNAs directing synthesis of secretory proteins, *Xenopus* oocytes secrete the correct translational products (Colman and Morser, 1979; Soreq et al., 1981; Mohun et al., 1981), and finally, in a number of cases, the injected mRNAs have been translated into biologically active products (Labarca and Paigen, 1977; Shulman and Revel, 1980; Soreq et al., 1981; Miskin and Soreq, 1981).

In the following we demonstrate that *Xenopus* oocytes synthesize and secrete catalytically active AChE upon microinjection with poly(A)-containing RNA prepared from whole rat brain, from dissected rat cerebellum and from *Torpedo* electric organ. We further define the stability and efficacy of the injected AChE-mRNA and, on the basis of the amounts of mRNA injected and AChE secreted, present calculations demonstrating that AChE-mRNA is a scarce mRNA species in both rat brain and *Torpedo* electric organ.

METHODS

mRNA was prepared from whole brain or cerebellum of 10-day-old Sprague–Dawley rats and from electric organ of *Torpedo ocellata*, as described elsewhere (Soreq et al., 1982). Microinjection into stage 6 selected single oocytes of *Xenopus laevis* frogs was as described previously (Soreq et al., 1981). Cholinesterase activity in rat brain homogenates was determined according to Ellman et al. (1961). All other cholinesterase determinations were carried out by the radiometric method of Johnson and Russell (1975).

RESULTS AND DISCUSSION

Rodent brain AChE-mRNA

When injected with poly(A)-containing mRNA from rat cerebellum (Soreq et al., 1982), *Xenopus* oocytes secrete into their incubation medium cholinesterase activity. The rate of degradation reaches the level of about 0.75 nmol per oocyte per h, whereas the cholinesterase secreted from control injected oocytes degrades acetylcholine (ACh) at a maximal rate of about 0.15 nmol per oocyte per h (Fig. 1).

The newly synthesized cholinesterase activity secreted by the oocytes appears to display the specificity of acetylcholinesterase (acetylcholine hydrolase, EC 3.1.1.7 AChE). Thus, >98% of the newly synthesized cholinesterase activity in the medium of mRNA-injected oocytes is inhibited by 10^{-4} M BW 284C51, a specific inhibitor of AChE (Austin and Berry, 1953). In contrast, the newly synthesized activity is not decreased in the presence of 10^{-4} M tetraisopropylpyrophosphoramide (iso-OMPA), a specific inhibitor of pseudocholinesterase (acylcholine hydrolase, EC 3.1.1.8; Austin and Berry, 1953). The endogenous oocyte enzyme may consist of two components, since it is completely inhibited by BW 284C51 and about 50% inhibited

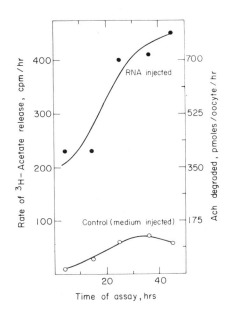

Fig. 1. Rate of ACh degradation by medium of microinjected oocytes. Oocytes were microinjected as described in the Experimental section with 200 ng cerebellar mRNA each, and incubated in Barth medium for 20 h. Cholinesterase activity was determined in duplicate samples of medium. Samples were incubated with [³H]ACh for different periods. The rate of ACh degradation was calculated for medium of mRNA-injected oocytes (●) and for control oocytes (○). Background degradation of ACh was subtracted.

by 10^{-4} M iso-OMPA. The observation that the newly synthesized enzyme is wholly BW 284C51-sensitive and insensitive to iso-OMPA, is compatible with the fact that AChE seems to be the predominant ACh-hydrolyzing enzyme in rat brain (Vijayan and Brownson, 1974). Thus, under our assay conditions, hydrolysis of ACh by extracts of whole rat brain is inhibited more than 90% by 10^{-4} M BW 284C51 and less than 10% by 10^{-4} M iso-OMPA. Moreover, we find that these extracts hydrolyze butyrylthiocholine at less than 10% of the rate at which they hydrolyze acetylthiocholine.

The newly synthesized cholinesterase, as well as the endogenous oocyte activity, is mostly secreted into the incubation medium (Fig. 2). The ratio of secreted to intracellular cholinesterase remained apparently unchanged throughout prolonged incubation of the oocytes (not shown).

Various studies on ganglia (Gisiger and Vigny, 1977) and on neuronal cells in culture (Kimhi et al., 1980) have shown that much of the AChE produced is secreted into the external medium. Our findings are, therefore, in line with earlier observations showing that *Xenopus* oocytes accumulate in vesicles (Mohun et al., 1981) and secrete into the medium exclusively secretory products, such as interferon (Soreq et al., 1981), milk proteins (Colman and Morser, 1979) and plasminogen activator (Miskin and Soreq, 1981), but not non-secretory proteins such as histones or globin (Colman and Morser, 1979). In the systems mentioned above, much of the AChE secreted is detected on sucrose gradients as oligomeric species (Gisiger and Vigny, 1977; Kimhi et al., 1980). Preliminary experiments suggest that the AChE secreted by oocytes microinjected with rat brain mRNA is also primarily in an

110

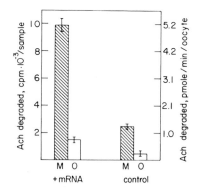

Fig. 2. Ratio of secreted to intracellular cholinesterase activity in oocytes microinjected with cerebellar mRNA. Oocytes were injected with 50 ng of rat cerebellum mRNA. Control oocytes were injected with Barth medium. Incubation was for 20 h. Cholinesterase activity was determined in triplicate in samples of oocyte homogenate (empty bars) or incubation medium (hatched bars) of microinjected oocytes. Mean values ±S.D. are presented.

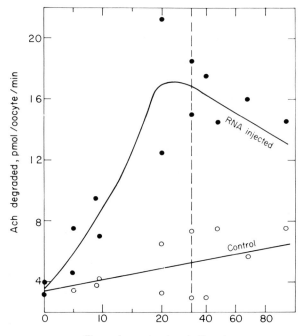

Fig. 3. Time dependence of cholinesterase secretion from microinjected oocytes. Oocytes were microinjected with rat brain mRNA as described in the Experimental section. At the times indicated on the abscissa, incubation medium was removed from the microinjected oocytes and assayed (24 h) for cholinesterase activity. Assays were carried out in triplicate. Pooled results of two experiments, performed with oocytes from different frogs, are presented. Background degradation of ACh was 3.0 and 4.3 pmol/min per sample for the two experiments. ●, Activity in medium of mRNA-injected oocytes; ○, activity in medium of control oocytes.

oligomeric form (Soreq et al., unpublished observations). It should be emphasized that different levels of newly synthesized and endogenous AChE were observed in the incubation medium of oocytes from different frogs. This variability between experiments might partially be explained by the heterogeneity in the proteolytic activities secreted by oocytes from different frogs (Soreq and Miskin, 1981).

The mRNA-induced AChE activity could clearly be detected as early as 5 h post-injection, similarly to the early appearance of interferon (Soreq et al., 1981) and plasminogen activator (Miskin and Soreq, 1981) in the medium of microinjected oocytes. AChE accumulates in the incubation medium of microinjected oocytes for over 20 h, and then decreases (Fig. 3). An average half-life of 10 ± 3 h (mean $\pm$ S.D.) for the AChE-mRNA could be calculated from 4 different experiments, and appears to be similar to the average in vivo half-life of polyadenylated mRNAs of mammalian origin (Littauer and Soreq, 1982).

Based on the observation that maximal levels of cholinesterase activity are detected in the oocyte incubation medium 20 h post-injection, increasing amounts of cerebellar mRNA were injected into oocytes and the amount of cholinesterase activity accumulating in the medium during this period was measured, in order to determine the range in which the level of newly synthesized cholinesterase corresponds linearly to the amount of microinjected mRNA. The mRNA-directed cholinesterase activity observed in the medium of oocytes microinjected with as little as 12.5 ng of non-fractionated poly(A)-containing mRNA per oocyte amounts to 6 pmol/oocyte/min. The level of induced enzyme increases with increasing amounts of poly(A)-containing mRNA, and 50 ng of mRNA appeared to saturate the capacity of the oocyte to synthesize AChE, at a level of about 12 pmol/oocyte/min. The limited capacity of the oocytes to express microinjected mRNA is in agreement with previous reports (Laskey et al., 1977). The level of excreted activity in the medium of oocytes injected with up to 50 ng of non-fractionated mRNA reflects, therefore, the abundance of AChE-mRNA in the injected mRNA population.

Torpedo electric organ AChE-mRNA

The production and excretion of AChE in oocytes has also been examined with mRNA prepared from the AChE-enriched electric organ of *Torpedo ocellata*. Electric organs were dissected from 8 cm long embryos of *Torpedo ocellata* (Fig. 4), in which the specific activity of the enzyme was determined to be 0.34 mmol/h/mg protein, similar to that reported for mature electric organ from *Torpedo marmorata* (Mellinger et al., 1978). When poly(A)-containing RNA from *Torpedo* electric organ was injected into the oocytes, it directed the secretion of cholinesterase capable of degrading 30 pmol of ACh per ng of injected mRNA per h.

In the linear range of dose response, one may assume that the injected AChE-mRNA is being translated fully. It is, therefore, possible to calculate the fraction which this particular mRNA species represents out of the total injected mRNA (Labarca and Paigen, 1977), by measuring the amount of its specifically directed and catalytically active protein product (Table I). Whereas the abundance of AChE-mRNA in rat brain is comparable to that of AChE in this tissue, the abundance of AChE-mRNA in *Torpedo* electric organ is much lower than that of its translation product (Table II). Implicit in the calculations presented in these tables is the assumption that elongation rates for biosynthesis of nascent polypeptide chains of

112

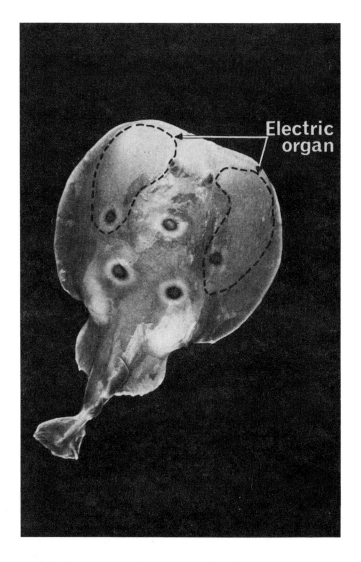

Fig. 4. *Torpedo ocellata* embryo. Embryos of *Torpedo ocellata* (8 cm long) were kept at $-70°C$ until used. The electric organ (area marked by arrow) was dissected on ice.

different proteins are approximately similar, and that the limiting factor in translation is the amount of mRNA. If so, the degradation rate of AChE protein in electric organ, but not in rat brain, is considerably slower than that of most other proteins. The bioassay described herein can be generally employed to monitor the level of AChE-mRNA in various tissues, in which the appearance of this scarce protein is correlated with physiological function. Furthermore, it can be exploited to investigate the post-translational processes involved in the formation of the various forms of this enzyme. Finally, a quantitative bioassay for AChE-mRNA is a necessary requirement for the preparation and amplification of a cDNA probe and the analysis of the genetic elements involved in the expression of this enzyme.

TABLE I

Abundance of AChE-mRNA in electric organ poly(A)-containing RNA

Twenty ng of poly(A)-containing mRNA were injected per oocyte. Incubation was for 20 h. Data presented are based on the average of two microinjection experiments. See details in text.

1. Turnover number of *Torpedo* AChE (Vigny et al., 1978)	$2.8 \times 10^{-17} \frac{mol}{h \times active\ site}$
2. Amount of cholinesterase activity synthesized and released during 1 h of linear secretion	$1.5 \times 10^{-12} \frac{mol\ ACh\ degraded}{h \times ng\ mRNA\ injected}$
3. Number of catalytic sites synthesized during 1 h of linear secretion	5×10^4
4. Rate of translation in oocytes (Gurdon et al., 1971; Chan et al., 1976)	10 cycles/h
5. Number of AChE-mRNA molecules capable of synthesizing the above number of AChE catalytic sites	5×10^3
6. Molecular weight of AChE catalytic subunit (Taylor et al., 1974)	$8 \times 10^4 \approx 800$ amino acid residues
7. Minimal molecular weight of AChE-mRNA	800 codon triplets, $\approx 8 \times 10^5$
8. Weight of a single AChE-mRNA molecule	1.3×10^9 ng
9. Weight of calculated number of AChE-mRNA molecules	7×10^{-6} ng
10. Estimated fraction of injected mRNA remaining at 10 h post-injection (Littauer et al., 1978)	~10%
11. Fraction of AChE-mRNA in injected mRNA	0.7×10^{-4}

SUMMARY

A novel technique for monitoring the level of the mRNA species which directs the synthesis of acetylcholinesterase (AChE) was developed, using microinjected *Xenopus* oocytes as a translation system.

When injected with poly(A)-containing RNA from whole rat brain or rat cerebellum and from electric organ of *Torpedo ocellata*, the oocytes synthesize and secrete catalytically active cholinesterase. The newly synthesized enzyme, which is mostly secreted into the oocytes' incubation medium, appears to be primarily AChE, since it is inhibited by the specific inhibitor BW 284C51. The AChE-mRNA displays

TABLE II

Abundance of AChE and AChE-mRNA in rat brain and Torpedo electric organ.

Specific activity of AChE was determined in homogenates of electric organ and of 10-day-old rat brain as described in the Experimental section. Tissue samples were dissolved in 1 M NaOH and protein was determined according to Lowry et al. (1951). Abundance of AChE-mRNA was calculated according to the scheme elaborated in Table I.

	Rat brain	*Torpedo electric organ*
AChE activity, mmol/h $\times$ g tissue	0.2	41.5
AChE fraction out of total protein	1×10^{-5}	2×10^{-3}
AChE-mRNA fraction out of total poly(A)-containing RNA	1×10^{-5}	0.7×10^{-4}

a half-life of about 10 ± 3 h in injected oocytes. The new enzymatic activity can be detected following injection of as little as 12.5 ng of poly(A)-containing RNA per oocyte, and there is a linear dependence of the oocytes ability to form cholinesterase on the amount of injected RNA. The abundance of AChE-mRNA in total non-fractionated rat brain mRNA was calculated to be about 1×10^{-5}, a value which is similar to the level of AChE protein determined in rat brain.

REFERENCES

Austin, L. and Berry, W.K. (1953) Two selective inhibitors of cholinesterase. *Biochem. J.*, 54: 695–700.

Blobel, G. and Dobberstein, B. (1976) Transfer of proteins across membranes. *J. Cell Biol.*, 67: 835–851.

Chan, L., Kohler, P.O. and O'Malley, B.W. (1976) Translation of ovalbumin mRNA in *Xenopus laevis* oocytes. Characterization of the system and effects of estrogen in injected mRNA populations. *J. clin. Invest.*, 57: 576–585.

Colman, A. and Morser, J. (1979) Export of proteins from oocytes of *Xenopus laevis. Cell*, 17: 517–526.

Ellman, G.L., Courtney, K.D., Andres, V. and Featherstone, R.M. (1961) A new and rapid colorimetric determination of AChE activity. *Biochem. Pharmacol.*, 7: 88–95.

Ghysdael, J., Hubert, H., Travniček, M., Bologneśi, D.P., Burny, A., Cleuter, Y. Kettman, G.F.R., Marbaix, G., Portetelle, D. and Chantrenne, H. (1977) Frog oocytes synthesize and completely process the precursor polypeptide to virion structural proteins after microinjection of avian myeloblastosis virus RNA. *Proc. nat. Acad. Sci. U.S.A.*, 74: 3230–3234.

Gisiger, V. and Vigny, M. (1977) A specific form of acetylcholinesterase is secreted by rat sympathetic ganglia. *FEBS Lett.*, 84: 253–256.

Gurdon, J.B., Lane, C.D., Woodland, H.R. and Marbaix, G. (1971) Use of frog eggs and oocytes for the study of messenger RNA and its translation in living cells. *Nature (Lond.)*, 233: 177–182.

Hall, Z.W. (1973) Multiple forms of acetylcholinesterase and their distribution in endplate and non-endplate regions of rat diaphragm muscle. *J. Neurobiol.*, 4: 343–361.

Jedrzejczyk, J., Silman, I., Lyles, J.M. and Barnard, E.A. (1981) Molecular forms of acetylcholinesterase and pseudocholinesterase inside and outside muscle endplates. *Biosci. Rep.*, 1: 45–51.

Johnson, C.D. and Russell, R.L. (1975) A rapid simple radiometric assay for cholinesterase suitable for multiple determinations. *Analyt. Biochem.*, 64: 229–238.

Kimhi, Y., Mahler, A. and Saya, D. (1980) Acetylcholinesterase in mouse neuroblastoma cells: Intracellular and released enzyme. *J. Neurochem.*, 34: 554–559.

Koenig, J. and Vigny, M. (1978) Neural induction of the 16S acetylcholinesterase in muscle cell cultures. *Nature (Lond.)*, 271: 75–77.

Labarca, C. and Paigen, K. (1977) mRNA directed synthesis of catalytically active mouse β-glucuronidase in *Xenopus* oocytes. *Proc. nat. Acad. Sci. U.S.A.*, 74: 4462–4465.

Lane, C.D. and Knowland, J. (1975) The injection of RNA into living cells: The use of frog oocytes for the assay of mRNA and the study of the control of gene expression. In R. Weber (Ed.), *The Biochemistry of Animal Development*, Vol. III, Academic Press, New York, pp. 145–181.

Lanks, K., Dorwin, J. and Papirmeister, B. (1974) Increased rate of acetylcholinesterase synthesis in differentiating neuroblastoma cells. *J. Cell Biol.*, 63: 824–830.

Laskey, R.A., Miles, A.D., Gurdon, J.B. and Partington, G.A. (1977) Protein synthesis in oocytes of *Xenopus laevis* is not regulated by the supply of messenger RNA. *Cell*, 11: 345–351.

Littauer, U.Z. and Soreq, H. (1982) The regulatory function of poly(A) and adjacent 3'-sequences in translatable RNA. *Progr. Nucleic Acid Res.*, 27: 53–83.

Littauer, U.Z., Soreq, H. and Cornelis, P. (1978) Polynucleotide phospnorylase as a probe for the regulatory function of the 3'-OH region of mRNA and viral RNA in translation. In P. Mildner and B. Reiss (Eds.), *Enzyme Regulation and Mechanisms of Action*, Pergamon, Oxford, pp. 233–243.

Lømo, T. and Slater, C.R. (1980) Control of junctional acetylcholinesterase by neural and muscular influences in the rat. *J. Physiol. (Lond.)*, 303: 191–202.

Lowry, O.H., Rosebrough, N.J., Farr, A.L. and Randall, R.J. (1951) Protein measurement with the Folin phenol reagent. *J. biol. Chem.*, 193: 265–275.

Massoulié, J. (1980) The polymorphism of cholinesterase and its physiological significance. *Trends Biochem. Sci.*, 5: 160–164.

Meedel, T.H. and Whittaker, J.R. (1979) Development of acetylcholinesterase during embryogenesis of the ascidian *Ciona intestinalis*. *J. exp. Zool.*, 210: 1–10.

Mellinger, J., Belbenoit, P., Ravaille, M. and Szabo, T. (1978) Electric organ development in *Torpedo marmorata chondriochthyes*. *Develop. Biol.*, 67: 167–188.

Miskin, R. and Soreq, H. (1981) Microinjected *Xenopus* oocytes synthesize active human plasminogen activator. *Nucleic Acid Res.*, 9: 3355–3364.

Mohun, T.J., Lane, C.D., Colman, A. and Wylie, C.C. (1981) The secretion of proteins in vitro from *Xenopus* oocytes and their accessory cells: a biochemical and morphological study. *J. Embryol. exp. Morph.*, 61: 367–383.

Nudel, U., Soreq, H., Littauer, U.Z., Huez, G., Marbaix, G., Hubert, H. and Leclercq, M. (1976) Globin mRNA species containing poly(A) segments of different lengths. *Europ. J. Biochem.*, 64: 115–121.

Rieger, F., Faivre-Bauman, A., Benda, P. and Vigny, M. (1976) Molecular forms of acetylcholinesterase: their de novo synthesis in mouse neuroblastoma cells. *J. Neurochem.*, 27: 1059–1063.

Rotundo, R.L. and Fambrough, D.M. (1980) Synthesis, transport and fate of acetylcholinesterase in cultural chick embryo muscle cells. *Cell*, 22: 583–594.

Rubin, L.L., Schuetze, S.M., Weill, C.L. and Fischbach, G.D. (1980) Regulation of acetylcholinesterase appearance at neuromuscular junctions in vitro. *Nature (Lond.)*, 283: 264–267.

Shulman, L. and Revel, M. (1980) Interferon-dependent induction of mRNA activity for (2'-5') oligo-isoadenylate synthetase. *Nature (Lond.)*, 288: 98–100.

Silman, I., Di Giamberardino, L., Lyles, J.M., Couraud, J.Y. and Barnard, E.A. (1979) Parallel regulation of acetylcholinesterase and pseudocholinesterase in normal, denervated and dystrophic chicken skeletal muscle. *Nature (Lond.)*, 280: 160–161.

Soreq, H., Sagar, M. and Sehgal, P.B. (1981) Translational activity and functional stability of human fibroblast β_1 and β_2 interferon mRNA species lacking 3'-terminal RNA sequences. *Proc. natl. Acad. Sci. U.S.A.*, 78: 1741–1745.

Soreq, H., Safran, A. and Zisling, R. (1982) Variations in gene expression during development of the rat cerebellum. *Develop. Brain Res.*, 3: 65–79.

Soreq, H. and Miskin, R. (1981) Secreted proteins in the medium of microinjected *Xenopus* oocytes are degraded by oocyte proteases. *FEBS Lett.*, 128: 305–310.

Taylor, P., Jones, J.W. and Jacobs, N.M. (1974) Acetylcholinesterase from *Torpedo*: characterization of an enzyme species isolated by lytic procedures. *Molec. Pharmacol.*, 10: 78–92.

Valle, G., Besley, J. and Colman, A. (1981) Synthesis and secretion of mouse immunoglobulin chains from *Xenopus* oocytes. *Nature (Lond.)*, 291: 338–340.

Vigny, M., Bon, S., Massoulie, J. and Leterrier, F. (1978) Active-site catalytic efficiency of acetyl-cholinesterase molecular forms in *Electrophorus*, *Torpedo*, rat and chicken. *Europ. J. Biochem.*, 85: 317–323.

Vijayan, V.K. and Brownson, R.H. (1974) Polyacrylamide gel electrophoresis of rat brain acetylcholines-terase: isoenzymes of normal rat brain. *J. Neurochem.*, 23: 47–53.

Walker, C.R. and Wilson, B.W. (1976) Regulation of acetylcholinesterase in chick muscle cultures after treatment with diisopropylphosphofluoridate: ribonucleic acid and protein synthesis. *Neuroscience*, 1: 509–513.

Adaptive Changes of Neurotransmitter Receptor Mechanisms in the Central Nervous System

JEAN-CHARLES SCHWARTZ, CATHERINE LLORENS CORTES, CHRISTIANE ROSE,
TAM THANH QUACH and HÉLÈNE POLLARD

*Unité 109 de Neurobiologie, Central Paul Broca de l'I.N.S.E.R.M., 2ter, Rue d'Alésia, 75014 Paris
(France)*

INTRODUCTION

The concept of adaptive changes in responsiveness to neurotransmitters is not a new one; the processes of hyper- and hyposensitivity of target-cells innervated by the peripheral nervous system have been known for a long time (for reviews see Trendelenburg, 1966; Fambrough, 1979). However, its extension to the CNS awaited the advent of suitable methods to quantify "responses" to neurotransmitters.

An important breakthrough was provided when it was shown that rats become progressively hyper-responsive to the behavioral actions of dopamine agonists following degeneration of the nigrostriatal dopaminergic neurons (Ungerstedt, 1971). This effect was interpreted as resulting from a process similar to that underlying the hypersensitivity of denervated muscle fibers to acetylcholine, and was followed by numerous observations showing that similar changes in responsiveness can be elicited by long-term (generally several weeks) interruptions of dopaminergic transmission by various procedures. Because the increased responsiveness of target-cells was observed under markedly artificial conditions (denervation or long-term disuse), it was not clear whether such changes could participate in the physiological regulation of synaptic transmission. However, that this might be the case was suggested by the observations that the spontaneous diurnal fluctuations of the activity of noradrenergic neurons ending in the pineal gland were accompanied by modulations in adrenergic receptor mechanisms which occurred in a matter of hours (Axelrod, 1974).

During the last decade the changes in responsiveness to CNS neurotransmitters have attracted the attention of a progressively increasing number of neuroscientists, as shown in recent reviews (Yarbrough and Phillis, 1975; Schwartz et al., 1978a; Olsen et al., 1980). The present article is not an attempt to extensively cover the literature on the subject but to: (a) describe the various experimental approaches that can be used; (b) discuss, using a few examples provided by studies of the catecholaminergic systems in brain (the most extensively studied ones in the respect), the characters and mechanisms of changes in responsiveness; (c) show that these changes are not restricted to catecholaminergic systems in brain; and (d) discuss one functional implication of these adaptive processes.

[117]

EVALUATION OF SENSITIVITY CHANGES

Generally the studies rely on comparing an index of "sensitivity" in controls and animals submitted to a pretreatment consisting of drug administration or brain lesions.

All methods allowing a quantification of receptor-mediated responses to CNS neurotransmitters, their agonists or antagonists can be used.

Quantification of responses on in vitro systems

When they can be used these methods present obvious advantages since they generally allow us a more precise quantification of responses than with living animals, and circumvent some of the difficulties associated with administration of the test agents ("blood–brain barrier" to neurotransmitters, lack of selective agonists, adaptive changes in the metabolic disposition of drugs, etc.).

The ability of several neurotransmitters to stimulate the formation of cAMP in brain slices or cell-free systems has been one of the most widely studied "responses". It has the advantage of being easily quantified because concentration–response curves can be established and both the apparent affinity of agonists and their maximal effect determined. However, this system is restricted to a few neurotransmitters, namely noradrenaline via β-receptors, dopamine via D_1-receptors, histamine via H_1- and H_2-receptors. In addition it must be realized that the stimulation of this "second messenger" formation only constitutes an early step in the chain of intracellular events leading to a final "response", and that its significance in neuro-neuronal transmission is not yet fully established.

Recently the glycogenolytic response to several neurotransmitters in brain slices, i.e. noradrenaline (via β_1-receptors), histamine (via H_1-receptors) and serotonin (Quach et al., 1978, 1980), has been used as a test-system. It offers several advantages: (a) responses mediated by new classes of receptors can be studied; (b) because the responses seem to be mediated by two distinct second messengers (cAMP for noradrenaline and calcium ions for histamine) the roles of the latter can be studied; and (c) in the case of glycogenolytic responses mediated by cAMP the changes in responsiveness can be analyzed at various steps between receptor stimulation and final response.

However, the in vitro models available to quantify the actions of neurotransmitters are still few and do not yet allow us to study the responses to all of these substances, which are identified in increasing numbers in the CNS.

Finally, with the development of suitable radioactive ligands for a large number of cerebral receptors, the adaptive changes occurring at the first step of the chain of events leading to the response, i.e. the recognition of the neurotransmitters, can be now studied. Radioreceptor assays have greatly contributed to our present understanding of the mechanisms involved in changes in responsiveness to neurotransmitters, but it should be noted that these changes might not (or only partially) involve this early step in the chain of events leading to a response.

Quantification of responses in vivo

Responses to neurotransmitters (as well as to effectors of their receptors) directly applied by microiontophoresis (or systemically administered) can be more or less quantified by evaluating the changes in firing rates they elicit. When iontophoresis is used quantification usually consists of the estimation of the threshold ejecting current for the response to be observed, but data are to be interpreted with caution because this value strongly depends, among other variables, on the characteristics and position of the micropipettes used. One important advantage of this method is that the effects can be evaluated on a class of identified neurons, e.g. by recording the changes in electrical activity of noradrenergic neurons at the level of their cell bodies in the locus coeruleus (Aghajanian, 1978) or of Purkinje neurons in cerebellum (Siggins and Schultz, 1979).

Changes in responsiveness of an identified class of target neurons can also be quantified by measuring the turnover rate of their neurotransmitter or even the neurotransmitter level when the latter reflects the turnover, as is the case for acetylcholine (Fibiger and Grewaal, 1974; Choi and Roth, 1978; Scatton and Worms, 1979). In some cases where the turnover rate of neurotransmitters is set by neuronal feed-back mechanisms involving their receptors, this rate can be taken as indirectly reflecting responses mediated by these receptors.

Cerebral receptor assays can be performed not only in vitro but also in the living animal following systemic administration of ^{3}H-labeled ligands, a method already used to investigate the mechanisms of dopamine receptor hypersensitivity in mouse striatum (Schwartz et al., 1978b).

Finally, in a large number of studies behavioral responses to neurotransmitter agonists have been used to assess changes in "receptor sensitivity". Studies of this type depend on the availability of a selective agonist (like apomorphine for dopamine receptors) and of behavioral tests in which the response is easily quantifiable (in terms of either threshold dose or complete dose–response curve).

RESPONSES MEDIATED BY β-ADRENERGIC RECEPTORS: HYPER- AND HYPOSENSITIVITY

Responses mediated by β-adrenergic receptors in brain display many advantages as a system for studying changes in responsiveness: (a) they are easy to quantify in in vitro systems and can also be studied in vivo by electrophysiological techniques; (b) the binding properties of β-adrenoreceptors can be studied with specific radioligands ([^{3}H]dihydroalprenolol or [^{125}I]hydroxybenzylpindolol); and (c) various steps between binding of agonists and final response can be studied separately in the glycogenolytic system. Responsiveness is rapidly and bidirectionally modified according to in vivo pretreatments.

Treatments triggering the development of hyper- or hyposensitivity

The general rule governing changes in sensitivity of β-adrenergic receptor-mediated systems seems to be: "decreased noradrenergic input triggers the development of hypersensitivity whereas increased noradrenergic input triggers the development of hyposensitivity".

This rule seems to apply to all in vitro or in vivo test systems used to quantify responses to noradrenaline, like cAMP accumulation (Dismukes and Daly, 1974;

Baudry et al., 1976) or [^{3}H]glycogen hydrolysis in slices (Quach et al., 1978), adenylate cyclase (Williams and Pirch, 1974; Dolphin et al., 1979) in homogenates, inhibition of Purkinje cell firing (Siggins and Schultz, 1979) to various brain regions (cerebral cortex, limbic forebrain, cerebellum) and to various animal species (rat, mouse, chick). Decreased noradrenergic inputs leading to hypersensitivity were obtained by chemical (6-hydroxydopamine) or electrolytic ablation of the ascending noradrenergic neurons, by impairment of storage of the neurotransmitter (reserpine), and by inhibition of its release by morphine (see below).

Conversely, hyposensitivity was observed to develop following a period of over-stimulation of β-adrenoreceptors obtained by administration of a direct agonist (isoprenaline in chick; Nahorski, 1977), an indirect agonist (amphetamine; Martres et al., 1975) or monoamine oxidase inhibitors (Vetulani et al., 1975). However the interpretation of hyposensitivity triggered by a large variety of tricyclic antidepressants raises some difficulties. Whereas the hyposensitivity elicited by agents like desipramine, known to inhibit noradrenaline uptake, is easily explained by their primary effect, this is less clear in the case of tricyclic antidepressants which do not share this property, like iprindole, mianserin or zimelidine (Sulser et al., 1978; Sulser, 1979). The long-term effects of the latter compounds could be explained either by a transsynaptic activation of noradrenergic neurons or, perhaps more interestingly, by a direct (but yet unidentified) action on the processes controlling the sensitivity of target-cells.

Characters of the changes in sensitivity

The opposite changes in sensitivity of target-cells seem to share several properties. Their time-courses are characterized by a progressive development while pretreatment continues and a duration which outlasts that of the triggering pretreatment. For instance, the enhanced responsiveness of the cAMP-generating system in rat cortical slices is already observed between 5 and 24 h after the beginning of reserpine administration, progressively develops during the following days and slowly decays in about two weeks after the end of treatment (Dismukes and Daly, 1974; Baudry et al., 1976). The hyposensitive state elicited by amphetamine

---

Fig. 1. Hypersensitivity elicited by reserpine: analysis of various steps of the glycogenolytic response to noradrenaline in mouse cortical slices. Mice pretreated with reserpine (5 mg/kg on day 1 and 2.5 mg/kg on day 2) were sacrificed 24 h after the last injection. Slices from cerebral cortex were prepared with a McIlwain apparatus and incubated for 20 min under identical conditions in oxygenated Krebs–Ringer medium for the various types of experiments. A: occupancy of β-adrenoreceptors by noradrenaline. Slices incubated in the presence of 10 nM [^{3}H]dihydroalprenolol (saturating concentration) and noradrenaline in increasing concentrations were homogenized before rapid filtration. Specific [^{3}H]dihydroalprenolol binding (inhibited by 10^{-4} M noradrenaline) was increased by 25% ($P < 0.01$) whereas K_i values for noradrenaline were $2.5 \pm 0.2\,\mu$M and $4.1 \pm 0.8\,\mu$M (n.s.) for reserpine-treated and controls, respectively. B: stimulation of cyclic AMP accumulation by noradrenaline. Characteristic values of the concentration–response curves were: $EC_{50} = 4.5 \pm 1.4\,\mu$M, maximal stimulation $= 674 \pm 7\%$ in controls and $EC_{50} = 3.7 \pm 0.6\,\mu$M, maximal stimulation $= 1120 \pm 69\%$ in reserpine-treated ($P < 0.005$, basal level not significantly modified). C: stimulation of [^{3}H]glycogen hydrolysis by dibutyryl-cAMP. Characteristic values of the concentration–response curves were: EC_{50}: $10.6 \pm 3.0\,\mu$M, maximal stimulation $68 \pm 5\%$ in controls and $EC_{50} = 5.4 \pm 2.0\,\mu$M, maximal stimulation $= 72 \pm 5\%$ in reserpine-treated (basal level not significantly modified). D: stimulation of [^{3}H]glycogen hydrolysis by noradrenaline. Characteristic values of the concentration–response curves were: $EC_{50} = 0.48 \pm 0.06\,\mu$M, maximal stimulation $= 72 \pm 3\%$ in controls, and $EC_{50} = 0.13 \pm 0.02\,\mu$M ($P < 0.002$), maximal stimulation $= 72 \pm 3\%$ in reserpine-treated (basal level not significantly modified).

treatment displays a similar time-course, with a half-time for decay of about 3 days (Martres et al., 1975; Baudry et al., 1976). Interestingly the time-course of these changes is similar to that of denervation hypersensitivity at the neuromuscular junction (Thesleff, 1973; Fambrough, 1979) but entirely different from that of the much more rapidly reversible processes of desensitization (Mukherjee and Lefkowitz, 1976). In addition both states are characterized by a change in maximal response without modification of the EC_{50} of noradrenaline (at least in the cAMP generating system). They could, therefore, be explained by opposite modifications in the number of β-adrenoreceptors. In agreement with this view, an enhanced number of sites recognizing β-adrenergic radioligands is associated with hypersensitivity

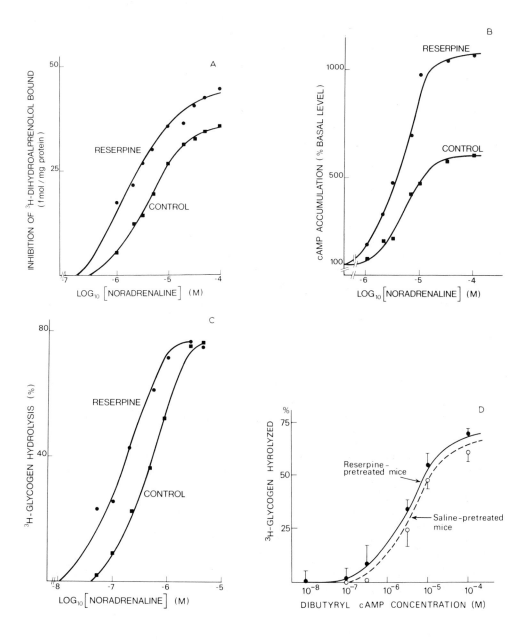

(Sporn et al., 1976; Nahorski, 1977; Llorens et al., 1978), whereas a decreased number accompanies hyposensitivity elicited by chronic administration of tricyclic antidepressants (Sulser et al., 1978). In all cases it was noticed that the percent change in cAMP response in slices was more marked than in the number of binding sites. This raises the question of relationships between receptor occupancy and final "response" that has been recently investigated in the glycogenolytic system.

Analysis of hypersensitivity in the noradrenaline-induced glycogenolytic response in brain slices

We have recently developed a convenient model to study the glycogenolytic action of neurotransmitters (Quach et al., 1978, 1980). [^{3}H]Glycogen accumulates in brain slices incubated in the presence of [^{3}H]glucose, and the glycogenolytic action of noradrenaline, histamine or serotonin is then evaluated by assaying the remaining [^{3}H]polymer isolated on filters (from which the excess of [^{3}H]glucose is eluted by ethanol). The glycogenolytic action of noradrenaline is selectively mediated by β_1-receptors, and its potentiation by phosphodiesterase inhibitors indicates that cAMP is involved. However the glycogenolytic response occurs at much lower concentrations of noradrenaline than those required for cAMP accumulation in the same preparation: labeling β_1-receptors in the slices with [^{3}H]dihydroalprenolol indicates that maximal glycogenolysis occurs for an occupancy of less than 10% of these sites by noradrenaline, whereas maximal stimulation of cAMP accumulation requires total occupancy.

In slices from reserpine-treated mice (two daily injections), the 20% increase in the number of β_1-receptors (Fig. 1A) is accompanied by: (a) a stronger increase (+100%) in maximal stimulation of cAMP accumulation (Fig. 1B), contrasting with the similar enhancement of [^{3}H]dihydroalprenolol binding sites and β-adrenergic-sensitive adenylate cyclase in a cell-free preparation (Dolphin et al., 1979); (b) a non-significantly modified glycogenolytic response to dibutyryl-cAMP (Fig. 1C); and (c) a 300% increase in responsiveness of the glycogenolytic system to noradrenaline (3-fold leftward shift of the concentration–response curve, Fig. 1D). Taken together these data indicate that the small increase in the number of receptors coupled to the cyclase is amplified by two processes: the small increase in cAMP formation results in a much larger increase in accumulation of the nucleotide (probably because the rate of its hydrolysis is not correspondingly increased), and then the amplification of the intracellular signal by the cascade leading to glycogen hydrolysis accounts for the shift in EC$_{50}$ regarding this final response (Fig. 1D).

RESPONSES MEDIATED BY DOPAMINE RECEPTORS

Changes in responsiveness are interesting to investigate in the dopaminergic system because it is one of the best suited to study relationships between receptors and behavioral responses, and also because these changes are likely to have clinical counterparts. From a behavioral point of view three types of changes can be distinguished: hyper- and hyposensitivity, triggered as in the case of β-adrenergic responses, and also behavioral facilitation, a state of increased responsiveness which paradoxically develops following agonist pretreatment.

Hypersensitivity

Hypersensitivity regarding behavioral responses mediated by dopamine receptors have long been known to develop after denervation or pharmacological interruption of dopaminergic transmission (Ungerstedt, 1971; Tarsy and Baldessarini, 1974). One striking observation made during the last few years is that hypersensitivity to apomorphine regarding stereotyped behaviors in mice develops after only a few hours of interrupted dopaminergic transmission (Costentin et al., 1975, 1977a; Hyttel and Möller-Nielsen, 1976). This behavioral state is temporarily accompanied by a decreased dopamine turnover, which probably reflects the increased responsiveness of the feedback system controlled by dopamine receptors (Martres et al., 1977). The development of α-methyl-p-tyrosine-induced hypersensitivity being prevented in mice pretreated with protein synthesis inhibitors, suggests that the process might be due to increased dopaminergic receptors as is the case for β-adrenoreceptors. The slow decay of this state of hypersensitivity ($t_{1/2} \simeq 2$ days) is also consistent with the half-life of receptors in other systems (Changeux and Danchin, 1976). Indeed, an increased number of [³H]haloperidol binding sites in striatum has been shown to accompany the hypersensitivity elicited by long-term interruption (3 weeks) of dopaminergic transmission (Burt et al., 1977; Creese et al., 1977). However, after short-term interruption elicited by a single administration of neuroleptics no significant change in binding sites assayed in vivo or in vitro can be detected (Schwartz et al., 1978b; Muller et al., 1980; Hyttel, 1980). This discrepancy with the behavioral and turnover data could be due to: (a) the existence of a short-term hypersensitivity process differing from that resulting from long-term interruption of neurotransmission and which would not involve, like the latter, a change in the number of receptors; (b) the existence of a high amplification factor between the changes in receptor number and of behavioral responsiveness; and (c) heterogenous changes in dopamine receptor number among various classes of target-cells.

Hyposensitivity

Following pretreatment with direct or indirect dopamine agonists animals become tolerant to a variety of behavioral actions of these agents. This hyposensitivity has been well studied in the case of the hypothermia elicited by stimulation of dopamine receptors located in the rostral hypothalamus (Sweatman and Jell, 1977; Costentin et al., personal communication).

In mice the development of tolerance to hypothermia, which can be observed after a single administration of a dopamine agonist, displays the following features: (a) the dose–response curve is shifted to the right without alteration of the maximal response; (b) tolerance develops in a matter of minutes and decays slowly over several weeks; and (c) its development is not impaired by protein synthesis inhibitors (Costentin et al., 1975; Schwartz et al., 1978b).

Tolerance to other actions of dopamine agonists has also been reported: hypokinesia (Costentin et al., 1977c), stereotypies (Worms and Scatton, 1977), and increase in striatal acetylcholine level (Scatton and Worms, 1979). This hyposensitive state is accompanied by an elevated turnover rate of dopamine in striatum and limbic structures (Worms and Scatton, 1977; De la Baume et al., 1979) which mirrors the opposite changes observed in dopamine hypersensitivity.

The mechanisms underlying these changes are still unclear; whereas a decrease in the dopamine-sensitive adenylate cyclase and number of dopaminergic binding sites has been reported (Quik and Iversen, 1978; Howlett and Nahorski, 1979), we have recently been unable to detect any significant change in subclasses of dopaminergic binding sites (Sokoloff et al., 1980a, b) of rats chronically treated with apomorphine (up to 14 daily 10 mg/kg injections).

Behavioral facilitation

This term refers to a paradoxical increase in responsiveness to the behavioral actions of dopamine agonists following chronic (or even acute) treatment with one of these agents. Thus the increased locomotor activity (Segal and Mandell, 1974; Costentin et al., 1977b, c), buccal stereotypies (Klawans and Margolin, 1975) and stereotyped climbing behavior (Martres et al., 1977) elicited by dopamine agonists are progressively and durably enhanced following a prior treatment which may consist of a single injection of apomorphine in low dosage. This process seems to differ from disuse hypersensitivity: (a) its development is not affected by protein synthesis inhibitors; (b) it is not accompanied by a change in dopamine turnover; and (c) only the responsiveness to dopamine agonists in low dosage is modified.

We have proposed that behavioral facilitation may correspond to a decreased responsiveness of dopamine autoreceptors (Martres et al., 1977; Schwartz et al., 1978b). Although this hypothesis has received some support from radioligand binding studies (Muller and Seeman, 1979) we have been unable to detect in rats chronically treated with apomorphine (see above) any change in striatal D_3 receptor binding sites localized, at least partly, on dopamine terminals (Sokoloff et al., 1980a, b).

CHANGES IN RESPONSIVENESS TO OTHER NEUROTRANSMITTERS AND UNANSWERED QUESTIONS

Most investigations on adaptive change in receptor mechanisms in CNS have so far been performed on catecholaminergic systems, which are the best known and for which the larger number of experimental tools are available. Nevertheless, it now appears that the observations made on these systems can, in fact, be extended to a variety of other neurotransmitters (or putative neurotransmitters). For example, changes towards either hyper- or hyposensitivity (or both) or modifications in the number of receptor binding sites have been reported regarding serotonin (Stewart et al., 1976; Wirz-Justice et al., 1978; Nelson et al., 1978; De Montigny and Aghajahian, 1978), acetylcholine (Bird and Aghajanian, 1975; Klein et al., 1979; Majocha and Baldessarini, 1980), histamine (for reviews see Schwartz et al., 1980) glutamate (Segal, 1977), GABA (Braestrup et al., 1979) and substance P (Wright and Roberts, 1978). These studies, the above list of which is far from complete, indicate that: (a) these processes are of general relevance, (b) they are usually triggered under the same conditions, e.g. hypersensitivity by decreased neurotransmission and the reverse for hyposensitivity; and (c) in some cases changes in responsiveness are accompanied by changes in receptor number, but the latter are generally of lower amplitude.

Because these modifications occur for excitatory as well as inhibitory neurotransmitters, for those known to use a cyclic nucleotide as second messenger as well as those which do not, it is difficult at present to understand how the target-cell receives its information to increase or decrease its responsiveness to a given neurotransmitter, i.e., at least in some cases, to modify the number of receptors. Furthermore, it is not yet known whether these changes affect a single class of receptors on the same target cell. Finally, whereas the increases in receptor number accompanying hypersensitivity could be due to an enhanced synthesis rate (hypersensitivity development being prevented by protein synthesis inhibitors), the mechanisms underlying the reverse situation are not clear. In view of their time course and of the lack of effect of protein synthesis inhibitors we have previously hypothesized that development of hyposensitivity in the CNS was due to an increased rate of receptor loss (Schwartz et al., 1978a). This hypothesis has recently received some support from Klein et al. (1979), who showed that the decrease in muscarinic receptors triggered by their sustained stimulation in a hybrid cell line of neuronal origin was due to an increased rate of receptor breakdown.

It is likely that simple experimental models like this one will teach us much during the forthcoming years about the mechanisms of receptor regulation.

POSSIBLE IMPLICATION OF RECEPTOR CHANGES IN THE DEVELOPMENT OF TOLERANCE TO AND DEPENDENCE ON OPIATES

It is clear that adaptive changes in receptor mechanisms in the CNS might account for the modified responsiveness to various pharmacological agents observed after chronic administration. One of the situations in which such adaptive changes might be important to assess is tolerance to and dependence on opiates. The realization that the actions of these agents was mediated by stimulation of specific receptors that can be easily studied with radioligands offered an opportunity to test the hypothesis that tolerance and addiction to morphine-like agents is the result of a modified number of opiate receptors. One model of addiction could have been that down-regulation of opiate receptors is triggered by exposure of target-cells to morphine-like drugs. In fact, it appears that the number and properties of [^{3}H]opiate binding sites are not modified in the brain of animals chronically treated with morphine (Simon and Hiller, 1978; Snyder and Simantov, 1977).

An alternative model postulates that a modified number of receptors to non-opioid neurotransmitters, whose release is acutely modified by administration of opiates, develops upon chronic treatment with morphine-like agents. Thus acute opiate administration results in an inhibition of noradrenergic transmission in brain mediated by opiate receptors located at the level of either nerve-endings (Montel et al., 1975; Llorens et al., 1978) or cell bodies in the locus coeruleus (Aghajanian, 1978). During long-term administration of morphine this primary inhibitory action might be progressively (and indirectly) compensated by an increased responsiveness of target-cells to noradrenaline and, therefore, could account for the tolerance to morphine. That hypersensitivity to noradrenaline develops in rats chronically treated with morphine has been shown by measuring the responsiveness of the cAMP-generating system in slices from cerebral cortex (Llorens et al., 1978). This change is apparently mediated by an increased number of β-adrenoreceptors as measured with

TABLE I

Effects of chronic treatments with morphine on the number of receptors in rat cerebral cortex

Rats were chronically treated with morphine pellets (70 mg of morphine base) during 10 days on the following schedule: one pellet on the first day, two on the 4th day, three on the 7th day. Rats were killed on the 11th day, 15 h after pellet removal. Binding studies were performed on aliquots of cerebral cortex particulate fractions. Concentrations used were: 6 nM [³H]dihydroergokryptine; 1.6 nM [³H]dihydroalprenolol; 1 nM [³H]quinuclidinylbenzylate and 5 nM [³H]mepyramine – these were incubated in the presence or absence of, respectively, 10^{-6} M phentolamine, 10^{-6} M alprenolol, 10^{-4} M oxotremorine, and 2×10^{-6} M triprolidine.

Receptor class	Radioligand	Change
α-Adrenergic	[³H]dihydroergokryptine	+28%
β-Adrenergic	[³H]dihydroalprenolol	+27%
Muscarinic	[³H]quinuclidylbenzylate	n.s.
H₁-Histaminergic	[³H]mepyramine	n.s.

[³H]dihydroalprenolol as ligand (Table I). This change is paralleled by the elevation of α-adrenoreceptors as evaluated with [³H]dihydroergokryptine, but its relative selectivity is indicated by the absence of significant modification in the binding of muscarinic and histaminergic radioligands (Table I) and the hardly significant change in dopaminergic binding sites (De la Baume et al., 1979).

The noradrenergic hypersensitivity developing after chronic administration of morphine and persisting after its interruption might be responsible for the abstinence symptoms which generally mirror those observed when the drug is acutely administered. In rats treated with morphine pellets during 10 days, the noradrenergic hypersensitivity decays after the pellet is withdrawn with a half-life (about 2 days) similar to that of the disappearance of the major behavioral symptoms of abstinence (Bläsig et al., 1973). That an increased noradrenergic transmission is implicated in the abstinence syndrome in humans is consistent with the observation that administration of clonidine, a drug inhibiting noradrenergic activity, dramatically alleviates the symptoms of opiate withdrawal in human addicts (Gold et al., 1978).

REFERENCES

Aghajanian, G.K. (1978) Tolerance of locus coeruleus neurones to morphine and suppression of withdrawal response by clonidine. *Nature (Lond.)*, 276: 186–188.

Axelrod, J. (1974) The pineal gland: a neurochemical transducer. *Science*, 184: 1341–1348.

Baudry, M., Martres, M.P. and Schwartz, J.C. (1976) Modulation in the sensitivity of noradrenergic receptors in the CNS studied by the responsiveness of the cyclic AMP system. *Brain Res.*, 116: 111–124.

Bird, S.J. and Aghajanian, G.K. (1975) Denervation supersensitivity in the cholinergic septohippocampal pathway: a microiontophoretic study. *Brain Res.*, 100: 355–370.

Bläsig, J., Herz, A., Reinhold, K. and Gansberger, S.S. (1973) Development of physical dependence on

127

morphine in respect to time and dosage and quantification of the precipitated withdrawal syndrome in rats. *Psychopharmacologia*, 33: 19–38.

Braestrup, C., Nielsen, M. and Squires, R.F. (1979) No change in rat benzodiazepine receptors after withdrawal from continuous treatment with lorazepam and diazepam. *Life Sci.*, 24: 347–350.

Burt, D.R., Creese, I. and Snyder, S.H. (1977) Antischizophrenic drugs: chronic treatment elevates dopamine receptor binding in brain. *Science*, 196: 326–328.

Changeux, J.-P. and Danchin, A. (1976) Selective stabilisation of developing synapses as a mechanism for the specification of neuronal networks. *Nature (Lond.)*, 264: 705–712.

Choi, R.L. and Roth, R.H. (1978) Development of supersensitivity of apomorphine-induced increases in acetylcholine levels and stereotypy after chronic fluphenazine treatment. *Psychopharmacology*, 17: 59–64.

Costentin, J., Protais, P. and Schwartz, J.C. (1975) Rapid and dissociated changes in the sensitivities of different dopamine receptors in mouse brain. *Nature (Lond.)*, 257: 405–407.

Costentin, J., Marçais, H., Protais, P., Baudry, M., De la Baume, S., Martres, M.P. and Schwartz, J.C. (1977a) Rapid development of hypersensitivity of striatal dopamine receptors induced by alpha-methyl paratyrosine and its prevention by protein synthesis inhibitors. *Life Sci.*, 21: 307–314.

Costentin, J., Marçais, H., Protais, P., Baudry, M., Martres, M.P. and Schwartz, J.C. (1977b) Facilitation d'un comportement moteur stéréotypé (verticalisation) par stimulation préalable des récepteurs dopaminergiques: hyposensibilité d'autorécepteurs? *C.R. Acad. Sci. (Paris)*, 284: 143–146.

Costentin, J., Marçais, H., Protais, P. and Schwartz, J.C. (1977c) Tolerance to hypokinesia elicited by dopamine agonists in mice: hyposensitization of autoreceptors? *Life Sci.*, 20: 883–886.

Creese, I., Burt, D.R. and Snyder, S.H. (1977) Dopamine receptor binding enhancement accompanies lesion induced behavioural supersensitivity. *Science*, 197: 596–598.

De la Baume, S., Patey, G., Marçais, H., Protais, P., Costentin, J. and Schwartz, J.C. (1979) Changes in dopamine receptors in mouse striatum following morphine treatments. *Life Sci.*, 24: 2333–2342.

De Montigny, C. and Aghajanian G.K. (1978) Tricyclic antidepressants: long term treatment increases responsivity of rat forebrain neurons to serotonin *Science*, 202: 1303–1305.

Dismukes, K. and Daly, J.W. (1974) Norepinephrine-sensitive systems generating adenosine 3'5'-mono-phosphate: increased responses in cerebral cortical slices from reserpine-treated rats. *Molec. Pharmacol.*, 10: 933–940.

Dolphin, A., Adrien, J., Hamon, M. and Bockaert, J. (1979) Identity of (^{3}H)dihydroalprenolol binding sites and β-adrenergic receptors coupled with adenylate cyclase in the central nervous system: pharmacological properties: distribution and adaptive responsiveness. *Molec. Pharmacol.*, 15: 1–15.

Fambrough, D.M. (1979) Control of acetylcholine receptors in skeletal muscle. *Physiol. Rev.*, 59: 165–277.

Fibiger, H.C. and Grewaal, D. (1974) Neurochemical evidence for denervation supersensitivity: the effect of unilateral substantia nigra lesions on apomorphine induced increases in neostriatal acetylcholine levels. *Life Sci.*, 15: 57–63.

Gold, M.S., Redmond, D.E. and Kleber, H.D. (1978) Clonidine blocks acute opiate-withdrawal symptoms. *Lancet*, II: 599–601.

Howlett, D.R. and Nahorski, S.R. (1979) Acute and chronic amphetamine treatments modulate striatal dopamine receptor binding sites. *Brain Res.*, 161: 173–178.

Hyttel, J. (1980) No evidence for increased dopaminergic receptor binding in super-responsive mice after a single dose of neuroleptics. *Advanc. Biochem. Psychopharmacol.*, 24: 167–174.

Hyttel, J. and Moller-Nielsen, I. (1976) Changes in catecholamine concentrations and synthesis rate in mouse brain during the "supersensitivity" phase after treatment with neuroleptic drugs. *J. Neurochem.*, 27: 313–317.

Klawans, H.L. and Margolin, D.I. (1975) Amphetamine-induced dopaminergic hypersensitivity in guinea pigs. *Arch. gen. Psychiat.*, 32: 725–732.

Klein, W.L., Nathanson, N. and Nirenberg, M. (1979) Muscarinic acetylcholine receptor regulation by accelerated rate of receptor loss. *Biochem. biophys. Res. Commun.*, 80: 506–512.

Llorens, C., Martres, M.P., Baudry, M. and Schwartz, J.C. (1978) Hypersensitivity to noradrenaline in cortex after morphine: relevance to tolerance. *Nature (Lond.)*, 274: 603–605.

Majocha, R. and Baldessarini, R.J. (1980) Increased muscarinic receptor binding in rat forebrain after scopolamine. *Europ. J. Pharmacol.*, 67: 327–328.

Martres, M.P., Baudry, M. and Schwartz, J.C. (1975) Subsensitivity of noradrenaline-stimulated cyclic AMP accumulation in brain slices of D-amphetamine-treated mice. *Nature (Lond.)*, 255: 731–733.

Martres, M.P., Costentin, J., Baudry, M., Marçais, H., Protais, P. and Schwartz, J.C. (1977) Long-term changes in the sensitivity of pre- and postsynaptic dopamine receptors in mouse striatum as evidenced by behavioural and biochemical studies. *Brain Res.*, 136: 319–337.

Montel, H., Starke, K. and Taube, H.D. (1975) Influence of morphine and naloxone on the release of NA from rat cerebellar cortex slices. *Naunyn-Schmiedeberg's Arch. Pharmacol.*, 288: 427.

Mukherjee, C. and Lefkowitz, R.J. (1976) Desensitization of β-adrenergic receptors by β-adrenergic agonists in a cell-free system: resensitization by guanosine 5'-(β-γ-imino)triphosphate and other purine nucleotides. *Proc. nat. Acad. Sci. U.S.A.*, 73: 1494–1498.

Muller, P. and Seeman, P. (1979) Presynaptic subsensitivity as a possible basis for sensitization by long-term dopamine mimetics. *Europ. J. Pharmacol.*, 55: 149–157.

Muller, P., Svensson, T.H. and Carlsson, A. (1980) Pre- and postsynaptic mechanisms in haloperidol-induced sensitization to dopaminergic agonists. *Advanc. Biochem. Psychopharmacol.*, 24: 69–74.

Nahorski, S.R. (1977) Altered responsiveness of cerebral β-adrenoceptors assessed by adenosine cyclic 3',5'-monophosphate formation and [³H]propranolol binding. *Molec. Pharmacol.*, 13: 679–689.

Nelson, D.L., Herbert, A., Bourgoin, S., Glowinski, J. and Hamon, M. (1978) Characteristics of central 5-HT receptors and their adaptive changes following intracerebral 5,7-dihydroxytryptamine administration in the rat. *Molec. Pharmacol.*, 14: 983–995.

Olsen, R.N., Reisine, T.D. and Yamamura, H.I. (1980) Neurotransmitter receptors – biochemistry and alterations in neuropsychiatric disorders. *Life Sci.*, 27: 801–808.

Quach, T.T., Rose, C. and Schwartz, J.C. (1978) [³H]Glycogen hydrolysis in brain slices: responses to neurotransmitters and modulation of noradrenaline receptors. *J. Neurochem.*, 30: 1335–1341.

Quach, T.T., Duchemin, A.M., Rose, C. and Schwartz, J.C. (1980) [³H]Glycogen hydrolysis elicited by histamine in mouse brain slices: selective involvement of H_1 receptors. *Molec. Pharmacol.*, 17: 301–308.

Quik, M. and Iversen, L.L. (1978) Subsensitivity of the rat striatal dopaminergic system after treatment with bromocriptine: effects on [³H]spiperone binding and dopamine-stimulated cyclic AMP formation. *Naunyn-Schmiedeberg's Arch. Pharmacol.*, 304: 141–145.

Scatton, B. and Worms, P. (1979) Tolerance to increases in striatal acetylcholine concentrations after repeated administration of apomorphine dipivaloyl ester. *J. Pharmacol.*, 31: 861–863.

Schwartz, J.C., Costentin, J., Martres, M.P., Protais, P. and Baudry, M. (1978a) Modulation of receptor mechanisms in the CNS: hyper- and hyposensitivity to catecholamines. *Neuropharmacology*, 17: 665–685.

Schwartz, J.C., Palacios, J.M., Barbin, G., Quach, T.T., Garbarg, M., Haas, H.L. and Wolf, P. (1978b) Histamine receptors in mammalian brain: characters and modifications studied electrophysiologically and biochemically. In T.O. Yellin (Ed.), *Histamine Receptors*, Spectrum, New York.

Schwartz, J.C., Pollard, H. and Quach, T.T. (1980) Histamine as a neurotransmitter in mammalian brain: neurochemical evidence. *J. Neurochem.*, 35: 26–33.

Segal, M. (1977) Supersensitivity of hippocampal neurons to acidic amino acids in decommissurized rats. *Brain Res.*, 119: 476–479.

Segal, D.S. and Mandell, A.J. (1974) Long-term administration of D-amphetamine: progressive augmentation of motor activity and stereotypy. *Pharmacol. Biochem. Behav.*, 2: 249–255.

Siggins, G.R. and Schultz, J.E. (1979) Chronic treatment with lithium or desipramine alters discharge frequency and norepinephrine responsiveness of cerebellar purkinje cells. *Proc. nat. Acad. Sci. U.S.A.*, 76: 5987–5992.

Simon, E.J. and Hiller, J.M. (1978) The opiate receptors. *Ann. Rev. Pharmacol. Toxicol.*, 18: 371–394.

Snyder, S.H. and Simantov, R. (1977) The opiate receptor and opioid peptides. *J. Neurochem.*, 28: 13–20.

Sokoloff, P., Martres, M.P. and Schwartz, J.C. (1980a) [³H]Apomorphine labels both dopamine post-synaptic receptors and autoreceptors. *Nature (Lond.)*, 288: 283–286.

Sokoloff, P., Martres, M.P. and Schwartz, J.C. (1980b) Three classes of dopamine receptors (D-2, D-3, D-4) identified by binding studies with [³H]apomorphine and [³H]domperidone. *Naunyn-Schmiedeberg's Arch. Pharmacol.*, 315: 89–102.

Sporn, J.R., Harden, T.K., Wolfe, B.B. and Molinoff, P.B. (1976) β-Adrenergic receptor involvement in 6-hydroxydopamine induced supersensitivity in rat cerebral cortex. *Science*, 194: 624–626.

Stewart, R.M., Growdon, J.H., Cancian, D. and Baldessarini, R.J. (1976) 5-Hydroxytryptophan-induced myoclonus: increased sensitivity to serotonin after intracranial 5,7-dihydroxytryptamine in the adult rat. *Neuropharmacology*, 15: 449–455.

Sulser, F. (1979) New perspectives on the mode of action of antidepressant drugs. *Trends Pharmacol. Sci.*. 1: 92–95.

Sulser, F., Vetulani, J. and Mobley, P.L. (1978) Commentary. Mode of action of antidepressant drugs. *Biochem. Pharmacol.*, 27: 257–261.

Sweatman, P. and Jell, R.M. (1977) Dopamine and histamine sensitivity of rostral hypothalamic neurones in the cat: possible involvement in thermoregulation. *Brain Res.*, 127: 173–178.

Tarsy, D. and Baldessarini, R.J. (1974) Behavioural supersensitivity to apomorphine following chronic treatment with drugs which interfere with the synaptic function of catecholamines. *Neuropharmacology*, 13: 927–940.

Thesleff, S. (1973) Functional properties of receptors in striated muscle. In H.P. Rang (Ed.), *Drug Receptors*, Macmillan, pp. 121–133.

Trendelenburg, U. (1966) Mechanisms of supersensitivity and subsensitivity to sympathomimetic amines. *Pharmacol. Rev.*, 18: 629–640.

Ungerstedt, U. (1971) Post-synaptic supersensitivity after 6-hydroxydopamine-induced degeneration of the nigro-striatal dopamine system. *Acta physiol. scand.*, 82, Suppl. 367: 69–93.

Vetulani, J. and Sulser, F. (1975) Action of various antidepressant treatment reduces activity of noradrenergic cyclic AMP-generating system in limbic forebrain. *Nature (Lond.)*, 257: 495–496.

Williams, B.J. and Pirch, J.H. (1974) Correlation between brain adenylcyclase activity and spontaneous motor activity in rats after chronic reserpine treatment. *Brain Res.*, 68: 227–234.

Wirz-Justice, A., Krauchi, K., Lichtsteiner, M. and Feer, H. (1978) Is it possible to modify serotonin receptor sensitivity? *Life Sci.*, 23: 1249–1254.

Worms, P. and Scatton, B. (1977) Tolerance to stereotyped behaviour and to decrease in striatal homovanillic acid levels after repeated treatment with apomorphine dipivaloyl ester. *Europ. J. Pharmacol.*, 45: 395–396.

Wright, D.M. and Roberts, M.H.T. (1978) Supersensitivity to a substance P analogue following dorsal root section. *Life Sci.*, 22: 19–24.

Yarbrough, G.G. and Phillis, J.W. (1975) Supersensitivity of central neurons. A brief review of an emerging concept. *J. Canad. Sci. Neurol.*, Aug: 147–152.

Polyribosomes Associated with Dendritic Spines in the Denervated Dentate Gyrus: Evidence for Local Regulation of Protein Synthesis During Reinnervation

OSWALD STEWARD and BARRY FASS

Departments of Neurosurgery and Physiology, University of Virginia School of Medicine, Charlottesville, VA 22908 (U.S.A.)

Evidence has been steadily accumulating in recent years that neurons of the mature mammalian central nervous system can dramatically remodel their synaptic connections either in response to denervating lesions or in response to patterns of activity (for a collection of reviews, see Cotman, 1978). Many of these observations of neuronal "plasticity" have involved the dendritic spine, where neurons of the mammalian brain, particularly cortical neurons, receive the majority of their excitatory synaptic inputs (Peters et al., 1976). Numerous studies have demonstrated alterations in spine size or number in response to denervation and reinnervation, and in response to alterations in afferent activity (Scheibel and Scheibel, 1968).

The maleability of spines is somewhat difficult to reconcile with classical notions of neuronal cell biology. A major tenet of cellular neurobiology is that the major synthetic activity of the neuron occurs in the cell body. Accordingly, the construction and maintenance of the detailed morphological specializations of the neuron (including the spine and associated postsynaptic membrane specialization) are thought to depend on the specific transport of already synthesized material from the cell body (see Grafstein and Forman, 1980). If spines are adjusted by mechanisms requiring the synthesis of proteins, the modification of spines would seemingly require an elaborate targeted transport system responsive to afferent activity. While such cellular processes are not inconceivable, they would seem to be relatively inefficient for providing materials for the adjustment of individual spines. Consequently, we were intrigued by ultrastructural observations which revealed presumed protein synthetic machinery (polyribosomal rosettes) selectively associated with dendritic spines in the dentate gyrus of the rat's hippocampal formation (Steward and Levy, 1982). This observation assumes special importance since the dentate gyrus is capable of dramatic injury-induced (Lynch et al., 1975; Cotman and Nadler, 1978), and stimulation-induced (Fifkova and Van Harreveld, 1977; Desmond and Levy, 1983) synaptic modifications which are accompanied by adjustments in affected spines. The present chapter summarizes our observations on the changes in the incidence of polyribosomes associated with dendritic spines during post-lesion reinnervation of the dentate granule cells.

Adult male Sprague–Dawley rats were prepared for electron microscopy 2, 4, 6, 8, 10, 12, 14 and approximately 200 days following unilateral lesions of the entorhinal cortex

[131]

(the major source of excitatory synaptic input to the dentate granule cells) (for more details see Steward, 1983). Such lesions extensively denervate the distal dendrites of the granule cells ipsilaterally (Matthews et al., 1976). Indeed, quantitative studies reveal that the lesions remove up to 95% of the synapses on the distal two-thirds of the granule cell's dendritic tree (Steward and Vinsant, 1983). Between approximately 6 and 12 days post-lesion the denervated dendrites are extensively reinnervated through the process of post-lesion synaptogenesis in surviving afferent systems (Lynch et al., 1975). While synaptogenesis does continue at a slower rate after 14 days post-lesion, the period of maximal growth is between 6 and 12 days. The electron microscopic analyses focused on the denervated portion of the granule cell dendrites before and during the period of post-lesion synaptogenesis. Since the projections from the entorhinal area are predominantly ipsilateral with only a very sparse crossed component (Steward et al., 1976), the dentate gyrus contralateral to the lesion served as the control.

As is the case with most mammalian neurons, there are relatively few polyribosomes or segments of rough endoplasmic reticulum in granule cell dendrites. The few polyribosomal clusters which are present decrease in frequency with distance from the soma. The remarkable aspect of the polyribosome clusters in granule cell dendrites was their frequent association with dendritic spines. As illustrated in Fig. 1A and B, polyribosome clusters are found at the intersection between the spine neck and the main dendritic shaft. Clusters containing many ribosomes were found in segments near the soma (Fig. 1A), while in more distal regions the number of ribosomes in the clusters was usually less (see Fig. 1B for a representative illustration of the picture most frequently encountered at mid-proximo-distal locations along the dendrite). Many polyribosome clusters were also found just under "mounds" jutting from the dendritic shaft (see Fig. 1C for a segment of dendrite exhibiting an unusually high density of these). Serial section analysis revealed that many of these mounds represent the base of spines which extend out of the plane of section (see Steward and Levy, 1982). Quantitative analyses reveal that at least 81% of the polyribosomes in mid-proximo-distal locations along the dendrites lay under identified or presumed spine bases (Steward and Levy, 1982). Very rarely, polyribosomes were also observed in spine necks or spine heads, although most of these clusters contained only two to three ribosomes, thus barely meeting the criteria for scoring.

Observations of denervated dendrites revealed changes in the distribution of polyribosome clusters within the denervated segments. First, polyribosomes associated with the spine neck/shaft intersection appeared much more frequently in denervated/reinnervated material than in the control, particularly between 6 and 8 days post-lesion. Second, spine heads with polyribosomes were encountered more frequently during the 6–10 day interval than in the control, with the polyribosome clusters often occupying a position immediately subjacent to the post-synaptic membrane specialization (see Fig. 1D). To provide a quantitative indication of the increased incidence of the polyribosomes at the spine neck/shaft intersections, 21–22 electron micrographs of identified intersections were taken at 10,000× on each side at each post-lesion interval. Intersections were identified as a dendritic shaft with a protrusion devoid of mitochondria and microtubules which was contacted by a presynaptic terminal or which contained a spine apparatus.

As illustrated in Fig. 2A, in control material (contralateral to the lesion) ap-

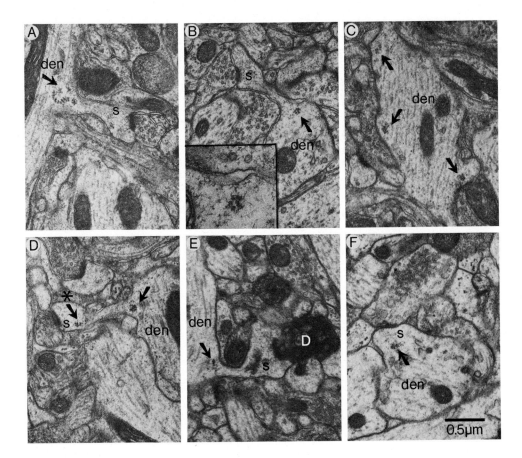

Fig. 1. Polyribosomes associated with dendritic spines. A–C: collections of polyribosomes in dendrites (den) from control material. A: the prominent collections which may be found in spines (s) relatively proximal to the soma. B: the typical appearance of the clusters at mid proximo-distal locations along the dendrite (inset 3× higher magnification). C: collections of polyribosomes at "mounds" in the dendrites which often represent the bases of spines which extend out of the plane of section. D–F: examples of polyribosomes associated with spines in denervated segments of dendrite (6 days post-lesion). D: a spine with collections of polyribosomes not only at the base (unlabeled arrow) but also in the spine head itself, just subjacent to the postsynaptic specialization. E: a spine with polyribosomes at the base which is apposed to a degenerating presynaptic terminal (D). F: a short stubby spine with associated polyribosomes apposed to an immature appearing presynaptic element with large vesicles adjacent to the site of contact.

proximately 12% of the spine neck/shaft intersections contained polyribosomes. On the side ipsilateral to the lesion, the proportion of the intersections containing polyribosomes increased dramatically after the lesions. Little change in incidence was apparent by day 4, but by day 6 incidence had increased almost 3-fold. The peak incidence occurred at 8 days post-lesion, when polyribosomes were found in almost 35% of the spine neck/dendritic shaft intersections (see Fig. 2A). As illustrated in Fig. 2B, the incidence of spine heads or necks with polyribosomes also increased. Again, the changes first appeared at 6 days post-lesion. The incidence of polyribosomes

134

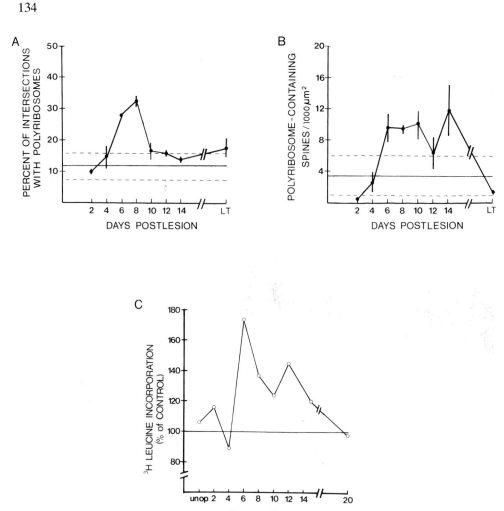

Fig. 2. A: time course of the changes in the incidence of polyribosomes at identified spine neck/dendritic shaft intersections in dendritic zones denervated following lesions of the ipsilateral entorhinal cortex (filled symbols). The incidence of polyribosomes from the control sides of the same animals is illustrated by the solid horizontal lines and the dashed lines indicate ± 1 S.D. around this mean. The bars indicate the range of values in the two animals analyzed at each survival interval. (From Steward, 1983, with permission.) B: the number of polyribosome-containing spines/1000 μm^2 is illustrated from the same material as in A. This is a separate population of spines than those with polyribosomes at the base. Spines were classified as polyribosome-containing if the polyribosomes lay in a spine head immediately subjacent to the postsynaptic membrane specialization or within the spine neck. In either case, spines were classified as polyribosome-containing only if the polyribosomes were well separated from the intersection of the spine and the dendritic shaft. The average incidence of polyribosome-containing spines in the control material is indicated by the solid line, and the dashed lines indicate ± 1 S.D. (From Steward, 1983, with permission.) C: the incorporation of leucine in the denervated neuropil is expressed as a percentage of the contralateral control. (From Fass and Steward, submitted.) At each post-lesion interval, animals were sacrificed 30 min after receiving intravenous injections of [3H]leucine, and their brains were prepared for autoradiography. Incorporation was evaluated by grain counting, and the grain density over the denervated neuropil ipsilateral to the lesion was expressed as a percentage of the grain density over the contralateral control.

at spine neck/shaft intersections and the incidence of polyribosome-containing spines decreased at longer post-lesion survival intervals (see Fig. 2A and B).

Because the principle criterion for the identification of the spine was the presence in the plane of section of the synaptic specialization itself, it was possible to define the nature of the presynaptic elements contacting spines with polyribosomes. As illustrated in Fig. 1D–F, spines with polyribosomes were apposed to both degenerating (Fig. 1E) and intact (Fig. 1D and F) presynaptic elements. A few were also found without contacts by any presynaptic element (empty spines). During the earlier post-lesion intervals (2–6 days) contacts with degenerating presynaptic elements were the rule, while after 6 days, the proportion apposed to intact presynaptic terminals increased. Particularly at 6 and 8 days (which previous evidence would suggest is very early in the period of lesion-induced synaptic proliferation), the "intact" synapses appeared quite immature and occasionally contained relatively large vesicles (Fig. 1F) reminiscent of those found in presumed axonal growth cones in developing animals (Vaughn and Sims, 1978).

The present observations assume special importance when considered within the context of other observations on the denervation and reinnervation of the dentate gyrus following entorhinal cortical lesions. As noted above, the reinnervation of the granule cells begins approximately 6 days post-lesion and continues at a rapid rate between 8 and 12 days. As is evident from Fig. 2A and B, the increase in the incidence of polyribosomes corresponds to the period of maximal growth. Given this fact, it is certainly tempting to speculate that these polyribosomes might be responsible for the synthesis of some protein or proteins critical to the preparation of the dendrite for reinnervation (such as degradation of obsolete contacts or the synthesis of new synaptic material) or perhaps even for some protein associated with the induction of the synaptogenesis itself. Other studies designed to analyze incorporation of protein precursors autoradiographically (after the method of Droz and Leblond, 1963) have revealed increased incorporation in the denervated neuropil (Fass and Steward, 1981, and submitted). Grain density in the autoradiographic preparations was higher in the denervated neuropil with respect to the contralateral control between 6 and 15 days post-lesion (see Fig. 2C). The parallel between the time course of increased incorporation and increased incidence of polyribosomes in spines certainly suggests that there might be a relationship between these two.

The increases in the incidence of polyribosomes and incorporation of protein precursors during the early part of the reinnervation period suggest a role for these processes in the reinnervation process. It is not clear whether the changes are in response to the reinnervation, or whether the reinnervation is in response to the reactive processes within the dendrite. Whatever the role of these processes during reinnervation, the strategic location of the polyribosomes certainly invites the speculation that they might make specific proteins for their associated postsynaptic specialization and, further, that their synthetic activity might be directly modified by functional activity at the synapse. Such notions provide new ways of thinking about how specialized regions of individual dendrites might be *locally* regulated rather than depending on the synthetic activities of the neuronal somata.

136

ACKNOWLEDGEMENTS

Thanks to Ms. S.A. Vinsant for her excellent technical help. Supported by NIH Grant NS-12333 to O.S. O.S. is the recipient of Research Career Development Award NS-00325.

REFERENCES

Cotman, C.W. (Ed.) (1978) *Neuronal Plasticity,* Raven Press, New York, 335 pp.

Cotman, C.W. and Nadler, J. (1978) Reactive synaptogenesis in the hippocampus. In C.W. Cotman (Ed.), *Neuronal Plasticity,* Raven Press, New York, pp. 227–271.

Desmond, N.L. and Levy, W.B. (1983) Synaptic correlates of associative potentiation/depression: an ultrastructural study in the hippocampus. *Brain Res.,* in press.

Droz, B. and Leblond, C.P. (1963) Axonal migration of proteins in the central nervous system and peripheral nerves as shown by radioautography. *J. comp. Neurol.,* 121: 325–346.

Fass, B. and Steward, O. (1981) Increases of protein-precursor incorporation in the denervated neuropil of rat dentate gyrus during sprouting. *Anat. Rec.,* 199: 80A.

Fifkova, E. and Van Harreveld, A. (1977) Long-lasting morphological changes in dendritic spines of dentate granule cells following stimulation of entorhinal area. *J. Neurocytol.,* 6: 211–230.

Grafstein, B. and Forman, D.S. (1980) Intracellular transport in neurons. *Physiol. Rev.,* 60: 1167–1283.

Lynch, G., Rose, G., Gall, C. and Cotman, C.W. (1975) The response of the dentate gyrus to partial deafferentation. In M. Santini (Ed.), *Golgi Centennial Symposium: Perspectives in Neurobiology,* Raven, New York, pp. 305–317.

Matthews, D.A., Cotman, C. and Lynch, G. (1976) An electron microscopic study of lesion-induced synaptogenesis in the dentate gyrus of the adult rat. II. Reappearance of morphologically normal synaptic contacts. *Brain Res.,* 115: 23–41.

Peters, A., Palay, S.L. and Webster, H. deF. (Eds.) (1976) *The Fine Structure of the Nervous System: The Neurons and Supporting Cells,* W.B. Saunders Co., Philadelphia, PA.

Scheibel, M.E. and Scheibel, A.B. (1968) On the nature of dendritic spines – report of a workshop. *Commun. Behav. Biol.,* Part A., 1: 231–265.

Steward, O. (1983) Alterations in polyribosomes associated with dendritic spines during the reinnervation of the dentate gyrus of the adult rat. *J. Neurosci.,* in press.

Steward, O. and Levy, W.B. (1982) Preferential localization of polyribosomes under the base of dentritic spines in granule cells of the dentate gyrus. *J. Neurosci.,* 2: 284–291.

Steward, O. and Vinsant, S.L. (1983) The process of reinnervation in the dentate gyrus of the adult rat: a quantitative electron microscopic analysis of terminal proliferation and reactive synaptogenesis. *J. comp. Neurol.,* in press.

Steward, O., Cotman, C.W. and Lynch, G. (1976) A quantitative autoradiographic and electrophysiological study of the reinnervation of the dentate gyrus by the contralateral entorhinal cortex following ipsilateral entorhinal lesions. *Brain Res.,* 114: 181–200.

Vaughn, J.E. and Sims, T.J. (1978) Axonal growth cones and developing axonal collaterals form synaptic junctions in embryonic mouse spinal cord. *J. Neurocytol.,* 7: 337–363.

Autoradiographic Localization of Binding Sites for Inhibitory Amino Acids and Their Antagonists in Cultured Rat CNS

ELISABETH HÖSLI and L. HÖSLI

Department of Physiology, University of Basel, Vesalgasse 1, CH-4051 Basel (Switzerland)

INTRODUCTION

From biochemical and electrophysiological studies there is considerable evidence that GABA, glycine, and possibly also β-alanine, are inhibitory transmitters in the mammalian CNS. The action of GABA is blocked by its antagonist bicuculline, whereas the effects of glycine and β-alanine are antagonized by strychnine (for refs. see Curtis and Johnston, 1974). Biochemical studies of binding to particulate fractions of CNS tissue have revealed a high density of GABA- and bicuculline-binding in the cerebellum (Enna et al., 1975; Möhler and Okada, 1977a; DeFeudis, 1979; De Feudis et al., 1980), whereas binding sites for glycine, β-alanine and strychnine were mainly observed in the spinal cord and brainstem (Snyder, 1975; DeFeudis et al., 1977; DeFeudis, 1979). Since nervous tissue cultures have proved to be a suitable model system to demonstrate binding sites for neurotransmitters by means of autoradiography, we have studied the cellular localization of binding of [^{3}H]GABA, [^{3}H]glycine, [^{3}H]β-alanine and their antagonists (+)[^{3}H]bicuculline and [^{3}H]strychnine, respectively, in cultures of rat cerebellum, brainstem and spinal cord.

MATERIALS AND METHODS

Explant cultures were prepared from the cerebellum, lower brainstem and spinal cord of fetal (17–18 days in utero) or newborn rats. The cultures were grown either in Maximov double-coverslip assemblies or in Roller tubes for 10–48 days at 35 °C (for details see Hösli et al., 1980). For the binding studies, the cultures were washed for 15 min to 1 h either in normal Na$^+$-containing Tyrode solution or in Na$^+$-free medium (Na$^+$ being replaced by choline and Tris). Afterwards, the cultures were incubated for 15 min to 1 h in normal medium (at 0 °C to block active transport processes; see DeFeudis, 1978) or in Na$^+$-free medium (35 °C) containing the labeled compounds. To provide estimates of the "specific" binding of the radioligands, unlabeled GABA, glycine, bicuculline and strychnine (10^{-3} M) were added to the pre- and incubation media (Hösli et al., 1980; Hösli and Hösli, 1981). After fixation and dehydration, Ilford L4 emulsion was placed over the cultures by the loop technique. The autoradiographs were stored for 3–5 weeks at 4 °C and then developed with a Kodak D19 developer.

[137]

Some cultures were also incubated with the benzodiazepine [³H]flunitrazepam using the method described by Möhler et al. (1980).

RESULTS AND DISCUSSION

Binding of [³H]GABA, [³H]muscimol, (+)[³H]bicuculline and [³H]flunitrazepam ([³H]FNZP)

In *cerebellar cultures*, binding sites for [³H]GABA, [³H]muscimol and (+)-[³H]bicuculline were found on many neurons (Hösli and Hösli, 1980a, b; Hösli et al., 1980). Large neurons which, from their size and shape seem to be Purkinje cells (Fig. 1A, B), as well as neurons appearing to be interneurons such as stellate, basket or Golgi cells (Fig. 1C), were labeled by the radioligands over the cell bodies and processes. [³H]FNZP was also bound to many cultured Purkinje cells (Fig. 1E) and interneurons (Fig. 1F), this being consistent with biochemical and autoradiographic binding studies on rat cerebellar slices (Möhler and Okada, 1977b; Young and Kuhar, 1979; Wamsley et al., 1981).

Many small neurons, probably granule cells, did not reveal binding sites for [³H]GABA and [³H]muscimol on their cell bodies, but were surrounded by a great number of fibers, probably dendrites and axons, which were intensely labeled (Hösli and Hösli, 1980a, b). Autoradiographic binding studies on cerebellar slices have also demonstrated a high density of GABA binding sites in the granule cell layer and it was suggested that granule cell dendrites might receive inhibitory terminals from the Golgi cells in the cerebellar glomeruli (Palacios et al., 1980; Wamsley et al., 1981).

Binding of all radioligands was also observed on fibers, probably unmyelinated axons, which were growing out from the explant (Fig. 1D), suggesting the existence of non-synaptic GABA receptors. This suggestion is supported by electrophysiological studies demonstrating that GABA causes a depolarization of unmyelinated axons (Brown and Marsh, 1978).

In *brainstem cultures*, there was a relatively great number of large- and medium-sized neurons showing binding sites for [³H]GABA, [³H]bicuculline and [³H]FNZP, whereas in *spinal cord cultures*, mainly small to medium-sized neurons, probably interneurons, were labeled (Fig. 2A, B; Hösli et al., 1980). It was often observed that labeled fibers approached large unlabeled neurons appearing to make contact with these cells (Hösli et al., 1980).

Fig. 1. A: cerebellar culture after incubation with [³H]GABA (10^{-8} M, Na⁺-free incubation medium). The cell bodies and processes of the (presumed) Purkinje cells are heavily labeled (culture 21 days in vitro). Bar = 30 μm. B: large cerebellar neurons, probably Purkinje cells, labeled by [³H]bicuculline methiodide (10^{-8} M, Na⁺-free incubation medium). Note intense labeling over the initial part of the axon (arrow)(culture 12 days in vitro). Bar = 50 μm. C: cerebellar neurons having the appearance of interneurons which show binding sites for [³H]GABA (10^{-8} M, Na⁺-containing incubation medium, culture 23 days in vitro). Bar = 30 μm. D: labeled fibers (probably unmyelinated axons) growing out from the explant of a cerebellar culture after incubation with [³H]muscimol (10^{-8} M, Na⁺-free incubation medium, culture 23 days in vitro). Bar = 30 μm. E: cerebellar culture after incubation with [³H]flunitrazepam (3 nM). The Purkinje cells show binding sites over their cell bodies, the primary and secondary dendrites (arrows) (culture 17 days in vitro). Bar = 50 μm. F: cerebellar interneurons labeled by [³H]flunitrazepam (3 nM, culture 17 days in vitro). Bar = 30 μm. (From Hösli et al., 1980, with permission.)

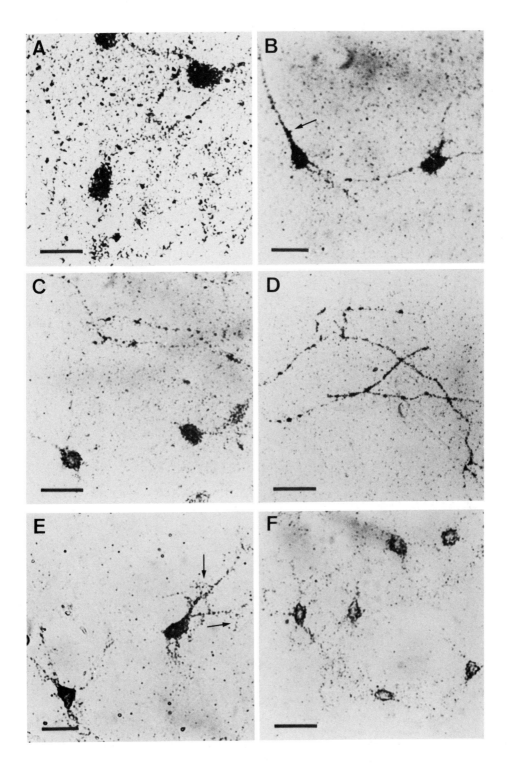

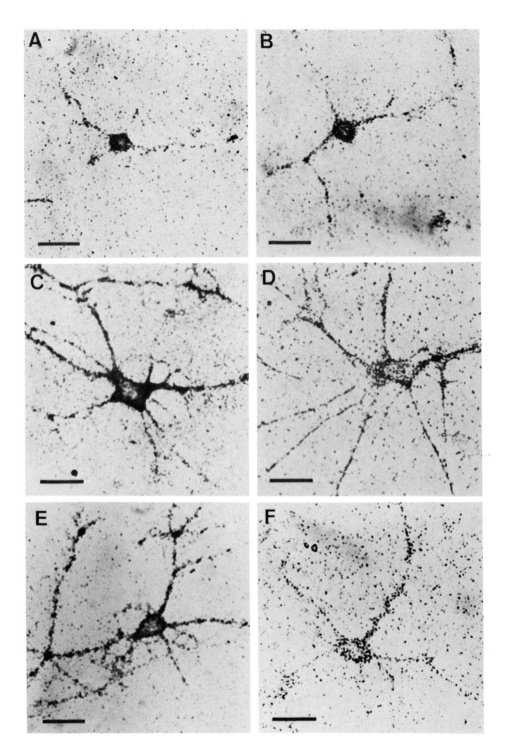

Binding of [³H]GABA, [³H]muscimol and [³H]bicuculline was markedly reduced or inhibited by adding unlabeled GABA or bicuculline (10^{-3} M) to the pre- and incubation media (Hösli and Hösli, 1980a, b; Hösli et al., 1980). Binding of [³H]FNZP was inhibited by adding the pharmacologically potent benzodiazepine Ro-11-7800 (Hösli et al., 1980).

Binding of [³H]glycine, [³H]β-alanine and [³H]strychnine

In contrast to the great number of binding sites for [³H]GABA and [³H]bicuculline on cultured *cerebellar* neurons, no, or only little, binding was observed for [³H]glycine, [³H]β-alanine and [³H]strychnine (Hösli and Hösli, 1981). In *brainstem* cultures, however, a relatively large number of medium-sized and large neurons were labeled by all radioligands (Fig. 2E; Hösli and Hösli, 1981). In *spinal cord cultures* mainly large neurons, probably motoneurons, showed binding sites for [³H]glycine and [³H]strychnine (Fig. 2C, D; Hösli and Hösli, 1981), whereas [³H]GABA and [³H]bicuculline were predominantly bound to interneurons (Fig. 2A, B). Our findings with [³H]glycine and [³H]strychnine are consistent with autoradiographic studies on brainstem and spinal cord sections, demonstrating high levels of glycine receptors in these regions (Palacios et al., 1981), as well as with electrophysiological investigations suggesting that glycine is an inhibitory neurotransmitter in the brainstem (Hösli and Tebēcis, 1970) and spinal cord (Curtis et al., 1968; Curtis and Johnston, 1974).

[³H]β-Alanine was bound to large and medium-sized neurons in brainstem and spinal cord cultures (Fig. 2F; Hösli and Hösli, 1981). However, binding of this amino acid was usually weaker than that of [³H]glycine, being consistent with biochemical studies on synaptosomal fractions from brainstem and spinal cord which have demonstrated that the B_{max} for highest-affinity β-alanine binding was an order of magnitude lower than that for glycine (DeFeudis et al., 1977). Adding unlabeled glycine and strychnine (10^{-3} M) to the incubation media markedly reduced binding with [³H]glycine, [³H]strychnine and [³H]β-alanine (Hösli and Hösli, 1981).

Glial cells

In contrast to uptake studies where almost all glial cells have accumulated amino acid transmitters (Fig. 3B) (for refs. see Hösli and Hösli, 1976, 1978), no binding sites for all radioligands studied were observed on glial elements (Fig. 3A, Hösli and Hösli, 1980a, b, 1981; Hösli et al., 1980, 1981a). Biochemical studies have also demonstrated that [³H]GABA and [³H]muscimol are not bound to subcellular particles prepared from cultured astroblasts (Ossola et al., 1979), whereas a great number of binding sites were observed on similar fractions prepared from neuron-enriched cultures (DeFeudis et al., 1980). Our finding that only neurons and not glial cells have binding sites for GABA,

---

Fig. 2. A and B: medium-sized spinal neurons, probably interneurons, showing binding sites for [³H]GABA (10^{-8} M, Na⁺-containing medium), and [³H]bicuculline methiodide (10^{-8} M, Na⁺-free incubation medium) respectively (cultures 18 days in vitro). C: spinal cord culture (30 days in vitro) after incubation with [³H]glycine (10^{-8} M, Na⁺-containing incubation medium). The cell body and processes of the large neuron, probably a motoneuron, are heavily labeled. D: large spinal neuron showing binding sites for [³H]strychnine (10^{-8} M, Na⁺-containing incubation medium). Culture 21 days in vitro. E: binding of [³H]glycine (10^{-8} M, Na⁺-free incubation medium) to a medium-sized brainstem neuron. Culture 20 days in vitro. F: brainstem neuron labeled with [³H]β-alanine (10^{-8} M, Na⁺-containing incubation medium). Culture 21 days in vitro. Bars = 30 μm. (A and B from Hösli et al., 1980; C–F from Hösli and Hösli, 1981, with permission.)

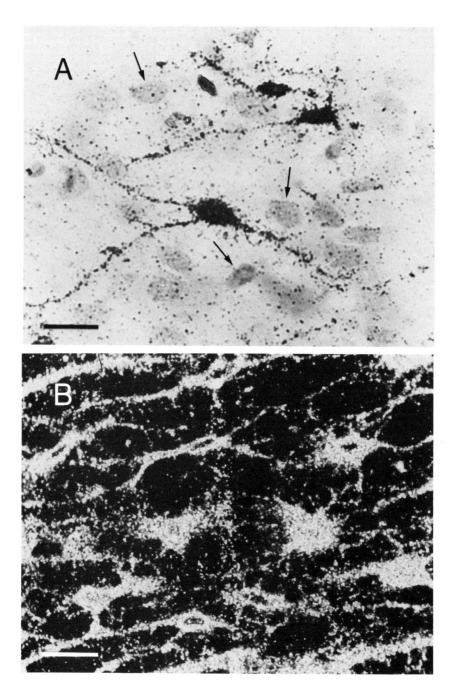

Fig. 3. Binding (A) and uptake (B) of [³H]GABA. A: large cerebellar neurons, resembling Purkinje cells, which are intensely labeled by [³H]GABA (10^{-8} M). Note that the glial cells (arrows) are almost free of label (culture 26 days in vitro, counterstained with cresyl violet). B: intensely labeled glial cells in the outgrowth zone of an 18-day-old cerebellar culture after incubation with [³H]GABA, 10^{-6} M for 10 min. Dark-field illumination. Bars = 30 μm. (A from Hösli et al., 1981a: B from Hösli and Hösli, 1976, with permission.)

glycine and β-alanine, are consistent with electrophysiological studies indicating that, unlike neurons, glial cells do not possess receptors for these amino acid transmitters (Hösli et al., 1981b).

SUMMARY

Autoradiographic binding studies have shown that in cerebellar cultures, many large neurons, probably Purkinje cells and interneurons, have binding sites for [³H]GABA, [³H]muscimol and [³H]bicuculline, whereas almost no labeling was found with [³H]glycine, [³H]β-alanine and [³H]strychnine. In brainstem cultures, all amino acids and their antagonists were bound to a relatively great number of neurons of varying size. In cultures from spinal cord, binding of [³H]GABA and [³H]bicuculline was mainly observed on small- and medium-sized neurons, whereas [³H]glycine, [³H]β-alanine and [³H]strychnine were usually bound to large cells, probably motoneurons.

No binding of any radioligand was observed on glial cells, whereas in uptake studies almost all glial elements show accumulation of the amino acids. The finding that only neurons but not glial cells show binding sites for GABA, glycine and β-alanine, is consistent with electrophysiological studies indicating that, unlike neurons, glial cells have no receptors for these neurotransmitters and that the amino acid-induced depolarization of glial elements is an indirect effect caused by the efflux of K^+ from neighboring neurons.

ACKNOWLEDGEMENT

We are grateful to Miss S. Zeugin for skillful technical assistance.

REFERENCES

Brown, D.A. and Marsh, S. (1978) Axonal GABA-receptors in mammalian peripheral nerve trunks. *Brain Res.*, 156: 187–191.

Curtis, D.R. and Johnston, G.A.R. (1974) Amino acid transmitters in the mammalian central nervous system. In *Reviews of Physiology, Vol. LXIX*, Springer-Verlag, Berlin, pp. 97–188.

Curtis, D.R., Hösli, L., Johnston, G.A.R. and Johnston, I.H. (1968) The hyperpolarization of spinal motoneurones by glycine and related amino acids. *Exp. Brain Res.*, 5: 235–258.

DeFeudis, F.V. (1978) Can the binding of GABA, glycine and β-alanine to synaptic receptors be determined in the presence of a physiological concentration of Na^+? *Experientia*, 34: 1314–1315.

DeFeudis, F.V. (1979) Binding and iontophoretic studies on centrally active amino acids – a search for physiological receptors. *Int. Rev. Neurobiol.*, 21: 129–216.

DeFeudis, F.V., Orensanz Muñoz, L.M., Moya, M.F., Latorre, A. and Fando, J.L. (1977) High-affinity, Na^+-independent, strychnine-sensitive binding sites for β-alanine in a synaptosome-enriched fraction of rat CNS. *Gen. Pharmacol.*, 8: 311–314.

DeFeudis, F.V., Ossola, L., Sarliève, L.L., Schmitt, G., Roussel, G., Rebel, G., Wolff, P., Varga, V. and Mandel, P. (1980) Receptors for [³H]muscimol and for [³H]GABA in neurone-enriched cultures. *Brain Res. Bull.*, 5, Suppl. 2: 201–208.

Enna, S.J., Kuhar, M.J. and Snyder, S.H. (1975) Regional distribution of postsynaptic receptor binding for gamma-aminobutyric acid (GABA) in monkey brain. *Brain Res.*, 93: 168–174.

Hösli, E. and Hösli, L. (1976) Autoradiographic studies on the uptake of ³H-noradrenaline and ³H-GABA in cultured rat cerebellum. *Exp. Brain Res.*, 26: 319–324.

144

Hösli, E. and Hösli, L. (1980a) Autoradiographic localization of ^{3}H-GABA and ^{3}H-muscimol binding in rat cerebellar cultures. *Exp. Brain Res.*, 38: 241–243.

Hösli, E. and Hösli, L. (1980b) Autoradiographic localization of GABA receptors in cultures of rat cerebellum. *Brain Res. Bull.*, 5, Suppl. 2: 149–154.

Hösli, E. and Hösli, L. (1981) Binding of [^{3}H]glycine, [^{3}H]β-alanine and [^{3}H]strychnine in cultured rat spinal cord and brain stem. *Brain Res.*, 213: 242–245.

Hösli, L. and Hösli, E. (1978) Action and uptake of neurotransmitters in CNS tissue culture. *Rev. Physiol. Biochem. Pharmacol.*, 81: 135–188.

Hösli, L. and Tebēcis, A.K. (1970) Actions of amino acids and convulsants on bulbar reticular neurones. *Exp. Brain Res.*, 11, 111–127.

Hösli, E., Möhler, H., Richards, J.G. and Hösli, L. (1980) Autoradiographic localization of binding sites for [^{3}H]γ-aminobutyrate, [^{3}H]muscimol, (+)[^{3}H]bicuculline methiodide and [^{3}H]flunitrazepam in cultures of rat cerebellum and spinal cord. *Neuroscience*, 5: 1657–1665.

Hösli, L., Hösli, E., Andrès, P.F. and Landolt, H. (1981a) GABA and glycine receptors in CNS cultures: autoradiographic binding and electrophysiological studies. In F.V. DeFeudis and P. Mandel (Eds.), *Amino Acid Neurotransmitters*, Raven Press, New York, pp. 437–443.

Hösli, L., Hösli, E., Andrès, P.F. and Landolt, H. (1981b) Evidence that the depolarization of glial cells by inhibitory amino acids is caused by an efflux of K$^+$ from neurones. *Exp. Brain Res.*, 42: 43–48.

Möhler, H. and Okada, T. (1977a) GABA receptor binding with [^{3}H](+)bicuculline-methiodide in rat CNS. *Nature (Lond.)*, 267: 65–67.

Möhler, H. and Okada, T. (1977b) Benzodiazepine receptor: demonstration in the central nervous system. *Science*, 198: 849–851.

Möhler, H., Battersby, M.K. and Richards, J.G. (1980) Benzodiazepine receptor protein identified and visualized in brain tissue by a novel type of photoaffinity label. *Proc. nat. Acad. Sci. U.S.A.*, 77: 1666–1670.

Ossola, L., DeFeudis, F.V. and Mandel, P. (1979) Lack of Na$^+$-independent [^{3}H]GABA binding to particulate fractions of cultured astroblasts of rat brain. *J. Neurochem.*, 34: 1026–1029.

Palacios, J.M., Scott Young, III, W. and Kuhar, M.J. (1980) Autoradiographic localization of γ-aminobutyric acid (GABA) receptors in the rat cerebellum. *Proc. nat. Acad. Sci. U.S.A.*, 77: 670–674.

Palacios, J.M., Wamsley, J.K., Zarbin, M.A. and Kuhar, M.J. (1981) GABA and glycine receptors in rat brain: autoradiographic localization. In P. Mandel and F.V. DeFeudis (Eds.), *Amino Acid Transmitters*, Raven Press, New York, pp. 445–451.

Synder, S.H. (1975) The glycine synaptic receptor in the mammalian central nervous system. *Brit. J. Pharmacol.*, 53: 473–484.

Wamsley, J.K., Palacios, J.M., Young, III, W.S. and Kuhar, M.J. (1981) Autoradiographic determination of neurotransmitter receptor distributions in the cerebral and cerebellar cortices. *J. Histochem. Cytochem.*, 29: 125–135.

Young, III, W.S. and Kuhar, M.J. (1979) Autoradiographic localisation of benzodiazepine receptors in the brains of humans and animals. *Nature (Lond.)*, 280: 393–395.

Principles of Functional Architecture
of the Central Nervous System

Rhythm Generator Circuits in a Simple Nervous System

GUNTHER S. STENT

Department of Molecular Biology, University of California, Berkeley, CA 94720 (U.S.A.)

THE LEECH NERVOUS SYSTEM

The comparatively simple central nervous system of the leech consists of a nerve cord of 32 segmentally iterated ganglia (Fig. 1). The rostral four and caudal seven segmental ganglia are fused, constituting a head and a tail ganglion, respectively. The other, unfused, or abdominal ganglia, are numbered rostrocaudally from 1 to 21. Each contains about 400 bilaterally paired neurons, as well as a few unpaired neurons. Sensory and effector neurons project their processes to targets outside the CNS via segmental nerves, whose roots emerge from the lateral edge of the ganglion. The anatomy of the leech ganglion is sufficiently stereotyped so that about one-quarter of the neurons of the segmental ganglion of the medicinal leech, *Hirudo medicinalis* have by now been identified according to various criteria, including function (Fig. 1). Thus, some cells have been classified as sensory, others as motor neurons, and yet others as interneurons, and their connectivity has been elucidated. These surveys have culminated in the description of sensory and motor pathways and of neuronal circuits controlling various reflexes, such as body shortening and raising the body wall into ridges. (A general account of leech neurobiology can be found in Muller et al., 1981.) The most complex behavioral routines of the leech of which accounts have so far been given in terms of networks of identified neurons are the heartbeat (Stent et al., 1979) and swimming rhythms (Stent et al., 1978).

HEARTBEAT RHYTHM

The "heart" of *Hirudo* consists of two contractile lateral vessels, or heart tubes, which form part of a closed circulatory system, comprising also a dorsal vessel and a ventral vessel, as well as minor, transverse channels and capillaries that irrigate the segmental body tissues (Fig. 2). The walls of the heart tubes are ringed by muscles. The periodic contraction of these heart muscles forms the heartbeat that circulates the blood through this vascular system. The heartbeat pattern is not bilaterally symmetric. On the *peristaltic* body side, the segmental heart-tube sections constrict in a rear-to-front sequence, producing a frontward peristalsis. On the *synchronic* body side the sections constrict almost simultaneously. Peristaltic and synchronic heartbeat modes are not permanent features of right and left sides; every few minutes the peristaltic side switches to the synchronic mode and the synchronic side switches to the peristaltic mode. The heartbeat rhythm is mediated by a set of rhythmically

148

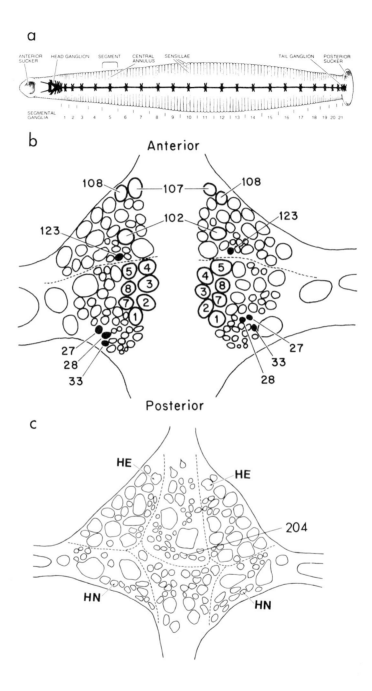

Fig. 1. a: schematic view of the segmental body plan of the leech and of its central nervous system, from the ventral aspect. The sensillae are circumferentially distributed segmental sensory organs containing mechano- and photoreceptors. b: dorsal aspect of the segmental ganglion of *Hirudo medicinalis*, showing the cell bodies of identified motor neurons (heavy outline) and of interneurons (solid black) related to the generation of the swimming rhythm. The cells are numbered according to the system of Ort et al. (1974). c: ventral aspect of the segmental ganglion of *H. medicinalis*, showing location of the cell bodies of the heart excitor motor neuron (HE), the heart interneuron (HN) and the swim initiator interneuron (204).

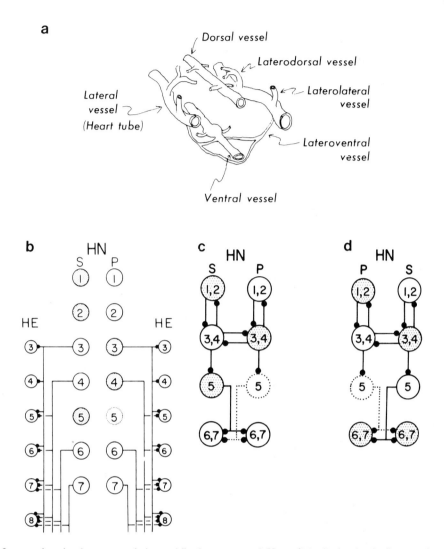

Fig. 2. a: major circulatory vessels in a midbody segment of *H. medicinalis*. b: circuit diagram showing inhibitory connections between HN and HE cells, with the left side beating in the synchronic (S) and the right side in the peristaltic (P) constriction mode. A line leaving an HN cell and ending with a solid circle upon an HE cell is an identified inhibitory synaptic link. HN cells with matching shading (white or stippled) are active roughly in phase; those with contrasting shading are active in antiphase. (The HN(5) cell shown in dotted outline is inactive.) c and d: simplified bilateral circuit diagram of inhibitory connections linking the HN cells. HN cells that are active in nearly the same phase and share the same connectivity pattern are represented as a single circle. c: left side beating in the S and right side in the P mode. d: left side beating in P and right side in the S mode. (After Peterson and Calabrese, 1982.)

active, excitatory motor neurons designated as *heart excitors*, or HE cells (Thompson and Stent, 1976a). Paired HE cells, which innervate the circular muscles of the ipsilateral segmental heart-tube, are present in segmental ganglia 3–19 of the nerve cord. The HE cell activity cycles, in which bursts of action potentials alternate with bursts of inhibitory synaptic potentials, are phase-locked in a manner that corresponds to the segmental heart-tube constriction pattern. Thus on the peristaltic side, the HE cell activity cycles maintain a frontward phase progression, whereas on the synchronic side the activity cycles are nearly in phase. Moreover, a right-left switch in heartbeat coordination mode is reflected in a corresponding phase transition in the HE cell activity cycles (Thompson and Stent, 1976a; Calabrese, 1977, 1979a). Since the characteristic activity pattern of HE cells occurs in a completely isolated nerve cord, it follows that the coordinated heartbeat rhythm is produced by a central rhythm generator that does not require sensory input for its patterned output.

The source of bursts of inhibitory synaptic potentials in HE cells is a set of bilateral pairs of rhythmically active *heart interneurons*, or HN cells (Thompson and Stent, 1979b). Heart interneurons have been identified in segmental ganglia 1–7 in the position shown in Fig. 1. Like the HE cell, the HN cell generates an impulse burst during its active phase and receives a burst of inhibitory synaptic potentials during its inactive phase. The manner in which HN cells of ganglia 3, 4, 6 and 7 are connected via inhibitory synapses to a series of ipsilateral HE cells in posterior ganglia is shown in Fig. 2, where also the phase relations of the activity cycles of the HN cells are indicated. It should be noted that of the HN(5) cell pair, only the cell on the synchronic side is rhythmically active, while its contralateral homologue on the peristaltic side is inactive. During transitions from peristaltic to synchronic coordination modes the phase of the activity cycles of the HN(6) and HN(7) cell pairs shifts, while the activity cycle phases of cells HN(1), HN(2), HN(3) and HN(4) remain invariant. However the transition is accompanied by the reactivation of the inactive HN(5) on the previously peristaltic side and its resumption of an activity cycle antiphasic to its ipsilateral cells HN(3) and HN(4).

We can now consider how the activity pattern of the HN cells imposes the peristaltic and synchronic activity modes on the HE cells. On the synchronic side, where all relevant HN activity cycles occur in nearly the same phase, the HE cell cycles would likewise occur in very nearly the same phase. But on the peristaltic side, where the activity cycles of the HN cells are out of phase, the HE cell cycles would form a peristaltic phase progression. This peristaltic progression is governed by three factors. First, the more anterior HN cell in each of the combined cell pairs of Fig. 2 is active in a somewhat earlier phase than is the posterior cell. Second, there exists an additional, bilaterally paired HN cell whose presence is known only by its synaptic effects on HE cells and other HN cells. This cell, called HN(X), is active in antiphase to the other HN cells on the synchronic side and is active in phase with HN(3) and HN(4) on the peristaltic side. Third, the inhibitory connections that link HN cells with HE cells manifest *presynaptic modulation*, or an increase in amplitude of the inhibitory synaptic potentials in the HE cell as the presynaptic HN cell is depolarized (Thompson and Stent, 1976c; Nicholls and Wallace, 1978). Since, moreover, each HN cell is linked via rectifying electric junctions to axons of anterior HN cells passing through the ganglion, the cyclical variations in membrane potential of each HN cell influence the amplitude of the inhibitory synaptic potentials evoked not only by its own impulses but also by impulses of the other HN cells to which that HN cell is electrically linked. Thus the blending of the inhibitory synaptic output of the set of HN cells can provide a reasonably quantitative account of the observed HE cell cycle phase relations on both peristaltic and synchronic sides, based on the pattern of HN–HE cell synaptic links shown in Fig. 2 and on the known relative phase relations of the HN cell activity cycles (Thompson and Stent, 1976c). The coordination of the HN cell activity rhythms is, in turn, produced by the network of inhibitory connections shown in Fig. 2 (Thompson and Stent, 1976c; Calabrese, 1977; Peterson and Calabrese, 1982). To a first approximation, the diagrams of Fig. 2 account for most of the observed phase relations of the HN and HE cell activity cycles responsible for generating the heartbeat.

If a rhythmically active neuron is part of a rhythm generator, then an evoked transient excitation or inhibition of that neuron *should shift the phase of the rhythm*. According to this criterion, the frontmost HN cells qualify as components of the rhythm generator: passage of depolarizing current into cells HN(1), HN(2), HN(3) or HN(4), causing impulses during their inactive phase, permanently shifts the phase of the heartbeat rhythm (Thompson and Stent, 1976b; Peterson and Calabrese, 1981). There is indirect evidence that HN cells can produce an endogenous polarization rhythm. They continue to be rhythmically active if deprived of inhibitory synaptic input by bathing the nerve cord preparation in chloride-free saline (Calabrese, 1979b). Moreover, the capacity to generate the rhythm is a property not only of the HN cell body but of several independent impulse-initiation sites located in the intersegmental HN cell axons (Thompson and Stent, 1976b, c; Calabrese, 1980). It should be noted, however, that there are also abundant reciprocal inhibitory connections within the HN cell network which could contribute to the generation of the rhythm, in accord with the "half center" oscillator model (McDougall, 1903; Brown, 1911; Harmon and Lewis, 1966).

SWIMMING RHYTHM

Hirudo swims by undulating its extended and flattened body in the dorsoventral plane, forming a wave that travels from head to tail. The moving crests of the body wave are produced by progressively phase-delayed contractile rhythms of the ventral body wall of successive segments and the moving troughs by similar, but antiphasic contractile rhythms of the dorsal body wall (Fig. 3). The forces exerted against the water by these changes in body form provide the propulsion that drives the leech forward. The period of the segmental contractile rhythm ranges from about 400 msec for fast to about 2000 msec for slow swimming (Kristan et al., 1974a). The periodic changes in length of the dorsal and ventral body wall segments are produced by the phasic local contraction of longitudinal muscles embedded in the body wall that are innervated by an ensemble of excitatory and inhibitory motor neurons in the corresponding segmental ganglion. It is the rhythmic impulse activity of this motor neuron ensemble that drives the local contraction and distension of the segmental musculature (Ort et al., 1974).

The motor neurons that participate in the swimming rhythm are located on the dorsal aspect of the segmental ganglion (Fig. 1). During swimming, these motor neurons produce impulse bursts in four phase angles of approximately 0°, 90°, 180° and 270°, as shown in Fig. 3. Inasmuch as the time taken for the body wave to travel from head to tail is about equal to the swim period (so that the body of the swimming leech forms one spatial wave length), the impulse burst phase of each of these motor neurons leads that of its serial homolog in the next posterior segmental ganglion by about 20° (Kristan et al., 1974b). The motor neurons of a completely isolated nerve cord, deprived of all sensory input from the body wall, can exhibit sustained episodes of swimming activity. Hence the basic swimming rhythm, like the

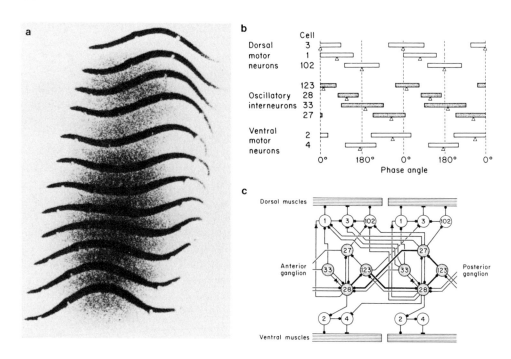

Fig. 3. a: the body wave of swimming *H. medicinalis*, as seen in a composite print of successive frames of a cinematographic record of a free-swimming specimen. The right-to-left displacement of the animal depicts its true progress in the water. The time occupied by this episode, which corresponds to one cycle period, is about 400 msec. b: summary phase diagram of the swimming activity cycles of the oscillatory interneurons and of a representative subset of the motor neurons. Each bar indicates the duration of the impulse burst of the cell, and the triangle under each bar points to the burst midpoint. The burst midpoint of cell 3 has been arbitrarily assigned the phase angle 0°. c: summary circuit diagram of identified synaptic connections between interneurons (shown as shaded circles), motor neurons (shown as plain circles), and longitudinal muscles responsible for the swimming rhythm. Meaning of symbols: T joint, excitatory synapse; filled circle, inhibitory synapse; diode, rectifying electrical junction. The connections forming the basic, 5-membered recurrent cyclic inhibition ring are shown as heavy lines.

heartbeat rhythm, is produced by a central rhythm generator whose oscillatory activity pattern is generated independently of any proprioceptive feedback (Kristan and Calabrese, 1976).

Four bilateral pairs of interneurons, designated as cells 27, 28, 33 and 123, were identified as the component elements of this swimming oscillator in each of the segmental ganglia (Fig. 1) (Friesen et al., 1978). During swimming episodes, these interneurons produce impulse bursts in four phase angles similar to those of the motor neuron activity cycles, as shown in Fig. 3, and their serial homologs in successive ganglia maintain a rostrocaudal phase lead of 20°. These interneurons are evidently part of the oscillator network, because transient passage of depolarizing current into any of them shifts the phase of the rhythm. The oscillator interneurons impose the swimming rhythm on the motor neurons via a set of identified excitatory and inhibitory connections (Poon et al., 1978) (Fig. 3). The oscillator interneurons do not possess an endogenous polarization rhythm; instead their impulse burst activity derives from their assembly into an oscillatory network. This network consists of both intraganglionic and interganglionic synaptic connections of serial homologs of

the four oscillatory interneurons, as shown in Fig. 3. The axons of three interneurons (cells 27, 38 and 33) project frontward along the nerve cord and make
inhibitory connections in several more anterior ganglia with serial homologs of one
or both cells with which they connect also in their own ganglion. The axon of the
fourth interneuron (cell 123) projects rearward and makes inhibitory connections in
several more posterior ganglia with serial homologs of a cell with which it does *not*
connect in its own ganglion.

Analysis of the interneuronal network of Fig. 3 has shown that it owes its oscillatory
character to recurrent cyclic inhibition (Székely, 1967; Friesen and Stent, 1977). This
network is topologically too complex to permit immediate recognition of its oscillatory
features and simple verbal explanation of how it manages to generate the observed
swimming rhythm. It is apparent, however, that the network includes a five-membered
recurrent cyclic inhibition ring formed by cells 28 and 123 of an anterior ganglion and
cells 28, 123 and 27 of a posterior ganglion. Two of the connections of that ring, namely
the interganglionic connections leading from the anterior cell 123 to the posterior cell 28
and from the posterior cell 27 to the anterior cell 28, incorporate a fixed conduction
delay, attributable to the time taken by impulses generated by an interneuron in one
ganglion to reach the synaptic terminals in another ganglion. To a first approximation,
therefore, the central swim oscillator can be thought of as an intersegmental network of
interlocking five-membered recurrent cyclic inhibition rings with two fixed delay lines.
In the absence of any other connections, this system would generate a crude version of
the swimming rhythm, in that in each ganglion, cells 28 and 123 would produce
antiphasic impulse bursts capable of driving the antiphasic rhythm of the motor neurons
to the dorsal and ventral longitudinal muscles and in that serial homologs of these two
interneurons in successive ganglia of the nerve cord would show a rostrocaudal phase
lead of about 20°. The actually identified, topologically more complex network of Fig. 3
can then be viewed as an elaboration of the basic five-membered intersegmental ring,
with additional cells and additional connections creating a set of subsidiary rings that
generate the actually observed four-phased segmental duty cycle. The cycle period of
this network can be shown to depend on two parameters: (1) the intersegmental travel
time taken by impulses conducted from ganglion to ganglion in the axons of the
oscillatory interneurons; and (2) the recovery time taken by each interneuron to reach
action potential threshold upon its release from inhibition (Friesen and Stent, 1977).

In order to test the properties of this complex cyclic network, an electronic analog
model of the interneurons and their intra- and interganglionic connections, as well as of
their output connections to the motor neurons, was constructed. This model consisted
of interconnected electronic "neuromime" elements, which mimic an excitable nerve
cell membrane and also provide for the simulation of both excitatory and inhibitory
synaptic currents. The analog model circuit produced a good approximation of the
observed interneuronal impulse burst relations shown in Fig. 3, and gives rise to an
appropriate rostrocaudal phase progression of the cycle phases in different ganglia of
the nerve cord (Friesen and Stent, 1977). This high degree of verisimilitude of the model
makes it appear that the network of Fig. 3 constitutes a major component of the central
swim oscillator.

Whereas the network of Fig. 3 can account for the steady-state generation of the
swimming rhythm, it does not provide an explanation for the transition from rest to
swimming. This transition appears to be controlled by an unpaired interneuron, designated as cell 204 (Fig. 1), present in each segmental ganglion that sends its axon both

154

frontward and rearward along the nerve cord (Weeks and Kristan, 1978). Passage of depolarizing current into cell 204 initiates and maintains the swimming rhythm, but does not shift the phase of an ongoing rhythm. Thus cell 204 is a swim-initiating interneuron, which does not form part of the network of oscillatory interneurons that generates the rhythm (Weeks and Kristan, 1978; Weeks, 1981a, b). Stimulation of cell 204 can initiate the swimming rhythm even in an isolated ganglion deprived of the *inter*ganglionic connections of the oscillatory interneurons (Weeks, 1981a). Since the present known *intra*ganglionic connections would not by themselves suffice for oscillatory activity, it would appear that the already quite complex swim generator network of Fig. 3 is still incomplete. That is to say, additional connections between or special properties of the identified neurons, or additional neurons, are still needed to account for the capacity of a wholly intraganglionic circuit to generate the basic swimming rhythm.

Inasmuch as the two identified neural circuits presented here pertain to the nervous system of the leech, one may ask whether these findings are generally applicable to central nervous oscillators generating rhythmic movements in animals of other species and phyla, particularly in the vertebrates. Although detailed cellular network analyses have thus far been possible only in a very few neurophysiologically favorable preparations, it is nevertheless significant that the mechanisms by which leech heartbeat and leech swimming circuits appear to generate their oscillations – endogenous rhythmic polarization and recurrent cyclic inhibition – were first proposed to account for generation of rhythmic movements in vertebrate animals. Moreover, the pattern of motor neuron activity in rhythmic movements of vertebrates is not necessarily more complex than the corresponding pattern in analogous movements of leeches. Therefore the very much greater number of neurons in the central nervous system of vertebrates does not necessarily imply a greater complexity of the central oscillators generating their rhythmic movements; it may only place greater obstacles in the way of identifying the underlying neuronal circuitry.

ACKNOWLEDGEMENTS

Supported by NIH Research Grant NS 12818 and NSF Grant BN577-19181.

REFERENCES

Brown, T.G. (1911) The intrinsic factors in the act of progression in the mammal. *Proc. roy. Soc. B*, 84: 308–319.

Calabrese, R.L. (1977) The neural control of alternate heartbeat coordination states in the leech, *Hirudo medicinalis. J. comp. Physiol.*, 122: 111–143.

Calabrese, R.L. (1979a) Neural generation of the peristaltic and non-peristaltic heartbeat coordination modes of the leech, *Hirudo medicinalis. Amer. Zool.*, 19: 87–102.

Calabrese, R.L. (1979b) The roles of endogenous membrane properties and synaptic interaction in generating the heartbeat rhythm of the leech, *Hirudo medicinalis. J. exp. Biol.*, 82: 163–176.

Calabrese, R.L. (1980) Control of impulse-initiation sites in a leech interneuron. *J. Neurophysiol.*, 44: 878–896.

Friesen, W.O. and Stent, G.S. (1977) Generation of a locomotory rhythm by a neural network with recurrent cyclic inhibition. *Biol. Cybernet.*, 28: 27–40.

Friesen, W.O., Poon, M. and Stent, G.S. (1978) Neuronal control of swimming in the medicinal leech. IV. Identification of a network of oscillatory interneurons. *J. exp. Biol.*, 75: 25–43.

Harmon, L.D. and Lewis, E.R. (1966) Neural modeling. *Physiol. Rev.*, 46: 513–591.

Kristan, W.B. and Calabrese, R.L. (1978) Rhythmic swimming activity in neurons of the isolated nerve cord of the leech. *J. exp. Biol.*, 65: 643–668.

Kristan, W.B., Stent, G.S. and Ort, C.A. (1974a) Neuronal control of swimming in the medicinal leech. I. Dynamics of the swimming rhythm. *J. comp. Physiol.*, 94: 97–119.

Kristan, W.B., Jr., Stent, G.S. and Ort, C.A. (1974b) Neuronal control of swimming in the medicinal leech. II. Identification, activity patterns and connectivity of motor neurons. *J. comp. Physiol.*, 94: 121–154.

McDougall, W. (1903) The nature of inhibitory processes within the nervous system. *Brain*, 26: 153–191.

Muller, K.J., Nicholls, J.G. and Stent, G.S. (Eds.) (1981) *Neurobiology of the Leech*. Cold Spr. Harb. Lab., Cold Spring Harbor, NY, p. 320.

Nicholls, J.G. and Wallace, B.G. (1978) Modulation of transmission at an inhibitory synapse in the central nervous system of the leech. *J. Physiol. (Lond.)*, 281: 157–170.

Ort, C.A., Kristan, W.B. and Stent, G.S. (1974) Neuronal control of swimming in the medicinal leech. II. Identification and connections of motor neurons. *J. comp. Physiol.*, 94: 121–154.

Peterson, E.L. and Calabrese, R.L. (1982) Dynamic analysis of a rhythmic neural circuit in the leech *Hirudo medicinalis*. *J. Neurophysiol.*, 47: 256–271.

Poon, M., Friesen, W.O. and Stent, G.S. (1978) Neuronal control of swimming in the medicinal leech. V. Connections between the oscillatory interneurons and the motor neurons. *J. exp. Biol.*, 75: 43–63.

Stent, G.S., Kristan, W.B., Jr., Friesen, W.O., Ort, C.A., Poon, M. and Calabrese R.L. (1978) Neuronal generation of the leech swimming movement. *Science*, 200: 1348–1357.

Stent, G.S., Thompson, W.J. and Calabrese, R.L. (1979) Neural control of heartbeat in the leech and in some other invertebrates. *Physiol. Rev.*, 59: 101–136.

Székely, G. (1967) Development of limb movements: embryological, physiological and model studies. In G. Wolstenholme and M. O'Connor (Eds.), *Ciba Foundation Symposium on Growth of the Nervous System*, Little, Brown, Boston, pp. 77–93.

Thompson, W.J. and Stent, G.S. (1976a) Neuronal control of heartbeat in the medicinal leech. I. Generation of the vascular constriction rhythm. *J. comp. Physiol.*, 111: 261–279.

Thompson, W.J. and Stent, G.S. (1976b) Neuronal control of heartbeat in the medicinal leech. II. Intersegmental coordination of heart motor neuron activity by heart interneurons. *J. comp. Physiol.*, 111: 281–307.

Thompson, W.J. and Stent, G. (1976c) Neuronal control of heartbeat in the medicinal leech. III. Synaptic relations of the heart interneurons. *J. comp. Physiol.*, 111: 309–333.

Weeks, J.C. (1981a) Neuronal basis of leech swimming: separation of swim initiation, pattern generation and intersegmental coordination by selective lesions. *J. Neurophysiol.*, 45: 698–723.

Weeks, J.C. (1981b) Synaptic pathways underlying swim initiation and pattern generation in the leech. I. Connections of a swim-initiating neuron (cell 204) with motor neurons and pattern-generating "oscillator" neurons. *J. comp. Physiol.*, in press.

Weeks, J.C. and Kristan, W.B. Jr. (1978) Initiation, maintenance and modulation of swimming in the medicinal leech by the activity of a single neuron. *J. exp. Biol.*, 77: 71–88.

A Constraint on Synaptic
Action in *Aplysia*:
Implications for Nervous System
Organization

MICHAEL M. SEGAL

Center for Neurobiology and Behavior, Physiology Department, College of Physicians and Surgeons, Columbia University, 722 W. 168th Street, New York, NY 10032 (U.S.A.)

A single neuron can have receptors to more than one neurotransmitter. For example, a neuron can receive synapses from cholinergic and adrenergic cells, and the cholinergic synapses can depolarize and the adrenergic synapses hyperpolarize by virtue of activating different types of receptors (Dun and Karczmar, 1978; Libet and Owman, 1974).

A single neuron can also have two types of receptor to the *same* neurotransmitter. For example, on a single neuron there can be acetylcholine (ACh) receptors that produce depolarization by opening Na^+ channels and ACh receptors that produce hyperpolarization by opening Cl^- channels (Blankenship et al., 1971). Can such a neuron receive two cholinergic synapses, with one depolarizing by opening only Na^+ channels and the other hyperpolarizing by opening only Cl^- channels? In other words, to what extent can neurons provide one type of receptor to one synaptic input, and a different type of receptor, for the same transmitter, to another input? Can a single postsynaptic cell recognize two inputs that use the same transmitter as "different" and provide one type of receptor to one input and a different type of receptor to the other input?

Several investigators have explored this question by iontophoresing neurotransmitters onto different regions of neurons. For some cells they have found different responses to a single neurotransmitter on different regions of the neuron (Alger and Nicoll, 1979; Andersen et al., 1980; Barker and Ransom, 1978; Gerschenfeld, 1977; Levitan and Tauc, 1972; Marder and Paupardin-Tritsch, 1978; Wilson and Wachtel, 1978). These experiments suggest that there are indeed instances in which a neuron provides one type of receptor to one input and a different type of receptor to another input that uses the same neurotransmitter. However, several investigators have suggested alternate explanations that could account for the topographic differences in response to iontophoresis, such as different responses to different concentrations of transmitter (Ger et al., 1979), or different chloride gradients in different regions of the neuron (Alger and Nicoll, 1979; Andersen et al., 1980).

Using extracellular stimulation of a whole nerve trunk, Libet and Tosaka (1969) found indirect evidence for the segregation of two types of ACh receptors to two different inputs in mammalian sympathetic ganglia. To search directly for segregation of different receptors to different synapses, John Koester and I have decided

[157]

to study neurons in the abdominal ganglion of *Aplysia californica* that receive convergent inputs from more than one cholinergic neuron (Segal and Koester, 1980). We tried to find a postsynaptic cell that receives one synaptic action from one cholinergic input and a different synaptic action from a different input.

Prior to our work, there were only two cholinergic neurons known to make synapses in the abdominal ganglion, L10 and Interneuron (Int) XIII (Audesirk, 1973; Eisenstadt et al., 1973; Giller and Schwartz, 1971; Stinnakre, 1970; Woodson and Schlapfer, 1979). It was known that the two neurons converge onto two types of follower cells, R15 and the RB cells, and that both presynaptic cholinergic neurons excite both types of follower cells (Audesirk, 1973; Kandel et al., 1967; Koester et al., 1974). We decided to expand on these two examples of convergence by identifying more presynaptic cholinergic neurons and looking for more postsynaptic cells receiving cholinergic synapses.

By using the specific cholinergic blocking drug hexamethonium (Ascher and Kehoe, 1975), we have determined that the neurons L16, L24 and Int XX are cholinergic (Segal and Koester 1980, 1982). We have also provided biochemical evidence that L16 and L24 are cholinergic by demonstrating that they convert injected [^{3}H]choline to ACh (Eisenstadt et al., 1973; Segal and Koester 1980, 1982). These three neurons that we studied bring to five the number of cholinergic neurons known to make synapses in the abdominal ganglion.

We have searched for synapses made by these five cholinergic neurons in the abdominal ganglion. The connections we have found, together with those previously known, are shown in Table I. For each postsynaptic cell, we found that all cholinergic inputs produce the same synaptic action. This finding holds even for cells such as L7 and RD$_G$, which have more than one type of ACh receptor and respond with the same type of two-component synaptic action to each of several presynaptic cholinergic neurons. Therefore, we have been unable to find an instance of a postsynaptic cell that provides one type of receptor to one cholinergic input and another type of receptor to another cholinergic input.

If all cholinergic inputs to a given cell produce the same type of synaptic action, then one would predict that all synaptic actions of different types are produced by non-cholinergic cells. Table II lists several postsynaptic cells in the abdominal ganglion in which the neurons L28, L32 and LE produce synaptic actions different from those produced by cholinergic inputs. We found that all three of these neurons, which produce synaptic actions different from those of cholinergic inputs, are non-cholinergic. We provided pharmacological evidence that L28, L32 and LE are non-cholinergic by applying the specific cholinergic blocking drug hexamethonium (Ascher and Kehoe, 1975) to the EPSPs made by these neurons to L7, and finding that none of the EPSPs were blocked by the drug (Segal and Koester, 1982). Furthermore, we provided biochemical evidence that L32 and LE cells are non-cholinergic by demonstrating that these cells convert only negligible amounts of injected [^{3}H]choline to ACh (Segal and Koester, 1982).

The experiments summarized in Tables I and II support the notion that each neuron we have studied provides the same type or types of receptors to all cholinergic inputs. We have been unable to find a postsynaptic cell that, for example, is depolarized by one cholinergic input and hyperpolarized by another cholinergic input. These data could be explained by a lack of segregation of different types of ACh receptors from each other on each postsynaptic cell. Although it is believed

TABLE I

Convergent cholinergic synapses in the abdominal ganglion

Postsynaptic	Presynaptic				
	L10	XIII	L24	L16	XX
L10		I_F[1]	I_F[2]	I_F[*]	
L11	I_F[3]	I_F[1]	I_F[2]		
LD$_{HI}$	I_F[4]		I_F[4]		
LB$_{VC}$	I_F[4]	I_F[2]			I_F[2]
L32	I_F[5]			I_F[5]	
L9$_G$	E[3]	E[1,6]	E[1]	—	E[2]
R15	E[3]	E[4,7]	—		—
RB	E[3]	E[4]	E[4]		
RD$_G$	I_F–I_S[2]	—	I_F–I_S[2]	—	I_F–I_S[2]
LD$_{G2}$	I_F–I_S[2]		I_F–I_S[2]		
L7	E–I_F[8]	E–I_F[1]	E–I_F[9]	E–I_F[2]	
LD$_{S1}$	E–I_F[2]		E–I_F[2]		

References are indicated by superscripts: [1]Segal and Koester, 1980; [2]Segal and Koester, 1982; [3]Kandel et al., 1967; [4]Koester et al., 1974; [5]Byrne, 1980; [6]Guthrie et al., 1979; [7]Audesirk, 1973; [8]Wachtel and Kandel, 1971; [9]Byrne and Koester, 1978; [*]J.H. Byrne, personal communication. E = excitation, I_F = fast inhibition, I_S = slow inhibition. A dash indicates no connection seen on at least two occasions.

TABLE II

Convergent synapses producing different synaptic actions

Postsynaptic	Presynaptic						
	Cholinergic				Unidentified transmitter		
	L10	XIII	L24	L16	L28	L32	LE
L14	—	—		I_F[5]	E–I_S[10]	E–I_S[5]	E[5]
LD$_{G2}$	I_F–I_S[2]		I_F–I_S[2]				E[*]
SOME LUQ	I_F–I_S[11]					E[*]	—
L7	E–I_F[8]	E–I_F[1]	E–I_F[9]	E–I_F[2]	E[10]	E[12]	E[13]
LD$_{S1}$	E–I_F[2]		E–I_F[2]				E[2]

References are indicated by superscripts as in Table I and in addition: [10]Hawkins et al., 1981; [11]Pinsker and Kandel, 1969; [12]Byrne, 1981; [13]Castellucci et al., 1970; [*]J.H. Byrne, personal communication. E = excitation, I_F = fast inhibition, I_S = slow inhibition, LUQ = left upper quadrant cells. A dash indicates no connection seen on at least two occasions.

that postsynaptic neurons concentrate receptors at synapses (Harris et al., 1971; Oswald and Freeman, 1981), it appears that the postsynaptic cells we have studied do not concentrate one type of ACh receptor at one cholinergic input, and another type of ACh receptor at another input on the same postsynaptic cell.

It is difficult to judge how generally this lack of receptor segregation will apply. The lack of receptor segregation exhibited by the neurons we have studied may simply reflect some peculiarity of the particular neurons we have studied, or of *Aplysia* neurons in general. There may be gross segregation of ACh receptors on the surface of certain neurons, with one type of ACh receptor on the cell body and another type on the dendrites. Since the vast majority of synapses in *Aplysia* are onto dendrites and not onto the soma (Rosenbluth, 1963; Schwartz and Shkolnik, 1981), the synapses we reported all could be dendritic synapses. Therefore, our sample may not include any synapses onto the cell body, a type that conceivably could produce a different synaptic action from that produced by synapses onto dendrites. Another possibility is that the two-component responses we observed are produced by complexes of two ionophore molecules connected to a single receptor molecule, thereby providing no opportunity for receptor segregation.

It will be important to test whether receptor segregation can occur on nerve cells, since a lack of such segregation could have important implications for our understanding of the organization of the nervous system.

The data in Table II suggest that in order for a neuron to produce a synaptic action different from that produced by cholinergic inputs, that second neuron will employ a different neurotransmitter. This could explain a need for two neurotransmitters in a nervous system. Moreover, a third neurotransmitter would also be needed if the first two presynaptic neurons produce the same synaptic action on a particular postsynaptic neuron while a third presynaptic neuron produces a different synaptic action. Therefore, if neurons do not segregate receptors so as to provide one type of receptor to one input and another type of receptor to another input using the same transmitter, then one could demonstrate a need for three (or more) neurotransmitters in a nervous system. It must be noted, however, that the presence of such a constraint on receptor segregation would not exclude the presence of other, different constraints, also requiring the presence of many neurotransmitters (Bloom, 1979; Gardner and Kandel, 1972; Sakharov, 1974).

A lack of segregation of different types of receptors for the same transmitter could also explain a need for certain interneurons found in neural circuits. In the mammalian spinal cord, I_A afferent sensory inputs monosynaptically excite motorneurons that innervate the same muscle, but their connections to motorneurons that innervate antagonist muscles are disynaptic, involving an interposed interneuron (Eccles, 1964). Sir John Eccles posed the question of why these interneurons are needed: why doesn't a I_A afferent fiber instead carry out direct excitation with one branch and direct inhibition with another branch? He suggested that there is a constraint such that a presynaptic neuron "...will function exclusively either in an excitatory or inhibitory capacity at all of its synaptic endings, i.e., there are functionally just two types of nerve cells, excitatory and inhibitory." (Eccles, 1957). According to this view, there is a constraint on the divergent branches of the presynaptic neuron requiring all synapses made by the neuron to have the same synaptic action on all follower cells. For the I_A afferents to produce different actions with different branches, Eccles (1957) suggested that an interneuron with a different transmitter would be required to carry out the change in synaptic action.

Although the view that each presynaptic neuron produces only a single type of synaptic action applies for this circuit in the spinal cord, it does not hold universally, as was shown by Eric Kandel and his colleagues for the neuron L10, which directly excites some follower cells and directly inhibits others (Kandel et al., 1967) (Table I). However, a need for this interneuron could arise instead from a constraint on receptor segregation applying to the postsynaptic neuron. If all I_A afferents use the same neurotransmitter, a motorneuron that is excited directly by one I_A input could not be inhibited directly by another I_A input without the motorneuron segregating excitatory receptors to one synapse and inhibitory receptors responding to the same transmitter to another synapse. If such receptor segregation does not occur, then an interneuron using a different neurotransmitter would be required for a I_A afferent to cause inhibition of a motorneuron that is directly excited by another I_A afferent. Therefore, the presence of an interneuron could allow different afferents to mediate opposite synaptic actions on the same motorneuron. It must be noted, however, that the presence of such a constraint requiring the existence of an interneuron would not exclude the presence of other constraints, such as the need for integration of I_A input, also requiring the existence of an interneuron.

Eccles (1957) suggested the constraint that "any one neurotransmitter substance always has the same synaptic action, i.e. excitatory or inhibitory, at all synapses on nerve cells," but that constraint turned out to be too broad. The data presented here suggest that there may be a more limited constraint: although synapses using the same neurotransmitter can produce *different* synaptic actions on *different* nerve cells, synapses using the same neurotransmitter will all produce the *same* synaptic action on *any particular* nerve cell. Although it is known that the broad constraint suggested by Eccles does not hold universally, it is not yet known how widely this more limited constraint for single neurons will apply.

It will be important to continue to search for such examples of receptor segregation. A constraint against segregation on a single cell of different receptors to the same neurotransmitter could help us understand some of the organizational principles of the nervous system, by explaining a need for many neurotransmitters and explaining a need for certain interneurons found in neural networks.

ACKNOWLEDGEMENTS

I thank J. Koester and D. Goldberg for reading an earlier version of this manuscript. This work was supported by NIH M.D.-Ph.D. Grant GM 07367, by NIH Research Grant NS 14385, and an I.T. Hirschl Career Scientist Award to J. Koester.

REFERENCES

Alger, B.E. and Nicoll, R.A. (1979) GABA-mediated biphasic inhibitory responses in hippocampus, *Nature (Lond.)*, 281: 315–317.

Andersen, P., Dingledine, R., Gjerstad, L., Langmoen, I.A. and Laursen, A.M. (1980) Two different responses of hippocampal pyramidal cells to application of gamma-amino butyric acid, *J. Physiol. (Lond.)*, 305: 279–296.

Ascher, P. and Kehoe, J.S. (1975) Amine and amino acid receptors in gastropod neurons. In L.L. Iversen, S.D. Iversen and S.H. Snyder (Eds.), *Handbook of Psychopharmacology, Vol. 4*, Plenum Press, New York, pp. 265–310.

162

Audesirk, G. (1973) Interaction of two circadian oscillators in the isolated central nervous system of *Aplysia. Physiologist*, 16: 256.

Barker, J.L. and Ransom, B.R. (1978) Amino acid pharmacology of mammalian central neurones grown in tissue culture. *J. Physiol. (Lond.)*, 280: 331–354.

Blankenship, J.E., Wachtel, H. and Kandel, E.R. (1971) Ionic mechanisms of excitatory, inhibitory, and dual synaptic actions mediated by an identified interneuron in abdominal ganglion of *Aplysia. J. Neurophysiol.*, 34: 76–92.

Bloom, F.E. (1979) Chemically coded transmitter systems. In M. Cuénod, G.W. Kreutzberg and F.E. Bloom (Eds.), *Development and Chemical Specificity of Neurons, Progr. in Brain Res.*, Vol. 51, Elsevier Biomedical, Amsterdam, pp. 125–131.

Byrne, J.H. (1980) Neural circuit for inking behavior in *Aplysia californica. J. Neurophysiol.*, 43: 896–911.

Byrne, J.H. (1981) Comparative aspects of neural circuits for inking behavior and gill withdrawal in *Aplysia californica, J. Neurophysiol.*, 45: 98–106.

Byrne, J. and Koester, J. (1978) Respiratory pumping: Neuronal control of a centrally commanded behavior in *Aplysia. Brain Res.*, 143: 87–105.

Castellucci, V., Pinsker, H., Kupfermann, I. and Kandel, E.R. (1970) Neuronal mechanisms of habituation and dishabituation of the gill withdrawal reflex in *Aplysia. Science*, 167: 1745–1748.

Dun, N.J. and Karczmar, A.G. (1978) Involvement of an interneuron in the generation of the slow inhibitory postsynaptic potential in mammalian sympathetic ganglia. *Proc. nat. Acad. Sci. U.S.A.*, 75: 4029–4032.

Eccles, J.C. (1957) *The Physiology of Nerve Cells*, Johns Hopkins Press, Baltimore, pp. 212–213.

Eccles, J.C. (1964) *The Physiology of Synapses*, Springer-Verlag, Berlin, pp. 202–207.

Eisenstadt, M., Goldman, J.E., Kandel, E.R., Koike, H., Koester, J. and Schwartz, J.H. (1973) Intrasomatic injection of radioactive precursors for studying transmitter synthesis in identified neurons of *Aplysia californica. Proc. nat. Acad. Sci. U.S.A.*, 70: 3371–3375.

Gardner, D. and Kandel, E.R. (1972) Diphasic postsynaptic potential: A chemical synapse capable of mediating conjoint excitation and inhibition. *Science*, 176: 675–678.

Ger, B.A., Katchman, A.N. and Zeimal, E.V. (1979) Biphasic acetycholine responses of molluscan neurones: their dependence on acetylcholine concentration. *Brain Res.*, 167: 426–430.

Gerschenfeld, H.M. (1977) Multiple receptor activation by single transmitters. In G.A. Cottrell and P.N.R. Usherwood (Eds.), *Synapses*, Blackie and Sons, Glasgow, pp. 157–176.

Giller, E. and Schwartz, J.H. (1971) Choline acetyltransferase in identified neurons of abdominal ganglion of *Aplysia californica. J. Neurophysiol.*, 34: 93–107.

Guthrie, P.B., Schlapfer, W.T. and Barondes, S.H. (1979) Long-term plasticities are different at different terminals of the same presynaptic neuron in *Aplysia. Soc. Neurosci. Abstr.*, 5: 741.

Harris, A.J., Kuffler, S.W. and Dennis, M.J. (1971) Differential chemosensitivity of synaptic and extrasynaptic areas on the neuronal surface membrane in parasympathetic neurons of the frog, tested by micro-application of acetylcholine. *Proc. roy. Soc. B*, 177: 541–553.

Hawkins, R., Castellucci, V.F. and Kandel, E.R. (1981) Interneurons involved in mediation and modulation of gill-withdrawal reflex in *Aplysia*. I. Identification and characterization. *J. Neurophysiol.*, 45: 304–314.

Kandel, E.R., Frazier, W.T., Waziri, R. and Coggeshall, R.E. (1967) Direct and common connections among identified neurons in *Aplysia. J. Neurophysiol.*, 30: 1352–1376.

Koester, J., Mayeri, E., Liebeswar, G. and Kandel, E.R. (1974) Neural control of circulation in *Aplysia*. II. Interneurons. *J. Neurophysiol.*, 37: 476–496.

Levitan, H. and Tauc, L. (1972) Acetylcholine receptors: Topographic distribution and pharmacological properties of two receptor types on a single molluscan neurone. *J. Physiol. (Lond.)*, 222: 537–558.

Libet, B. and Tosaka, T. (1969) Slow inhibitory and excitatory postsynaptic responses in single cells of mammalian sympathetic ganglia. *J. Neurophysiol.*, 32: 43–50.

Libet, B. and Owman, C. (1974) Concomitant changes in formaldehyde-induced fluorescence of dopamine interneurones and in slow inhibitory postsynaptic potentials of the rabbit superior cervical ganglion, induced by stimulation of the preganglionic nerve or by a muscarinic agent. *J. Physiol. (Lond.)*, 237: 635–662.

Marder, E. and Paupardin-Tritsch, D. (1978) The pharmacological properties of some crustacean neuronal acetylcholine, γ-aminobutyric acid, and L-glutamate responses. *J. Physiol. (Lond.)*, 280: 213–236.

Oswald, R.E. and Freeman, J.A. (1981) Alpha-bungarotoxin binding and central nervous system nicotinic acetylcholine receptors. *Neuroscience*, 6: 1–14.

Pinsker, H. and Kandel, E.R. (1969) Synaptic activation of an electrogenic sodium pump. *Science*, 163: 931–935.

Rosenbluth, J. (1963) The visceral ganglion of *Aplysia californica*. *Z. Zellforsch.*, 60: 213–236.

Sakharov, D.A. (1974) Evolutionary aspects of transmitter heterogeneity. *J. Neural Transm.*, Suppl. XI: 43–59.

Schwartz, J.H. and Shkolnik, L.J. (1981) The giant serotonergic neuron of *Aplysia*: A multitargeted nerve cell. *J. Neurosci.*, 1: 606–619.

Segal, M.M. and Koester, J. (1980) Different cholinergic synapses converging onto neurons in *Aplysia* produce the same synaptic action. *Brain Res.*, 199: 459–465.

Segal, M.M. and Koester, J. (1982) Convergent cholinergic neurons produce similar postsynaptic actions in *Aplysia*: Implications for neural organization. *J. Neurophysiol.*, 47: 742–759.

Stinnakre, J. (1970) Action de l'hemicholinium sur une synapse centrale d'*Aplysie*, *J. Physiol. (Paris)*, Suppl. 3, 62: 452–453.

Wachtel, H. and Kandel, E.R. (1971) Conversion of synaptic excitation to inhibition at a dual chemical synapse. *J. Neurophysiol.*, 34: 56–68.

Wilson, W.A. and Wachtel, H. (1978) Prolonged inhibition in burst firing neurons: synaptic inactivation of the slow regenerative inward current. *Science*, 202: 772–775.

Woodson, P.B.J. and Schlapfer, W.T. (1979) The amplitude of post-tetanic potentiation of the EPSP RC1–R15 in *Aplysia* is modulated by environmental parameters. *Brain Res.*, 173: 225–242.

Organizational and Cellular Mechanisms Underlying Chemical Inhibition of A Vertebrate Neuron

H. KORN and D.S. FABER

Inserm U3, CHU Pitié Salpêtrière, 91 Blvd. de l'Hôspital, Paris B (France) and Division of Neurobiology, Department of Physiology, SUNY at Buffalo, Buffalo, NY (U.S.A.)

INTRODUCTION

Little is known so far about the cellular principles underlying integration in the vertebrate central nervous system (CNS) because few neuronal constellations permit meaningful comparison between anatomical and functional data; while the former have accumulated in the past, the latter have been obtained infrequently, primarily due to technical limitations. It can be expected, however, that investigations of basic networks may allow us to unravel some operative rules before generalization is attempted for higher brain functions. Such models should include morphologically well-defined post synaptic elements and their associated excitatory and inhibitory inputs. For instance, spinal motoneurons and neocortical pyramidal cells, with their excitatory afferents and intercalated inhibitory interneurons (see Eccles, 1969) are imbedded in elementary circuits of this nature. As we show here, analyses of apparently quite disparate arrays, such as those which involve the mammalian Purkinje cells (Pc) and the Mauthner cell (M-cell) of teleosts indicate common patterns which might be present in the other structures as well. This work has been made possible by the fact that both experimental materials, particularly that of the M-cell, are well suited for electrophysiological investigations and for extensive histological correlations (Eccles et al., 1967; Faber and Korn, 1978). Because of these advantages and in order to fill at least some gaps in the present understanding of inhibitory synaptic interactions, we have focused our attention in two quite different directions that have so far been, by necessity, relatively unapproachable: (1) the processing by a single neuron of opposing excitatory and inhibitory drives, particularly when the former activates both the output cell and the units regulating its excitability through a feedforward inhibition, and (2) the cellular processes underlying quantal release of inhibitory transmitter and postsynaptic conductance changes, including the kinetics of activated chloride channels. This second type of study was otherwise only achieved on isolated preparations such as the skeletal neuromuscular junction, and it remained to be seen whether concepts so derived were valid for the central assemblies of nerve cells.

[165]

REGULATION OF M-CELL EXCITABILITY

The best model for exploring the properties of inhibition in the vertebrate brain at diverse levels, including even the molecular one, is provided by the M-cell. As for other examples in the vertebrate CNS (Eccles, 1969), a strong recurrent collateral pathway controls its responsiveness. And, as will be shown below, this system has a number of similarities with that of the Renshaw cells, which mediates a negative feedback on spinal motoneurons (Eccles et al., 1954; Renshaw, 1946). Although it is somewhat difficult to compare the two circuits functionally, since in the former the controlled element may be likened to a "command cell", it still may be significant that in both, collateral and afferent inputs converge on the same interneurons. As these two networks are presently understood, the major difference is that the inhibition acting on the Mauthner cell is more complex, involving at least two distinct mechanisms (Furukawa and Furshpan, 1963). One is the classic type mediated chemically. The other is electrical, depending on an extracellular current and signalled by a large extracellular positivity named the "extrinsic hyperpolarizing potential" (EHP).

Impulses in single intrinsic cells generate the two types of inhibitions (Korn and Faber, 1976); they can be identified by the presence of a passive hyperpolarizing potential, or PHP, synchronous with the M-cell spike (Faber and Korn, 1973). This property has allowed secure identification of the interneurons so that simultaneous pre- and postsynaptic intracellular recordings can be achieved. To date no other central formation has provided such an opportunity.

For M-cell studies, teleosts have been used and handled according to techniques now standard in our laboratories (Korn and Faber, 1975). Presynaptic recordings were often performed with HRP-filled microelectrodes for intracellular staining of their processes (Korn et al., 1981b). KCl-filled electrodes in the M-cell permitted the Cl^--ion injections necessary to displace away from resting potential the driving force for inhibitory postsynaptic potentials (IPSPs); thus, these responses appeared as depolarizations.

SPECIFIC FINDINGS

A number of observations relevant to the role of inhibition in neuronal integration have been collected, and three points that might have general significance are specifically pinpointed here.

(1) Relatively low threshold activation of inhibitory interneurons

The complexity of a "simple" network influencing the excitability of a central neuron is exemplified by Fig. 1. Only one type of interneuron, i.e. a collateral one which is part of a pool of such cells, is drawn along with its input and output connections. The point relevant to our discussion is that all the excitatory afferent pathways monosynaptic to the M-cell also converge on the inhibitory elements, with a consequent disynaptic control of M-cell membrane potential. That this pattern of connectivity may have complex functional implications has been further deduced from activation of a selected input, as shown below.

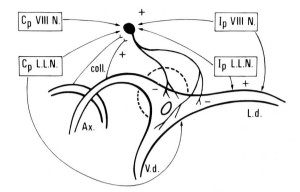

Fig. 1. Scheme illustrating that pathways excitatory to the M-cell also indirectly inhibit this target neuron, through monosynaptic activation of common interneurons. One cell of the collateral network is shown projecting to the axon cap, soma, and proximal dendrites of the ipsilateral M-cell. This inhibitory interneuron (−) receives excitatory (+) inputs from collaterals (coll.) of both M-axons (Ax.) and, bilaterally, from fibers of the lateral line and posterior eighth nerves. With the exception of the contralateral eighth nerve, all of these sensory systems are also excitatory to the M-cell. This diagram is not meant to imply, however, that branches of the same sensory fibers innervate both the M-cell and the collateral interneurons.

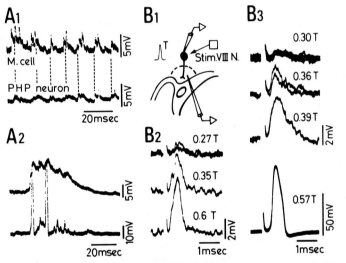

Fig. 2. Evidence that an eighth nerve excitation of the intrinsic interneurons underlies low-threshold inhibition of the M-cell. A_1 and A_2: Simultaneous intracellular recordings from the M-cell (upper traces) and two different PHP neurons (lower traces) of spontaneous (A_1) and sound-evoked (A_2) "synaptic noise". Vertical lines in A_1 indicate common synaptic inputs. B_1–B_3: evidence that low-threshold electrical inhibition of the M-cell following ipsilateral eighth nerve stimulation is mediated through excitation of presynaptic inhibitory interneurons (PHP neurons). B_1: recordings of responses to eighth nerve stimulations at different intensities (1.0T defines threshold for orthodromic activation of the M-cell) were obtained extracellularly from the axon cap in order to monitor the extrinsic hyperpolarizing potentials (EHPs) which reflect activation of inhibitory interneurons (see text), and intracellularly from those cells. B_2: potentials in the axon cap; at a stimulus intensity of 0.27T, the lowest strength producing an EPSP in the M-cell (not shown), a small EHP was detectable, and it increased as a function of stimulus intensity. B_3: stimulus–response characteristics of a PHP-exhibiting neuron in the same experiment. Subthreshold EPSPs were recorded between 0.30T and 0.39T, and with 0.42T or higher, the cell fired impulses at a latency comparable to that of the EHPs recorded in B_2, as shown for 0.57T. (From Faber and Korn, 1978, with permission.)

The simultaneous recordings from the M-cell and PHP neurons in Fig. $2A_1$ and A_2 show that excitatory inputs are common to the two. It is already evident from the auditory responses in A_2 that the latter units are more readily excited by physiological stimuli. In addition, a helpful feature of this model is that, unlike other systems where excitation and inhibition cannot always be quantified separately, the latter can here be distinguished in extracellular recordings (Fig. $2B_1$); it is represented by the positive EHPs (Fig. $2B_2$) which signal firing of the inhibitory interneurons, and it can be measured alone. When the strength of VIIIth nerve stimulation was expressed relative to that necessary to orthodromically activate the M-cell (1.0T), EHPs already appeared following much weaker stimuli. In confirmation, EPSPs and spikes were also observed in PHP cells at similar low intensities (Fig. $2B_3$). In fact, the M-cell typically does not fire under these experimental conditions until the inhibitory process has saturated (see Fig. 30, Faber and Korn, 1978).

A comparable design can be readily seen in a quite different structure, the rat cerebellar cortex, where the parallel fibers, which are excitatory to the Purkinje cells (Pc), also project to the inhibitory basket cells (Bc), as shown in Fig. 3. A comparison of the records in A_1 and A_2 demonstrates that the basket cells are the units more easily fired following activation of this input through a Loc stimulus. Accordingly, there is a powerful low-threshold suppression of the Purkinje cell impulses (A'_1 and A'_2). This, in fact, represents but one of many surprising analogies between these phylogenetically remote local circuits (see also Korn and Axelrad, 1980). It may thus be generally true that (a) *inhibition dominates excitation*, possibly reflecting the small size and greater excitability of the inhibitory cells, and (b) *integration is a process which includes overcoming a background inhibitory activity*.

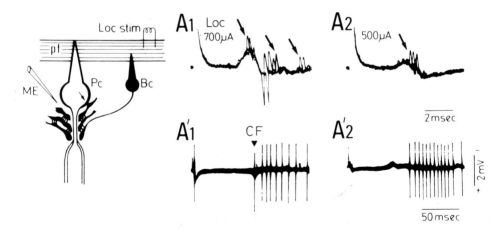

Fig. 3. Evidence that the functional organization of the inhibitory network impinging on cerebellar Purkinje cells is comparable to that of the M-cell. The diagram shows a Purkinje cell (Pc), one of its associated basket cells (Bc), a beam of parallel fibers (pf) presynaptic to both neurons and surface electrodes (Loc stim) for their orthodromic stimulation. The microelectrode (ME) is close to the brush-like structure formed around the initial segment of the Purkinje cell by terminal axons of several basket cells, one of which establishes an inhibitory synapse (arrow.) A_1–A'_2: extracellular recordings, at fast and slow sweeps, of basket cell spikes (arrows) and Purkinje cell action potentials (large spikes). A Loc stimulus of 700 μA activated both sets of neurons (A_1) and produced a long-lasting inhibition of the Pc's spontaneous firing (A'_1). Note that a weaker shock which excited the Bc only (A_2) still depressed the Pc's excitability (A'_2). (From Axelrad and Korn, unpublished.)

(2) Relation between IPSP conductance change and activated Cl⁻-channel lifetime

Central IPSPs are known to be long-lasting, reflecting either a prolonged elevation of transmitter concentration in the synaptic cleft or a long mean open time, τ_c, of inhibitory channels. The last hypothesis would imply that the inhibitory conductance change decays exponentially with a time constant equal to τ_c (Magleby and Stevens, 1972; Anderson and Stevens, 1973). This analytical approach, initially restricted to peripheral junctions, was applied by us to the M-cell (Faber and Korn, 1980). First, using simultaneous intracellular recordings (Fig. 4A), the time course of unitary IPSPs evoked by single presynaptic impulses (Fig. 4B) was shown to be the same as that of the underlying conductance change (Fig. 4C). This finding may be valid for most central neurons, where the membrane time constant is generally much less than that of the IPSP decay (see also Dingledine and Langmoen, 1980). This decay was strictly exponential, with a mean time constant, τ_{IPSC}, of 6.5 msec. Second, we further exploited the unique property of the M-cell that its membrane time constant is so short that measured potential changes are direct indications of

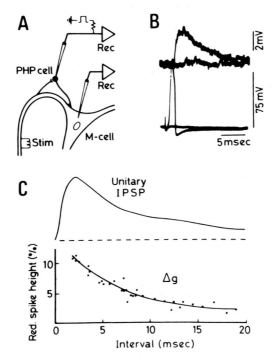

Fig. 4. The conductance change underlying unitary IPSPs recorded in the M-cell lasts throughout the decay phase of the response. A: experimental arrangement used for simultaneous intracellular recordings (Rec) from and stimulation of the M-cell and presynaptic inhibitory interneuron (PHP cell), both neurons having been identified by their responses to antidromic activation of the M-axon (Stim). B: typical unitary IPSP recorded in an M-cell injected with Cl⁻ (upper trace) after a single presynaptic impulse (lower trace). Stimulus current straddled the threshold for spike initiation. C: comparison of the IPSP decay (upper tracing) and of the underlying conductance change (Δg), the latter evaluated from the reduction in the amplitude of a test antidromic spike (not shown). Each data point is a computed average of at least five successive measurements and is expressed as the percentage decrease relative to control. (From Faber and Korn, 1980 © 1980, American Association for the Advancement of Science, with permission.)

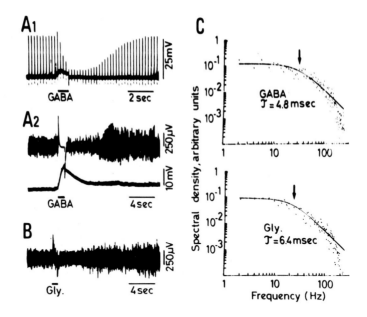

Fig. 5. Analysis of M-cell potential fluctuations induced by iontophoretic applications of GABA and glycine indicates a mean channel lifetime consistent with the time constant of unitary IPSP decay. A_1 and A_2: responses evoked by GABA. A_1: prolonged conductance change after drug application shown by the reduction in antidromic spike height (ac coupled recording). A_2: example of increased voltage variance (upper trace) during the tail of a GABA-induced depolarization (lower trace). B: enhanced noise attributable to glycine. C: power density spectra of amino acid-induced potential fluctuations obtained during the trials illustrated in A_2 and B. In each the data points fit a single Lorentzian curve, with the cutoff frequencies (arrows) providing mean channel open times of 4.8 and 6.4 msec, respectively. (From Faber and Korn, 1980, © 1980 American Association for the Advancement of Science, with permission.)

postsynaptic currents, which can then be estimated without resorting to voltage clamp. Specifically, we analyzed the statistical properties of membrane potential fluctuations due to iontophoretic applications of γ-aminobutyric acid (GABA) and glycine, the putative inhibitory transmitter. In Cl⁻-loaded M-cells, both produce depolarizations associated with marked conductance changes and an enhanced membrane noise (Fig. 5A₁, B). The power spectral densities of the drug-induced fluctuations approximated single Lorentzians (Fig. 5C), and the calculated mean channel lifetime averaged 7.15 msec. Since the two independent measurements of τ were essentially the same, we concluded that *single-shot receptor activation fully accounts for the duration of unitary IPSPs*. This result, which extends to the CNS concepts derived from the neuromuscular junction raises, however, an important question for future investigations, namely that of the mechanism for rapidly eliminating the inhibitory transmitter from the synaptic cleft.

(3) Quantal nature of evoked transmission and its significance

The rules governing transmitter output at central terminals have not yet been unraveled, primarily because of the inability to control presynaptic events and the contamination due to postsynaptic noise. In contrast to most other neurons in the brain and spinal cord, statistical treatment of fluctuating PSPs could be achieved with the M-cell and, in addition, morphofunctional correlations based upon reconstruction of HRP-filled interneurons were possible (Korn et al., 1981a). Using a basic deconvolution model to eliminate the contribution of background noise, it could be shown that binomial predictions of the form $p_x = \binom{n}{x} p^x (1 - p)^{n-x}$ provide a better description of IPSP variations than the Poisson (in this construction, n and p are the number of available units and the probability of release, respectively, and x is the number of quanta actually released). In the example illustrated here the binomial n equalled 9 (Fig. 6A), which also was the number of terminal boutons visualized in the camera lucida reconstruction of the injected cell (Fig. 6C and D). Examples of averaged unitary and full-sized IPSPs are shown in B_1 and B_2. This striking equivalence is further demonstrated for another case in Fig. $7A_1$–A_3, and its functional meaning could be definitely established, after it was demonstrated that all injected terminals studied at the electron microscope level contain morphologically well-defined chemically mediating synaptic complexes (Fig. 7B; see Triller and Korn, 1981). Thus, the identity between the binomial and histological n's, summarized in the plot of Fig. 7D, allowed us to conclude that *each bouton functions in an all-or-none manner* and that the quantum defined by binomial terms is the basic unit processed by the postsynaptic neuron.

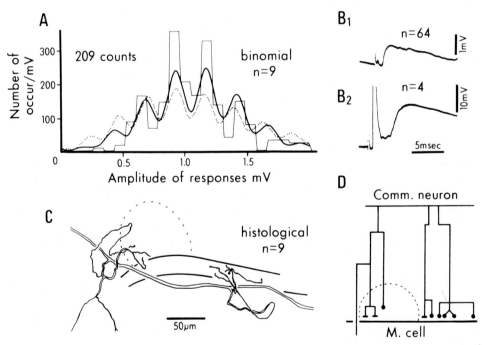

Fig. 6. Evidence that the binomial parameter n is equivalent to the number of presynaptic terminal boutons. A: comparison of observed IPSP amplitude variations (step-wise plot for 209 responses) with the best fits obtained assuming Poisson (dashed line) and binomial (continuous curve) equations. B_1 and B_2: on-line computer-averaged unitary and collateral IPSPs, respectively. C and D: camera lucida reconstruction (C) and schematic representation (D) of the terminals established by the HRP-filled investigated interneuron. Note that the binomial term n had a value of 9, which was equal to its histological counterpart, i.e. the number of synaptic knobs. (Korn, Triller, Mallet and Faber, unpublished.)

172

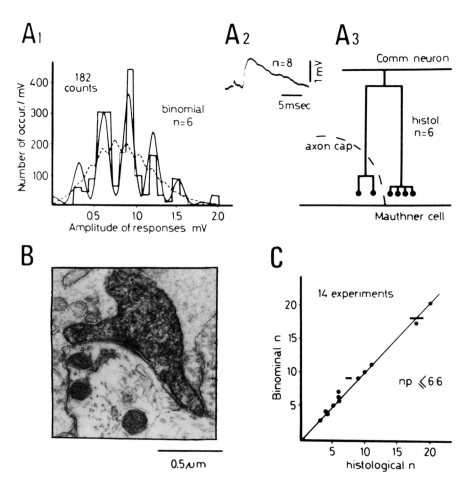

Fig. 7. Correlated statistical properties of postsynaptic responses and presynaptic morphological features. A_1: observed IPSP amplitude variations (stepwise plot for 182 responses) and best fits obtained with the Poisson (dashed line) and binomial (continuous curve) equations. Only the binomial passed the Kolmogorov test ($P > 0.05$); its corresponding parameters were $n = 6$, $p = 0.46$, and $q = 310 \mu V$. A_2: sample computer-averaged unitary IPSP. A_3: schematic representation of the terminals established on the M-cell by the investigated inhibitory interneuron, showing a total of six synaptic boutons (histological n). B: electron micrograph, from another preparation, of an HRP-filled bouton synapsing on an M-cell cap dendrite. Note the synaptic vesicles, the presynaptic differentiation, and the postsynaptic density (arrow) characterizing chemically transmitting junctions. C: one-to-one correspondence between the binomial (ordinate) and histological (abscissa) n's as determined in 14 experiments for which the product np was less than or equal to 6.6. Horizontal bars indicate range of possible values in two cases. The correlation suggests that for these cells the quantal unit corresponds to the transmitter released by a single bouton. (From Korn et al., 1981a, with permission.)

The above result raised the question of how much transmitter is released by each synaptic knob. We were able to address this issue at the M-cell since the IPSP driving force could be reliably evaluated in a simple manner (Faber and Korn, 1981). As a consequence, the conductance change corresponding to a single quantum is about $3-5 \times 10^{-8}$ S. If we assume a single channel conductance of 25 pS, the number of channels opened per quantum would be about 1000 to 2000. Keeping in mind the vesicular theory, these calculations have led to the hypothesis that *a single bouton can only release the contents of one vesicle* (Korn et al., 1981b).

GENERAL COMMENTS

Two notions with possible broad significance come to mind when considering the material reviewed here. One is that the results pertaining to both noise and quantal analysis are remarkably similar to those obtained at neuromuscular junctions; they even expand upon them by pointing to a new basic concept, *the binary release from a single synapse.* Thus, our data explicitly emphasize the unity of the nervous system, since apparently diverse excitable cells continue to share some basic operational features. Similarly, some of the laws established for inhibitory synapses onto the M-cell should be found valid for other central systems, when adequately explored.

Second, as has been remarked elsewhere (see Eccles, 1969), the integrative properties of the central nervous system depend upon the magnitude and temporal features characterizing, at each cellular level, the interplay between excitation and inhibition. As far as the final output of a network is concerned, the addition of inhibition converts the simple to the sophisticated.

ACKNOWLEDGEMENTS

Work supported by DGRST 81E0576 and INSERM Grant 81.60.42. We are indebted to Mrs. J. Nicolet for patient and skillful technical assistance.

REFERENCES

Anderson, C.R. and Stevens, C.F. (1973) Voltage clamp analysis of acetylcholine produced end-plate current fluctuations at frog neuromuscular junction. *J. Physiol. (Lond.),* 235: 655–691

Dingledine, R. and Langmoen, I.A. (1980) Conductance changes and inhibitory actions of hippocampal recurrent IPSPs. *Brain Res.,* 185; 277–287.

Eccles, J.C. (1969) *The Inhibitory Pathways of the Central Nervous System,* Thomas, Springfield, IL, 135 pp.

Eccles, J.C., Fatt, P. and Koketsu, K. (1954) Cholinergic inhibitory synapses in a pathway from motor-axon collaterals to motoneurons. *J. Physiol. (Lond.),* 126: 524–562.

Eccles, J.C., Ito, M. and Szentagothai, J. (1967) *The Cerebellum as a Neuronal Machine,* Springer Verlag, New York, 335 pp.

Faber, D.S. and Korn, H. (1973) A neuronal inhibition mediated electrically. *Science,* 179: 577–578.

Faber, D.S. and Korn, H. (1978) Electrophysiology of the Mauthner cell: Basic properties, synaptic mechanisms and associated networks. In D. Faber and H. Korn (Eds.), *Neurobiology of the Mauthner Cell,* Raven Press, New York, pp. 47–131.

Faber, D.S. and Korn, H. (1980) Single-shot channel activation accounts for duration of inhibitory postsynaptic potentials in a central neuron. *Science,* 208: 612–615.

Faber, D.S. and Korn, H. (1981) Transmission at a central inhibitory synapse. I. Magnitude of the unitary postsynaptic conductance change and kinetics of channel activation. *J. Neurophysiol.,* in press.

Furukawa, T. and Furshpan, E.J. (1963) Two inhibitory mechanisms in the Mauthner cell of goldfish, *J. Neurophysiol.,* 26: 759–774.

Korn, H. and Axelrad, H. (1980) Electrical inhibition of Purkinje cells in the cerebellum of the rat. *Proc. nat. Acad. Sci. U.S.A.,* 77: 6244–6247.

Korn, H. and Faber, D.S. (1975) An electrically mediated inhibition in goldfish medulla. *J. Neurophysiol.,* 38: 452–471.

Korn, H. and Faber, D.S. (1976) Vertebrate central nervous system: Same neurons mediate both electrical and chemical inhibitions. *Science*, 194: 1166–1169.

Korn, H., Faber, D.S., Mallet, A. and Triller, A. (1981a) Possible significance of binomial parameters, n, p and q at a central inhibitory synapse. *Neurosci. Abstr.*, 7: 477.

Korn, H., Triller, A., Mallet, A. and Faber, D.S. (1981b) Fluctuating responses at a central synapse: n of binomial fit predicts number of stained presynaptic boutons. *Science*, 213: 898–901.

Magleby, K.L. and Stevens, C.F. (1972) The effect of voltage on the time course of end-plate currents. *J. Physiol. (Lond.)*, 223: 151–171.

Renshaw, B. (1946) Central effects of centripetal impulses in axons of spinal ventral roots. *J. Neurophysiol.*, 9: 191–204.

Triller, A. and Korn, H. (1981) Morphologically distinct classes of inhibitory synapses arise from the same neurons: Ultrastructural identification from crossed vestibular interneurons intracellularly stained with HRP. *J. comp. Neurol.*, 203: 131–155.

Crossed Vestibulo-Vestibular Interneurons in Teleost Fish: Morphological Basis For a Near Simultaneous Inhibition of Target Cells on Both Sides of the Brainstem

ANTOINE TRILLER and JOSSELINE NICOLET

INSERM U3, CHU Pitié-Salpêtrière, 91 Boulevard de l'Hôpital, 75634 Paris Cedex 13 (France)

INTRODUCTION

Crossed vestibular inhibition first described in mammals by Shimazu and Precht (1966), also occurs in many species ranging from reptiles to mammals, but was not observed in frog and toadfish (refs. in Korn et al., 1977). During a study of the inhibitory pathways of the Mauthner cell (M-cell) of a teleost, two classes of interneurons were individualized. Their identification was made possible by intracellular injection of horseradish peroxidase (HRP) after they had been physiologically identified by the presence of an intracellularly recorded passive hyperpolarizing potential (Faber and Korn, 1973) induced by the firing of their adjacent M-cell. Interneurons of the first group are part of the recurrent collateral network of the M-cell (Korn and Faber, 1975; Korn et al., 1978); they have some similarities with the Renshaw cells. The second group is composed of commissural vestibulovestibular neurons (Triller and Korn, 1978; Zottoli and Faber, 1979, 1980). Activation of this last set of neurons by the VIIIth nerve produces ipsi- and contralateral inhibition of the M-cell. Their direct intracellular activation produces a monosynaptic Cl⁻-dependent unitary IPSP in the two M-cells. As these neurons indeed inhibit at least some of their target (here the M-cells), the identification of the fibers mediating the commissural inhibition could be more firmly established. Furthermore, in a recent study of the neurons inhibiting the M-cell of teleosts, it was demonstrated that each bouton established on the M-cell by the commissural and recurrent collateral interneurons functions as an independent all-or-none unit (Korn et al., 1981; see also Korn and Faber, this volume). This result has prompted the investigation of the ultrastructure of these endings to determine if they were morphologically different from those found at other central chemically transmitting synapses.

The morphology of these commissural cells was investigated at both light and electron microscopic levels on cells which had been physiologically identified at the unitary level prior to the intracellular injection of HRP (for technique, see Triller and Korn, 1981).

[175]

RESULTS

Neuronal morphology

The general outlook of all these cells is similar and is summarized in Fig. 1A, which is a camera lucida reconstruction of one of them. The somata, located in the

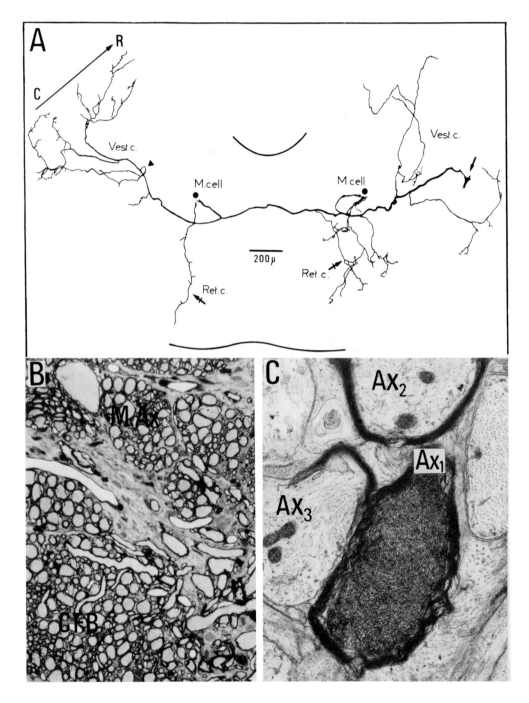

stato-acoustical area, issue axons with a thin initial segment which enlarge rapidly and course toward the contralateral vestibular complex. On its way, this process sends many collaterals within the vestibular nuclei and in the reticular formation and to the M-cell on both sides of the brainstem. When crossing the midline, these axons contribute in part to the bulbar or acoustical commissure (Bartelmez, 1915; Ariëns Kappers et al., 1936) confirming the hypothesis of Mano et al., (1968), who suggested that commissural pathways are mainly formed by axons of inhibitory interneurons.

The measurements of HRP-injected fibers at the level of the decussation give internal diameters (since the myelin is not visible with this technique) as large as $10 \, \mu m$ (m = 5.7 μm; S.D. = 1.8; n = 13). The commissural fiber bundle could easily be identified on parasagittal $1 \, \mu m$-thick plastic sections (Fig. 1B) stained with toluidine blue. Measurements of internal and external (which includes the myelin sheath) diameters give respective values of m = 7.8 μm (S.D. = 2.5; n = 44) and m = 9.5 μm (S.D. = 3.02; n = 44), allowing the computation of the ratio g (axon/total fiber diameter), which was 0.76 (S.D. = 0.08; n = 44). This last value is close to that calculated at other central myelinated fibers (Bernstein, 1966; Waxman, 1978) and close to the theoretical value of 0.6 for maximum conduction velocity (Rushton, 1951). The injected axons remain myelinated until their thinnest processes, at the vicinity of the axon cap (Fig. 1C) or within the reticular formation and the vestibular complex (not illustrated here). Because of the short distance between the two M-cells (about 1 mm) and between the vestibular complexes (about 2 mm), the commissural interneurons probably inhibit their ipsi- and contralateral target cells almost simultaneously. Considering that the fine ramifications are of equal length on both sides of the brain, the delay for inhibition between the two sides of the brainstem can be calculated. In fact, conduction velocity/diameter ratio of Hursh (1939) (corrected to 5.7 and a Q_{10} factor of 2.5, see Paintal, 1978) or either the ratio of 2.5 (Cragg and Thomas, 1957) or 2.5 (Tasaki, 1953) determined in cold-blooded animals, can be applied to the larger axons of the commissure fiber bundle. Then the computation gave delays as short as 0.04–0.05 msec for inhibition reaching the two M-cells and of 0.08–0.10 msec for inhibition reaching the two vestibular complexes.

Ultrastructure of identified terminals

Since the physiological effects of crossed vestibular interneurons on the Mauthner

---

Fig. 1. Axonal morphology of vestibulo-vestibular commissural inhibitory interneurons. A: camera lucida reconstruction of a PHP-exhibiting neuron intracellularly stained by horseradish peroxidase; prior to dye injection, this cell had been identified as inhibitory to the M-cell and belonging to the commissural pathway. The soma of the cell is located in the region of the vestibular complex (Vest. c.) and its axon crosses the midline before ending in the region of the contralateral vestibular nuclei. Note that this process emits numerous ramifications; their terminals reach the Mauthner cells (M-cell), the reticular formation (Ret. c., crossed arrows) on both sides. Profuse collaterals are also distributed within the vestibular regions whether ipsi- or contralateral to the injected cell body (arrow). The overall caudal to rostral (C→R) extension of this one plane representation is of about 700 μm. From a tench, *Tinca tinca*. B: parasagittal view of the brainstem showing the commissural fiber bundle (CFB) and the nearby M-cell axon (M-Ax) just before its decussation (this light micrograph was obtained from a 1 μm-thick plastic section, stained with toluidine blue). ×480. C: electron micrograph of a cross-sectioned HRP-filled axon (Ax_1) of about 2 μm in diameter including its myelin sheath and of two non-injected neighboring axons (Ax_2, Ax_3). This stained process, located in the immediate vicinity of the axon cap, represents the preterminal part of a secondary axonal ramification. ×19,000. B and C are from goldfish, *Carassius auratus*.

cell are well documented (see Introduction) we shall focus our description on the HRP-filled axon terminals synapsing on this target. Close to the level of the M-cell, the commissural fiber separates in two groups of terminal branchlets: one penetrates the axon cap (AC) and then contacts the M-cell axon hillock; the other group

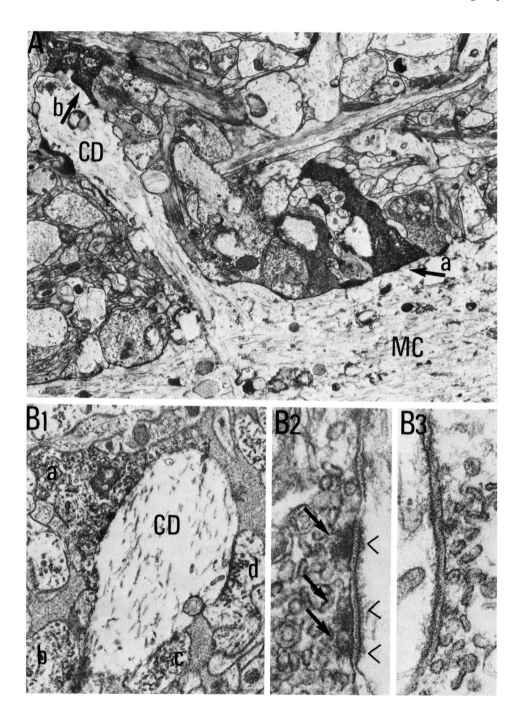

bypasses this region before synapsing on the M-cell soma and on the initial portion of its main dendrites. These boutons have the morphological features of un-myelinated club endings (UCEs) in the AC (Fig. 2A) and of small vesicle boutons (SVBs) outside of it (Nakajima, 1974). This distribution of the terminals of these interneurons is similar to that of the inhibitory cells of the recurrent collateral network (Korn et al., 1978). Although UCEs and SVBs are easily distinguished with morphological criteria, their synaptic apparatus exhibit common ultrastructural characteristics (Triller and Korn, 1981). These boutons (one of them is illustrated in Fig. $2B_1$ and B_2) contain a pleiomorphic population of vesicles which can be characterized by their "elongation index" which is the ratio of the maximum to the minimum diameters (D/d) and it ranged (for labeled boutons) from 1.4 to 1.5 (the larger its value, the more elongated is the vesicle); the mean diameter of the vesicles ($\sqrt{Dd}$) ranged from 40 to 46 nm and their surface area ($\pi Dd/4$) from 13 to $15 \cdot 10^2$ nm^2. Similar morphometrical study of unlabeled equivalent boutons (as for instance the one illustrated in Fig. $2B_3$) shows vesicles inclined to be more spherical in HRP-filled terminals. In boutons where the reaction product of HRP was moderate, the presynaptic dense projections (PDPs) were well visible (Fig. $2B_2$), and even seemed to be enhanced. These structures appear roughly triangular in trans-versal sections with their base facing the plasma membrane and their vertex directed toward the cytoplasm. The width of the base ranged between 55 and 100 nm, their height was from 50 to 70 nm and the distance between the centers of two PDPs varied between 70 and 170 nm. These values are comparable to those obtained in other axonal systems with different techniques (Pfenninger et al., 1969). The width of the synaptic cleft is 20–25 nm and the postsynaptic density is formed by a fuzzy continuous band of electron-dense material facing the presynaptic grid, the synaptic grid itself occupying only a small area of the whole contact. All these morphological features exhibited by these synaptic complexes are therefore similar to those of the chemically transmitting synapses of the symmetrical Gray type II (refs. in Peters et al., 1976).

CONCLUSION

Previous electrophysiological study has shown the existence of a vestibular ipsi-

---

Fig. 2. Morphological characteristics of the synaptic boutons established by interneurons on the Mauthner cell within the axon cap. A: electron micrograph obtained through the peripheral part of the Mauthner cell axon cap visualizing two terminals belonging to a second order vestibular neuron: one of them (arrow a) contacts the soma of the Mauthner cell (MC) and the second one (arrow b) impinges on a cap dendrite (CD). ×6600. B_1–B_3: ultrastructural features of unmyelinated club endings synapsing on a cap dendrite. B_1: a cap dendrite (CD) is contacted by one HRP-filled bouton (a) and three other unlabeled profiles (b, c and d) which are also unmyelinated club endings, one of them (d) establishes a complete active zone with the postsynaptic element (×21,000). B_2: higher magnification of the contact between the bouton labeled "a" in B_1 and the cap dendrite. Since this ending is lightly labeled, its organelles are easily identified although membranous and paramembranous components are enhanced by the enzymatic reaction product. This profile is filled with a pleiomorphic population of vesicles. Three presynaptic dense projections (arrows) facing a postsynaptic thickening (V shaped triangles) are also visible within the plane of section. The synaptic cleft (about 20 nm wide) is filled with an uneven electrondense material (×98,000). B_3: higher magnification of the synaptic complex established between the bouton which is labeled "d" in B_1 and the adjacent cap dendrite. This ending contains a pleiomorphic population of vesicles which is slightly more elongated than those of the HRP-stained profile (×98,000).

and contralateral monosynaptic inhibition of the Mauthner cell (Faber and Korn, 1978). The present observation brings substantial morphological evidence about this commissural pathway. The role of such a widespread and quasi-instantaneous medullary inhibition in teleost fish remains unclear: it can be speculated however (Faber and Korn, 1978) that activation of the VIIIth nerve at low stimulus intensities provides a general inhibition of their postsynaptic target to both sides of the brainstem. In contrast, at higher stimulus intensities, the first activated M-cell produces a tail flip while the contralateral one is inhibited almost at once by commissural PHP-exhibiting cells which also prevent other neurons projecting down the spinal cord from firing, thus leading to a better efficiency of the escape reaction.

Concerning the morphology of the synapse (Gray type II) associated with elongated vesicles, established on the M-cell, a satisfactory correlation is found with its inhibitory function though caution is required for its generalization (Nakajima, 1974). In a recent study (Triller and Korn, 1982) we have shown that almost all the terminals which are issued from this set of neurons and also from others, contain only one presynaptic grid. This, added to the fact that this type of terminal boutons behaves in an all-or-none manner (Korn et al., 1981), indicates that the active zone is a non-reducible release unit.

SUMMARY

This report deals with the relation that was found between the morphology and the function of a set of neurons that are known to inhibit the M-cell, in this case second order vestibulo-vestibular interneurons. Two main conclusions are to be drawn.

(1) Part of the acoustical commissure is constituted by the axons of these cells. Computations taking into account their diameter and the distance between the target cells indicate that they are responsible for a widespread and almost simultaneous inhibition on both sides of the brainstem.

(2) Investigation of the ultrastructure of the HRP-labeled boutons, in the present case those contacting the M-cell, indicates that they contain a pleiomorphic population of vesicles and establish Gray type II symmetrical synaptic contacts similar to other studied inhibitory synapses. Comparison with adjacent unstained equivalent terminals reveals that HRP allows a good morphometric analysis of synaptic organelles, although vesicles are slightly less elongated in enzyme-filled profiles.

ACKNOWLEDGEMENTS

The author is grateful to Dr. C. Sotelo (INSERM U106, CMC Foch, Suresnes, France) for providing facilities and kind criticism during this work. I am indebted to D. Le Cren for his skillful photographic assistance.

REFERENCES

Ariëns Kappers, C.U., Hubber, G.C. and Crosby, E.C. (1936) *The Comparative Anatomy of the Nervous System of Vertebrates. Including Man, Vol. 1*, Hafner, New York.

Bartelmez, G.W. (1915) Mauthner's cell and the nucleus motorius tegmenti. *J. comp. Neurol.*, 25: 87–128.

Bernstein, J.J. (1966) Relationship of cortico-spinal tract growth to age and body weight in the rat. *J. comp. Neurol.*, 127: 207–218.

Cragg, B.G. and Thomas, P.K. (1957) The relationship between conduction velocity and the diameter and internodal length of peripheral nerve fibers. *J. Physiol. (Lond.)*, 136: 606–614.

Faber, D.S. and Korn, H. (1973) A neuronal inhibition mediated electrically. *Science*, 179: 577–578.

Faber, D.S. and Korn, H. (1978) Electrophysiology of the Mauthner cell: Basic properties, synaptic mechanisms and associated networks. In D.S. Faber and H. Korn (Eds.), *Neurobiology of the Mauthner Cell*, Raven Press, New York, pp. 47–131.

Hursh, J.B. (1939) Conduction velocity and diameter of nerve fibers. *Amer. J. Physiol.*, 127: 131–139.

Korn, H. and Faber, D.S. (1975) An electrically mediated inhibition in goldfish medulla. *J. Neurophysiol.*, 38: 452–471.

Korn, H., Sotelo, C. and Bennett, M.V.L. (1977) The lateral vestibular nucleus of the toadfish *Opsanus tau*: Ultrastructural and electrophysiological observations with special reference to electrotonic transmission. *Neuroscience*, 2: 851–884.

Korn, H., Triller, A. and Faber, D.S. (1978) Structural correlates of recurrent collateral interneurons producing both electrical and chemical inhibitions of the Mauthner cell. *Proc. roy. Soc. B*, 202: 533–538.

Korn, H., Triller, A., Mallet, A. and Faber, D.S. (1981) Fluctuating responses at a central synapse: n of binomial fit predicts number of stained presynaptic boutons. *Science*, 213: 898–901.

Mano, N., Oshima, T. and Shimazu, H. (1968) Inhibitory commissural fibers interconnecting the bilateral vestibular nuclei. *Brain Res.*, 8: 378–382.

Nakajima, Y. (1974) Fine structure of the synaptic endings on the Mauthner cell of the goldfish. *J. comp. Neurol.*, 156: 375–402.

Paintal, A.S. (1978) Conduction properties of normal peripheral mammalian axons. In S.G. Waxman (Ed.), *Physiology and Pathobiology of Axons*, Raven Press, New York, pp. 131–144.

Peters, A., Palay, S.L. and Webster, H.F. (1976) *The Fine Structure of the Nervous System: The Neurons and Supporting Cells*, W.B. Saunders Co., Philadelphia, pp. 80–86.

Pfenninger, K., Sandri, C., Akert, K. and Eugster, C.H. (1969) Contribution to the problem of structural organization of the presynaptic area. *Brain Res.*, 12: 10–18.

Rushton, W.A.H. (1951) A theory of the effect of fibre size in medullated nerve. *J. Physiol. (Lond.)*, 115: 101–122.

Shimazu, H. and Precht, W. (1966) Inhibition of central vestibular neurons from the contralateral labyrinth and its mediating pathway. *J. Neurophysiol.*, 29: 467–492.

Tasaki, I. (1953) *Nervous Transmission*, Charles C. Thomas, Springfield, IL, pp. 81–85.

Triller, A. and Korn, H. (1978) Mise en évidence électrophysiologique et anatomique de neurones vestibulaires inhibiteurs commissuraux chez la tanche (*Tinca tinca*). *C.R. Acad. Sci. (Paris) D*, 286: 89–92.

Triller, A. and Korn, H. (1981) Morphologically distinct classes of inhibitory synapses arise from the same neurons: ultrastructural identification from crossed vestibular interneurons intracellularly stained with HRP. *J. comp. Neurol.*, 203: 131–155.

Triller, A. and Korn, H. (1982) Transmission at a central inhibitory synapse. III – Ultrastructure of physiologically identified HRP-stained terminals. *J. Neurophysiol*, 48: 708–736.

Waxman, S.G. (1978) Variations in axonal morphology and their functional significance. In S.G. Waxman (Ed.), *Physiology and Pathobiology of Axons*, Raven Press, New York, pp. 169–190.

Zottoli, S.J. and Faber, D.S. (1979) Morphological and electrophysiological characterization of a discrete class of statoacoustical interneurons in a vertebrate brain. *Neurosci. Abstr.*, 5: 749.

Zottoli, S.J. and Faber, D.S. (1980) An identifiable class of statoacoustical interneurons with bilateral projections in the goldfish medulla. *Neuroscience*, 5: 1287–1302.

Mosaics and Territories of Cat Retinal Ganglion Cells

H. WÄSSLE, L. PEICHL and B.B. BOYCOTT

Max-Planck-Institut für Hirnforschung, Duetschordenstr. 46, D-6000 Frankfurt (71) (F.R.G.) and (B.B.B.)
Medical Research Council Cell Biophysics Unit, King's College, 26–29 Drury Lane, London WC2B 5RL
(U.K.)

INTRODUCTION

When nerve cells have to overlay a planar surface with their dendrites so that every point is covered by at least one dendritic field, there are more or less economic ways to design such a cell assembly. If the cells would be arrayed in a precisely square (Fig. 1A) or hexagonal (Fig. 1B) array with a minimal intercell spacing "a", circular dendritic fields of radius "$a/\sqrt{2}$" or "$a/\sqrt{3}$" respectively would provide an at least one-fold coverage. If the cells would be distributed randomly (Fig. 1C and D), the one-fold coverage could be either achieved by rather large dendritic fields of uniform size (Fig. 1C) or by an interaction between neighbouring cells, which adjust the dendritic field size to the local intercell spacing (Fig. 1D).

TOPOGRAPHY OF ON- AND OFF-CENTER ALPHA CELLS

Ganglion cells of the retina are a good model system to study the organization of such a sheet of neurons because their cell bodies and their dendritic fields are each basically confined to a single layer. In the cat retina several different morphological (Boycott and Wässle, 1974) and physiological classes (Cleland and Levick, 1974) of ganglion cells are described. With neurofibrillar staining methods it was possible to stain all α-ganglion cells (see Fig. 2A) to their whole extent, i.e. cell body and dendritic tree (Wässle et al., 1981c). It was shown that the ON–OFF dichotomy of their physiological correlate, the brisk-transient (Y) cells, corresponds to a differing branching level of α-cell dendrites in the inner plexiform layer: all OFF-center cells have their dendritic branches close to the inner nuclear layer, all ON-center cells have their branching plane 10 μm nearer towards the ganglion cell layer (Nelson et al., 1978; Peichl and Wässle, 1981). On this basis the physiological type (ON- or OFF-center) of every single α-cell could be determined in flat mount preparations of the cat retina, and a functionally homogeneous population of neurons became accessible to investigation.

Fig. 3A shows all α-cells stained in a small field of retina. The dendritic fields of neighbouring α-cells overlap strongly and a complex plexus of dendritic branches is formed. Fig. 3B isolates the ON-population and a homogeneous overlay of that field with dendritic branches becomes apparent. The cell bodies are distributed non-

[183]

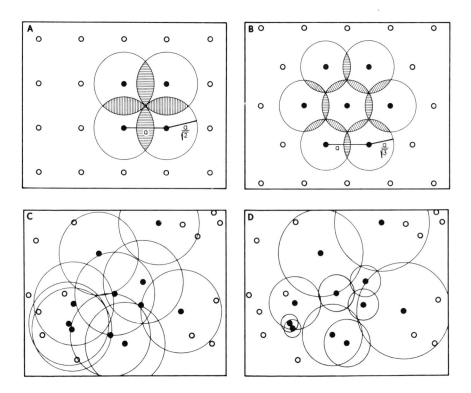

Fig. 1. A: square lattice of cell bodies. The smallest circular dendritic fields, which could provide a one-fold coverage have a radius of $a/\sqrt{2}$. In the hatched area the dendrites of two cells overlap. B: hexagonal array of cell bodies. In this instance at least one-fold coverage is ensured by dendritic fields of radius $a/\sqrt{3}$. C: random distribution of cell bodies with dendritic fields of uniform sizes. Rather large dendritic fields are necessary to ensure one-fold coverage everywhere. But at the same time this has the consequence of multiple coverage in other areas. D: random distribution of cell bodies with adjustment of the dendritic fields to the local intercell spacing.

randomly: this was shown by analyzing their nearest neighbour-distribution which is Gaussian (Wässle et al., 1981c; Wässle and Riemann, 1978). The degree of dendritic overlap is rather small, especially the area occupied by the cell body of a neuron is not covered by the dendritic branches of surrounding cells. The same arrangement is found for OFF-cells (Fig. 3C). Dendritic fields were defined by connecting the outermost dendritic tips of every ON-α-cell by a smooth closed curve (Fig. 3D). The dendritic fields are rather irregularly shaped and in some cases there is a clear

Fig. 2. Whole mount preparations of the cat retina viewed from the vitreal side. The focus was taken at the ganglion cell layer. A: ganglion cell layer stained by the Gros-Schultze-reduced silver method. This method stains all α-cells to their whole extent, i.e. cell body, dendritic tree and axon. The cell bodies of other ganglion cells are only faintly stained. B: ganglion cell layer retrogradely labeled after HRP injection into the ipsilateral LGN. All α-cells, all β-cells and less than half of the γ-cell population were labeled. Some eight-α-cells can be distinguished by their large cell bodies and dendritic trees. The medium-sized cell bodies with densely branched dendritic trees are partly stained β-cells. The small cell bodies with hardly any dendrites stained are labeled γ-cells. The scale bar in A and B represents 100 μm.

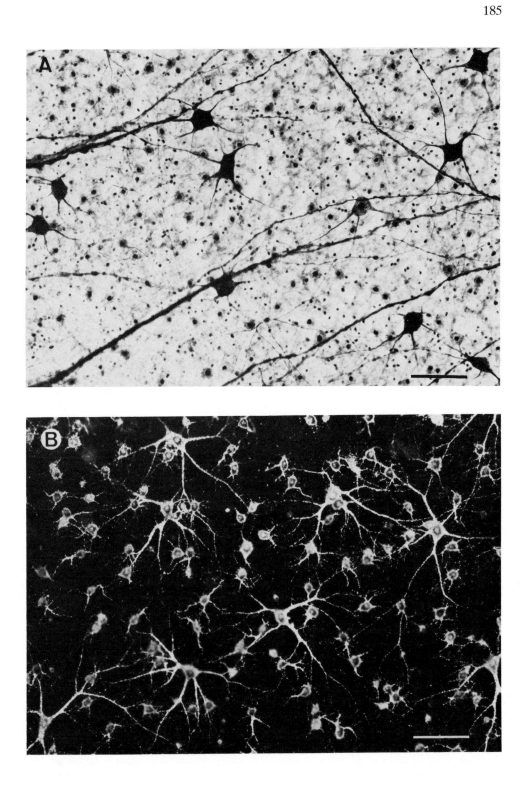

186

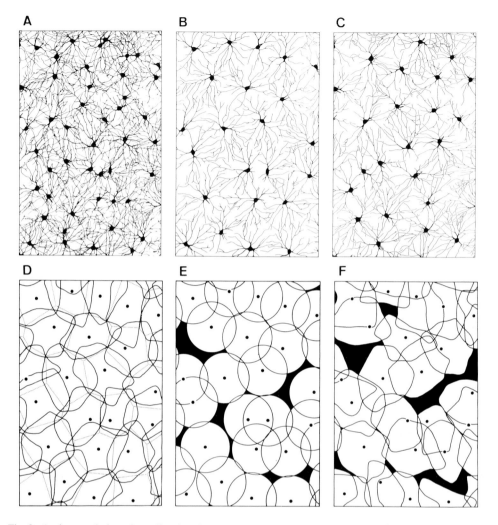

Fig. 3. A: the population of α-cells taken from an area 1.7×1.2 mm of a Bodian-stained cat retinal whole mount (eccentricity 4 mm). B: same field as in A, but only ON-α-cells are shown. C: same field as in A, but only OFF-α-cells are shown. D: solid curves are the contours of the ON-α-cells shown in B and the dots indicate the cell body locations. The dotted polygons are Dirichlet domains, which were constructed for each cell body as described in the text. E: coverage of the retina with hypothetical circular dendritic fields based on the mosaic of ON-α-cells; the black areas are not covered. F: every ON-α-cell dendritic field is substituted by its right-left mirror image with the cell body unchanged.

correlation between the dendritic tree of a cell and the space not occupied by neighbours.

The concept of Dirichlet domains (Honda, 1978), which cover the area by convex polygons without leaving gaps, is introduced in Fig. 3D for comparison. Around every cell body a circle of 500 μm diameter was constructed and the intersecting lines of neighbouring circles are drawn. Dirichlet domains subdivide the area into small territories surrounding every cell with the property that every point in a particular territory has a shorter distance to its own cell body than to any other.

Thus the Dirichlet domains would describe a dendritic growth model in which the dendrites grow out of the cell bodies at the same time and rate, and stop growing when they touch dendrites of neighbouring cells. It can be seen that the Dirichlet domains are a rather good approximation of the dendritic fields in Fig. 3D although they do not account for overlapping dendritic fields. Basic features like the orientation of the long axis nearly always agree when comparing dendritic field and Dirichlet domain. This implies that there might be some mutual regulation of the dendritic growth of neighbouring ganglion cells of the same type.

Another test for the correlation between the dendritic field and the available "territory" is shown in Fig. 3E. Circular fields of the average dendritic field diameter (399 μm) were constructed around every single ON-cell perikaryon. Such uniform dendritic fields leave gaps, the coverage is consequently incomplete and not very homogeneous (Fig. 3E). The same holds for Fig. 3F, where every dendritic field is replaced by its mirror image with the cell body in its original position. In this case, too, the coverage is very inhomogeneous, uncovered gaps are found next to areas where the dendritic fields of several ganglion cells overlap.

We infer from these observations that some kind of interaction between cell positions and dendritic fields must occur during development. This process must be highly specific, because it involves only a very narrow functional group: ON-center cells interfere with neighbouring ON-center cells but not with OFF-center cells and vice versa (Wässle et al., 1981b).

How economic is the way in which ganglion cells subdivide the retina into dendritic domains? Every point of Fig. 3D is covered by an average of 1.4 ON-α-cells (average dendritic field area × density). If the cells were arrayed in a square lattice with circular dendritic fields, the geometrical constraints given in Fig. 1A would require an average coverage of 1.57 in order to guarantee a one-fold coverage everywhere. An arrangement of the ganglion cells in a hexagonal lattice (Fig. 1B) would require an average coverage of 1.21. This shows that although the ganglion cells are distributed less precisely than in a geometric lattice, their dendritic trees cover the given field of Fig. 3 in a way which is more economic than in a square array and close to the theoretical limit possible in a hexagonal lattice.

TOPOGRAPHY OF ON- AND OFF-CENTER BETA CELLS

A multiple injection of horseradish peroxidase (HRP) into one lateral geniculate nucleus (LGN) gave a homogeneous staining of ganglion cells in the retina (Fig. 2B). The filling of dendrites in HRP-labeled cells was good enough to enable classification of the cells into α, β and γ-cells. But observation of the dendritic morphology of HRP and Golgi-stained β-cells shows that HRP stains only the first part of the dendritic tree of the cells (Fig. 4A). Fortunately this was sufficient to reveal their differing branching levels and therefore to separate ON- and OFF-β-cells (Fig. 4B and C).

The mosaic formed by ON- and OFF-β-cells was analyzed by measuring the distance to the nearest neighbour of each cell (Wässle and Riemann, 1978). As a first step we measured from the position of every β-cell the distance to the next β-cell independent of its physiological type. The histogram in Fig. 4D shows the nearest neighbour distances obtained. For the great majority of cells (129 out of 136) the

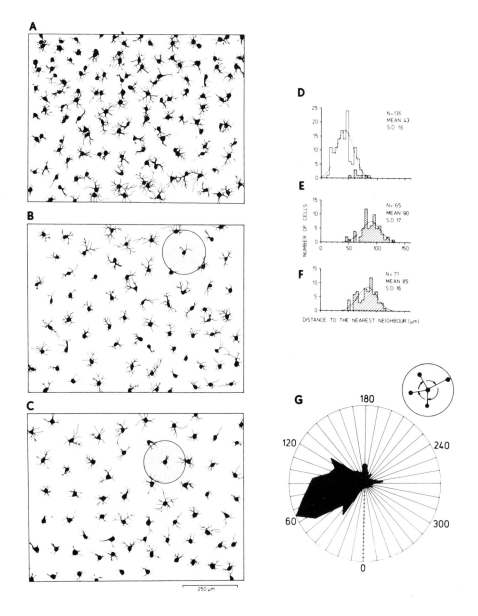

Fig. 4. Analysis of the β-cell mosaic. A: this is a drawing of all β-cells from a field containing Fig. 2B. The β-cells fill the field rather homogeneously and are often grouped into pairs. B: same field as in A, but only OFF-β-cells are shown. C: same field as in A, but only ON-β-cells are shown. The stippled fields in B and C indicate the dendritic field of a β-cell from Golgi-stained material at the same eccentricity. Thus neighbouring dendritic fields would overlap and it is only the limitations of the HRP staining that show the β-cell dendritic fields as isolated. D: histogram showing the distribution of the distances from each cell to its nearest neighbour, taken from the heterogeneous ON-OFF-β-cell population in A. The hatched bins indicate the few cases where neighbours were either both ON or OFF. E: nearest neighbour histogram for the population of ON-β-cells in C. F: nearest neighbour histogram for the OFF-β-cells in B. G: as explained by the inset this diagram shows for each OFF-β-cell the angles between all neighbours found within a circle of 110 μm radius.

nearest neighbour is of the opposite type, which confirms the qualitative impression (Fig. 4A) that ON- and OFF-cells are grouped into pairs. The overall histogram can be approximated by a Gaussian although it is skewed to lower distances. The ratio mean/S.D. is 2.72; this is low and indicates the mosaic to be rather imprecise. There is a large scatter of nearest neighbour distances.

Restricting the analysis to the ON- and OFF-populations then independent mosaics of distinctive regularity become apparent (Fig. 4E and F). The nearest neighbour histograms are Gaussian and are closely similar for both ON- (Fig. 4E) and OFF-β-cells (Fig. 4F). For the ON-β-cells the ratio mean/S.D. is 5.19 and for the OFF-β-cells 5.28. This shows that ON- and OFF-β-cells each form a regular mosaic and that, as with α-cells (Wässle et al., 1981a), and the two types of horizontal cells (Wässle et al., 1978), these mosaics are independent. Such superimposition of two regularities does not create a random overall β-cell distribution, but, as in this instance, a rather sloppy regularity.

The idea that ON- and OFF-cells are independently arrayed was tested in the following way. The ON-mosaic and a mirror image of the OFF-mosaic were superimposed and the resulting nearest neighbour histogram of this uncorrelated array was compared with the histogram in Fig. 4D: Both the mean and the standard deviation closely agreed indicating that the mosaics have a similar form. No statistical significant difference between the histograms was observed (sign reversal test, $P > 0.17$).

Crystalline regular two-dimensional patterns can exhibit square or hexagonal packing (Fig. 1A and B), which means 90 or 60 degrees angular symmetry. The polar diagram in Fig. 4G tests the angular symmetry of the β-cell mosaic. Each OFF-β-cell was connected by lines to all neighbours within a circle of 220 μm diameter. The angles between these lines are shown in Fig. 4G. For square packing angles mainly of 90° would be expected, for hexagonal packing angles mainly of 60° should be found. In fact a rather broad angular distribution that forms a continuum between 60° and 90° is found. This shows the lack of angular symmetry in the β-cell mosaic.

To obtain a coverage factor for β-cells it is necessary to take the dendritic field dimensions from the Golgi data and the cell densities from the HRP labeled material. The shrinkage of the retina produced by the two methods is near enough the same, so both sets of data can be combined without conversion factors. The average dendritic field diameter of all β-cells at 6 mm eccentricity was 200 μm. The coverage factor (dendritic field area × density) for OFF-β-cells was 3.1, that of ON-β-cells was 2.83. Thus at every point in Fig. 4A the dendritic trees of 6 β-cells would be seen to overlap were the cells completely stained.

The distance to the nearest neighbour for both ON- and OFF-center cells was about 90 μm, which agrees well with the dendritic field radius of 100 μm. As can be seen in Fig. 4B and C the perikarya of the nearest neighbours are positioned at the perimeter of the dendritic tree. Thus, unlike the α-cells, the dendritic fields of β-cells are completely covered by their immediate neighbours. This does not mean that there might be no mechanism of mutual regulation of dendritic growth of neighbouring β-cells. The two dendritic fields inserted in Fig. 4B and C suggest a stop of the dendritic growth at the position of the cell body of the neighbours. But at the present no more detail can be given because of the lack of sufficient dendritic staining in the HRP material.

CONCLUSIONS

Two-dimensional sheets of neurons are not only found in the retina; arrangement in layers is common in many parts of the central nervous system. The multilamellar structure of the cerebral cortex is an example and it would be interesting to see whether identical functional units there exhibit the same kinds of territorial attributes and regular intercell spacings.

SUMMARY

Ganglion cells have to cover the retina with their dendritic fields so that every point of visual space is "seen" by at least one ganglion cell of each physiological type.

Using neurofibrillar methods it was possible to stain all α-ganglion cells so that their dendritic network could be analyzed. Both subpopulations of α-cells, corresponding physiologically to ON-center and OFF-center brisk-transient (Y) cells (Cleland and Levick, 1974), achieve a uniform and independent coverage of the retina. The cell bodies are arrayed in a regular mosaic and the dendritic fields adapt to the available space.

The spatial distribution of ON- and OFF-β-cells was studied from HRP-labeled material. ON-β-cells form a regular lattice with regular inter-cell spacings; OFF-β-cells are also regularly arrayed. The two lattices are superimposed independently of each other and of the α-cells.

REFERENCES

Boycott, B.B. and Wässle, H. (1974) The morphological types of ganglion cells of the domestic cat's retina. *J. Physiol. (Lond.)*, 240: 397–419.

Cleland, B.G. and Levick, W.R. (1974) Brisk and sluggish concentrically organized ganglion cells in the cat's retina. *J. Physiol. (Lond.)*, 240: 421–456.

Honda, H. (1978) Description of cellular patterns by Dirichlet domains: the two-dimensional case. *J. theoret. Biol.*, 72: 523–543.

Nelson, R., Famiglietti, E.V. and Kolb, H. (1978) Intracellular staining reveals different levels of stratification for ON- and OFF center ganglion cells in cat retina. *J. Neurophysiol.*, 41: 472–483.

Peichl, L. and Wässle, H. (1981) Morphological identification of on- and off-centre brisk transient (Y) cells in the cat retina. *Proc. roy. Soc. B*, 212: 139–156.

Wässle, H. and Riemann, H.J. (1978) The mosaic of nerve cells in the mammalian retina. *Proc. roy. Soc. B*, 200: 441–461.

Wässle, H., Peichl, L. and Boycott, B.B. (1978) Topography of horizontal cells in the retina of the domestic cat. *Proc. roy. Soc. B*, 203: 269–291.

Wässle, H., Boycott, B.B. and Illing, R.B. (1981a) Morphology and mosaic of on- and off-beta cells in the cat retina and some functional considerations. *Proc. roy. Soc. B.*, 212: 177–195.

Wässle, H., Peichl, L. and Boycott, B.B. (1981b) Dendritic territories of cat retinal ganglion cells. *Nature*, 292: 344–345.

Wässle, H., Peichl, L. and Boycott, B.B. (1981c) Morphology and topography of on- and off-alpha cells in the cat retina. *Proc. roy. Soc. B.*, 212: 157–175.

The Organization of Amacrine Cell Types
Which Use Different Transmitters
in Chicken Retina

IAN G. MORGAN

Department of Behavioural Biology, Research School of Biological Sciences, Australian National University, PO Box 475, Canberra City ACT 2601 (Australia)

INTRODUCTION

Ramón y Cajal (1893) described 15 different morphological types of amacrine cell in the chicken retina in Golgi-stained material. The amacrine cell types differ in the locations of their cell bodies within the inner nuclear layer, or sometimes in the ganglion cell layer, and in the patterns of their dendrite arborizations within the inner plexiform layer. The different types of amacrine cell appear likely to be involved in specific relationships with specific ganglion cell types, in view of the often complementary patterns of organization of the dendrites of the two groups of cells.

TRANSMITTER-SPECIFIC AMACRINE CELL TYPES

A corresponding diversity of transmitters is used by the amacrine cells (for review see Bonting, 1974). In birds, acetylcholine (Baughman and Bader, 1977), γ-amino-butyric acid (Marshall and Voaden, 1974a), glycine (Marshall and Voaden, 1974b), dopamine (Ehinger, 1967), an indoleamine-like compound (Floren, 1979; Floren and Hansson, 1980) and taurine (Lake et al., 1978) have been implicated. More recently, neuropeptides have also been localized to amacrine cell types in chickens and pigeons. These include amacrine cells reacting with antisera directed against Met- and Leu-enkephalin (Brecha et al., 1979; Morgan, Oliver and Chubb, unpublished results), substance P (Karten and Brecha, 1980), somatostatin (Brecha et al., 1981; Buckerfield et al., 1981), neurotensin (Brecha et al., 1981), glucagon and vasoactive intestinal peptide (Stell et al., 1980) and cholecystokinin octapeptide (Osborne et al., 1982).

The basic morphological features of these amacrine cell types have been defined (Fig. 1), in the case of the amacrine cells which appear to contain peptides by immunohistochemistry and in the case of the classical transmitters by autoradio-graphic localization of high affinity uptake systems, histochemical techniques and chemically-induced fluorescence. Poor resolution, particularly of those techniques involving autoradiographic localization of high affinity uptake systems, has often made it difficult to fully define cell morphologies.

In only one case is it claimed that there is a good fit between an amacrine cell

[191]

192

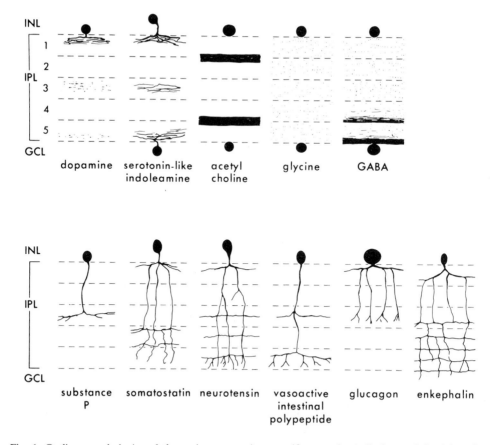

Fig. 1. Outline morphologies of the various transmitter-specific amacrine cell classes defined in avian retinas. The diagrams are based on information in the following papers: dopamine (Ehinger, 1967); serotonin-like indoleamine (Floren, 1979); acetylcholine (Baughman and Bader, 1977); glycine (Marshall and Voaden, 1974); GABA (Marshall and Voaden, 1974a); substance P (Karten and Brecha, 1980); somatostatin (Brecha et al., 1981; Buckerfield et al., 1981); neurotensin (Brecha et al., 1981); vasoactive intestinal polypeptide and glucagon (Stell et al., 1980); enkephalin (Brecha et al., 1979; Morgan et al., unpublished results).

type defined in terms of its putative transmitter (substance P-like immunoreactivity) and a morphological amacrine cell type (type J) defined so many years ago by Ramón y Cajal (1893). Unfortunately, this fit involves the one peptide-containing amacrine cell type over which there is some dispute, since we have been consistently unable to find amacrine cells showing substance P-like immunoreactivity in both chickens and pigeons by immunohistochemical and radioimmunoassay techniques, although in other studies we have detected substance P-like immunoreactivity in chicken spinal cord and in a range of mammalian retinas. Even if the substance P-immunoreactive amacrine cell type reported by Karten and Brecha (1980) contains an immunologically cross-reactive molecule rather than authentic substance P (cf. Eskay et al., 1981), it will be important to establish which molecule has been detected by Karten and Brecha (1980), for it is certainly defining a unique amacrine cell type.

SYNAPTIC INTERACTIONS OF TRANSMITTER-SPECIFIC AMACRINE CELL TYPES

Amacrine cells make their synaptic connections in the inner plexiform layer, with bipolar cells, ganglion cells and interplexiform cells. Amacrine cells may receive synaptic input from bipolar cells, interplexiform cells and other amacrine cells. In addition, in birds, some amacrine cells receive synaptic input from the centrifugal fibers reaching the retina from the isthmo-optic nucleus (Dowling and Cowan, 1966). In turn, amacrine cells may make synapses onto bipolar cells, ganglion cells, interplexiform cells and other amacrine cells. Not all amacrine cell types show all these potential interconnections. To help define the bipolar cell input to the amacrine cell types, and their interactions with ganglion cells, we have used two chemical lesioning techniques.

Intravitreal injections of colchicine – Destruction of ganglion cells

In birds, section of the optic nerve leads to retrograde degeneration of the ganglion cell bodies in the retina. This has not proven to be a useful routine tool in our hands, since it leads to a variable amount of retinal degeneration due to the disruption of the retinal blood supply. I have developed a simple and reliable chemical lesioning technique for eliminating the retinal ganglion cells, intravitreal injection of colchicine (Morgan, 1981). The biochemical profile of the lesioned retina is given in Table I. In addition to the expected loss of transmitter receptors associated with the ganglion cell dendrites, levels of some amacrine cell transmitters or related pre-synaptic activities decrease. So far reductions have been noted for GABA, glycine and choline acetyltransferase which are found in amacrine cells that

TABLE I

Levels of amacrine cell transmitter-related activities in lesioned chicken retinas

Activity	Control activity/retina	% change	
		40 nmol kainic acid	1 µg colchicine
Choline acetyltransferase	530 nmol/h	−68	−20
High affinity choline uptake	48 pmol/min	−75	−15
Acetylcholinesterase	240 nmol/min	−61	−54
Muscarinic acetylcholine receptors	1077 fmol	−60	−4
Nicotinic acetylcholine receptors	2481 fmol	−80	−50
Dopamine	40 pmol	−7	not determined
GABA	0.054 µmol	−92	−45
GABA receptors (K_d 0.5 nM)	6.0 pmol	−26	−53
Benzodiazepine receptors	1.63 pmol	−88	−51
Glycine	0.107 µmol	−51	−29
Glycine receptors	9.8 pmol	−48	−42
Somatostatin	12.2 ng	−81	+11
Met-enkephalin	5.41 ng	−68	−4

194

in other species appear to directly synapse onto ganglion cells (Straschill and Perwein, 1969, 1973; Masland and Ames, 1976; Miller et al., 1977; Caldwell et al., 1978; Negishi et al., 1978). The levels of the two putative peptide transmitters examined did not change. These results have been in part confirmed in retinas which have suffered selective loss of ganglion cells after optic nerve section. The most likely interpretation of these findings is that receptor activities are lost as a simple result of the degeneration of ganglion cell dendrites on which they are located. The loss of presynaptic amacrine cell transmitter-related activities is a result either of down-regulation of the amacrine cells which have partially lost their target cells, or of loss of amacrine cell synapses as appears to be the case in rat retinas after optic nerve section (West and Chernenko, 1978). The more sensitive and unequivocal technique for examining amacrine cell–ganglion cell interaction is that involving receptor loss, and it is therefore important to confirm our predictions about the peptide-immunoreactive cells by looking for loss of retinal enkephalin-receptors (Medzihradsky, 1976; Howells et al., 1980).

Intravitreal injection of kainic acid – Elimination of amacrine and bipolar cells

Schwarcz and Coyle (1977) showed that intravitreal injections of kainic acid in young chickens led to marked destruction of cells in the inner nuclear layer of the retina. We have examined this phenomenon in more detail (Ehrlich and Morgan, 1980; Morgan and Ingham, 1981; Ingham and Morgan, 1983). Intravitreal injections of 20–60 nmol of kainic acid lead to loss of amacrine cells, displaced amacrine cells and approximately two-thirds of the bipolar cells, leaving the photoreceptors, Muller glial, horizontal and ganglion cells alive (Fig. 3). Recently it has been show that pretreatment with anesthetic doses of barbiturates and benzodiazepines protects the amacrine cells from the excitotoxic effects of kainic acid, while the bipolar cells still succumb (Imperato et al., 1981).

Since the benzodiazepines and other anesthetics are believed to prevent the "distant" effects of kainic acid mediated by hyperactivity in cells directly affected by kainic acid (Ben-Ari et al., 1979), this suggests the picture of kainic acid effects on retinal cell classes shown in Fig. 2. Kainic acid may interact directly with bipolar cell

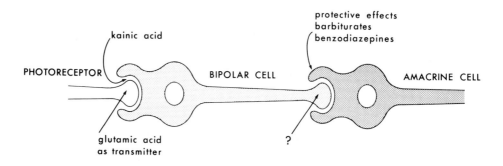

MODES OF ACTION OF KAINIC ACID

Fig. 2. Modes of action of kainic acid. The light dotted cell is killed off by direct effects of kainic acid, and in the retina would be a bipolar cell. The dark dotted cell is killed by the distant effects of kainic acid, and in the retina would be an amacrine cell.

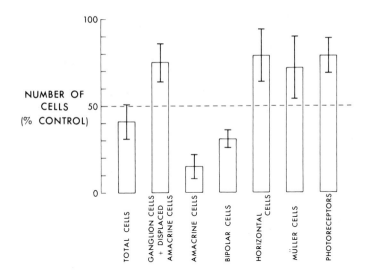

Fig. 3. This figure gives the percentage of cells surviving in each of the major classes of retinal cells after intravitreal injection of 20–60 nmol kainic acid, as judged from counts of cell nuclei in 1 μm sections through the central retina ± the standard deviation. Three standard strips of 100 μm width were counted through the thickness of each retina (n = 8 for experimentals; n = 5 for controls).

dendritic receptors (and with those of horizontal cells, see Morgan and Ingham, 1981), presumably due to the nature of the photoreceptor transmitter (Wu and Dowling, 1978; Neal et al., 1979). The death of amacrine cells after exposure to kainic acid may in fact be due to kainic acid-induced hyperactivity in the bipolar cells. This implies that only those amacrine cell types which receive input from bipolar cells would be sensitive to intravitreal kainic acid.

This lesioning technique has been used to localize transmitters to amacrine and bipolar cells, although the new techniques for selectively destroying bipolar cells have not yet been exploited by us. Loss of transmitter receptors after intravitreal kainic acid has been used to throw some light upon the involvement of amacrine cell transmitters in synaptic inputs to other amacrine cells and bipolar cell terminals. The results of this approach are summarized in Table I.

The basic patterns of amacrine cell organization in chicken retina derived from our studies are remarkably consistent with the knowledge of amacrine cell organization obtained with other vertebrates. Dopaminergic amacrine cells (Dowling and Ehinger, 1978; Adolph et al., 1980) and interplexiform cells (Dowling and Ehinger, 1978b; Dowling et al., 1981) from several species have been shown morphologically not to receive bipolar cell input, while dopamine levels (Table I) and tyrosine hydroxylase activities (Schwarcz and Coyle, 1977) in chicken are relatively resistant to kainic acid treatment. There is also morphological evidence for the survival of dopaminergic cells after kainic acid injections in chickens (Ingham and Morgan, 1983), goldfish (Yazulla and Kleinschmidt, 1980) and rats (Lessell et al., 1980). By contrast, rat GABAergic amacrine cells are believed to receive bipolar cell input (Wood et al., 1976), and are sensitive to kainic acid (Goto et al., 1981), as are those of chicken (Table I: Schwarcz and Coyle, 1977). The loss of receptors and activities after intravitreal injections of colchicine is consistent with the known GABAergic, gly-

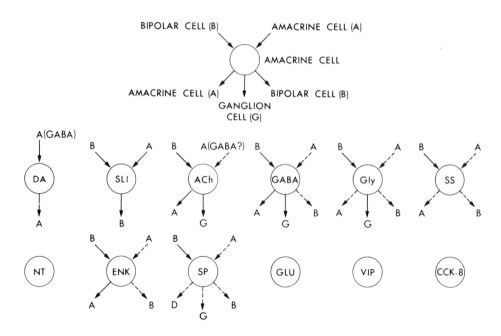

Fig. 4. Schematic picture of the inputs to and outputs from amacrine cells based on studies carried out on a range of vertebrates using electrophysiological, morphological and biochemical procedures. A full arrow indicates a confirmed connection, a dashed arrow an uncertain connection, and absence of an arrow indicates that the connection does not appear to exist.

cinergic and cholinergic inputs to ganglion cells in other species. Equally, lack of change in levels of enkephalin after ganglion cell destruction is consistent with the indirect electrophysiological effects of opiates on ganglion cells reported in other species (Dick et al., 1980; Djamgoz et al., 1981).

Pooling the available information on all vertebrates which have been examined, a picture of possible synaptic inputs to and outputs from transmitter-specific amacrine cell types can be constructed (Fig. 4). None of the data available on chicken retina amacrine cells is in conflict with this general picture. However, it is clearly important to test these biochemically and physiologically based predictions by electron microscopic techniques.

PERSPECTIVES

Two problems emerge from the characterization of amacrine cell types already achieved. Firstly, it is necessary to determine how the different amacrine cell types interact with each other. Electron microscopy, coupled with immunohistochemistry, autoradiography of transmitter uptake systems and specific cell degeneration holds out some promise. Pharmacological manipulation of transmitter levels, turnover and release (Massey and Neal, 1979; Morgan and Kamp, 1980) has already been successfully applied in a few cases, giving evidence of GABAergic inputs to cholinergic and dopaminergic amacrine cells.

The second question concerns the interaction of the amacrine cell types with specific ganglion cell types suggested in the Golgi studies of Ramón y Cajal (1893). There has been little progress in defining functionally-specific and transmitter-specific ganglion cell classes in birds. However, in several species (cat, Nelson et al., 1978; rabbit, Bloomfield and Miller, 1981; turtle, Marchiafava and Weiler, 1980; goldfish, Famiglietti et al., 1977) ON-center and OFF-center ganglion cell dendrites seem to be anatomically segregated in the inner and outer parts of the inner plexiform layer respectively. If this pattern of organization exists for the chicken retina, then it is clear from Fig. 1 that the dendrites of the two different ganglion cell classes must exist in quite different synaptic environments. Cholinergic, GABAergic, glycinergic and perhaps serotoninergic displaced and normally placed amacrine cells appear to provide some symmetry, but dopaminergic amacrine cells and those using peptide transmitters appear to be asymmetrically distributed, and therefore to be differentially involved in the ON-center and OFF-center ganglion cell response system.

ADDENDUM

Osborne (personal communication) has shown that the amacrine cells which react with antisera directed against serotonin are destroyed by kainic acid in the chicken, which is consistent with the bipolar input to the amacrine cells possessing a high affinity uptake system for serotonin described morphologically in mud-puppy (Adolph et al., 1980) and rabbit (Ehinger and Holmgren, *Cell Tiss. Res.*, 197 (1979) 175–194). Osborne has also demonstrated that chicken amacrine cells which contain substance P-like immunoreactivity are destroyed after intravitreal injections of kainic acid. In the goldfish somatostatin-immunoreactive amacrine cells receive bipolar cell input (Marshak et al., *Neurosci. Abstr.* 7 (1981) 203.5), in agreement with their sensitivity to kainic acid in chicken. However, these cells appear to contact both amacrine and ganglion cells, which may mean that the lack of depression of amacrine cell transmitter levels after destruction of the ganglion cells is not a completely reliable indicator of lack of amacrine cell–ganglion cell contacts.

REFERENCES

Adolph, A., Dowling, J.E. and Ehinger, B. (1980) Monoaminergic neurons of the mud puppy retina. *Cell Tiss. Res.* 210: 269–282.

Baughman, R.W. and Bader, C.R. (1977) Biochemical characterization and cellular localization of the cholinergic system in the chicken retina. *Brain Res.*, 138: 469–485.

Ben-Ari, Y., Tremblay, E., Ottersen, O.P. and Naquet, R. (1979) Evidence suggesting epileptogenic lesions after kainic acid: pretreatment with diazepam reduces distant but not local damage. *Brain Res.*, 165: 362–365.

Bloomfield, S.A. and Miller, R.L. (1981) Functional stratification of ON and OFF pathways in the rabbit retina. *ARVO Abstr.*, 20: (April) p. 13.

Bonting, S.L. (Ed.) (1976) *Transmitters in the Visual Process*, Pergamon Press, Oxford.

Brecha, N., Karten, H.J. and Laverack, C. (1979) Enkephalin-containing amacrine cells in the avian retina: Immunohistochemical localization. *Proc. nat. Acad. Sci. U.S.A.*, 76: 3010–3014.

Brecha, N., Karten, H.J. and Schenker, C. (1981) Neurotensin-like and somatostatin-like immunoreactivity within amacrine cells of the retina. *Neuroscience*, 6: 1329–1340.

Buckerfield, M., Oliver, J., Chubb, I.W. and Morgan, I.G. (1981) Somatostatin-like immunoreactivity in amacrine cells of the chicken retina. *Neuroscience*, 6: 685–693.

Caldwell, J.H., Daw, N.W. and Wyatt, H.J. (1978) Effects of picrotoxin and strychnine on rabbit retinal ganglion cells: lateral interactions for cells with more complex receptive fields. *J. Physiol. (Lond.)*, 176: 277–298.

Dick, E., Miller, R.F. and Behbehani, M.M. (1980) Opioids and substance P influence ganglion cells in amphibian retina. *ARVO Abstr.*, 19: 132.

Djamgoz, M.B.A., Stell, W.K., Chin, C.-A. and Lam, D.M.K. (1981) An opiate system in the goldfish retina. *Nature (Lond.)*, 292: 620–623.

Dowling, J.E. and Cowan, W.M. (1966) An electron microscopic study of normal and degenerating centrifugal fiber terminals in the pigeon retina. *Z. Zellforsch.*, 71: 14–28.

Dowling, J.E. and Ehinger, B. (1978a) Synaptic organization of the dopaminergic neurons in the rabbit retina. *J. comp. Neurol.*, 180: 203–220.

Dowling, J.E. and Ehinger, B. (1978b) The interplexiform cell system. I. Synapses of the dopaminergic neurons of the goldfish retina. *Proc. roy. Soc. B*, 201: 7–26.

Dowling, J.E., Ehinger, B. and Floren, I. (1981) Fluorescence and electron microscopical observations on the amine-accumulating neurons of the Cebus monkey retina. *J. comp. Neurol.*, 192: 665–685.

Ehinger, B. (1967) Adrenergic nerves in the avian eye and ciliary ganglion. *Z. Zellforsch.*, 82: 577–588.

Ehrlich, D. and Morgan, I.G. (1980) Kainic acid destroys displaced amacrine cells in post-hatch chicken retina. *Neurosci. Lett.*, 17: 43–49.

Eskay, R.L., Furness, J.F. and Long, R.T. (1981) Substance P activity in the bullfrog retina: localization and identification in several vertebrate species. *Science*, 212: 1049–1051.

Famiglietti, E.V., Kaneko, A. and Tachibana, M. (1977) Neuronal architecture of ON and OFF pathways to ganglion cells in carp. *Science*, 198: 1267–1269.

Floren, I. (1979) Indoleamine accumulating neurons in the retina of chicken and pigeon. A comparison with the dopaminergic neurons. *Acta ophthalmol.*, 57: 198–210.

Floren, I. and Hansson, H.C. (1980) Investigations into whether 5-hydroxytryptamine is a neurotransmitter in the retina of rabbit and chicken. *Invest. Ophthalmol., Vis. Sci.*, 19: 117–125.

Goto, M., Inomata, N., Ono, H., Saito, K.-I. and Fukuda, H. (1981) Changes of electroretinogram and neurochemical aspects of GABAergic neurons of retina after intraocular injection of kainic acid in rats. *Brain Res.*, 211: 305–314.

Howells, R.D., Groth, J., Hiller, J.M. and Simon, E.J. (1980) Opiate binding sites in the retina: properties and distribution. *J. Pharmacol. exp. Ther.*, 215: 60–64.

Imperato, A., Porceddu, M.L., Morelli, M., Fossarello, M. and Di Chiara, G. (1981) Benzodiazepines prevent kainate-induced loss of GABAergic and cholinergic neurons in the chick retina. *Brain Res.*, 213: 205–210.

Ingham, C.A. and Morgan, I.G. (1983) Dose-dependent effects of intravitreal kainic acid on specific cell types in chicken retina. *Neuroscience*, in press.

Karten, H.J. and Brecha, N. (1980) Localization of substance P immunoreactivity in amacrine cells of the retina. *Nature (Lond.)*, 283: 87–88.

Lake, N., Marshall, J. and Voaden, M.J. (1978) High affinity uptake sites for taurine in the retina. *Exp. Eye Res.*, 27: 713–718.

Lessell, S., Craft, J.L. and Albert, D.M. (1980) Kainic acid induces mitoses in mature retinal neurones in rats. *Exp. Eye Res.*, 30: 731–735.

Marchiafava, P.L. and Weiler, R. (1980) Intracellular analysis and structural correlates of the organization of inputs to ganglion cells in the retina of the turtle. *Proc. roy. Soc. B*, 208: 103–113.

Marshall, J. and Voaden, M. (1974a) An autoradiographic study of the cells accumulating $^{3}H\gamma$-aminobutyric acid in the isolated retinas of pigeons and chickens. *Invest. Ophthalmol., Vis. Sci.*, 13: 602–607.

Marshall, J. and Voaden, M.J. (1974b) A study of γ-[^{3}H]aminobutyric acid and [^{3}H]glycine accumulation by the isolated pigeon retina utilizing scintillation radioautography. *Biochem. Soc. Trans.*, 2: 268–270.

Masland, R.H. and Ames, A. III, (1976) Responses to acetylcholine of ganglion cells in an isolated mammalian retina. *J. Neurophysiol.*, 39: 1220–1235.

Massey, S.C. and Neal, M.J. 1979) The light-evoked release of acetylcholine from the rabbit retina in vivo and its inhibition by γ-aminobutyric acid. *J. Neurochem.*, 32: 1327–1329.

Medzihradsky, F. (1976) Steroespecific binding of etorphine in isolated neural cells and in retina, determined by a sensitive microassay. *Brain Res.*, 108: 212–219.

Miller, R.L., Dacheux, R.F. and Frumkes, J.E. (1977) Amacrine cells in *Necturus* retina: evidence for independent γ-aminobutyric acid and glycine-releasing neurons. *Science*, 198: 148–150.

Morgan, I.G. (1981) Sensitivity of chick retina ganglion cells to colchicine during development. *Neurosci. Lett.*, 24: 255–260.

Morgan, I.G. and Ingham, C.A. (1981) Kainic acid affects both plexiform layers of chicken retina. *Neurosci. Lett.*, 21: 275–280.

Morgan, W.W. and Kamp, C.W. (1980) A GABAergic influence on the light-induced increase in dopamine turnover in the dark-adapted rat retina in vivo. *J. Neurochem.*, 34: 1082–1086.

Neal, M.J., Collins, G.G. and Massey, S.C. (1979) Inhibition of aspartate release from the retina of the anaesthetized rabbit by stimulation with light flashes. *Neurosci. Lett.*, 14: 241–245.

Negishi, K., Kato, S., Teranishi, T. and Laufer, M. (1978) An electrophysiological study of the cholinergic system in the carp retina. *Brain Res.*, 148: 85–93.

Nelson, R., Famiglietti, E.V. and Kolb, H. (1978) Intracellular straining reveals different levels of stratification for on- and off-center ganglion cells in cat retina. *J. Neurophysiol.*, 41: 472–483.

Osborne, N.N., Nicholas, D.A., Dockray, G.J. and Cuello, A.C. (1982) Cholecystokinin and substance P immunoreactivity in retinas of rats, hogs, lizards and chicks. *Exp. Eye Res.*, 34: 639–649.

Ramón y Cajal, S. (1893) La rétine des vertébrés, *La Cellule*, 9: 17–257.

Schwarcz, R. and Coyle, J.T. (1977) Kainic acid; Neurotoxic effects after intraocular injection. *Invest. Ophthalmol., Vis. Sci.*, 16: 141–148.

Stell, W., Marshak, D., Yamada, T., Brecha, N. and Karten, H. (1980) Peptides are in the eye of the beholder. *Trends Neurosci.*, 3: 292–295.

Straschill, M. and Perwein, J. (1969) The inhibition of retinal ganglion cells by catecholamines and γ-aminobutyric acid. *Pflügers Arch.*, 312: 45–54.

Straschill, M. and Perwein, J. (1973) The effect of iontophoretically applied acetylcholine upon the cat's retinal ganglion cell. *Pflügers Arch.*, 339: 289–298.

West, R.W. and Chernenko, G.A. (1978) Lack of synaptic reorganization in inner plexiform layer (IPL) of retina following ganglion cell degeneration. *Experientia*, 34: 1082–1083.

Wood, J.G., McLaughlin, J.B. and Vaughan, J.E. (1976) Immunocytochemical localization of GAD in electron microscopic preparations of rodent CNS. In E. Roberts, T.N. Chase and D.B. Tower (Eds.), *GABA in Nervous System Function*, Raven Press, New York, 1976, pp. 133–148.

Wu, S.M. and Dowling, J.E. (1978) L-Aspartate: Evidence for a role in cone photoreceptor synaptic transmission in the carp retina. *Proc. nat. Acad. Sci. U.S.A.*, 75: 5205–5209.

Yazulla, S. and Kleinschmidt, J. (1980) The effects of intraocular injection of kainic acid on the synaptic organization of the goldfish retina. *Brain Res.*, 182: 287–301.

Brain Cell Surface Glycoproteins
Identified by Monoclonal Antibodies

C. GORIDIS, M. HIRN, O.K. LANGLEY, S. GHANDOUR and G. GOMBOS

Centre d'Immunologie INSERM-CNRS de Marseille-Luminy, Case 906, F-13288 Marseille Cédex 9 and (O.K.L., S.G. and G.G.) Centre de Neurochimie du CNRS, F-67084 Strasbourg Cédex (France)

INTRODUCTION

In the developing brain, processes such as the migration of neuroblasts, the growth of axons or the generation of synaptic connections seem to involve inter-action between cell surfaces. Very little is known about the underlying molecular mechanisms, but most hypotheses imply the existence of molecules, differing in kind or quantity from cell to cell, which mediate the necessary recognition events. Antibodies directed against neural cell surface components have been widely used in the search for molecules characteristic of certain cells or developmental stages.

Many of the limitations inherent to the immunological approach have been removed by the introduction of somatic hybridization techniques (Köhler and Milstein, 1975) which allow the isolation of lymphocyte clones secreting antibodies specific for individual molecules even though a complex mixture of antigens was used for immunization. Most authors using the hybridoma technique for generating antibodies to brain cell membranes concentrated on obtaining antibodies specific for a given cell type, and striking examples for the feasibility of this approach have been reported (Barnstable, 1980; Vulliamy et al., 1981; Zipser and McKay, 1981). However, molecules involved in cell interactions need not be exclusive to a class of neurons or glial cells. For instance, the adhesive molecule CAM is expressed by all neurons (Rutishauser et al., 1981) and the antigen described by Trisler et al. (1981) which appears to specify positional information in the developing retina is present on all cells in a given segment. Since glycoproteins of the plasma membrane, which are among the molecules most prominently exposed at the cell surface, are likely candidates for the hypothesized cell interaction molecules, we tried to derive monoclonal antibodies to surface glycoproteins present on developing brain cells. This communication describes observations on two monoclonal antibodies that recognize cell-surface glycoproteins on immature and adult mouse brain cells.

DERIVATION OF MONOCLONAL ANTIBODIES

The two monoclonal antibodies (mAb) described which we have named anti-BSP-2 (anti-brain cell surface protein-2) and anti-BSP-3 (in this nomenclature BSP-1 is defined by a rabbit antibody to a 140,000 molecular weight glycoprotein, see below), were derived from two separate fusions of hyperimmune rat spleen cells with the

[201]

mouse myeloma NS1-Ag 4.1. In the case of the BSP-2 antibody, rats had been immunized with high-molecular weight concanavalin-A binding proteins from neonatal mouse cerebrum (Hirn et al., 1981a), BSP-3 antibody was obtained after immunization with primary cultures of 4-day-old (P4) mouse cerebella (Hirn et al., 1982).

It cannot be emphasized too strongly that the screening procedure is the key to success in production of mAb. We used a battery of indirect trace radioactive binding assays to select relevant antibodies. First, anti-cell surface antibodies were detected by their binding to live monolayers of cerebellar cells (Hirn et al., 1981b). To rule out the possibility that the antigens were present only in vitro, positive hybridoma supernatants were retested on high-speed pellets prepared from mouse cerebellum. To discard antibodies recognizing antigens present on all mouse tissues, supernatants were then screened by binding assays on liver membranes and on thymocytes. Finally, those antibodies were selected which immunoprecipitated labeled material from iodinated, detergent-solubilized brain glycoproteins. This last test may seem superfluous, especially when a glycoprotein fraction has been used for immunization. However, mAb, although fully reactive in binding tests to intact cells and membranes, are often barely capable of recognizing their antigens after detergent-solubilization. On the intact membrane, the low affinity of some monoclonal antibodies can probably be compensated by multivalent binding, impossible after dispersion in detergent. Alternatively, the unique determinant recognized by a mAb may be altered by detergent-solubilization. Be it as it may, screening on solubilized antigens gives the assurance that the antibody recognizes its antigen in the presence of detergent, a prerequisite for all immunochemical studies of membrane components.

LOCALIZATION OF THE ANTIGENS

The mAb anti-BSP-2 and -3 were initially detected by their reactivity with live monolayers of cerebellar cells. Their binding to unfixed cerebellar cells proved that the antigens were present at the cell surface. The tissue distribution of the antigens was studied by absorption with membranes from various tissues (Hirn et al., 1981a, c). Both antigens were detectable in mouse forebrain and cerebellum. Whereas BSP-2 was not found outside the brain, BSP-3 was also detected in the small intestine. The antigens were present in P2-cerebellum (Fig. 1), when relatively undifferentiated cells predominate in the cerebellar cortex and long before the onset of the massive synaptogenesis characteristic of later phases of cerebellar development. On a protein basis, membranes from neonatal cerebellum contained more BSP-2 antigen than adult cerebellum. By contrast, BSP-3 was more concentrated in the adult tissue.

The cell type expressing the antigen in cultures from young postnatal mouse cerebellum was determined by immunofluorescent staining using double-labeling with established markers (Raff et al., 1979) for cell type identification (Hirn et al., 1981a, 1982). BSP-2 appeared to be confined to tetanus-toxin[+] cells of neuronal morphology and was never observed on astrocytes (GFAP[+]). In contrast, BSP-3 labeled preferentially GFAP[+] cells, and neurons were much more weakly stained. Fibronectin[+] fibroblasts were negative for both antibodies. However, in sections of

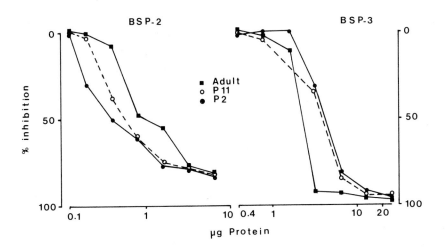

Fig. 1. Quantitative absorption of anti-BSP-2 and -3 by membranes from mouse cerebella of different ages. Antibody solution was diluted so as to be limiting in the assay and absorbed with serial dilutions of crude membranes. Residual activity was determined using the radioactive binding assay on monolayers of cerebellar cells.

adult cerebellum no differences were detected at either the light or electron microscope levels in the localisation of the two antigens. Dense immunoperoxidase precipitate was found over the plasma membrane of Purkinje cell bodies and dendrites, which extended beneath synaptic boutons on their perikarya (Fig. 2). However, their cytoplasm and nuclei were free of label. By contrast, the cytoplasm

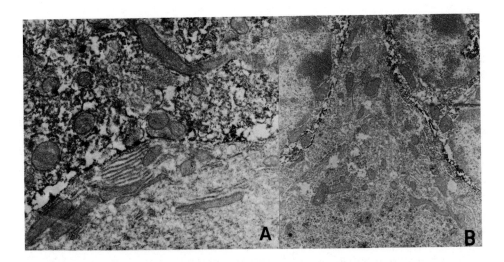

Fig. 2. Electron microscopic localisation of BSP-2 (A) and -3 (B) in sections from adult mouse cerebellum as revealed by immunoperoxidase technique. A: Purkinje cell dendrite. Peroxidase precipitate is limited to the Purkinje cell surface membrane, the surrounding glial and neuronal processes and parallel fibers. Not counterstained, ×27,100. B: Purkinje cell and adjacent granular layer. Immunolabel is associated with the Purkinje cells plasma membrane, the surrounding astroglial processes and with granule cells. Not counterstained, ×19,800.

of granule cells was heavily labeled as well as their plasma membranes. Both antibodies labeled astrocytes, predominantly over their plasma membranes but also intracellularly. Oligodendrocytes, endothelial cells and the leptomeninges were never found to be labeled. This similarity of staining obtained with two antibodies directed against different antigens could question the specificity of the reaction. However, normal rat serum never gave such staining and a rat mAb of the same class specific for endothelial cells (Ghandour et al., 1981) failed to label astrocytes or neurons. It is unclear at present why anti-BSP-2 does not label astrocytes in culture. Different culture conditions may be required for expression of BSP-2 by astrocytes or astrocytes of young postnatal cerebella have not yet acquired the antigen.

IMMUNOCHEMICAL IDENTIFICATION OF THE ANTIGENS

The nature of the molecules with which anti-BSP-2 and -3 react on the surface of cultured cerebellar cells was determined by immunoprecipitation and gel electrophoretic analysis of the labeled antigen from detergent lysates of surface-iodinated cerebellar cultures. Immunoprecipitates prepared with BSP-2 antibody contained three labeled polypeptides of 180,000, 140,000 and 120,000 apparent mol. wt. BSP-3 reacted with a single iodinated polypeptide of 48,000 dalton (Hirn et al., 1981a, 1982). A comparison with the overall pattern of iodinatable polypeptides showed that the 48,000 mol. wt. protein was a relatively minor component whereas heavily labeled bands occurred in the 120,000–180,000 mol. wt. region. Especially the 140,000 mol. wt. surface proteins seemed to be heterogenous. We have prepared a rabbit antiserum against a glycoprotein of 140,000 dalton (BSP-1) which is the major high mol. wt. protein shed into the culture medium by cerebellar cultures and tissue slices (Goridis et al., 1980). This antibody stains the surface of cultured cerebellar neurons in a manner very similar to anti-BSP-2. Sequential immunoprecipitation experiments, however, showed that the antigens recognized by the two antibodies were not identical (Fig. 3). Lectin-binding studies and metabolic labeling experiments with radioactive sugars confirmed the glycoprotein nature of the BSP-3 antigen and the three bands immunoprecipitated by anti-BSP-2 (Hirn et al., 1981a, 1982). The antibodies seem to recognize the protein part of the antigens since neuraminidase digestion and periodate oxidation of the glycan chains, although causing slight shifts in electrophoretic mobility, did not affect antibody recognition.

These earlier experiments did not clarify whether the three BSP-2 bands carried all the antigenic determinant or were co-precipitated since they formed a three-chain complex. The recent refinement of blotting techniques in which antibodies are reacted with polypeptide chains after gel electrophoretic separation and transfer to cellulose sheets (Towbin et al., 1979; Burnette, 1981) allows for the identification of individual antigenic polypeptides provided that the determinant stays intact or recovers after denaturation. When the membrane proteins from adult or late postnatal cerebellum were separated according to mol. wt., transferred to nitrocellulose sheets and reacted with anti-BSP-2, the same triplet of 180,000, 140,000 and 120,000 mol. wt. immunoprecipitated from surface-iodinated cultures was revealed by the mAb (Fig. 4). Clearly, the three bands are structurally related and all carry the BSP-2 determinant. This experiment further shows that the BSP-2 antigens expressed in cultures from young postnatal cerebellum and in the adult cerebellum

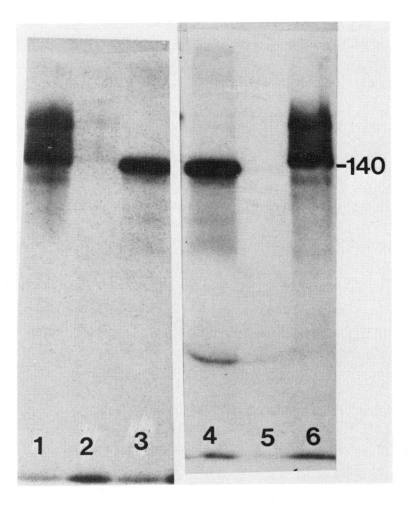

Fig. 3. Gel electrophoretic analysis of sequential immunoprecipitation experiments demonstrating the non-identity of BSP-1 and -2 antigens. A lysate of surface-iodinated cerebellar cultures was divided into two aliquots. One aliquot was depleted of BSP-1 by two cycles of immunoprecipitation, the second aliquot was depleted of BSP-2. The BSP-1 or -2 antigens left in solution were then immunoprecipitated with the other antibody. Lanes 1 and 4: molecules precipitated by anti-BSP-2 and anti-BSP-1, respectively, in the first cycle of immunoprecipitation. Lanes 2 and 5: after a second cycle no molecules are left reacting with either anti-BSP-2 or anti-BSP-1. Lanes 3 and 6: these lysates cleared of BSP-2 or -1 antigens still contain the molecules recognized by the other antibody.

in vivo are very similar if not identical. Surprisingly, however, very different results were obtained, when neonatal cerebella were analysed (Fig. 4): the pattern of BSP-2-reactive polypeptide chains was dominated by very high mol. wt. material. Preliminary results on the developmental time course suggest that the adult pattern of cerebellar BSP-2 antigens emerges around postnatal day 8.

Further studies are needed to clarify the relation between the different BSP-2 polypeptides present in adult and developing cerebellum. The differences in apparent mol. wt. between the neonatal and adult antigens seem too important to be

206

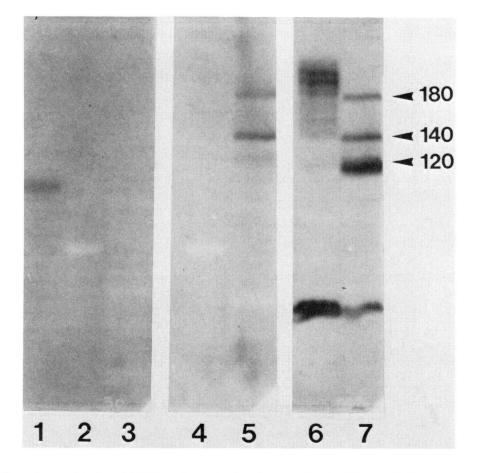

Fig. 4. Immunodetection of BSP-2-reactive molecules after separation in SDS gels. Crude membranes were prepared from cerebellum and liver of adult mice or from P2-cerebellum and either extracted with NP40 or dissolved directly in SDS. Equal amounts of the reduced proteins were fractionated on 7% polyacrylamide gels in the presence of SDS and transferred to nitrocellulose paper. The blot thus obtained was reacted with monoclonal rat antibody and radioiodinated rabbit anti-rat Ig and labeled bands revealed by autoradiography. The heavily labeled low mol. wt. band in lanes 6 and 7 most probably represents actin which is known to react with Ig non-specifically and which is contained in SDS extracts in relatively higher amounts. Lane 1: dansylated mol. wt. marker (94,000 dalton). Lanes 2–4: Specificity controls. NP40 extracts of liver (2 and 4) and adult cerebellar (3) membranes reacted with anti-BSP-2 (4) and irrelevant monoclonal rat antibody (2 and 3). Lane 5: NP40 extract from adult cerebellum. Lane 6: SDS extract from P2 cerebellum. Lane 7: SDS extract from adult cerebellum.

accounted for by changes in glycosylation, although this possibility cannot be completely excluded. The different chains could be created by proteolytic cleavage from a common precursor or coded for by genes derived from gene duplication. It is unlikely that the bands are created artifactually by proteolysis occurring during membrane preparation or cell lysis, since protease inhibitors are present throughout and since the patterns persisted after incubation of lysates 1 h at 37 °C even in their absence. Alternatively, the proteins may exist in different aggregation states not dissociated by sodium dodecylsulfate and mercaptoethanol, as has been reported for gap junction proteins (Henderson et al., 1979).

The different electrophoretic mobility of BSP-2 in neonatal and adult cerebellum could reflect a relative enrichment of neonatal cerebellum in some cell types rather than a maturation occurring on cells of the same lineage. Although this possibility cannot be excluded, some evidence for the structural identity of neuronal and astroglial BSP-2 antigens has been obtained. The triplet immunoprecipitated from iodinated primary cultures, where anti-BSP-2 stained only neurons, should represent neuronal BSP-2. On the other hand, a clone of transformed astrocytic cells (kindly provided by Dr. B. Pessac) contained BSP-2-reactive polypeptides of identical mol. wt. (unpublished results).

Fucosylated or surface-iodinatable proteins of a mol. wt. similar to BSP-2 and -3 have been detected among synaptic membrane proteins (Gurd, 1979; Fu et al., 1981) and surface proteins of cerebellar cultures (Goridis et al., 1978; Goridis et al., 1980; Rohrer and Schachner, 1980). Among immunologically defined surface proteins from rodent brain, the NS4 (Goridis et al., 1978) and D2 (Jorgensen, 1979) antigens may be related to BSP-2 although D2 has a rather different immunohistochemical localization (Jorgensen and Möller, 1980). However, experiments reported in this communication show that brain cell surface proteins in the 140,000 mol. wt. region are heterogenous. It is very well possible that these high mol. wt. glycoproteins of the brain cell surface will eventually be shown to consist of a family of structurally related polypeptides with shared and unshared antigenic determinants, in a manner similar to some glycoproteins of immunocompetent cells (Coffman and Weissman, 1981; Dalchau and Fabre, 1981; Klein et al., 1981).

CONCLUSIONS

Very little is known of the biochemistry, localisation and function of the major cell surface proteins on neural cells. This communication demonstrates that mono-clonal antibodies are valuable tools for characterizing individual surface proteins. Although not useful as specific markers for a given cell type, the anti-BSP-2 and -3 mAb have permitted studies of the biochemical identity and the cellular and subcellular occurrence of two glycoproteins expressed at least in part at the cell surface. Without the use of mAb, results such as the differences in subcellular localization between Purkinje and granule cells and the structural changes during cerebellar development could not have been ascribed to the same antigen. The fact that mAb are directed against unique determinants often creates difficulties. An antibody reacting with the intact membrane and useful in immunohistochemistry may not recognize its determinant after solubilization or denaturation of the protein and vice versa. A judicious choice of immunizing material (solubilized proteins vs intact cells or membranes) and screening methods (e.g. immunoprecipitation, eventually binding to membranes fixed in the way used in electron microscopy) may contribute to selecting mAb useful for immunochemistry *and* ultrastructural studies.

The long term goal of our research is the identification of brain cell surface proteins possibly involved in cell-cell interaction phenomena during histogenesis. Evidence for the implication of BSP-2 or -3 in such processes is still lacking. The presence of the antigens in the immature cerebellum and, in the case of BSP-2, the biochemical differences between the antigenic polypeptides in neonatal and adult cerebellum are suggestive evidence of their functional significance in developmental processes.

208

REFERENCES

Barnstable, C.J. (1980) Monoclonal antibodies which recognize different cell types in the rat retina. *Nature (Lond.)*, 286: 231–235.

Burnette, W.N. (1981) Western blotting: Electrophoretic transfer of proteins from sodium dodecylsulfate-polyacrylamide gels to unmodified nitrocellulose and radiographic detection with antibody and radioiodinated protein A. *Analyt. Biochem.*, 112: 195–203.

Coffman, R.L. and Weissman, J.L. (1981) B220: A B cell-specific member of the T200 glycoprotein family. *Nature (Lond.)*, 289: 681–683.

Dalchau, R. and Fabre, J.W. (1981) Identification with a monoclonal antibody of a predominantly B lymphcoyte-specific determinant of the human leucocyte common antigen. *J. exp. Med.*, 153: 753–765.

Fu, S.C., Cruz, T.F. and Gurd, J.W. (1981) Development of synaptic glycoproteins: effect of postnatal age on the synthesis and concentration of synaptic membrane and synaptic junctional fucosyl and sialyl glycoproteins. *J. Neurochem.*, 36: 1338–1351.

Ghandour, S., Langley, K., Gombos, G., Hirn, M., Hirsch, M. and Goridis, C. (1981) A surface marker for murine vascular endothelial cells defined by monoclonal antibody. *J. Histochem. Cytochem.*, 30: 165–170.

Goridis, C., Joher, M.A., Hirsch, M. and Schachner, M. (1978) Cell surface proteins of cultured brain cells and their recognition by anticerebellum (anti-NS-4) serum. *J. Neurochem.*, 31: 531–539.

Goridis, C., Hirsch, M., Dosseto, M. and Baechler, E. (1980) Identification and characterisation of two surface glycoproteins on cultured cerebellar cells. *Brain Res.*, 182: 397–414.

Gurd, J.W. (1979) Molecular and biosynthetic heterogeneity of fucosyl glycoproteins associated with rat brain synaptic junctions. *Biochim. biophys. Acta*, 555: 221–229.

Henderson, D., Eibl, H. and Weber, K. (1979) Structure and biochemistry of mouse hepatic gap junctions. *J. molec. Biol.*, 132: 193–218.

Hirn, M., Pierres, M., Deagostini-Bazin, H., Hirsch, M. and Goridis, C. (1981a) Monoclonal antibody against cell surface glycoprotein of neurons. *Brain Res.*, 214: 433–439.

Hirn, M., Demierre, M. and Goridis, C. (1981b) A radioimmunoassay for detecting antibodies to brain cell surface antigens. *Brain Res. Bull.*, 7: 441–444.

Hirn, M., Pierres, M., Deagostini-Bazin, H., Hirsch, M., Goridis, C., Ghandour, S., Langley, K. and Gombos, G. (1982) A new brain cell surface glycoprotein identified by monoclonal antibody. *Neuroscience*, 7: 239–250.

Jorgensen, O.S. (1979) Polypeptides of the synaptic membrane antigens D1, D2 and D3. *Biochim. biophys. Acta*, 581: 153–162.

Jorgensen, O.S. and Moller, M. (1980) Immunocytochemical demonstration of the D2 protein in the presynaptic complex. *Brain Res.*, 194: 419–429.

Köhler, G. and Milstein, C. (1975) Continuous cultures of fused cells secreting antibody of predefined specificity. *Nature (Lond.)*, 256: 495–497.

Klein, J., Juretic, A., Baxevanis, N.C. and Nagy, Z. (1981) The traditional and a new version of the mouse H-2 complex. *Nature (Lond.)*, 291: 455–460.

Raff, M.C., Fields, K.L., Hakomori, S.I., Mirsky, R., Pruss, R.M. and Winter, J. (1979) Cell-type specific markers for distinguishing and studying neurons and the major classes of glial cells in culture. *Brain Res.*, 174: 283–308.

Rohrer, H. and Schachner, M. (1980) Surface proteins of cultured mouse cerebellar cells. *J. Neurochem.*, 35: 792–803.

Rutishauser, U., Thiery, J.P., Brackenbury, R. and Edelman, G.M. (1978) Adhesion among neural cells of the chick embryo. III. Relationship of the surface molecule CAM to cell adhesion and the development of histiotypic pattern. *J. Cell Biol.*, 79: 371–381.

Towbin, H., Staehelin, T. and Gordon, J. (1979) Electrophoretic transfer of proteins from polyacrylamide gels to nitrocellulose sheets: Procedure and some applications. *Proc. nat. Acad. Sci. U.S.A.*, 76: 4350–4354.

Trisler, G.D., Schneider, M.D. and Nirenberg, M. (1981) A topographic gradient of molecules in retina can be used to identify neuron position. *Proc. nat. Acad. Sci. U.S.A.*, 78: 2145–2149.

Vulliamy, T., Rattray, S. and Mirsky, R. (1981) Cell-surface antigen distinguishes sensory and autonomic peripheral neurons from central neurons. *Nature (Lond.)*, 291: 418–420.

Zipser, B. and McKay, R. (1981) Monoclonal antibodies distinguish identifiable neurones in the leech. *Nature (Lond.)*, 289: 549–554.

Functional Organization
of the Visual Cortex

CHARLES D. GILBERT and TORSTEN N. WIESEL

Department of Neurobiology, Harvard Medical School, Boston, MA 02115 (U.S.A.)

INTRODUCTION

Although the cortex is in many ways a uniform structure, different regions of cortex are devoted to very different purposes, ranging from sensory perception to motor control to higher intellectual functions. Within the sensory cortex, one finds a further spatial segregation of the modalities. The focus of this paper is the primary visual cortex, which, though only one of a number of cortical visual areas (Hubel and Wiesel, 1965; Allman and Kaas, 1975; Palmer et al., 1978; Van Essen and Zeki, 1978; Zeki, 1978), bears many structural similarities to all other areas of cortex.

Each visual area has a functional organization that follows several rules, including retinotopic order, columnar ordering of specific receptive field features and laminar segregation of functional cell types. With regard to retinotopic order, certain areas devote more space to particular parts of the visual field more than others, and some have less rigidly organized maps than others. Area 17 has the most precise topographic organization, where a small part of the visual field is mapped onto a small part of the cortical area. Within that part, looking at a finer level of resolution, one finds that the cortex follows a columnar organization. This was discovered through the study of single cell responses, which showed that cells in area 17 respond optimally to bars or edges having a particular orientation and that they tend to prefer stimulation of one eye over the other (Hubel and Wiesel, 1962). Cells that share the same orientation preference or the same ocular preference are clustered together into columns, running from pia to white matter. When viewed from the surface, the ocular dominance columns and orientation columns each form an irregular striped pattern, and the two systems run in different directions, as illustrated in Fig. 1.

A small set of cells is responsible for analyzing a particular spot in the visual field, for responding to contours of a particular orientation and for having a particular ocular preference. These cells lie in a narrow column of cortex that runs from the pia to the white matter, crossing the cortical layers. In each layer cells receive unique inputs, have unique receptive field properties, and have distinct projections out of the immediate cortical area. From this one gets the impression that no two cells are functionally alike. To produce such a functional diversity, there exists within the cortex a stereotyped set of connections running between layers and across the cortical columns. These connections are responsible for producing the transformation of receptive field properties from the relatively simple structure of the receptive fields of cells in the lateral geniculate nucleus (the source of input to the

[209]

210

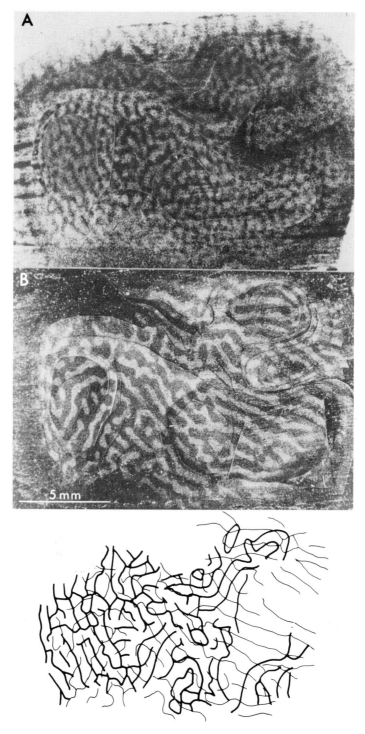

Fig. 1. Orientation columns (A) and ocular dominance columns (B) reconstructed from tangential sections of monkey visual cortex. Ocular dominance columns were demonstrated by autoradiography following transynaptic transport of [³H]proline from the eye. Orientation columns were demonstrated by autoradiography following selective uptake of [¹⁴C]deoxyglucose after stimulation with moving vertical stripes. Third panel shows superimposed orientation (heavy lines) and ocular dominance (fine lines) columns. (Reprinted from Hubel et al., 1978, with permission.)

cortex) to the more complex structure of cortical cell receptive fields. The distribution of the cortical afferents, the intrinsic connections of the cortex, and the pattern of connections between cortical areas will be dealt with in this paper.

CORTICAL AFFERENTS AND EFFERENTS

The cortex receives input from a number of structures, including several nuclei in the thalamus, other cortical areas and diffuse projections from the brainstem. Area 17 receives its strongest input from the lateral geniculate nucleus (LGN), but there are other thalamic nuclei that also project to it, including the medial interlaminar nucleus and the lateral posterior/pulvinar complex (Rezak and Benevento, 1976; Graybiel and Berson, 1981). The LGN is a layered structure, with each set of layers giving rise to a projection that has a distinct laminar distribution (Hubel and Wiesel, 1972; LeVay and Gilbert, 1976). In the cat, one can further subdivide the projection of a single geniculate lamina into the projection produced by each of several types of principal cell that reside together within the layer. The distribution of the terminals of each geniculate cell type becomes important when considering the distribution of different functional classes of cortical cell, in that each class is influenced by the thalamic input that it receives.

Fig. 2 shows the projections of particular thalamic nuclei in the cat and monkey. The dorsal laminae of the LGN in the cat project to layer 4 and to the upper half of layer 6. In these laminae there is a mixture of at least two functional (X- and Y-cells) and morphological (type 1 and 2 cells) classes of principal cell. (Guillery, 1966; Enroth-Cugell and Robson, 1966; Cleland et al., 1971; Wilson et al., 1976). These cells have concentric center/surround receptive fields, and can be on- or off-centered. The X/Y classification scheme is based on the linearity of spatial summation of receptive fields, although there are also differences in conduction velocity, receptive field size and phasic versus tonic response. X- and Y-cells have distinct cortical projections, with Y-cells projecting to layer 4ab and X-cells projecting to layer 4c (Ferster and LeVay, 1978; Gilbert and Wiesel, 1979). Thus the dorsal layers of the

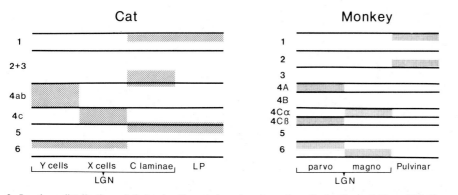

Fig. 2. Laminar distribution of thalamic afferents in cat and monkey. Projections of X- and Y-afferents (Ferster and LeVay, 1978; Gilbert and Wiesel, 1979), C laminae (LeVay and Gilbert, 1976) and latero-posterior nucleus (LP; Miller et al., 1980) in the cat; magno- and parvocellular layers of the monkey's lateral geniculate nucleus (Hubel and Wiesel, 1972; Hendrickson et al., 1978) and pulvinar (Ogren and Hendrickson, 1977; Rezak and Benevento, 1979) (with permission).

lateral geniculate nucleus, which contain a mixture of X- and Y-cell types, keep the input from these two populations segregated upon their arrival in the cortex. The segregation of functionally different inputs into different cortical laminae is seen for other inputs as well: the C-laminae project to two bands bracketing layer 4, outside the projection zones of the X- and Y-cells (LeVay and Gilbert, 1976).

There is also a segregation of the cortical afferents in a plane parallel to the cortical surface, one which gives rise to the ocular dominance columns mentioned above. Cells in the LGN are driven by one eye only. They have a clustered projection in the cortex, with patches of dense innervation separated by non-innervated spaces, which, more than likely, correspond to and form the basis of the two sets of ocular dominance columns.

The thalamic afferents to the cortex, though they have been divided into several functional classes, nevertheless tend to share the concentric antagonistic center/surround receptive field organization. In marked contrast, the cells in the cortex, and consequently the outputs of the cortex, have oriented receptive fields which exhibit a rich variety of other features. Cells in different layers have very distinct and specialized receptive fields, allowing a single cortical area to participate in a number of different functions. This is reflected in the sites of projection of cells in different cortical layers: cells in the superficial layers project to other cortical areas, cells in layer 5 project to the superior colliculus and cells in layer 6 project to the LGN, forming a substantial recurrent loop to the nucleus that provides the cortex with its input (Gilbert and Kelly, 1975; Lund et al., 1975).

RECEPTIVE FIELD PROPERTIES OF STRIATE CORTICAL CELLS

In addition to orientation specificity and ocular dominance, a number of other features can be attributed to cortical receptive fields. For one, there are different receptive field classes. Simple cells have distinct on and off, mutually antagonistic subregions, and show considerable specificity in their response to the position of the stimulus within the receptive field. Complex cells, on the other hand, have uniform receptive fields, and are more generalized in responding to the stimulus placed anywhere within the receptive field. Both simple and complex cells show a wide range of receptive field size; many have the property of end-inhibition, showing a reduction in response as the length of the stimulating bar is increased beyond the receptive field; and they can show directionality, responding more to movement of the bar in one direction than in the opposite direction. It has also been shown that they can be sensitive to the disparity between the positions of the stimulus on the two retinae, a phenomenon thought to constitute the mechanism of stereoscopic depth perception.

Cells bring together particular combinations of these properties to suit given functions, and consequently one sees particular receptive field types restricted to given layers (Hubel and Wiesel, 1962; Gilbert, 1977). Complex cells in the superficial layers tend to have small, end-inhibited receptive fields. These cells participate in cortico-cortical connections, and this set of properties is appropriate for the higher resolution, pattern recognition function that the cortex serves. In layer 5 one finds complex cells with large fields that are sensitive to the movement of a small stimulus in a particular direction. These cells project to the superior colliculus, and their fields are well suited to the eye tracking function of that structure. Cells in layer 6 tend to have very long receptive fields, showing summation for increased length of the stimulating bar up to large values. It is known that these cells are responsible for the recurrent projection from cortex to LGN, but the role of this receptive field property in influencing geniculate function is not known. However, it is clear that this property is restricted to cells in layer 6.

Besides viewing receptive fields as being designed to suit the function of the structure to which cells project, it is also of interest to see how they reflect the properties of their inputs. Simple cells are found in layer 4 and in the upper half of layer 6, which is precisely the distribution of afferents from the dorsal layers of the lateral geniculate nucleus. This supports the hypothesis originally advanced by Hubel and Wiesel that simple cells constitute the first stage in cortical processing, with their on and off subregions derived from the centers of on and off geniculate cell receptive fields. Complex cells, on the other hand, tend to lie outside the X- and Y-cell afferent zones, and, as will be discussed later, receive most of their input from other cortical cells, thus representing later stages in cortical processing.

CORTICAL MICROCIRCUITRY AND RECEPTIVE FIELD SPECIALIZATION

Our understanding of the cortical circuit has, as one might expect, changed along with the development of techniques to visualize the morphology of neurons. The Golgi technique provided the first detailed view of the structure of individual neurons. Those who pioneered the use of the technique focused primarily on the dendritic morphology of cells and based their classification scheme accordingly. More recently people have emphasized the morphological diversity of the axonal arbor. The technique of intracellular injection of horseradish peroxidase (HRP) has greatly enhanced the ability to see the full axonal arbor, and has revealed that cells possess a considerably more lavish network of axonal collaterals, both in density and extent, than had been previously thought to exist.

Within the cortex there is a wide variety of cells, as judged by their dendritic and axonal morphology. Whether or not a cell projects to a distant site, it invariably gives rise to an intricate and dense set of connections within the same cortical area in which it resides. Although at first sight these connections seem hopelessly complicated, they do tend to be stereotyped for cells in a given layer or sublayer, so that one can summarize the principal connections in a circuit of a half dozen or so elements (Fig. 3). By comparing the receptive field properties of the cell population whose axons terminate in a particular layer with the properties of the cells that are on the receiving end, one can get an idea of the functional role of the connection between the two cell groups (Gilbert and Wiesel, 1979).

Within a single cortical area, such as area 17, it appears that information is processed through a number of stages. In addition, information from the different types of cortical input (X- and Y-cells) is processed separately and in parallel, at least for the first two steps. The stages, in the cat, are as follows: The geniculate input arrives in two principal channels, with the X input going to layer 4c and the Y input going to layer 4ab. The cells in layer 4 project upward to layer 2 + 3. From there the

214

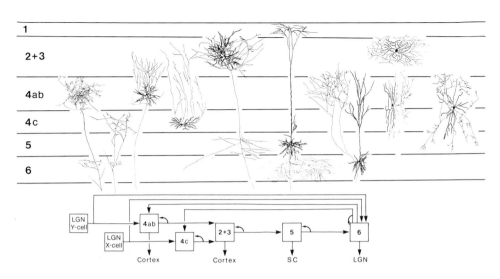

Fig. 3. Schematic diagram of the intracortical connections of the cat's striate cortex. The spiny stellate and pyramidal cells are presumably responsible for most of the excitatory connections, and their intracortical and efferent connections are summarized in the block diagram. Smooth stellate cells, several types shown at upper right, are presumed to mediate inhibitory interactions in the cortex.

cells project to layer 5, layer 5 cells project to layer 6, and layer 6 cells close a loop, projecting up to layer 4. As described above, at each stage the loop is tapped for output to other cortical and subcortical structures.

Each stage is important for developing particular receptive field properties. In both the X and Y afferent zones one finds simple cells. The simple cells in 4c have much smaller receptive fields than those in 4ab, presumably reflecting differences in the receptive field size and extent of the axonal arbor of their respective inputs.

The projection from layer 4 to layer 2+3 represents a projection from simple cells to complex cells, supporting the idea advanced by Hubel and Wiesel that complex cells represent the second stage of processing in cortex after the arrival of input from the geniculate. Although it has been clearly established that the X- and Y-pathways remain segregated as far as layer 4, it is not known if this segregation is further maintained in layer 2+3, but preliminary evidence suggests that it is. Among superficial layer cells, different populations are responsible for projections to different cortical areas. This is once again reflected in differences in receptive field size, with upper layer 2+3 complex cells having smaller receptive fields than those lower in the layer. The pyramidal cells in the superficial layers have axons that arborize in two layers, one set in layer 2+3 and one set in layer 5. The collaterals in layer 5 run for quite a distance in the horizontal direction, parallel to the pial surface. This may account for the principal difference in receptive field properties between superficial layer and layer 5 cells. Layer 5 cells have much larger receptive fields, though they are also complex. The extent of the collaterals of layer 2+3 pyramidal cells in layer 5 allows individual layer 5 cells to collect input from a relatively wide area of cortex, and hence from a relatively large part of the visual field, enabling them to construct large receptive fields.

Cells in layer 5 have axons that arborize quite extensively in layer 6, making the longest-ranging intracortical connections. The extent of these connections accounts for the very long receptive fields that one sees for layer 6 cells.

Layer 6 cells provide as dense an input for layer 4 cells as the input from the LGN. The role of this projection is not known. Cells in layer 4 are responsible for developing many of the receptive field features seen among cortical cells in general: orientation selectivity, directional preference and end-inhibition. It may well be that one or more of these features are produced through the input from layer 6 cells.

Further evidence is required to definitively attribute a given function to a given connection. It is in this context that neurochemistry will play a significant role. Once a particular transmitter is found to be associated with a particular connection it will be possible to employ pharmacological techniques to investigate the role of that connection. This approach has already been employed in studying the role of the inhibitory connections. Smooth stellate cells are thought to be inhibitory, due to the fact that they selectively take up GABA, an inhibitory transmitter (Hökfelt and Ljundahl, 1972), and are stained with immunohistochemical stains for glutamic acid decarboxylase, the GABA synthetic enzyme (Ribak, 1978). They also tend to make symmetric synapses, which are associated with inhibitory connections, while the pyramidal cells make asymmetric synapses, which are associated with excitatory connections (LeVay, 1973). By iontophoresing a GABA inhibitor, bicuculline, while recording from cortical cells, it has been found that GABA inhibition may play an important role in the production of orientation selectivity and directional preference (Sillito, 1975).

Some advances have already been made in associating other transmitters with particular cell types. The acidic amino acids aspartate and glutamate, which appear to be excitatory, are associated with layer 6 pyramidal cells (Baughman and Gilbert, 1981). Different peptides are located in different smooth stellate cells. Vasoactive intestinal polypeptide (VIP), for example, is associated with one class, the bipolar cell (Fuxe et al., 1977). It is likely that many different transmitters are employed in the cortex, and that it will soon be possible to differentiate cortical cell classes according to the transmitters they release.

The above summary of the intracortical pathway neglects many features of cortical connectivity whose functional significance is as yet unknown. Take, first, the variety of connections of smooth stellate cells. These appear to specialize in their post-synaptic targets: One class of cells, the chandelier cell, makes symmetric synapses exclusively upon the initial segments of the axons of pyramidal cells (Somogyi, 1977). Another class, the bipolar cell, forms asymmetric (excitatory) synapses with apical dendrites of pyramidal cells (Peters and Kimerer, 1981), and a third class, the basket cell, forms inhibitory synapses with cell bodies (Marin-Padilla, 1974). The purpose of these specialized contacts is unknown. Another mystery of cortical organization is the apical dendrite of the pyramidal cell. What does this enable pyramidal cells to do that stellate cells are incapable of doing? One suggestion, since pyramidal cells are responsible for the outflow of signals from the cortex, is that apical dendrites serve to synchronize this outflow for cells lying in the same vertical cortical column, either through dendritic bundling or electrical synapses or by receiving a common input from a given bipolar cell. Any definitive description of the microcircuitry of cortex will have to take account of these aspects of synaptic and morphological specialization.

INTERCOLUMNAR COMMUNICATION

The columnar functional organization of the cortex arises from different mechanisms. While the ocular dominance columns are produced by the pattern of afferent input, the orientation columns depend on intrinsic cortical connections. Looking at the projections of individual neurons and of populations of neurons, it is clear that cells make use of extensive intercolumnar connections in processing information. Single cells have axon collaterals reaching distant parts of the areas in which they reside. The distribution of their axonal fields is not uniform or circularly symmetric. Rather, the overall distribution of the axonal field tends to be asymmetric, extending much more in certain directions than others, and the terminal branches occur in discrete clusters. The relationship between these clusters and the orientation or ocular dominance columns has not yet been established.

The projections between cortical areas have a similar quality. The distribution of cells in area 17 that project to areas 18 or 19 is a clustered one. This has been demonstrated by retrograde transport of HRP (Gilbert and Kelly, 1975). Using anterograde techniques for tracing connections, one also sees that a particular site in area 17 makes a patchy projection to other cortical areas (Wong-Riley, 1979; Montero, 1980). Similarly, for the recurrent projections from areas 18 and 19 to area 17, the connections go from clusters of cells to patches of terminals. In the visual system the function of the projection clusters or bands has not been established. While the patchiness in the projection from the geniculate to the cortex is known to separate the input from the two eyes, the cortico-cortical projection patches constitute a distinct phenomenon, unrelated to ocular dominance or orientation columns (Gilbert and Wiesel, 1980). The recurrent afferents from other cortical areas are patchy, and these patches are superimposed with the clusters of cells that project to those areas. Cells projecting to different cortical areas have different laminar distributions, and they are arranged in patterns of patches which are distinct from one another (Gilbert and Wiesel, 1981).

The functional significance of these connections has undergone substantial scrutiny in the past few years. It has been shown that this pattern of connectivity is universal, seen in cortical areas serving all modalities, including visual, somatosensory (Jones et al., 1978) and auditory (Imig and Reale, 1980), and also in frontal cortex (Goldman and Nauta, 1977). For some areas callosal projections as well as ipsilateral associational cortical projections form bands of terminals (Imig and Brugge, 1978; Jones et al., 1978). In the auditory cortex there has been some success in determining a functional correlate of these projection bands. There, they seem to be associated with the aural interaction columns – in one set of columns cells respond better to stimulation of both ears than to one ear alone (summation columns), and in the intervening set of columns the response to binaural stimulation is less than that to monaural stimulation (suppression columns). The callosal connection bands appear to project to the summation columns.

The functional role of the patches and stripes in the visual cortex has yet to be determined. One speculation is that these geometric arrangements allow for a spatial segregation of inhibition and excitation, and is required to produce the functional properties of cortical cells (Blakemore and Tobin, 1972). To determine the role of the projection patches it will be important to determine if each set of patches receives distinct inputs and contains unique cell types, just as the cortical layers do.

In summary, the cortex can be seen to adhere to a number of rules that endow it with a highly organized structure. The functional significance of some of the patterns of organization have been clearly demonstrated, while that of other patterns has not been worked out, and they represent tantalizing clues to the mechanism of operation of the cortex.

REFERENCES

Allman, J.M. and Kaas, J.H. (1975) The dorsomedial cortical visual area: a third tier area in the occipital lobe of the owl monkey (*Aotus trivirgatus*). *Brain Res.*, 100: 473–487.

Baughman, R.W. and Gilbert, C.D. (1981) Aspartate and glutamate as possible neurotransmitters in the visual cortex. *J. Neurosci.*, 1: 427–439.

Blakemore, C. and Tobin, E. (1972) Lateral inhibition between orientation detectors in the cat's visual cortex. *Exp. Brain Res.*, 15: 439–440.

Cleland, B.G., Dubin, M.W. and Levick, W.R. (1971) Sustained and transient neurons in the cat's retina and lateral geniculate nucleus. *J. Physiol. (Lond.)*, 267: 473–496.

Enroth-Cugell, C. and Robson, J.G. (1966) The contrast sensitivity of retinal ganglion cells in the cat. *J. Physiol. (Lond.)*, p. 187: 517–552.

Ferster, D. and LeVay, S. (1978) The axonal arborization of lateral geniculate neurons in the striate cortex of the cat. *J. comp. Neurol.*, 182: 923–944.

Fuxe, K., Hokfelt, T., Said, S.I. and Mutt, V. (1977) Vasoactive intestinal polypeptide and the nervous system: immunohistochemical evidence for localization in central and peripheral neurons, particularly intracortical neurons of the cerebral cortex. *Neurosci. Lett.*, 5: 241–246.

Gilbert, C.D. (1977) Laminar differences in receptive field properties in cat primary visual cortex. *J. Physiol. (Lond.)*, 268: 391–421.

Gilbert, C.D. and Kelly, J.P. (1975) The projections of cells in different layers of the cat's visual cortex. *J. comp. Neurol.*, 163: 81–106.

Gilbert, C.D. and Wiesel, T.N. (1979) Morphology and intracortical projections of functionally identified neurons in cat visual cortex. *Nature (Lond.)*, 280: 120–125.

Gilbert, C.D. and Wiesel, T.N. (1980) Interleaving projection bands in cortico-cortical connections. *Neurosci. Abstr.*, 6: 315.

Gilbert, C.D. and Wiesel, T.N. (1981) Projection bands in visual cortex. *Neurosci. Abstr.* 7: 356.

Graybiel, A.M. and Berson, D.M. (1981) On the relation between transthalamic and transcortical pathways in the visual system. In Schmitt, Worden, Adelman and Dennis. (Eds.), *The Organization of the Cerebral Cortex*, MIT Press, Cambridge, MA, pp. 285–319.

Goldman, P.S. and Nauta, W.J.H. (1977) Columnar distribution of corticocortical fibers in the frontal association, limbic and motor cortex of the developing rhesus monkey. *Brain Res.*, 122: 393–413.

Guillery, R.W. (1966) A study of Golgi preparations from the dorsal lateral geniculate nucleus of the adult cat. *J. comp. Neurol.*, 128: 21–50.

Hendrickson, A.E., Wilson, J.R. and Ogren, M.P. (1978) The neuroanatomical organization of pathways between the dorsal lateral geniculate nucleus and visual cortex in old world and new world primates. *J. comp. Neurol.*, 182: 123–136.

Hökfelt, T. and Ljundahl, A. (1972) Autoradiographic identification of cerebral and cerebellar cortical neurons accumulating labeled gamma-aminobutyric acid (3H-GABA). *Exp. Brain Res.*, 14: 354–362.

Hubel, D.H. and Wiesel, T.N. (1962) Receptive fields, binocular interaction and functional architecture in the cat's visual cortex. *J. Physiol. (Lond.)*, 160: 106–154.

Hubel, D.H. and Wiesel, T.N. (1965) Receptive fields and functional architecture in two non-striate visual areas (18 and 19) of the cat. *J. Neurophysiol.*, 28: 229–289.

Hubel, D.H. and Wiesel, T.N. (1972) Laminar and columnar distribution of geniculocortical fibers in the macaque monkey. *J. comp. Neurol.*, 146: 421–450.

Hubel, D.H., Wiesel, T.N. and Stryker, M.P. (1978) Anatomical demonstration of orientation columns in macaque monkey. *J. comp. Neurol.*, 177: 361–380.

Imig, T.J. and Brugge, J.F. (1978) Sources and terminations of callosal axons related to binaural and frequency maps in primary auditory cortex of the cat. *J. comp. Neurol.*, 182: 637–660.

Imig, T.J. and Reale, R.A. (1980) Patterns of cortico-cortical connections related to tonotopic maps in cat auditory cortex. *J. comp. Neurol.*, 192: 293–332.

Jones, E.G., Coulter, J.D. and Hendry, S.H.C. (1978) Intracortical connectivity of architectonic fields in the somatic sensory, motor and parietal cortex of monkeys. *J. comp. Neurol.*, 181: 291–348.

Jones, E.G., Coulter, J.D. and Wise, S.P. (1979) Commissural columns in the sensory-motor cortex of monkeys. *J. comp. Neurol.*, 188: 113–136.

LeVay, S. (1973) synaptic patterns in the visual cortex of the cat and monkey. Electron microscopy of Golgi preparations. *J. comp. Neurol.*, 150: 53–86.

LeVay, S. and Gilbert, C.D. (1976) Laminar patterns of geniculocortical projection in the cat. *Brain Res.*, 113: 1–19.

Lund, J.C., Lund, R.D., Hendrickson, A.E., Bunt, A.H. and Fuchs, A.F. (1975) The origin of efferent pathways from the primary visual cortex, area 17, of the macaque monkey as shown by retrograde transport of horseradish peroxidase. *J. comp. Neurol.*, 164: 287–304.

Marin-Padilla, M. (1974) Three-dimensional reconstruction of the pericellular nests (baskets of the motor (area 4) and visual (area 17), areas of the human cerebral cortex). A Golgi study. *Z. Anat. Entwickl.-Gesch.*, 144: 123–135.

Miller, J.W., Buschmann, M.B.T. and Benevento, L.A. (1980) Extrageniculate thalamic projections to the primary visual cortex. *Brain. Res.*, 189: 221–227.

Montero, V.M. (1980) Patterns of connections from the striate cortex to cortical visual areas in superior temporal sulcus of macaque and middle temporal gyrus of owl monkey. *J. comp. Neurol.*, 189: 45–59.

Ogren, M.P. and Hendrickson, A.E. (1977) The distribution of pulvinar terminals in visual areas 17 and 18 of the monkey. *Brain Res.*, 137: 343–350.

Palmer, L.A., Rosenquist, A.C. and Tusa, R.J. (1978) The retinotopic organization of lateral suprasylvian visual areas in the cat. *J. comp. Neurol.*, 177: 237–256.

Peters, A. and Kimerer, L. (1981) Bipolar neurons in rat visual cortex: combined Golgi-electron microscopic study. *J. Neurocytol.*, 10: 921–946.

Rezak, M. and Benevento, L.A. (1979) A comparison of the organization of the projections of the dorsal lateral geniculate nucleus, the inferior pulvinar and adjacent lateral pulvinar to primary visual cortex (area 17) in the macaque monkey. *Brain Res.*, 169: 19–40.

Ribak, C.E. (1978) Aspinous and sparsely-spinous stellate neurons in the visual cortex of rats contain glutamic acid decarboxylase. *J. Neurocytol.*, 7: 461–478.

Sillito, A.M. (1975) The contribution of inhibitory mechanisms to the receptive field properties of neurones in the striate cortex of the cat. *J. Physiol. (Lond.)*, 250: 305–329.

Somogyi, P. (1977) A specific 'axo-axonal' interneuron in the visual cortex of the rat. *Brain Res.*, 136: 345–350.

Van Essen, D.C. and Zeki, S.M. (1978) The topographic organization of rhesus monkey prestriate cortex. *J. Physiol. (Lond.)*, 277: 273–290.

Wilson, P.D., Rowe, M.H. and Stone, J. (1976) Properties of relay cells in cat's lateral geniculate nucleus: A comparison of W-cells with X- and Y-cells. *J. Neurophysiol.*, 39: 1193–1209.

Wong-Riley, M. (1979) Columnar cortico-cortical interconnections within the visual system of the squirrel and macaque monkeys. *Brain Res.*, 162: 201–217.

Zeki, S.M. (1978) Uniformity and diversity of structure and function in rhesus monkey prestriate visual cortex. *J. Physiol. (Lond.)*, 277: 273–290.

The Relationship Between Wavelength and Color Studied in Single Cells of Monkey Striate Cortex

S. ZEKI

Department of Anatomy, University College London, Gower Street, London WC1E 6BT (U.K.)

The study of color vision is technically no more difficult, or easy, than the study of other branches of sensory physiology. But it presents a formidable problem conceptually. Here, more than any other branch of sensory physiology, there is a schism between our perceptions and physical reality. Indeed, in terms of physical reality, color vision is perhaps the greatest of all sensory illusions. The most refined measuring instruments may tell us that the amounts of different wavelengths of light reflected off two surfaces, one red and the other green, are identical. Yet our nervous system reports them to be different in color (Land, 1977). This is fortunate, for the amount of light of different wavelengths reflected off any surface varies continuously during the day. If the color of objects and surfaces were to vary accordingly, then color vision would lose its significance as a biological signalling mechanism. If an orange, for example, were to appear red in one set of circumstances, green in another, and yellow in a third, then the presence of an orange would no longer be signalled by its color but by some other attribute. Because of the biological value of maintaining the constancy of colors, the nervous system has elaborated a set of rules which makes, within very wide limits, the amount of light of different wavelengths reflected off a surface irrelevant in determining its color. Indeed, to the nervous system, it is physical reality that is an illusion!

This illusory relationship between the physical reality and the perceptual reality is perhaps the root cause of much of the difficulty in studying color vision. Here I want to address myself to but one problem that has been the source of much confusion, namely the relationship between wavelength and perceived color as studied in single cells of the primate visual cortex.

It is now almost three centuries ago that Newton (1704) stated unambiguously that light itself is not colored. He wrote:

"The homogeneal Light and Rays which appear red, or rather make Objects appear so, I call Rubrifick or Red-making; those which make Objects appear yellow, green, blue and violet, I call Yellow-making, Green-making, Blue-making, and Violet-making and so of the rest. And if at any time I speak of Light as coloured or as endued with colours, I would be understood to speak not philosophically or properly, but grossly, and accordingly to such Conceptions as vulgar People in seeing all these Experiments would be apt to frame. *For the Rays to speak properly are not coloured. In them there is nothing else than a certain Power and Disposition to stir up a Sensation of this or that Colour.*" (my italics).

However, even though light itself has no color, it is common knowledge that the visible spectrum appears colored to us, short-wave lights looking blue, middle-wave lights green and long-wave lights red. Between the physical reality of the colorless wavelengths of light and our perceptual reality of it as colored is a gulf so great that we suppose intuitively that light itself *is* colored and interpret our physiological results accordingly, without probing into the more fundamental question of why, if light itself is colorless, the visible spectrum looks colored to us (Land, 1981). Because middle wave light looks green, we suppose it to be green and because green objects have a higher reflectance for middle wave than for short and long wave light, we also suppose that the excess of middle wave light reflected off a surface makes it look green. Newton (1704) himself so believed. He wrote: "Every Body reflects the rays of its own Colour more copiously than the rest, *and from their excess and predominance in the reflected Light has its Colour*" (my italics). In other words, to Newton, a red surface looks red because it reflects more long than middle or short wave light and a green surface green because it reflects more middle than short or long wave light. It is but one logical step from acceptance of this Newtonian equation of excess wavelength = color, to the further supposition that a cell in the nervous system that responds to middle-wave light only is a "green" cell responding best, or perhaps even only, to green surfaces, and a cell responsive to long-wave light only is a "red" cell. This is perhaps what all neurophysiologists have assumed, either implicitly or explicitly. A further supposition is that a cell giving an ON response to long-wave light and an OFF response to middle wave light is a "Red-ON, green-OFF" cell. Such cells have been thought to provide a neuro-physiological basis for Hering's Opponents Theory of Color Vision (see, for example, Boynton, 1979).

There is thus a chain of logical steps leading from our perception of the visible spectrum as colored to our supposition that the spectral selectivity of a cell is a guide to its color preference. It is worth examining the truth of the steps in this chain.

If Newton's supposition that the excess of wavelengths in the light reflected off a surface determines its color is true, then a green surface that reflects more long wave than middle or short wave light should look red, not green. In fact, as Land (1974, 1977) has shown in a series of rigorously controlled experiments, the color of a surface in a *complex, multi-colored scene* is independent, within very wide limits, of the wavelength composition of the light reflected off it. Thus, a green surface continues to look green even if it reflects more long wave than middle or short wave light and a white surface continues to look white even if it reflects the identical amount of long, middle and short wave light that a green surface reflects. Hence the second part of Newton's statement is not true for the perception of colors in a *complex, multi-colored scene*, i.e. in most natural situations. The predominance of light of any waveband reflected off a surface does not determine the color of that surface. One step in our logical chain is thus untrue. It necessitates a re-examination of the subsequent steps. This is that a cell that responds to, say, long wave light only is necessarily a "red" cell, responding best, or only, to red surfaces, and a cell that is responsive to middle wave light only is a "green" cell. Such cells have been found in monkey striate cortex, (Lennox- Buchthal, 1965; Dow, 1973; Gouras, 1974; Michael, 1978). They are commonly called opponent color cells and designated as R^+ if responsive to long wave lights only, G^+ if responsive to middle wave lights only and R^+G^- if they give an on response to long wave lights and an off response to middle wave lights. Let us suppose that they are indeed "color coded" cells and test that supposition.

To do this, we isolated single, wavelength selective cells in monkey striate cortex (V1). The first step was to plot their receptive field and wavelength sensitivity curve (action spectra) in the traditional manner (see Zeki, 1977, 1978). Next the cells were studied using the same experimental paradigm as Land (1974, 1977) used in his perceptual experiments on color vision. The only difference is that whereas Land was studying the responses of human observers, we were studying the responses of single cells. Specifically, "Color Aid" papers of different color and of the size of the cells' receptive field were placed in the receptive field against a black velvet cloth; alternatively different colored rectangles of a multicolored Mondrian display were placed in the receptive field in such a way that the rectangle coincided with the borders of the receptive field. In practice, for narrow band cells *in V1*, it makes little difference whether one uses a small colored patch in a multi-colored display, or a piece of colored paper in isolation. The description given below can thus be applied to either situation. The screen facing the animal, including the receptive field, could be illuminated with three 350 W projectors, each equipped with a band-pass filter, one passing long wave light only, another middle-wave light only and the third short-wave light only (see Land and McCann, 1971). A rheostat attached to each projector allowed variations in the intensity of light coming from each. The amount of light reflected off the area in the cell's receptive field when each projector was turned on alone could be read by means of a Gamma Scientific telephotometer, equipped with an equal energy filter. In the description given below, whenever I refer to color, I mean color as perceived by human observers since there is no device, besides the human visual system, that can measure color. With such an experimental paradigm we are in a position to test rigorously the proposition that excess wavelengths = perceived color and that therefore wavelength selective cells are necessarily "color coded". Here, the description is restricted to wavelength selective cells in monkey striate cortex.

Proposition I: Light of long wavelengths appears red to human observers and light of middle wavelengths appears green. We suppose therefore that a wavelength selective cell in monkey striate cortex that responds to long wave light only will respond to red surfaces and one that responds to middle wave light only will respond to green surfaces. Since a surface will continue to appear red (or green) to human observers even in spite of wide ranging variations in the amounts of long, middle and short wave-bands in the light reflected off that surface, we suppose further that a cell selective for long wavelengths will respond to a red surface *as long as it appears red to human observers*, i.e. regardless of the wavelength composition of the light reflected off it.

Fig. 1 shows the responses of a cell in monkey striate cortex. Its wavelength sensitivity curve (action spectrum) was plotted by shining monochromatic light of different wavelengths onto the receptive field, and noting the minimum intensity at every wavelength which elicits a response from the cell. The action spectrum so plotted showed that the cell was responsive to long wave light only. (That it did not respond to light of other wavelengths or to white light suggests that it must have received an opponent input from light of other wavelengths, perhaps at some antecedent stage of the visual pathways.) Because long wave light looks red to us, one might suppose that it will respond to a red surface only. To test this, a red area of a multicolored Mondrian display was put in the receptive field of the cell and the

222

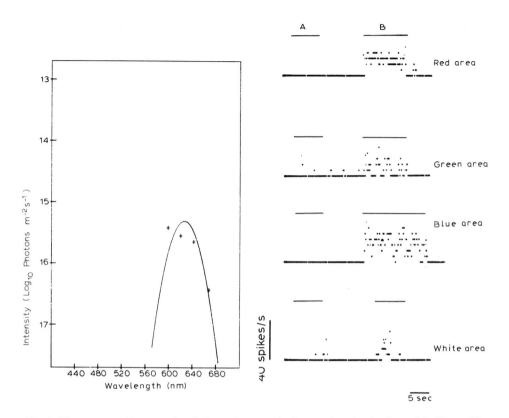

Fig. 1. The response (shown as the discharge frequency) of a wavelength selective cell in V1 to different colored areas of the Mondrian display (right). In column A, each area when placed in the cell's receptive field, was made to reflect 69, 33 and $6\,mW \cdot Sr^{-1} \cdot m^{-2}$ of long, middle and short wave light. In column B, the amount of long wave light was increased, without entailing a change in perceived color, until the cell responded. The action spectrum of the cell is shown to the left, a parabola being drawn through the experimentally determined points. The reaction of this cell, as well as those of Figs. 2 and 3, were studied with monocular stimulation.

display illuminated with all three projectors. By varying the intensities of the three projectors, the red area was made to reflect 69, 33 and $6\,mW \cdot Sr^{-1} \cdot m^{-2}$ of long, middle and short wave light. *The area appeared a vivid red to human observers.* When the shutters were opened, the cell did not respond (trace IA). Next, the amount of long wave light coming off the red area was increased, *but the area still looked a vivid red to human observers.* Now the cell gave a response to the same red surface (trace IB). Similar responses were obtained from other cells whose wavelength sensitivity was restricted to long wavelengths. When the reaction of cells sensitive to middle wave light only, to green areas placed in their receptive field, was studied, identical responses were obtained. In other words, the cells responded or not to the green area depending upon the amount of middle wave light reflected off it even though the area always looked green to human observers.

Proposition I is therefore false. A long wavelength selective cell in monkey striate cortex does not respond to a red area per se. It may respond to it or not depending upon the amount of long wave light reflected off its surface, *and regardless of its color,* just as a middle-wavelength selective cell may or may not respond to a green area placed in its receptive field depending upon the amount of middle wave light reflected off its surface. *Thus the responses of these wavelength-selective cells cannot be correlated with the perceived color.*

Proposition II: Even though a cell which is responsive to long wave light only may or may not respond to a red area, depending upon the amount of long wave light reflected off it, it is still selective to color in that it will not respond to an area which appears, say, white or yellow or blue to human observers, no matter how intense the amount of long wave light reflected off these areas.

Fig. 1 shows the responses of the wavelength selective cell, responsive to long wave light only, to the white, green and blue areas of a Mondrian display. Each area, when placed in the cell's receptive field, was made to reflect 69, 33 and 6 mW $\cdot$ Sr^{-1} $\cdot$ m^{-2} of long, middle and short wave light although each area retained its color. The cell did not respond to any of the areas, *including* the red one. However, *it could be made to respond to each area if the amount of long wave light was sufficiently increased, even though with such increases the color of the area in the cell's receptive field did not change.*

All the wavelength selective cells in V1 that were tested (34) behaved in a similar way, i.e. regardless of their action spectrum, they either did not respond, or responded, to an area of any color placed in their receptive field when the amount of long, middle and short wave light reflected off the areas was identical. If the cell did not respond, it could be induced to do so by increasing the amount of light of its preferred wavelength reflected off the area in its receptive field, without changing its perceived color. If it did respond, its response could be reduced or abolished by decreasing the amount of its preferred wavelength in the reflected light, without changing the color. The cells were thus unable to distinguish between the colors. Proposition II is therefore false.

Proposition III: A cell that gives an ON response to middle wave light and an OFF response to long wave light (or vice versa) is a red ON-green OFF cell (or vice versa), being excited by a red surface and inhibited by a green one. Its responses can be correlated with the perception, by humans, of red and its after image and it is this activity in many cells which is the basis of the psychophysically observed colored after images.

Fig. 2 shows the responses of a long wave light OFF, middle wave light ON cell (see inset for its action spectrum). When a red area of the Mondrian display was placed in the receptive field and made to reflect more long than middle wave light, the cell did not give a response when the shutters were opened, but responded when they were closed, i.e. it gave an OFF response (trace B). But when the red area was made to reflect more middle wave than long wave light, *and still looked red to human observers*, the cell responded at ON but not at OFF (trace A). I emphasize that for human observers the after image produced by viewing the red area in either of the two conditions mentioned above was green. Hence the responses of the cell could not be correlated either with the perceived color or the color of the after-image produced by viewing that area. Next the green area of the Mondrian display was placed in the receptive field of the cell and arranged to reflect more middle than long wave light. The area looked green to human observers and its after image was red. The cell responded at ON but not at OFF (trace C). When the same green area was

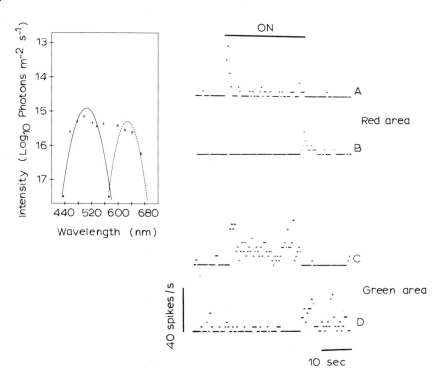

Fig. 2. The responses of a wavelength-selective, ON–OFF, cell in V1 (see inset for its action spectrum) to the red and green areas of the Mondrian display. A: the cell gave an ON response to the *Red* area when this was made to reflect 83, 103 and 11 mW · Sr^{-1} · m^{-2} of long, middle and short wave light, and appeared red. B: the cell gave an OFF response to the *red* area when it was made to reflect 83, 40 and 11 mW · Sr^{-1} · m^{-2} of long, middle and short wave light and still appeared red. D: the cell gave an OFF response to the *green* area when this was made to reflect 80, 40 and 20 mW · Sr^{-1} · m^{-2} of long, middle and short wave light and looked green. C: the cell gave an ON response to the *green* area when it was made to reflect 40, 80 and 20 mW · Sr^{-1} · m^{-2} of long, middle and short wave light. In the action spectrum, + = on response, 0 = off response.

made to reflect more long than middle wave light, *and the area still looked green to human observers*, the cell responded at OFF but not at ON (trace D). In the latter instance, the after image produced by viewing the green area was still red. Other cells with frank opponent inputs behaved in the same manner. Thus the responses of the cells could not be correlated with color but only with the "excess and pre-dominance" of light of the relevant wavelength. Proposition III is therefore false.

These experiments show:

(a) that the perceived color of a surface does not depend upon the wavelength composition of the light reflected off that surface (Land 1974, 1977). The reaction of the wavelength selective cells in V1, by contrast, does depend upon that composition, the cells responding, or not, to a surface of *any* color depending upon the amount of light of their preferred wavelength that is present in the light reflected off a surface, *and independently of its color*;

(b) that the Newtonian equation of excess wavelength = perceived color is not, in general, true perceptually but that the notation excess of relevant wavelength = response from a wavelength selective cell of V1 is true, (but see below);

(c) that it follows from (a) and (b) that the *wavelength selective cells of V1 are not "color-coded"*;

(d) that since the perceived color of a surface is independent of the wavelength composition of the light reflected off it, *so is the after image*. In other words, that the after image also does not obey the rule excess wavelength = perceived color = color of after image;

(e) that it follows from (d) that the responses of these opponent input cells of V1 cannot be the direct basis of the colored after-image; and

(f) that the action spectrum of a cell is not necessarily a guide to which colors it will respond to.

There are, of course, cells in the visual cortex of the rhesus monkey whose responses do correlate with the perceived color. The responses of these cells, by definition, are independent of the wavelength composition of the light reflected off a surface, and correlate with the color alone. Such cells have been found in V4 (Zeki, 1980) and need not be further described here. They too have narrow action spectra. If one were to restrict one's study of wavelength selective cells to a study of their action spectra, one might well reach the conclusion that there is no difference between cells in V1 and in V4. More sophisticated studies, reported here, reveal a radical difference.

I have alluded above to the fact that perceptually, the Newtonian notation of excess wavelength = color is not, *in general*, true. There is however, one situation in which it is true, one which we may call the Newtonian context. If one were to look at a small patch in a void, so that one can only see that small patch and nothing else, and illuminate that patch with three projectors, the perceived color of that patch, *no matter what its color is in normal surroundings*, will depend upon the wavelength composition of the light reflected off it. Thus, if a red patch is viewed in this Newtonian void, and intensities so arranged that the patch reflects more middle than short or long wave light, the patch will appear perceptually *green*. If a patch of paper which appears green in normal surroundings is viewed in a Newtonian void and the intensities from the projectors so arranged that the green patch is made to reflect twice the amount of long wave than of middle or short wave light, it will appear perceptually gray. Since in this Newtonian situation our perception of colors is determined by the excess of wavelengths in the reflected light, it seemed interesting to ask whether the response of the wavelength selective cells in V1 is also always determined by the presence of an excess of light of their preferred wavelength in the light reflected off a surface in their receptive field.

This would appear to be so for the cell of Fig. 1, since for that cell to respond the amount of long wave light reflected off the surface in its receptive field had to be far in excess of middle and short wave light. But this was not so for the cell of Fig. 3. This wavelength selective cell was responsive to middle wave light only. However, when a green or red patch was put in its receptive field and arranged to reflect 69, 33 and 6 mW $\cdot$ Sr^{-1} $\cdot$ m^{-2} of long, middle and short wave light, the cell responded to either area with almost equal vigor and without distinction. When these two areas, reflecting the above amounts of light, were viewed in isolation, they looked pinkish gray, not green. Hence, although the equation, excess wavelength = perceived color in the Newtonian void is true, this is not necessarily so for the wavelength cell of V1 described above since it responded when the amount of middle wave light, to which it was selective, was less than the amount of long wave light. We thus modify (b) above and write:

"Sufficient amount of light of relevant wavelength = response from a wavelength selective cell in V1".

226

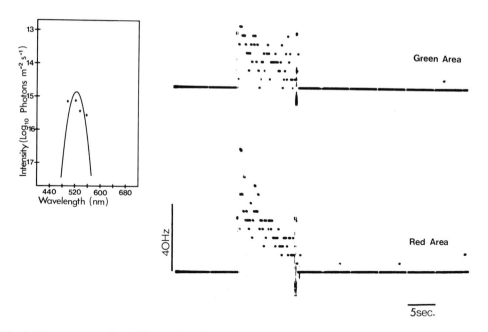

Fig. 3. The responses of a middle-wavelength selective cell in V1 (see inset for its action spectrum) to the red and green areas of a Mondrian display. Each area, when placed in the cell's receptive field, was made to reflect 69, 33 and 6 mW · Sr^{-1} · m^{-2} of long, middle and short wave light.

The term sufficient can be defined operationally, in terms of a cell's response, since some middle wave selective cells give a response if the amount of middle wave light is less than the amount of long wave light (as in Fig. 3) whereas for others the amount of middle wave light has to be in excess.

The interest in viewing patches of color in isolation arises from the fact that there may be similarities between this perceptual situation and the responses of cells in V1. When we view a patch in isolation our perception of its color depends upon the wavelength composition of the light reflected off it alone, and is unaffected by anything in the surround. The striate cortex of the monkey receives a "point-to-point" projection from the retina. Anatomical work (Fisken et al., 1973) shows that the lateral connections of each small region of the striate cortex are limited to 1–2 mm. In other words, the cells in each part of the striate cortex "look" at a small part of the field of view and are not influenced by what goes on elsewhere, at least not by the activity of cells lying beyond 1–2 mm (Hubel and Wiesel, 1977). Since our perception of colors as constant depends upon comparing reflectances from extensive parts of the field of view, it follows that the wavelength selective cells in V1 which are unable, because of their restricted connections, to make such comparisons, can react to the wavelength composition alone, and not to color. This is, of course, speculative and it is possible that the double-opponent cells that Michael (1978) has found in monkey striate cortex do respond to colors as such. It is, however, striking that the lateral connections in V4, where *color*-coded cells have been found (Zeki, 1980), are much more widespread than those in V1 (Zeki, unpublished results).

My aim in this work was to show that the wavelength sensitivity curves of the wavelength selective cells cannot predict whether a cell is color coded or not. It follows that to give an adequate description of the neurophysiology of color vision, a much more detailed study is required, one in which the reaction of cells to colors in natural situations is taken into account.

ACKNOWLEDGEMENT

This work was supported by the Science Research Council.

REFERENCES

Boynton, R.M. (1979) *Human Color Vision*, Holt Rinehart and Winston, New York.

Dow, B.M. (1973) Functional classes of cells and their laminar distribution in monkey visual cortex. *J. Neurophysiol.*, 37: 927–946.

Fisken, R.A., Garey, L.J. and Powell, T.P.S. (1973) Patterns of degeneration after instrinsic lesions of the visual cortex (area 17) of the monkey. *Brain Res.*, 53: 208–213.

Gouras, P. (1974) Opponent-colour cells in different layers of foveal striate cortex. *J. Physiol.*, *(Lond.)*, 238: 583–602.

Hubel, D.H. and Wiesel, T.N. (1977) Functional architecture of macaque monkey visual cortex. *Proc. roy. Soc. Lond. B*, 198: 1–59.

Land, E.H. (1974) The retinex theory of color vision. *Proc. roy. Inst. Gt. Brit.*, 47: 23–58.

Land, E.H. (1977) The retinex theory of color vision. *Sci. Amer.*, 237: 108–128.

Land, E.H. (1981) "*Why is the Spectrum Colored?*" *The Sack Lecture*, Cornell University.

Land, E.H. and McCann, J.J. (1971) Lightness and Retinex Theory. *J. Opt. Soc. Amer.*, 61: 1–11.

Lennox-Buchtal, M.A. (1965) Spectral sensitivity of single units in the cortical area corresponding to central vision in the monkey. *Acta physiol. scand.*, 65: 101–104.

Michael, C.R. (1978) Color vision mechanisms in monkey striate cortex: simple cells with dual opponent color receptive fields. *J. Neurophysiol.*, 41: 1233–1248.

Newton, I. (1704) *Opticks*, *(Book 1, Part 2, Proposition 10)*, Dover Publications, New York, 1952.

Zeki, S.M. (1977) Color coding in the superior temporal sulcus of rhesus monkey visual cortex. *Proc. roy. Soc. B*, 197: 195–223.

Zeki, S.M. (1978) Uniformity and diversity of structure and function in rhesus monkey prestriate visual cortex. *J. Physiol. (Lond.)*, 277: 273–290.

Zeki, S. (1980) The representation of colours in the cerebral cortex. *Nature (Lond.)*, 284: 412–418.

Subsystems Within the Visual Association Cortex as Delineated by their Thalamic and Transcortical Affiliations

DAVID M. BERSON and ANN M. GRAYBIEL

Division of Biology and Medicine, Brown University, Providence, RI 02912 and (A.M.G.) Department of Psychology and Brain Science, Massachusetts Institute of Technology, Cambridge, MA 02139 (U.S.A.)

INTRODUCTION

Studies of the neurobiological basis of vision are being focused increasingly on the visual association cortex. This intensification of interest in the extrastriate visual areas has prompted a reexamination of fiber pathways distributing visual information to these areas and permitting interactions among them. For nearly a century, it has been recognized that the association areas receive visual signals, either directly or indirectly, from corticocortical fibers originating in the primary visual cortex (see Diamond, 1979 for review). This cascade of transcortical fiber projections leading out from the striate cortex has been repeatedly confirmed with modern neuroanatomical methods (Jones and Powell, 1970; Heath and Jones, 1971; Rockland and Pandya, 1979) and figures prominently in much of our current thinking about the processing of visual information by the forebrain (see, e.g., Geschwind, 1965; Hubel and Wiesel, 1965; Jones and Powell, 1970).

It has been known since the retrograde degeneration studies of the 1930s (Waller and Barris, 1937; Walker, 1938), however, that the association areas also receive ascending inputs from the thalamus. These arise from nuclei of the lateral group lying outside the lateral geniculate body. More recently, it has been shown that these so-called extrageniculate thalamic nuclei receive fibers from the superior colliculus (e.g., Graybiel 1972b; Harting, et al., 1973) and the pretectum (e.g., Benevento and Ebner, 1970; Graybiel, 1972b), two brainstem areas to which the retina projects directly. An important implication of such anatomical findings is that the extrastriate cortex has access to visual information independent – and fundamentally different – from that carried by the retino-geniculo-striate pathway and its transcortical extensions.

Many questions raised by the discovery of these alternate ascending conduction routes have yet to be resolved. Prominent among these is how the transcortical association and ascending extrageniculate pathways are combined and integrated at the level of the visual cortex. We report here preliminary results indicating that, at least in the cat, these two sets of connections are systematically related. Viewed together, the anatomical findings strongly suggest the existence of three relatively distinct, though interacting, subsystems within the visual association cortex.

[229]

ORGANIZATION OF PARALLEL EXTRAGENICULATE
CHANNELS IN THE CAT

In the cat, the extrageniculate regions sending thalamocortical fibers to the visual association cortex lie mainly in the complex formed by the lateral posterior (LP) and pulvinar nuclei. It is, by now, well established that the LP–pulvinar complex is composed of three main subdivisions which can be recognized on the basis of certain afferent fiber inputs (Fig. 1A). The lateral posterior nucleus contains a medial division (LPm) receiving fibers from the superficial layers of the superior colliculus, and a lateral division (LPl) getting an input from the striate cortex. The third zone, more or less coextensive with the "pulvinar" of classical descriptions, receives an ascending projection from the pretectal area (see Graybiel, 1972b). First recognized on the basis of these afferent fiber inputs, the zones have subsequently been shown to be distinguishable in several other respects, including their connections with the extrastriate cortex (Updyke, 1977, 1979; Berson and Graybiel, 1978a, b; Symonds et al., 1978; Hughes, 1980), their content of acetylcholinesterase (Graybiel and Berson, 1980) and their physiological attributes (Fish and Chalupa, 1979; Mason, 1981).

Using modern axon transport techniques, we have examined the distribution within the areas of the visual cortex (Fig. 1B) of thalamocortical fibers arising in each of the three main zones of the LP–pulvinar complex. We have found that each subdivision sends its heaviest projections to a largely distinct set of areas in the association cortex (Fig. 2; see also Berson and Graybiel, 1978b and Graybiel and Berson, 1981a, b). The tectorecipient zone (LPm) sends fibers to the lateral division

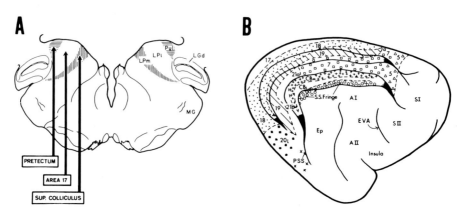

Fig. 1. Semi-schematic diagrams illustrating location of: A, main subdivisions of the LP–pulvinar complex, and B, some areas of the visual and association cortex in the cat. In A, the three main extrageniculate zones of the LP–pulvinar are illustrated diagrammatically on an outline drawing of a transverse section through the posterior thalamus. Sources of afferent fiber projection used to define the zones are shown at left. In B, cortical areas are shown schematically on a lateral view of the right cerebral hemisphere which has been depicted as if the lips of the lateral and suprasylvian sulci were drawn apart. Areas of visually responsive cortex are delineated largely on the basis of work of Tusa and colleagues (see Tusa and Palmer, 1980). B is modified slightly from Graybiel and Berson, 1981b. Abbreviations for this and following figures: CBm, CBl, medial and lateral divisions of the Clare–Bishop area; EVA, ectosylvian visual area; LGd, dorsal lateral geniculate nucleus; LPl, LPm, lateral and medial divisions of lateral posterior nucleus; MG, medial geniculate body; PSS, posterior suprasylvian sulcal area; S.S. Fringe, suprasylvian fringe.

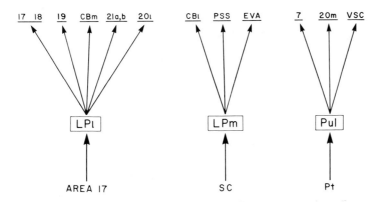

Fig. 2. Schematic diagram illustrating clustering of visual association areas into "families" based on their main input from the subdivisions of the LP–pulvinar complex. Auxiliary thalamocortical pathways (see text) are not illustrated here. Abbreviations: Pt, pretectal area; SC, superior colliculus; VSC, ventral splenial cortex; others as in Fig. 1.

of the Clare-Bishop area (CBl), to the ectosylvian visual area (EVA: see Olson and Graybiel, this volume) and to an area lying just rostral to area 20 at the foot of the posterior suprasylvian sulcus (called here area PSS). The striate-recipient zone (LPl) projects to areas 17, 18 and 19; areas 21a and 21b; the medial division of the Clare–Bishop complex (CBm); the part of area 20 lying on the lateral surface of the hemisphere (20l); and probably to the splenial visual area. The pulvinar sends its densest projections to area 7, to the ventral splenial cortex (VSC; see Graybiel and Berson, 1981b), and to a part of area 20 lying on the medial wall of the hemisphere (20m)*. These dominant thalamocortical pathways, schematically summarized in Fig. 2, can be used to define three main classes or "families" of extrastriate areas, members of each family sharing a common extrageniculate thalamic input.

Closer scrutiny of the thalamocortical pathways indicates that the segregation between these families of areas is incomplete. In addition to their predominant thalamic input, many cortical areas receive projections from one (or in some cases several) additional zones of the LP–pulvinar complex. For example, area 19, besides its input from LPl, receives less prominent inputs from the pulvinar and from a part of LPm adjoining LPl (Berson and Graybiel, in preparation). Nevertheless, we have almost always found such thalamocortical pathways to be less dense or extensive than the principal pathways shown in Fig. 2 and for this reason we consider them as "auxiliary", though undoubtedly of specific functional importance. The relatively weak projection from the LP – pulvinar complex to area 17 represents a more familiar example of such auxiliary conduction routes**.

Available evidence from this laboratory and others (Updyke, 1977, 1979; Berson and Graybiel, 1978a; Berson and Graybiel, in preparation) suggests that virtually all of these thalamocortical connections are reciprocated by corticothalamic pathways.

*For location of cortical areas considered here, see Fig. 1B and also Tusa and Palmer (1980) and Graybiel and Berson (1981a, b).

**In the present context, however, the striate cortex may still be considered a member of the "LPl-family" of cortical areas, for LPl provides area 17 with its main source of input from the *extrageniculate* visual thalamus.

Accordingly, each extrastriate area sends axons primarily to one extrageniculate zone, but may send auxiliary projections to others.

Beside the three main zones in the LP–pulvinar complex, several other regions in the lateral group of thalamic nuclei may channel visual information to the association cortex. Among these is the so-called lateral medial nucleus (LM; see Olson and Graybiel, this volume), which adjoins LPm ventromedially and which may receive ascending input from the deep collicular layers. A second such zone, lying in the caudal part of the lateral intermediate nucleus, receives ascending fiber projections from the pretectal region (Graybiel and Berson, 1980). The input–output relations of these thalamic zones have not been worked out in detail and the possibility remains that their thalamocortical projections, particularly those of LM, may be used to define additional "families" of visual cortical areas. Preliminary evidence does suggest that thalamocortical fibers originating in these zones are distributed at least partly to cortical areas which also receive input from the main zones of the LP–pulvinar complex proper (see Berson and Graybiel, 1978a and Olson and Graybiel, this volume).

TRANSCORTICAL AFFILIATIONS OF THE STRIATE AND EXTRASTRIATE CORTEX

Our most recent experiments have probed the relationship between the clusters of areas defined by their shared thalamic input and the systems of association fibers interconnecting various areas of visually responsive cortex. We have used mainly the autoradiographic method, making large deposits of radioactive amino acids in order to label as fully as possible the transcortical efferent projections of single cortical areas. The preliminary findings bolster the impression gained from the thalamocortical studies that the visual cortex contains at least three subsystems or families of areas because cortical areas having a common thalamic input have proved to be heavily linked by association fibers.

This relationship first became apparent in examining the transcortical projections of areas receiving their main extrageniculate input from LPl (i.e. members of the "LPl-family"). In agreement with earlier reports (e.g., Polley and Dirkes, 1963; Hubel and Wiesel, 1965; Kawamura, 1973), we found that the striate cortex sends dense projections to area 19 and CBm, and we also found at least weak projections to area 21. All of these extrastriate areas are members of the LPl-family (Fig. 3). Area 18, another LPl-family member, is known to receive projections from area 17 as well (e.g., Polley and Dirkes, 1963; Hubel and Wiesel, 1965; Gilbert and Kelly, 1975), though for technical reasons we have not been able to analyze this connection in our material. In fact, we have identified only one cortical target of efferent striate projections outside the LPl-family – a restricted part of the lateral division of the Clare–Bishop area (dashed arrow in Fig. 3).

The extrastriate members of the LPl-family show a similar pattern of dense within-family transcortical projection. Area 19 sends association fibers back to areas 17 and 18 as well as to the medial division of the Clare–Bishop area, area 21a (and probably area 21b), the splenial visual area and the lateral part of area 20. As shown in the schematic diagram of Fig. 4, all of these cortical areas appear to receive their main extrageniculate thalamic input from LPl. A similar arrangement appears to hold for

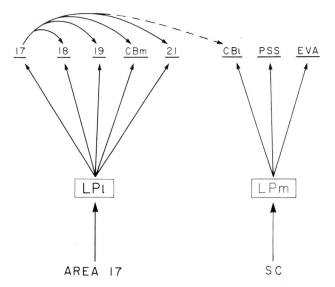

Fig. 3. Schematic diagram illustrating close correspondence between distributions of transcortica projections of area 17 and thalamocortical projections of the striate-recipient zone of LP (LPl). Except for the restricted projection to the lateral division of the Clare–Bishop area (dashed arrow), the striate cortex does not send fibers to the main cortical targets of LPm or pulvinar.

CBm; it projects to most of the areas in the LPl-family, including areas 17, 18, 19, 20_l and probably area 21a as well. Both areas 19 and CBm have more restricted projections to cortical areas receiving their main thalamic input from LPm ("LPm-family"; see below), but appear to lack almost completely connections with the "pulvinar-family" areas.

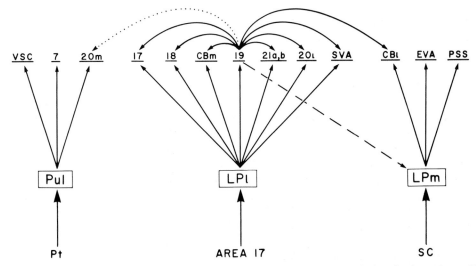

Fig. 4. Schematic diagram illustrating close correspondence between transcortical projections of area 19 and thalamocortical projections of LPl. Note that the projection to the lateral division of the Clare–Bishop area is paralleled by a restricted projection to the source of its main thalamic input, LPm (dashed arrow). Dotted arrow indicates extremely limited projection to pulvinar-family cortex. Abbreviation: SVA, splenial visual area; others as in Figs. 1 and 2.

Our evidence on the transcortical affiliations of LPm- and pulvinar-family members is less complete, but here too the pattern seems to be one of extensive within-family and restricted between-family connectivity. Of the cortical regions receiving thalamic input from LPm (the lateral division of the Clare–Bishop complex, CBl; the ectosylvian visual area, EVA; and the cortex at the rostral end of area 20, here called PSS), we have found that CBl projects to both EVA and PSS and Olson and Graybiel (this volume) have found that EVA projects to CBl and PSS. By contrast, projections from CBl and EVA to members of the LPl family are restricted or weak, and those to the pulvinar cortex, if they exist at all, are too weak to be traced by autoradiography.

In a similar pattern, area 7, a member of the pulvinar family, projects to the ventral splenial cortex and the medial part of area 20, both of which receive projections from the pulvinar. Cortical areas in the LPm-family apparently receive no such projection. Deposits of radiolabel in area 7 do elicit some labeling in LPl-family areas, but we are unsure of the significance of this because the injection sites may involve the adjacent LPl-family area, CBm.

This close correspondence between thalamocortical and corticocortical connectivity is reflected in the experimental results illustrated in Fig. 5. In each pair of cases, a direct comparison is made between the transcortical projections of a particular extrastriate area and the thalamocortical projections of the extrageniculate region to which it is predominantly connected. The first pair of diagrams compares the cortical distribution of fibers arising in area 19 with those from LPl (and the adjacent part of LPm); the second pair compares the efferent projections of CBl and LPm; and the last pair those of area 7 and the pulvinar (and adjacent lateral intermediate nucleus).

The similarities in corticocortical and thalamocortical connectivity among members of the same cortical family may extend to corticofugal projections as well. Yeterian and van Hoesen (1978), for example, have shown in the monkey that cortical areas linked by association fibers project to overlapping zones within the striatum.

PATHWAYS FOR INTERACTION AMONG FAMILIES

As has been mentioned above, the transcortical fiber projections of particular areas of the visual cortex, though primarily distributed to areas in the same family cluster, may extend to areas lying in other families. This is reminiscent of the pattern

---

Fig. 5. Illustration of the close correspondence of certain patterns of corticocortical and thalamocortical projection as visualized by the autoradiographic method. For each pair (A–B, C–D, and E–F), results of a case of tracer deposit in the visual association cortex (A, C and E) are compared with those of a case of deposit in the thalamic region most heavily interconnected with that cortical area (B, D and F). Area of dense cortical deposit is depicted by solid black, weaker deposit by cross-hatching. Thalamic deposits appear as dense stippling in B.4, D.4 and F.4. For each pair of cases, anterograde cortical labeling is diagramatically shown at five closely matched transverse levels. Comparisons of patterns of ipsilateral corticopetal fiber projection are made between area 19 (A) and LPl and the adjacent part of LPm (B); between the lateral division of the Clare–Bishop complex (C) and LPm (D); and between area 7 (E) and the pulvinar (F). Note close correspondence of thalamic injection sites in B, D and F to sites of anterograde thalamic labeling in A, C and E and similar areal distribution of anterograde cortical labeling in each pair. Abbreviations: C, cingulate gyrus; others as in Figs. 1 and 2.

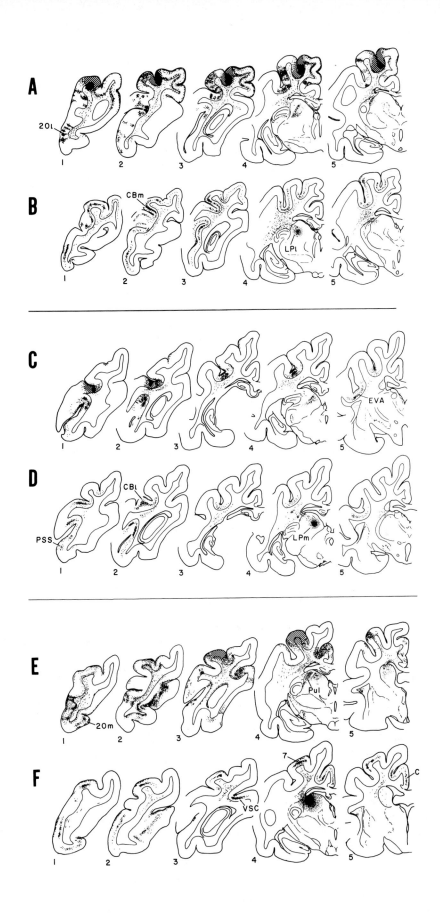

seen in the corticothalamic projections: individual visual areas, though sending their principal (i.e. heaviest) corticothalamic projection to a single extrageniculate subdivision, may have auxiliary connections with one or more additional subdivisions. The similarity may be more than coincidental, for there appears to be some congruence between an area's extra-family transcortical affiliations and its auxiliary thalamic connections. Thus, for example, two areas of the LPl-family, areas 19 and CBm, send transcortical fibers to CBl, a member of the LPm-family; at the same time, these extrastriate areas have restricted "auxiliary" connections with LPm itself (see Berson and Graybiel, in preparation). This congruence between corticothalamic and corticocortical "escape routes" from the main family cluster is schematically illustrated in Fig. 4.

The existence of these bridging pathways means that the anatomical segregation between families is relative, rather than absolute. One function of such incomplete segregation may be to allow the striate cortex indirect access to the frontal and limbic lobes. Areas to which the striate cortex sends direct projections (LPl-family members) appear to lack association connections with these cortical regions, while at least one member of the pulvinar family (area 7) has strong connections with both area 6 and the cingulate gyrus (unpublished observations).

Just how signals from the retino-geniculo-striate pathway are funneled to more distal cortical regions by means of these cross-family connections remains to be worked out in detail. Nonetheless, there are hints that this transcortical cascade leading out from the striate cortex may be organized similarly in cats and primates. Rockland and Pandya (1979) have demonstrated in the monkey that "rostrally directed" transcortical projections (i.e. those leading out from the striate cortex) terminate within the middle layers of the cortex, while "caudally directed" association fibers terminate predominantly in layer I. We have observed a similar distinction in the cat, both among the members of the LPl-family itself and in their transcortical associations with members of different families. Projections arising in the striate cortex terminate heavily in the granular layer of areas 19 and CBm, whereas the return projections terminate most densely in the molecular and infragranular layers of area 17. Similarly, the projections from area 19 and CBm to the LPm-family cortex (CBl) are densely distributed in the granular layer, whereas the weak return projections appear to terminate primarily in layer I.

CONCLUSIONS

The picture that is emerging for the cat, then, is compatible with the classical view in which visual signals reach the association cortex by means of direct and indirect transcortical projections originating in the striate cortex. But, according to the view proposed here, this transcortical cascade operates within the context of relatively independent thalamocortical subsystems. Cortical areas in each subsystem are linked by the receipt of a common extrageniculate input-channel and are further bonded together by a dense network of corticocortical connections. A simplified view of this anatomical arrangement is presented in schematic form in Fig. 6. The anatomy alone, of course, provides little help in evaluating the functional role played by each of these subsystems. Their existence nevertheless seems likely to reflect some fundamental division of labor in the analysis of visual information by the forebrain.

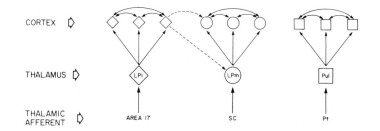

Fig. 6. Schematic diagram illustrating hypothetical subsystems within the visual association cortex inferred from connections described in text. Cortical areas within a single "family" receive principal extrageniculate input from a single thalamic subdivision and are heavily interconnected by transcortical projections (solid arrows). Communication between cortical subsystems may be effected either by transcortical projection (upper dotted arrow) or by corticothalamic crossover (lower dotted arrow).

ACKNOWLEDGEMENTS

We are pleased to acknowledge the technical assistance of Mr. Henry F. Hall, Ms. Elaine Yoneoka and Ms. Dianne Sahagian. Supported by Grants R01 EY02866-01 and 1-P30-EY02621 from the National Institutes of Health, BNS75-18758 and 78-10549 from the National Science Foundation and NGR 22-009826 from the National Aeronautics and Space Administration.

REFERENCES

Benevento, L.A. and Ebner, F.F. (1970) Pretectal, tectal, retinal and cortical projections to thalamic nuclei of the opossum in stereotaxic coordinates. *Brain Res.*, 18: 171–175.

Berson, D.M. and Graybiel, A.M. (1978a) Parallel thalamic zones in the LP–pulvinar complex of the cat identified by their afferent and efferent connections. *Brain Res.*, 147: 139–148.

Berson, D.M. and Graybiel, A.M. (1978b) Thalamo-cortical projections and histochemical identification of subdivisions of the LP–pulvinar complex in the cat. *Neurosci. Abstr.*, 4: 620.

Diamond, I.T. (1979) The subdivisions of neocortex: a proposal to revise the traditional view of sensory, motor, and association areas. In J.M. Sprague and A.N. Epstein (Eds.), *Progress in Psychobiology and Physiological Psychology, Vol. 8*, Academic Press, New York, pp. 1–43.

Fish, S.E. and Chalupa, L.M. (1979) Functional properties of pulvinar-lateral posterior neurons which receive input from the superior colliculus. *Exp. Brain Res.* 36: 245–257.

Geschwind, N. (1965) Disconnexion syndromes in animals and man. Part I. *Brain*, 88: 237–294.

Gilbert, C.D. and Kelly, J.P. (1975) The projections of cells in different layers of the cat's visual cortex. *J. comp. Neurol.*, 163: 81–106.

Graybiel, A.M. (1972a) Some ascending connections of the pulvinar and nucleus lateralis posterior of the thalamus in the cat. *Brain Res.*, 44: 99–125.

Graybiel, A.M. (1972b) Some extrageniculate visual pathways in the cat. *Invest. Ophthalmol.*, 11: 322–332.

Graybiel, A.M. and Berson, D.M. (1980) Histochemical identification and afferent connections of subdivisions in the LP-pulvinar complex and related nuclei in the cat. *Neuroscience*, 5: 1175–1238.

Graybiel, A.M. and Berson, D.M. (1981a) Families of related cortical areas in the extrastriate visual system: summary of an hypothesis. In C.N. Woolsey (Ed.), *Multiple Cortical Sensory Areas: Somatic, Visual and Auditory*, The Humana Press, Clinton, NJ, in press.

Graybiel, A.M. and Berson, D.M. (1981b) On the relation between transthalamic and transcortical pathways in the visual system. In F.O. Schmitt, F.G. Worden and F. Dennis (Eds.), *The Organization of the Cerebral Cortex*, MIT Press, Cambridge, MA, pp. 286–319.

238

Harting, J.K., Hall, W.C., Diamond, I.T. and Martin, G.F. (1973) Anterograde degeneration study of the superior colliculus in *Tupaia glis*: evidence for a subdivision between superficial and deep layers. *J. comp. Neurol.*, 148: 361–386.

Heath, C.J. and Jones, E.G. (1971) The anatomical organization of the suprasylvian gyrus of the cat. *Ergebn. Anat. Entwickl-Gesch.*, 45: 1–64.

Hubel, D.H. and Wiesel, T.N. (1965) Receptive fields and functional architecture in two nonstriate visual areas (18 and 19) of the cat. *J. Neurophysiol.*, 28: 229–289.

Hughes, H.C. (1980) Efferent organization of the cat pulvinar complex, with a note on bilateral claustrocortical and reticulocortical connections. *J. comp. Neurol.*, 193: 937–965.

Jones, E.G. and Powell, T.P.S. (1970) An anatomical study of converging sensory pathways within the cerebral cortex of the monkey. *Brain*, 93: 793–820.

Kawamura, K. (1973) Corticocortical fiber connections of the cat cerebrum. III. The occipital region. *Brain Res.*, 51: 41–60.

Mason, R. (1981) Differential responsiveness of cells in the visual zones of the cat's LP–pulvinar complex to visual stimuli. *Exp. Brain Res.*, 43: 25–33.

Polley, E.H. and Dirkes, J.M. (1963) The visual cortical (geniculocortical) area of the cat brain and its projections. *Anat. Rec.*, 145: 345.

Rockland, K.S. and Pandya, D.N. (1979) Laminar origins and terminations of cortical connections of the occipital lobe in the rhesus monkey. *Brain Res.*, 179: 3–20.

Symonds, L., Rosenquist, A., Edwards, S. and Palmer, L. (1978) Thalamic projections to electrophysiologically defined visual areas in the cat. *Neurosci. Abstr.*, 4: 647.

Tusa, R.J. and Palmer, L.A. (1980) Retinotopic organization of areas 20 and 21 in the cat. *J. comp. Neurol.*, 193: 147–164.

Updyke, B.V. (1977) Topographic organization of the projections from cortical areas 17, 18 and 19 onto the thalamus, pretectum, and superior colliculus in the cat. *J. comp. Neurol.*, 173: 81–122.

Updyke, B.V. (1979) Projections from lateral suprasylvian cortex to the lateral posterior complex in the cat. *Anat. Rec.*, 193: 707–708.

Walker, A.E. (1938) *The Primate Thalamus*. University of Chicago Press, Chicago.

Waller, W.H. and Barris, R.W. (1937) Relationships of thalamic nuclei to the cerebral cortex in the cat. *J. comp. Neurol.*, 67: 317–341.

Yeterian, E.H. and van Hoesen, G.W. (1978) Cortico-striate projections in the rhesus monkey. I. The organization of certain cortico-caudate connections. *Brain Res.*, 139: 43–63.

An Outlying Visual Area
in the Cerebral Cortex of the Cat

CARL R. OLSON and ANN M. GRAYBIEL

Department of Psychology and Brain Science, Massachusetts Institute of Technology, Cambridge, MA 02139
(U.S.A.)

The visual cortex has been shown in both primates and non-primates to include a large number of extrastriate areas in addition to the classically defined visual areas 17, 18 and 19. Not all of these extrastriate areas contain full representations of the visual field, but, whether their maps are partial or complete, the areas abut one another, often with mirror reversals at their borders. As a consequence, the striate and extrastriate areas together form a zone of exclusive visual reponsiveness in the posterior neocortex that is continuous even though having separate areas within it. The arrangement of these visual areas into a continuum has obvious advantages in keeping transcortical association pathways short and also has suggested that the multiple maps might have evolved by a process akin to gene duplication (Kaas, 1977). We have recently discovered a visual area which appears anomalous in that it lies at a distance from the striate and extrastriate areas, in the anterior part of the cat's cerebral cortex, and yet, like the posterior visual areas, is a zone containing unimodal visually responsive neurons. We have undertaken both to define the limits of this outlying visual area in electrophysiological mapping experiments and to analyze its pattern of connections using neuroanatomical tracers.

The area we have studied is located in the depths of the cat's anterior ectosylvian sulcus, near the classic auditory and somatic sensory fields. The cortex in this region had been thought to have polysensory association functions because auditory, somatosensory and visual evoked responses could be recorded through macroelectrodes placed at the surface of the sulcus (Bignall et al., 1966). Certain properties of the visual evoked response had nevertheless been taken to indicate that this response originates in a distinct population of cells (Guiloff et al., 1971) and we have confirmed this suggestion in microelectrode experiments in which we recorded from neurons along numerous closely spaced penetrations through the sulcal cortex. The visually responsive zone we have defined lies in a discrete part of the buried pocket of anterior ectosylvian sulcal cortex extending from the ventral bank of the sulcus at caudal levels to the dorsal bank rostrally. The location of this zone, which we have termed the ectosylvian visual area, or EVA, is shown in Fig. 1A–C.

Altogether, EVA occupies about 20 mm^2 of sulcal cortex and is bounded on different sides by at least three non-visual areas. This arrangement is evident in results from a representative mapping experiment, displayed in Fig. 2, where symbols indicating the sensory properties of recorded cells are projected onto a map of the surface of the unfolded sulcal cortex. The zone containing visually responsive neurons (solid circles) is bounded rostrally by somatosensory cells (open triangles),

240

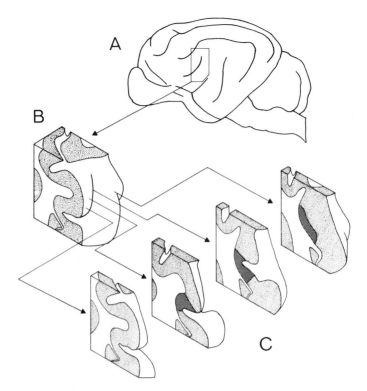

Fig. 1. Schematic serial dissection demonstrating the location of EVA. A: lateral view of left hemisphere (box encloses caudal part of anterior ectosylvian sulcus). B: block of cortex enclosed by box (block is rotated so that lateral face appears at the right; stippling indicates cut surface of gray matter). C: slabs formed by sectioning the block with frontal cuts placed 1.3 mm apart (EVA is cross-hatched).

caudally and dorsally by auditory units (open squares) and laterally by neurons not responsive to standard forms of sensory stimulation (horizontal line segments). Areas of polysensory responsiveness (half-filled symbols) were found rarely, mainly along the borders between areas. We conclude that most of the cortex in this part of the anterior ectosylvian sulcus, far from having polysensory functions, is specialized for processing information coded in terms of specific sensory modalities.

In the course of mapping out EVA, we characterized in a qualitative way the visual-response properties of single neurons and unit clusters at hundreds of sites in the area. We found that units in EVA are markedly unlike those in areas 17, 18 and 19 but possess properties resembling, for the most part, the properties of cells in other outlying extrastriate visual areas, notably areas in the Clare–Bishop complex. Neurons in EVA characteristically respond to stimulation through either eye, prefer moving to flashed stimuli, and respond optimally to a small spot swept rapidly through the receptive field in a particular preferred direction. Their receptive fields are large, averaging around 20° in diameter. As in the most rostral subdivisions of the Clare–Bishop complex (Palmer et al., 1978), there is a major preponderance of neurons whose receptive fields are centered beneath the horizontal midline of the visual field. EVA appears to be organized roughly along retinotopic lines, but the pattern of organization is remarkably coarse and variable, and consists primarily in a tendency for ventrally located cells to have central receptive fields and for cells

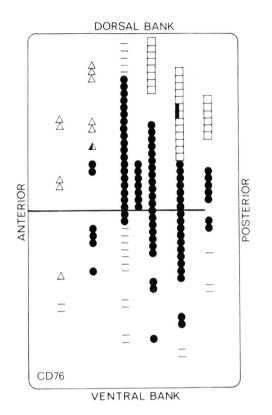

Fig. 2. Symbols representing the sensory properties of neurons recorded in one cat are projected onto a map of the cortex of the left anterior ectosylvian sulcus. Filled circles, exclusively visual response; triangles, somatosensory (if half-filled, then also visual); squares, auditory (if half-filled, then also visual); line segments, not responsive. The large rectangle represents a 5×10 mm area of cortex at the caudal extreme of the sulcus. The cortical surface is presented as if it has been exposed to lateral view by retracting the dorsal and ventral banks of the sulcus upward and downward respectively.

located dorsally to have receptive fields in some part of the visual-field periphery.

We were especially anxious to determine the fiber connections of EVA because its electrophysiological properties suggested it would be associated with the extrageniculate visual thalamus (the LP–pulvinar complex) and with the extrastriate cortex, whereas its position would indicate connections with auditory and perhaps somatic sensory structures. Previous findings had been equivocal on this subject. Work on the thalamic connections had linked the anterior ectosylvian cortex both to the visually responsive medioventral part of the nucleus lateralis posterior nearest the posterior nuclear group (LPm; Graybiel, 1970, 1972a, b; Berson and Graybiel, 1978; Graybiel and Berson, 1981a, b) and to the thalamic region medial to LPm that is called the LM–Sg complex (Graybiel and Berson, 1980, 1981b). At the cortical level, the same anterior ectosylvian sulcal cortex had been shown to receive input from the visually-responsive lateral part of the Clare–Bishop complex (CBl) (Squatrito et al., 1981; Berson and Graybiel, this volume). Despite this evidence for vision-related inputs from thalamus (LPm) and cortex (CBl), the anterior ectosylvian cortex was considered because of its position to be part of the auditory association cortex and to have functions only complexly related to the mapping of visual space (Graybiel, 1972b). A similar suggestion was made about the LM–Sg complex, which was known to receive deep collicular input, on account of its projection to the anterior ectosylvian cortex, the suprasylvian fringe and the insula (Graybiel and Berson, 1981a).

With the electrophysiology as a guide we have been able to analyze the fiber connections of EVA in axon transport experiments by placing in the center of the area small deposits of anterograde or retrograde tracer substance ([³H]amino acids and horseradish peroxidase) and examining the resulting distributions of transported tracer. In this way we knew we were dealing with connections of the electrophysiologically defined visually responsive part of the anterior ectosylvian sulcus. These experiments definitively establish that EVA is reciprocally connected with both LPm and the LM–Sg complex of the thalamus but show that its connections with LM–Sg are considerably stronger than those with LPm. This dual thalamic linkage can be seen in Fig. 3C and D, and is discussed further below. These experiments further showed that the LM–Sg connections involve only part of the LM–Sg complex. Anterograde and retrograde labeling in LM–Sg was invariably distributed in a patchy and irregular pattern, and involved mainly the lateral part of LM–Sg, regardless of the part of EVA injected.

This result intrigued us because the LM–Sg complex is known to be chemo-architecturally heterogeneous, consisting of a system of acetylcholinesterase-rich blotches, especially concentrated medially, which lie against a background of low acetylcholinesterase activity (Graybiel and Berson, 1980). When we compared the histochemical and tracer distributions in serial sections, we consistently found that after injections into EVA, most of the labeled fibers and cell bodies in LM–Sg lay in the pale parts of the complex and avoided its acetylcholinesterase-rich parts. From this result we conclude that the subdivisions of the LM–Sg visible in the acetylcholinesterase stain are functionally significant. Because the patches of labeling tend to interdigitate with the enzyme-positive patches we further think it likely that the subdivision of LM–Sg interconnected with EVA is genuinely irregular and broken in morphology. This conclusion is strengthened by another, still preliminary, finding, namely, our observation that tracers injected into the auditory association cortex of the posterior ectosylvian gyrus are transported selectively to those parts of LM–Sg which are not interconnected with EVA, i.e. to the acetylcholinesterase-rich patches.

When we looked at the transcortical connections of EVA in the same cases, we learned that it is related to a number of areas of extrastriate cortex, but that there are no direct connections between EVA and the classic visual areas 17, 18 and 19. The strongest extrastriate ties are with the lateral division of the Clare–Bishop complex and parts of the posterior suprasylvian cortex and area 20; there are weaker reciprocal pathways linking EVA to the medial division of the Clare–Bishop complex. Thus the corticocortical connections of EVA, far more than its main thalamic input from LM–Sg, are predictive of its physiologically demonstrated exclusive visual responsiveness.

Berson and Graybiel, in this volume and elsewhere (Graybiel and Berson, 1981a, b) have proposed a system of classification by which the cortical areas related to vision are divided into families. An area is assigned to a family on the basis of the extrageniculate visual subdivision with which it is most heavily interconnected. According to their scheme, the well known extrageniculate visual areas of the cat are divided into three families, one related to the lateral division of the lateroposterior

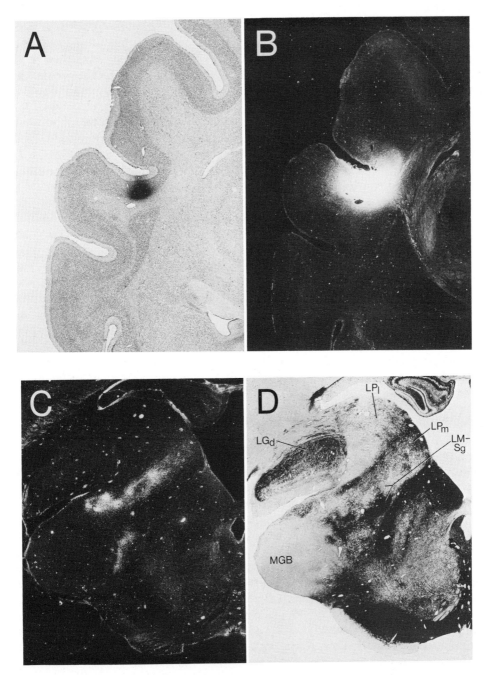

Fig. 3. Corticothalamic projection arising from EVA. A and B: silver grains mark site in EVA at which [³H]amino acids were deposited under electrophysiological guidance (A, bright-field; B, dark-field). Survival time, 1 week. Autoradiographic exposure time, 5 weeks. C: terminal field in frontal section through left thalamus (same case; dark-field). D: section immediately adjacent to that shown in C, stained for acetylcholinesterase activity to reveal the major thalamic subdivisions at this level. Note the complementary distribution of the two large terminal fields in C and of the cholinesterase-dense patch in D which separates them. LGd, dorsal nucleus of the lateral geniculate body; LPl, lateral division of the nucleus lateralis posterior; LPm, medial division of the nucleus lateralis posterior; LM–Sg, nucleus lateralis medialis–suprageniculate nucleus complex; MGB, medial geniculate body.

nucleus (LPl), another to its medial division (LPm) and a third to the pulvinar. Since EVA is weakly connected to LPm, as indicated by encroachment of label transported from it into parts of LPm lying adjacent to LM–Sg, we might properly regard EVA as having an affiliation with the LPm family. However, the major thalamic connections of EVA are with the LM–Sg complex and this has led us to assign EVA to a distinct family of areas receiving input from LM–Sg. We think there may be other visual areas in this LM–Sg-related family, because studies in other laboratories (Updyke, 1981) as well as in our own have indicated that some laterally and rostrally disposed parts of the suprasylvian sulcal cortex are interconnected with LM–Sg. The suggestion that LM–Sg defines a family cluster is in agreement with the surmise of Graybiel and Berson (1981a). Like these authors, we have also found evidence for connections between the LM–Sg family and limbic or pre-limbic cortex. However, in contrast to their previous interpretation of these connections as representing links between auditory association cortex and the limbic system, we now can place at least some of these firmly in the domain of outlying visual pathways.

A further proposal in the classification by families is that cortical areas within a given extrastriate cluster are more heavily interconnected than cortical areas belonging to different families (Berson and Graybiel, this volume, and Graybiel and Berson, 1981a, b). EVA partly but by no means fully fits this generalization. On one hand, EVA is not detectably connected with members of the pulvinar family or with lower-order members of the LPl-family (17, 18, 19), and is very densely connected with LPm family cortex (e.g. the lateral Clare–Bishop area) as would be predicted on the basis of its direct connections with LPm. On the other hand, EVA apparently projects only weakly to the suprasylvian fringe, though this cortical area appears to be a member of the LM–Sg family and it does, in contrast, project across family lines to an important member of the LPl family, namely, the medial Clare–Bishop area (CBm). The apparent discrepancy involving the suprasylvian fringe may have an explanation in the heterogeneity of LM–Sg: the acetylcholinesterase-poor part may define an LM family, the second acetylcholinesterase-rich part an Sg family. This cannot be the case for the LPl-cortex discrepancy, however, which therefore represents a clear exception to the rule of high intrafamily-low interfamily connectivity. This particular interfamily pathway is relatively weak as indicated by the facts: (a) that HRP deposited in EVA is transported only to a scattering of cell bodies in CBm while densely labeling cell bodies in CBl, and (b) that [^{3}H]amino acid injections apparently restricted to CBm do not produce detectable labeling of EVA while comparable injections into CBl do (see Berson and Graybiel, this volume). Both the relative weakness of the CBm–EVA connections and the fact that they represent links with higher-order rather than lower-order members of the LPl family suggest that ordering by family is embedded in a hierarchical pattern of trans-cortical connectivity (cf. Berson and Graybiel, this volume, and Graybiel and Berson, 1981a, b).

The findings we have presented indicate that EVA is a cortical visual area of particularly high order. Physically distant from primary visual cortex, it is also connectionally distant, in the sense that it lacks direct connections either to areas 17, 18 and 19 or to regions of the thalamus upon which they project. Any flow of visual information between these areas and EVA thus must occur by way of synapses in intermediate cortical zones to which both are connected, for example, the Clare–

Bishop complex, or by way of a corticotectocortical loop involving descending projections from areas 17, 18 and 19 to the superior colliculus and ascending projections from the colliculus to LPm and from LPm to the Clare–Bishop complex. In harmony with this connectional analysis, functional study has revealed a number of traits which sharply differentiate EVA from primary visual cortex, notably the great size of the receptive fields of its neurons and the coarseness of its retinotopic organization. In these properties as well as in its physical and connectional distance from area 17, EVA resembles primate higher-order visual areas such as inferotemporal cortex (Desimone and Gross, 1979). We hope that further study of EVA will throw some light on the basic questions of why there are multiple visual areas and how they are organized into hierarchical and family systems.

ACKNOWLEDGEMENTS

This work was supported by NIH Grants 5 F32 EY05316-02, 5-R01-EY02866-03, EY 02621; and a Johnson and Johnson Postdoctoral Fellowship.

REFERENCES

Berson, D.M. and Graybiel, A.M. (1978) Thalamo-cortical projections and histochemical identification of subdivisions of the LP–pulvinar complex in the cat. *Neurosci. Abstr.*, 4: 620.

Bignall, K.E., Imbert, M. and Buser, P. (1966) Optic projections to nonvisual cortex of the cat. *J. Neurophysiol.*, 29: 396–409.

Desimone, R. and Gross, C.G. (1979) Visual areas in the temporal cortex of the macaque. *Brain Res.*, 178: 363–380.

Graybiel, A.M. (1970) Some thalamocortical projections of the pulvinar-posterior system of the thalamus in the cat. *Brain Res.*, 22: 131–136.

Graybiel, A.M. (1972a) Some ascending connections of the pulvinar and nucleus lateralis posterior of the thalamus of the cat. *Brain Res.*, 44: 99–125.

Graybiel, A.M. (1972b) Some fiber pathways related to the posterior thalamic region in the cat. *Brain Behav. Evol.*, 6: 363–393.

Graybiel, A.M. and Berson, D.M. (1980) Histochemical identification and afferent connections of subdivisions in the LP–pulvinar complex and related thalamic nuclei in the cat. *Neuroscience*, 5: 1175–1238.

Graybiel, A.M. and Berson, D.M. (1981a) On the relation between trans-thalamic and trans-cortical pathways in the visual system. In F.O. Schmitt, F.G. Worden and F. Dennis (Eds.), *The Organization of the Cerebral Cortex*, MIT Press, Cambridge, MA, pp. 286–319.

Graybiel, A.M. and Berson, D.M. (1981b) Families of related cortical areas in the extrastriate visual system: Summary of an hypothesis. In C.N. Woolsey (Ed.), *Multiple Cortical Sensory Areas: Somatic, Visual and Auditory*, The Humana Press, Clinton, NJ.

Guiloff, R.D., Lifschitz, W.S., Ormeno, G.O. and Adrian, H.A. (1971) Visual evoked potentials in cortical auditory and anterior ectosylvian areas of cat. *Vision Res.*, Suppl., 3: 339–364.

Kaas, J.H. (1977) Sensory representations in mammals. In G.S. Stent (Ed.), *Function and Formation of Neural Systems*, Dahlem Konferezen, Abakon Verlag, Berlin, pp. 65–80.

Palmer, L.A., Rosenquist, A.C. and Tusa, R.J. (1978) The retinotopic organization of the lateral suprasylvian areas in the cat. *J. comp. Neurol.*, 177: 237–256.

Squatrito, S., Galletti, C., Maioli, M.G. and Battaglini, P.P. (1981) Cortical visual input to the orbito-insular cortex in the cat. *Brain Res.*, 221: 71–79.

Updyke, B.V. (1981) Projections from visual areas of the middle suprasylvian sulcus onto the lateral posterior complex and adjacent thalamic nuclei in cat. *J. comp. Neurol.*, 201: 477–506.

Compartmental Organization of the Mammalian Striatum

ANN M. GRAYBIEL

Department of Psychology and Brain Science, Massachusetts Institute of Technology, Cambridge, MA 02139 (U.S.A.)

By far the most striking architectural characteristic of the mammalian cerebral hemisphere is its division into tissue of cortical and subcortical types. This distinction has dominated views about the level of sophistication and neural processing in different parts of the telencephalon, and has also influenced ideas about the evolution of the cerebral hemispheres from an apparently more primitive striatal type to the exquisitely differentiated neocortical type found in higher mammals, especially man (Herrick, 1926, 1956; Romer, 1962). Because the cerebral cortex is the largest subdivision of the human brain, and disproportionately so by comparison with other species, the view naturally arose that the specialized structure of cortex somehow forms a necessary prerequisite for the complex mental capacities unique to the human. The fact that there is very little cortical tissue in the telencephalon of non-mammalian vertebrates, but instead a large noncortical "striatal" mass, led to the parallel assumption that the striatum is the highest integrative subdivision in these forms. Thus for years it was thought that the great development of the striatum in birds was related to their highly evolved instinctive patterns of behavior. The term, striatum, was applied to this non-cortical mass in birds and other non-mammals mainly because the tissue looked like the striatum (caudate-putamen) of mammalian species. With rough equivalence of the striatum in these different forms assumed, the cortical rind of mammals thus appeared to be a new and greatly modified form of telencephalic tissue overlying a more primitive core. The final link in the reasoning was that in mammals, sophisticated forms of behavior come to be under the control of the neocortex, while the striatum is left in charge of simpler generalized functions, for example, the control of tone.

Three lines of evidence have led to major modifications in this view. First, it became possible to define the mammalian striatum by its histochemistry: it is rich in dopamine and in acetylcholinesterase (Dahlström and Fuxe, 1964; Jacobowitz and Palkovits, 1974). When histochemical methods were applied to the non-mammalian forebrain, it turned out that only a small part of the entire striatal mass is equivalent, in terms of its histochemistry, to the mammalian caudate nucleus and putamen (Fig. 1; see Parent and Olivier, 1970; Karten and Dubbeldam, 1973). Second, with the development of reliable methods for tracing central nervous pathways, Karten and other comparative neuroanatomists were able to show that much of the large remaining part of the non-mammalian striatum has fiber connections very much like those of the neocortex (Karten, 1969). The implication of these findings was that the uniqueness of the neocortex cannot simply lie in its connections, for example, its connections with the thalamus. This raised a fundamental question, still unanswered, about how the

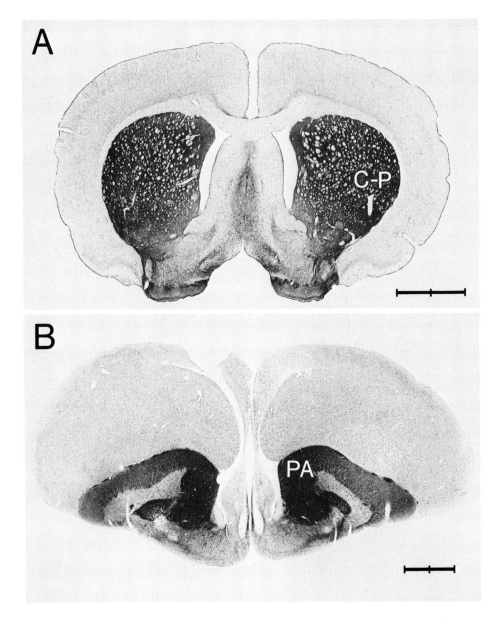

Fig. 1. Transverse sections through the forebrain of rat (A) and pigeon (B) stained for acetylcholinesterase activity. Note relatively small size of the acetylcholinesterase-positive region in the bird's brain; this region (the paleostriatum augmentatum, PA) is the only part of the avian striatum histochemically indentifiable as the counterpart of the mammalian striatum (caudoputamen, C-P). Bars = 2 mm.

architecture of a tissue is related to the connections it is allowed and not allowed to make.

Finally, and most recently, it has become clear that the striatum of mammals has a more complex structure than was evident before. As reviewed below, the caudoputamen has a compartmental organization reflected in the patterning both of its histochemistry and its input-output connections. Apparently, just as we had distinguished too sharply between the mammalian and non-mammalian forebrain, so we may also have overdrawn the contrast between neocortex and striatum in mammals.

The first hints of compartmental ordering in the striatum of adult mammals were given already in comments on the cytoarchitecture of the striatum: though lacking distinguishable layers, the caudate nucleus and putamen were described by Papez (1929), for example, as being "composed of tubular clusters of large quantities of small radiating cells with short axon cylinders . . . [and] within the clusters, large branching cells". Recent work by Mensah (1977), Goldman-Rakic (1982), and our own group (see Fig. 2 and Graybiel and Hickey, 1982; Graybiel, 1982) has confirmed the occurrence of such cluster patterns. However, as Goldman-Rakic (1981) has emphasized (see also Graybiel and Ragsdale, 1980, and Fig. 2A), it is only in fetal and neonatal brains that the clustering of cell bodies of striatal neurons is as obvious as inhomogeneities in the distributions of neurotransmitter-related compounds and receptors described below.

It was in the immature striatum that a striking histochemical differentiation of the caudoputamen was first demonstrated. Two groups of investigators showed that formaldehyde-induced catecholamine fluorescence, mainly attributable to dopamine, was organized in patches in the striatum of young animals and only become uniform later in development (Olson et al., 1972; Tennyson et al., 1972). The other characteristic histochemical marker for striatal tissue, acetylcholinesterase, was also shown to occur in patches in the caudoputamen of neonates (Butcher and Hodge, 1976). Recently we have shown that there is an exact spatial correspondence between the dopaminergic and acetylcholinesterase-containing patches (Fig. 3), so that the acetylcholinesterase and dopamine likely coexist in the same mesostriatal fibers (Graybiel et al., 1981a).

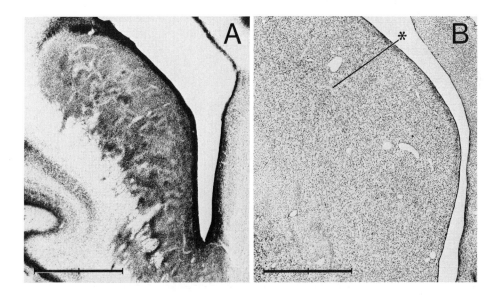

Fig. 2. A: clustering of neurons in the developing striatum; Nissl-stained transverse section through caudate nucleus of an E63 kitten fetus. B: Nissl-stained transverse section through the caudate nucleus of adult cat; typical lack of striking cytoarchitectural differentiation is evident but some cluster-patterns (e.g. asterisk) are visible nonetheless. Bars = 2 mm.

250

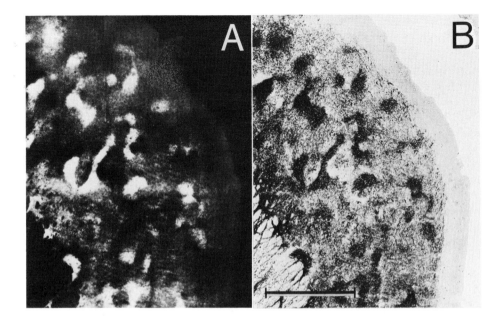

Fig. 3. A: demonstration by the glyoxylic acid histofluorescence method of the so-called dopamine islands in the caudate nucleus of an E54 kitten fetus. B: same section photographed a second time following post-fixation and staining for acetylcholinesterase activity. Note precise correspondence of patches in A and B. Refer to Graybiel et al. (1981a). Bar = 1 mm.

The compartmental ordering in the immature striatum was assumed to reflect developmental processes finally leading to uniformity or near uniformity of tissue organization in the adult, because not only dopamine and acetylcholinesterase activity, but also afferent fibers and projection neurons, were thought to have a homogeneous distribution in the mature caudoputamen. A series of findings in the past ten years have made it clear, however, that this view is incorrect. For the dopaminergic innervation, Fuxe and colleagues showed that the apparent homogeneity of histofluorescence in Falck–Hillarp preparations of adult caudoputamen could be changed to a patch pattern resembling that in the neonate by pretreatment with a tyrosine hydroxylase inhibitor (Olson et al., 1972). For the acetylcholinesterase activity, we found that with brief incubation times a mosaic of small zones of low acetylcholinesterase activity appeared in the otherwise acetylcholinesterase-rich striatal tissue (Fig. 4); we came to call these "striosomes" (Graybiel and Ragsdale, 1978, 1979). When the afferent connections of the striatum were studied by means of the autoradiographic technique, corticostriatal (Künzle, 1975; Goldman and Nauta, 1977; Jones et al., 1977) and thalamostriatal (Kalil, 1978; Royce, 1978) fibers and, very recently, amygdalostriatal fibers (Kelly and Nauta, 1981) were found to terminate in clusters and patches or to avoid small patches of striatum. Similarly, with retrograde tracers, we found that striatal projection neurons are distributed in mosaic patterns (Graybiel et al., 1979). Finally, when techniques were developed to demonstrate opiate receptors in histological material, one of the most striking findings reported was of the patchy distribution of receptors in the caudoputamen (Pert et al., 1976; Young and Kuhar, 1979). We have made the corresponding

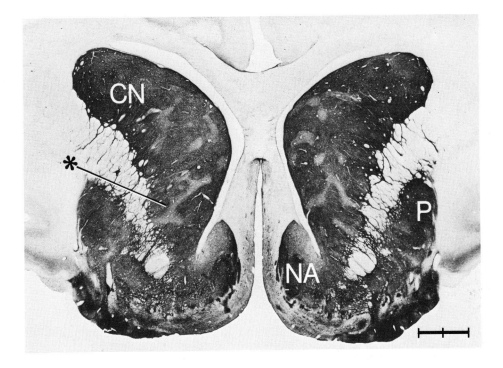

Fig. 4. Acetylcholinesterase-poor zones (called striosomes) visible in a thiocholine-stained transverse section through the caudate nucleus (CN) of adult cat. Note branching patterns of the zones, e.g., at asterisk. P, putamen; NA, nucleus accumbens septi. Bar = 2 mm.

observation that enkephalin-like immunoreactivity follows a comparable organization into patch-patterns (Graybiel et al., 1981b).

With such overwhelming evidence for compartmentalization in the striatum, the question clearly becomes one of how the different patchworks are related to one another, and what the functional consequences of the compartmental ordering might be. We have approached the matter of correlations by comparing the histochemical and immunohistochemical patterns in the striatum to patterns of afferent and efferent fiber distribution visible after appropriate injections of anterograde or retrograde tracer substances (Graybiel et al., 1979, 1981b; Ragsdale and Graybiel, 1981; Graybiel, 1981). The findings suggest that in the adult striatum of the cat acetylcholinesterase-poor striosomes are related in a systematic way to each of the other distributions: afferent fibers just fill or just avoid the striosomes (Fig. 5A); HRP-labeled projection neurons mainly (though not necessarily exclusively) avoid them (Fig. 5B); and Met-enkephalin-like immunoreactivity (and, for some striosomes, substance P-like immunoreactivity) is richest in these zones (Fig. 5C). In a related correlative study in the rat, Herkenham and Pert (1981) have reported that opiate receptor patches also just match the acetylcholinesterase-poor striosomes.

We have a great deal still to learn about this compartmental organization at the anatomical level. We do not know, for example, whether there are multiple striosomal organizations of which we have clearly identified only one, the acetylcholinesterase-poor striosomes. We do not know how the large neurons and various classes of medium

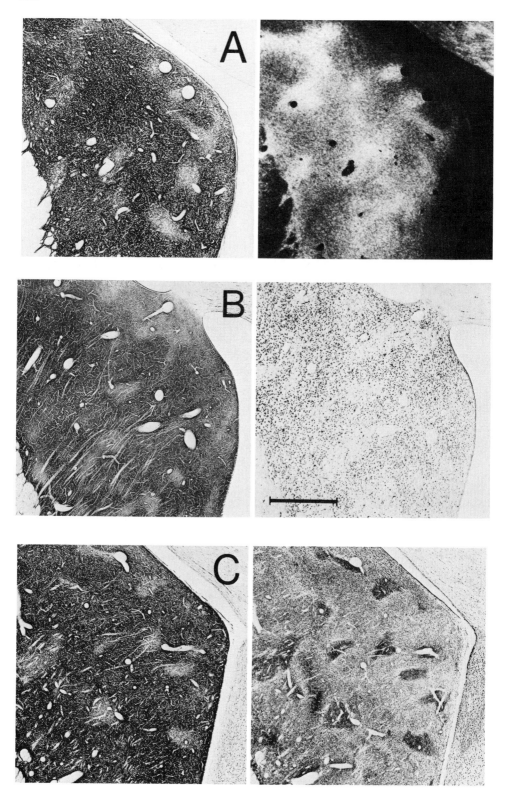

sized neurons are arranged with respect to the striosomes, nor the rules governing which afferents are engaged or kept apart from striatal interneurons or projection neurons by means of the striosomal ordering. The ultrastructural characteristics of the striosomes also remain to be defined. Nevertheless, the correlational work already done suggests that the striosomes comprise a key architectural unit of the striatum by means of which afferent and efferent connections are separated or brought together and within which modulation of transmission by particular neuropeptides can occur. A study of the physiological properties of these regions would clearly be of great interest.

If this compartmental ordering of the striatum is compared to that of the neocortex, a formal similarity is apparent (Fig. 6). In the neocortex (see, e.g., Lund, 1981; Gilbert and Wiesel, 1981; Jones, 1981; Emson and Hunt, 1981), afferent fibers of a particular type terminate only in certain cortical layers (and sometimes only in certain columns or slabs within these layers). Each cortical efferent projection pathway originates from cells within similarly restricted layers or sublayers. And at least some layers (and certain patches within layers) are characterized by distinctive histochemistries. For the striatum there apparently are comparable specifications: input fibers either terminate in the striosomes or just avoid them (Fig. 6); the output cells and probably interneurons are organized with respect to the striosomes; and the histochemistry of the striosomes is distinctive. Thus, at the macroscopic level, at least, the striosomes in the caudoputamen and the layers and columns of the neocortex appear to share a significance in representing structural counterparts of an ordered channeling of information through each tissue.

It is not yet clear whether the analogy should be extended to the functional level, with striosomes representing intrinsic processing units of the striatum in the manner of the physiologically defined columns of the neocortex. The striatum lacks the apical dendritic organization of the neocortex and, at the functional level, this may well be a crucial difference between striatum and cortex in terms of the relative functional potential and evolutionary advantage of their tissue arrangements. For these apical dendrites may represent a mechanism for coordinated sampling across multiple compartments that gives the cortex a computational capacity superior to that of any other part of the brain.

Fig. 5. Examples from correlational studies demonstrating correspondence, in the cat's caudate nucleus, of acetylcholinesterase-poor striosomes and (A) figures formed by corticostriatal afferent-fiber terminations, (B) regions of weak retrograde labeling after injection of horseradish peroxidase into the pallidum, and (C) regions of high Met-enkephalin-like immunoreactivity. For each pair, serially adjoining sections are shown with the acetylcholinesterase-stained section on the left. On the right, A shows autoradiogram of the contralateral frontocaudate projection (see Ragsdale and Graybiel, 1981); B shows tetramethylbenzidine staining (Mesulam, 1978) of striatal neurons sending axons to (or through) the ipsilateral internal pallidum (entopeduncular nucleus) (see Graybiel et al., 1979; Graybiel and Ragsdale, 1979); and C shows peroxidase–antiperoxidase immunohistochemical preparation (Sternberger, 1979), following incubation with antiserum raised against the neuropeptide, Met-enkephalin (see Graybiel et al., 1981b). Photomicrographs at same scale. Bar = 1 mm.

254

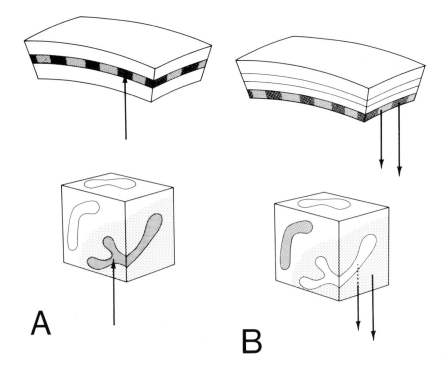

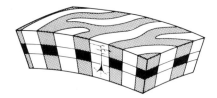

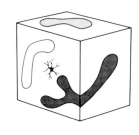

Fig. 6. Three schematic drawings comparing the compartmental organizations of the neocortex (above) and striatum (below). A: patterns of afferent-fiber termination in relation to layers and "columns" in neocortex, and in relation to striosomes in caudoputamen. B: patterns of efferent-cell organization in the two structures. In C, functional subdivisions (columns, slabs) are shown for the neocortex, but the functional subdivisions drawn for the striatum are hypothetical. Note presence of apical dendrites orientated along columns in the neocortex, and the absence of an apical dendritic organization in the striatum.

ACKNOWLEDGEMENTS

The work described was supported by the National Science Foundation (BNS 78-10549 and BNS 81–12125), the National Institutes of Health (Biomedical Research Support Grant 5-S07-RR07047-14) and the Scottish Rite Foundation. It is a pleasure to aknowledge the help of Mr. Henry F. Hall, who made the photographs.

REFERENCES

Butcher, L.L. and Hodge, G.K. (1976) Postnatal development of acetylcholinesterase in the caudate-putamen and substantia nigra of rats. *Brain Res.*, 106: 223–240.

Dahlström, A. and Fuxe, K. (1964) Evidence for the existence of monoamine-containing neurons in the central nervous system. *Acta physiol. scand.*, 62, Suppl. 232: 1–55.

Emson, P.C. and Hunt, S.P. (1981) Anatomical chemistry of the cerebral cortex In F.O. Schmitt, F.G. Worden and F. Dennis (Eds.), *The Organization of the Cerebral Cortex.*, MIT Press, Cambridge, MA, pp. 325–345.

Gilbert, C.D. and Wiesel, T.N. (1981) Laminar specialization and intracortical connections in cat primary visual cortex. In F.O. Schmitt, F.G. Worden and F. Dennis (Eds.), *The Organization of the Cerebral Cortex*, MIT Press, Cambridge, MA, pp. 163–191.

Goldman, P.S. and Nauta, W.J.H. (1977) An intricately patterned prefronto-caudate projection in the rhesus monkey. *J. comp. Neurol.*, 171: 369–386.

Goldman-Rakic, P.S. (1981) Prenatal formation of cortical input and development of cytoarchitectonic compartments in the neostriatum of the rhesus monkey. *J. Neurosci.*, 1: 721–735.

Graybiel, A.M. (1982) Correlative studies of histochemistry and fiber connections in the central nervous system. In S.L. Palay and V. Chan-Palay (Eds.), *Cytochemical Methods in Neuroanatomy*, Alan Liss, New York, pp. 45–67.

Graybiel, A.M. and Hickey, T.L. (1981) Chemospecificity of ontogenetic units in the striatum demonstrated by combining [^{3}H]thymidine neuronography and histochemical staining. *Proc. nat. Acad. Sci. U.S.A.*, 79: 198–202.

Graybiel, A.M. and Ragsdale, C.W. (1978) Histochemically distinct compartments in the striatum of human, monkey and cat demonstrated by acetylthiocholinesterase staining. *Proc. nat. Acad. Sci. U.S.A.*, 75: 5723–5726.

Graybiel, A.M. and Ragsdale, C.W. (1979) Fiber connections of the basal ganglia. In M. Cuénod, G.W. Kreutzberg and F.E. Bloom (Eds.), *Development and Chemical Specificity of Neurons, Progr. Brain Res.*, Vol. 51, Elsevier/North-Holland, Amsterdam, pp. 239–283.

Graybiel, A.M. and Ragsdale, C.W. (1980) Clumping of acetylcholinesterase activity in the developing striatum of the human fetus and young infant. *Proc. nat. Acad. Sci. U.S.A.*, 77: 1214–1218.

Graybiel, A.M., Ragsdale, C.W. and Edley, S.M. (1979) Compartments in the striatum of the cat observed by retrograde cell labeling. *Exp. Brian Res.*, 34: 188–195.

Graybiel, A.M., Pickel, V.M., Joh, T.H., Reis, D.J. and Ragsdale, C.W. (1981a) Direct demonstration of a correspondence between the dopamine islands and cholinesterase patches in the developing striatum. *Proc. nat. Acad. Sci. U.S.A.*, 78: 5871–5875.

Graybiel, A.M., Ragsdale, C.W., Yoneoka, E.S. and Elde, R.P. (1981b) An immunohistochemical study of enkephalins and other neuropeptides in the striatum of the cat with evidence that the opiate peptides are arranged to form mosaic patterns in register with the striosomal compartments visible by acetylcholinesterase staining. *Neuroscience*, 6: 377–397.

Herkenham, M. and Pert, C.B. (1981) Mosaic distribution of opiate receptors, parafascicular projections and acetylcholinesterase in rat striatum. *Nature (Lond.)*, 291: 415–418.

Herrick, C.J. (1926) *Brains of Rats and Men*. Univ. of Chicago Press, Chicago.

Herrick, C.J. (1956) *The Evolution of Human Nature*. Univ. of Texas Press/Harper Brothers, New York.

Jacobowitz, D.M. and Palkovits, M. (1974) Topographic atlas of catecholamine and acetylcholinesterase-containing neurons in the rat brain. I. Forebrain (telencephalon, diencephalon). *J. comp. Neurol.*, 157: 13–28.

Jones, E.G. (1981) Anatomy of cerebral cortex: columnar input-output organization. In F.O. Schmitt, F.G. Worden and F. Dennis (Eds.), *The Organization of the Cerebral Cortex*, MIT Press, Cambridge, MA, pp. 199–235.

Jones, E.G., Coulter, J.D., Burton, H. and Porter, R. (1977) Cells of origin and terminal distribution of corticostriatal fibers arising in the sensory-motor cortex of monkeys. *J. comp. Neurol.*, 173: 53–80.

Kalil, K. (1978) Patch-like termination of thalamic fibers in the putamen of the rhesus monkey: an autoradiographic study. *Brain Res.*, 140: 333–339.

Karten, H.J. (1969) The organization of the avian telencephalon and some speculations on the phylogeny of the amniotic telencephalon. *Ann. N.Y. Acad. Sci.*, 167: 164–179.

Karten, H.J. and Dubbledam, J.L. (1973) The organization and projections of the paleostriatal complex in the pigeon (*Columbia livia*). *J. comp. Neurol.*, 148: 61–90.

Kelly, A.E., Domesick, V.B. and Nauta, W.J.H. (1981) The amygdalostriatal projection in the rat. *Anat. Rec.*, 199: 134A.

Künzle, H. (1975) Bilateral projections from precentral motor cortex to the putamen and other parts of the basal ganglia. *Brain Res.*, 88: 195–210.

Lund, S.J. (1981) Intrinsic organization of the primate visual cortex, area 17, as seen in Golgi preparations. In F.O. Schmitt, F.G. Worden and F. Dennis (Eds.), *The Organization of the Cerebral Cortex*, MIT Press, Cambridge, MA, pp. 105–124.

Mensah, P.L. (1977) The internal organization of the mouse caudate nucleus: evidence for cell clustering and regional variation. *Brain Res.*, 137: 53–66.

Mesulam, M.-M. (1978) Tetramethyl benzidine for horseradish peroxidase neurohistochemistry: a non-carcinogenic blue reaction-product with superior sensitivity for visualizing neural afferents and efferents. *J. Histochem. Cytochem.*, 26: 106–117.

Olson, L., Seiger, Å. and Fuxe, K. (1972) Heterogeneity of striatal and limbic dopamine innervation: highly fluorescent islands in developing and adult rats. *Brain Res.*, 44: 283–288.

Papez, J.W. (1929) *Comparative Neurology*, Thomas Y. Crowell Co., New York, p. 319.

Parent, A. and Olivier, A. (1970) Comparative histochemical study of the corpus striatum. *J. Hirnforsch.*, 12: 73–81.

Pert, C.B., Kuhar, M.J. and Snyder, S.H. (1976) Opiate receptor: autoradiographic localization in rat brain. *Proc. nat. Acad. Sci. U.S.A.*, 73: 3729–3733.

Ragsdale, C.W. and Graybiel, A.M. (1981) The fronto-striatal projection in the cat and monkey and its relationship to inhomogeneities established by acetylcholinesterase histochemistry. *Brain Res.*, 208: 259–266.

Romer, A.S. (1962) *The Vertebrate Body*, W.B. Saunders Co., Philadelphia.

Royce, G.J. (1978) Autoradiographic evidence for a discontinuous projection to the caudate nucleus from the centromedian nucleus in the cat. *Brain Res.*, 146: 145–150.

Sternberger, L.A. (1979) *Immunocytochemistry*, Wiley and Sons, New York.

Tennyson, V.M., Barrett, R.E., Cohen, G., Côté, L., Heikkila, R. and Mytilineou, C. (1972) The developing neostriatum of the rabbit: correlation of fluorescence histochemistry, electron microscopy, endogenous dopamine levels, and [³H]dopamine uptake. *Brain Res.*, 46: 251–285.

Young, W.S. and Kuhar, M.J. (1979) A new method for receptor autoradiography: [³H]opioid receptors in rat brain. *Brain Res.*, 179: 255–270.

An Electrophysiological Analysis of
Some Afferent and Efferent Pathways of
the Rat Prefrontal Cortex

A.M. THIERRY, J.M. DENIAU, G. CHEVALIER, A. FERRON and J. GLOWINSKI

Groupe NB INSERM U 114, Collège de France, 11, place Marcelin Berthelot, 75231 Paris Cedex 05; and (J.M.D. and G.C.) Laboratoire de Physiologie des Centres Nerveux, Université Pierre et Marie Curie, 4, place Jussieu, 75230 Paris Cedex 5 (France)

INTRODUCTION

In the rat, the prefrontal cortex may be defined as the mesocortical zone receiving converging projections from the mediodorsal nucleus of the thalamus (MD) and from the dopamine (DA) cell group localized in the ventromedial mesencephalic tegmentum (VMT) (Divac et al., 1978). It is composed of two subfields: a medial region, the pregenual medial wall of the hemisphere in reciprocal connection with the lateral part of the MD; and a lateral region on the dorsal bank of the rhinal sulcus which is reciprocally connected with the medial part of the MD (Leonard, 1969). A great number of cortical and subcortical structures receive efferents from prefrontal cortex and differences have been demonstrated anatomically as regards its medial and lateral projections (Beckstead, 1979). These projections involve other portions of the cortex (presubiculum, retrosplenial, perirhinal and entorhinal cortex) and subcortical structures related to the limbic system (midline thalamic nuclei, hypothalamus and the paramedian mesencephalic tegmentum) or the extrapyramidal system (striatum, substantia nigra (SN) and deep layers of the superior colliculus (CS)). The medial and lateral areas of the prefrontal cortex can also be distinguished on a functional basis since in the rat distinct behavioral deficits have been observed to result from their lesioning (Kolb, 1977). In the present report we will review results from recent studies aimed at further characterization of: (a) the afferents to medial prefrontal cortex originating from the VMT, and (b) the efferents from medial prefrontal cortex projecting to diencephalic and mesencephalic structures.

VENTROMEDIAL MESENCEPHALIC TEGMENTUM
AFFERENTS TO THE MEDIAL PREFRONTAL CORTEX

The VMT contains the DA neurons initially described by Dahlström and Fuxe (1964) as the A10 cell group. These cells are distributed in the ventral tegmental area of Tsai, the paranigral nucleus and the caudal linearis nucleus. The A10 cell group innervates not only the prefrontal cortex but also other cortical and subcortical limbic structures (Lindvall and Björklund, 1978).

In a first series of experiments we sought to determine: (1) whether all VMT cells

[257]

which innervate the prefrontal cortex share similar electrophysiological properties, and (2) whether these projection neurons also send axon collaterals to limbic structures such as the septum and nucleus accumbens.

(1) Does a single population of VMT neurons project to prefrontal cortex?

VMT cells were identified on the basis of their antidromic activation from prefrontal cortex in ketamine-anesthetized rats (see Deniau et al. (1980) for technical details). The antidromicity of the spike potentials was tested according the three criteria: fixed latency, collision with spontaneous spikes, ability to follow high frequency stimulations. The distribution of the latencies of the mesocortical antidromic responses suggested at least two groups of neurons on the basis of their conduction velocity (Fig. 1). One group was characterized by long latencies and a slow conduction velocity (m = 0.55 m/sec); the other by short latencies and a fast conduction velocity (m = 3.2 m/sec). It is likely that these two groups of VMT cells correspond to DA and non-DA neurons respectively. Indeed, axons of the DA neurons have been described as thin unmyelinated fibers (Fuxe et al., 1964; Hökfelt, 1978) and the conduction velocity of unmyelinated axons is generally considered to be less than 1 m/sec (Hursch, 1939; Waxman and Bennett, 1972; Swadlow and Waxman, 1976).

To test this possibility, a similar analysis was performed after previous unilateral destruction of the DA ascending systems with 6-hydroxydopamine (6-OHDA). Two microinjections of 6-OHDA were made, one lateral to the VMT and the other in the vicinity of the DA ascending pathway (Thierry et al., 1980). Such lesioning induced a 69% decrease of the activity of the biosynthetic enzyme, tyrosine hydroxylase, in the ipsilateral VMT. In lesioned rats, the proportion of fast and slow conducting neurons was significantly different from that in the controls (Fig. 1). Whereas the population of slow conducting neurons was greatly reduced, there was no apparent decrease in the number of fast conducting neurons. This demonstration of a double axonal projection (DA and non-DA) from VMT to prefrontal cortex was confirmed by the results of a combined retrograde fluorescent tracing and fluorescent histochemical study (Albanese and Bentivoglio, 1981).

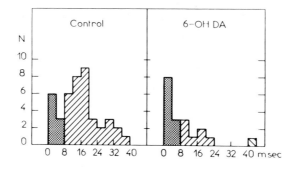

Fig. 1. Distribution of the latencies of antidromic spikes elicited in the VMT after prefrontal cortex stimulation in control and 6-OHDA-lesioned rats. The conduction velocity of the fibers could be estimated by taking into account the approximative distance (11.5 mm) between the recording and stimulating sites. Dotted columns, fast conducting neurons; hatched columns, slow conducting neurons.

(2) Are VMT afferents of prefrontal cortex collateralized to limbic structures?

The VMT is the locus of origin not only for the DA innervation of cerebral cortex (mesocortical system) but also for that of several limbic structures such as septum and nucleus accumbens (mesolimbic system). Much experimental evidence hints at important differences in the utlilization of DA between these two systems (see Glowinski, 1982). It was therefore of interest to explore the possibility that VMT cells which project to prefrontal cortex might also project to the septum and/or nucleus accumbens. However, among 28 VMT cells antidromically driven from prefrontal cortex none could also be driven from the nucleus accumbens and only 3 from the septum. These data were in agreement with the recent results of Albanese et al. (1981) indicating that a very low percentage of VMT neurons is simultaneously labeled with two different fluorescent dyes injected one in the septum and the other in the prefrontal cortex.

EFFERENTS OF THE MEDIAL PREFRONTAL CORTEX

This series of experiments was designed to investigate whether a given neuron of prefrontal cortex projects solely to one or to multiple subcortical regions. Cortical cells projecting to the MD, VMT, SN or CS were identified by the antidromic technique when a given neuron could be antidromically driven from more than one of these structures, evidence of axonal branching was sought by the collision test (Fig. 2). The mean conduction velocity of the cortical cells projecting to the various structures analyzed was relatively slow (m = 1 m/sec). A great number of cortical

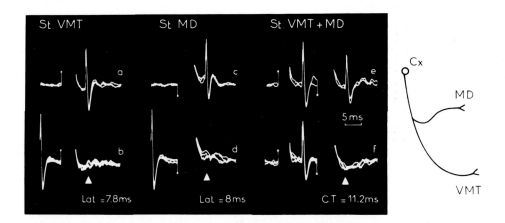

Fig. 2. Demonstration of the axonal branching of a prefrontal neuron activated antidromically from VMT and MD. The antidromic responses triggered either from the VMT (trace a) or MD (trace c) are suppressed by collision with a spontaneous spike (trace b and d, respectively). Traces e and f illustrate the collision test between the two antidromically evoked spikes. The collision time is the greatest interval between the two stimulations with which blockade of the second spike may be obtained (trace f). Axonal branching is demonstrated since the collision time (CT = 11.2 msec) is superior to the difference in the latencies of the two antidromic responses (0.2 msec) plus the refractory period of the axon at the second site stimulated (1.5 msec).

neurons were antidromically invaded following stimulation of more than one region. The existence of 6 branching patterns was established: VMT–MD; VMT–CS; VMT–SN; MD–SN; MD–CS and SN–CS. Furthermore, in some cases a single cortical cell could be shown to project to three different structures (VMT–SN–CS; MD–SN–CS). Sixty-four percent of the cortical neurons antidromically driven from the VMT were also driven either from the MD, the SN or the CS.

CONCLUDING REMARKS

(1) As previously shown for the nigrostriatal (Deniau et al., 1978; Guyenet and Aghajanian, 1978), the VMT–septum (Thierry et al., 1980) and the VMT–nucleus accumbens projections (Berger et al., 1978; Thierry et al., 1980; Yim and Mogenson, 1980), the present data demonstrate the existence of parallel DA and non-DA projections from the VMT to prefrontal cortex. In the case of all these projections, the non-DA pathway appears to be characterized by a higher conduction velocity than the DA pathway. Even though GABA has been suggested to be the transmitter for the non-DA nigrostriatal projections, that or those in the non-DA mesolimbic and mesocortical systems remain to be identified.

(2) The preliminary results thus far available do not indicate an important collateralization of the mesocortical DA and non-DA projection to subcortical limbic structures.

(3) In contrast, many neurons of the prefrontal cortex sending efferents to the MD, VMT, SN and CS distribute axonal branches to more than one of these subcortical regions. It was of interest that such neurons were mainly located in deep layers of the cortex, which are the ones receiving a dense DA innervation (Berger et al., 1976). Although it has not yet been demonstrated that DA regulates the activity of these cells, their axonal branching toward various subcortical structures might provide the beginning of an explanation for the involvement of cortical DA in complex behavior such as the spatial delayed alternation performance (Brozoski et al., 1979; Simon, 1981).

ACKNOWLEDGMENTS

We wish to thank Dr L. Descarries for his helpful comments on this manuscript. A. Ferron was the recipient of fellowships from the Conseil de la Recherche en Santé du Québec and the Fondation Simone et Cino del Duca.

REFERENCES

Albanese, A. and Bentivoglio, M. (1981) Dopaminergic and non-dopaminergic mesocortical neurons in the rat. *Neurosci. Lett.*, Suppl. 7: S397.

Albanese, A., Minciachi, D., and Bentivoglio, M. (1981) Multiple retrograde fluorescent tracing of the efferent projections of the ventral tegmental area in the rat. *Neurosci. Lett.*, Suppl. 7: S45.

Beckstead, R.M. (1979) An autoradiographic examination of cortico-cortical and subcortical projections of the mediodorsal-projection (prefrontal) cortex in the rat. *J. comp. Neurol.*, 184: 43–62.

Berger, B., Thierry, A.M., Tassin, J.P. and Moyne, M.A. (1976) Dopaminergic innervation of the rat prefrontal cortex: a fluorescence histochemical study. *Brain Res.*, 106: 133–145.

Berger, B., Nguyen-Legros, J. and Thierry, A.M. (1978) Demonstration of horseradish peroxidase and fluorescent catecholamines in the same neuron. *Neurosci. Lett.* 9: 297–302.

Brozoski, T.J., Brown, R.M., Rosvold, H.E. and Goldman, P.S. (1979) Cognitive deficit caused by regional depletion of dopamine in prefrontal cortex of rhesus monkey. *Science*, 205: 929–932.

Dahlström, A. and Fuxe, K. (1964) Evidence for the existence of monoamine containing neurons in the central nervous system. I. Demonstration of monoamines in the cell bodies of brain stem neurons. *Acta physiol. scand.*, 62, Suppl. 232: 1–55.

Deniau, J.M., Hammond, C., Riszk, A. and Feger, J. (1978) Electrophysiological properties of identified output neurons of the rat substantia nigra (pars compacta and pars reticulata): evidence for the existence of branched neurons. *Exp. Brain Res.*, 32: 409–422.

Deniau, J.M., Thierry, A.M. and Feger, J. (1980) Electrophysiological identification of mesencephalic ventromedial (VMT) neurons projecting to the frontal cortex, septum and nucleus accumbens. *Brain Res.*, 189: 315–326.

Divac, I., Björklund, A., Lindvall, A. and Pasingham, R.E. (1978) Converging projections from the mediodorsal thalamic nucleus and mesencephalic dopaminergic neurons to the neocortex in three species. *J. comp. Neurol.*, 180: 59–72.

Fuxe, K., Hökfelt, T. and Nilsson, O. (1964) Observations on the localization of dopamine in the caudate nucleus of the rat. *Z. Zellforsch.*, 63: 701–706.

Glowinski, J. (1982) In vivo regulation of nigro-striatal and mesocortico-prefrontal dopaminergic neurons. In H.F. Bradford (Ed.), *Neurotransmitter Interaction and Compartmentation*, Plenum, New York, pp. 219–233.

Guyenet, P. and Aghajanian, G.K. (1978) Antidromic identification of dopaminergic and other output neurons of the rat substantia nigra. *Brain Res.*, 150: 69–84.

Hökfelt, T. (1978) In vitro studies on central and peripheral monoamine neurons at the ultrastructural level. *Z. Zellforsch.*, 91: 1–74.

Hursch, J.B. (1939) Conduction velocity and diameter of nerve fibers. *Amer. J. Physiol.*, 127: 131–139.

Kolb, B. (1977) Studies on the caudate putamen and the dorsomedial thalamic nucleus of the rat: implications for mammalian frontal lobe functions, *Physiol. Behav.*, 18: 237–244.

Leonard, C.M. (1969) The prefrontal cortex of the rat. I. Cortical projection of the mediodorsal nucleus II. Efferent connections. *Brain Res.*, 12: 321–343.

Lindvall, O. and Björklund, A. (1978) Organization of catecholamine neurons in the rat central nervous system. In L.L. Iversen, S.D. Iversen and S. Snyder (Eds.), *Handbook of Psychopharmacology*, Vol. 9, Plenum, New York, pp. 139–231.

Simon, H. (1981) Neurones dopaminergiques A10 et système frontal. *J. Physiol. (Paris)*, 77: 81–95.

Swadlow, H.A. and Waxman, S.G. (1976) Variations in conduction velocity and excitability following simple and multiple impulses of visual callosal axons in the rabbit. *Exp. Neurol.*, 53: 128–150.

Immunocytochemical Characterization of the Dopaminergic and Noradrenergic Innervation of the Rat Neocortex During Early Ontogeny

B. BERGER, C. VERNEY, M. GAY and A. VIGNY

INSERM U.134, Laboratoire de Neuropathologie Charles Foix, Hôpital Salpêtrière, 75651 Paris Cedex 13; (C.V.) INSERM U.154, Hôpital Saint Vincent de Paul, 74 avenue Denfert-Rochereau, 75674 Paris Cedex 14 and (A.V.) Institut de Biologie physico-chimique, 12 rue Pierre Curie, 75005 Paris (France)

INTRODUCTION

Several studies have suggested that monoamines, and especially catecholamines, could play an important role in the development and differentiation of the cerebral cortex (Butler et al., 1981; for review see Hamon and Bourgoin, 1981). However, the mechanism and precise time of their action are far from being ascertained. In this perspective, a morphological analysis of the time of arrival and cytoarchitectonic distribution of the different aminergic pathways in the developing cerebral cortex was a prerequisite. Indeed, such a study has been undertaken by several groups in the last ten years, especially in the rat (Dupin et al., 1976; Kristt, 1979; Levitt and Moore, 1979; Lidov et al., 1978; Loren et al., 1976; Schlumpf et al., 1980; Seiger and Olson, 1973). However, the techniques used to visualize the early catecholaminergic innervation have not allowed the differentiation between noradrenergic and dopaminergic pathways. Thus, in order to reveal specifically the noradrenergic system, most studies were carried out on neocortical areas where no dopaminergic innervation occurs. Yet, the ontogeny of the cortical dopaminergic innervation seemed all the more worthy of analysis. Indeed, the neocortical dopaminergic system, the so-called mesocortical system, discovered by biochemical analysis in 1973 (Thierry et al., 1973) and visualized by histochemistry in 1974 (Berger et al., 1974; Lindvall et al., 1974), has been shown in these last years to be involved in cognitive functions (Simon et al., 1980) and to exert a prominent role in primate cortical function (Brozoski et al., 1979).

In the present work, we have tried to visualize independently the dopaminergic and noradrenergic innervation of the early developing rat neocortex by immunocytochemistry using antibodies raised against tyrosine hydroxylase (TH), the first enzyme in the synthetic pathway of catecholamines, and against dopamine-β-hydroxylase (DBH), the enzyme which converts dopamine to norepinephrine. The distribution of TH-like and DBH-like immunoreactive fibers was strikingly different until postnatal day 2, indicating that at least under our experimental conditions noradrenergic axons and terminals were not visualized during this period in the developing neocortex using TH immunocytochemistry. Thus, we provisionally considered TH as a selective marker

[263]

of the cortical dopaminergic innervation during late prenatal and early postnatal development.

The preparation of antibodies against TH (Berger et al., 1982) and DBH (Grzanna et al., 1977) is described in detail elsewhere, as well as the immunocytochemical techniques used to visualize DBH (Verney et al., 1982). To reveal TH-like immunoreactivity, the animals were perfused with 4% paraformaldehyde in phosphate buffer, or the brains fixed by immersion in the fixative for the youngest embryos (E16–E17). After 2–4 h fixation, followed by 48 h rinsing in buffer + sucrose 5%, cryostat sections obtained in sagittal, coronal or horizontal planes were submitted either to Nissl staining or to immunofluorescence or immunoperoxidase (PAP) technique. Antibody against TH was used at 1/400 and 1/1600 dilution respectively.

TYROSINE HYDROXYLASE-LIKE IMMUNOREACTIVITY

Sparse TH-like immunoreactive fibers were first observed in the just forming intermediate zone of the frontal cortex on embryonic day 16 (E16). They became numerous at E17. From E18 to E20, large bundles of positive fibers running through the striatum, as well as ventrally and rostrally to it, progressively reached the rhinal cortex, the olfactory tubercle and the anterior olfactory nucleus, the intermediate zone of the medial frontal and most rostral cingular cortex. From E21 to postnatal day 2 (P2), deep TH-like positive axons increased in number extending into the developing cortical layers: they progressively invaded the cortical plate of the medial frontal and supragenual and entorhinal cortex (Figs. 1 and 2). At P1, some TH-containing axons were also observed in the marginal zone of the anterior frontal pole. However, almost no TH-like-positive fibers were observed in the lateral frontal cortex until postnatal day 3. Thus, from E16 to P2, cortical TH-like immunoreactivity was primarily observed in areas known to receive a dopaminergic innervation in adult animals. On the contrary, from postnatal day 3 on, TH-like-positive axons and terminals were progressively detected in all layers of the whole neocortex.

DOPAMINE-β-HYDROXYLASE-LIKE IMMUNOREACTIVITY

Contrary to the pattern of TH-like immunoreactivity, DBH was first observed in two axonal bundles: a dense superficial one, visualized in the marginal zone as dispersed dots at E19 and thick varicose fibers at E21; and a deeper plexus of thin non-varicose fibers detected at birth in the deep intermediate zone (Figs. 2 and 3).

Figs. 1–3. Three photomontages of rat frontal cortex at birth. Sagittal section. × 300.

Fig. 1. TH-like immunoreactivity (PAP technique) observed in dark field. From the bulk of fibers running through the intermediate zone (IZ), some diverge towards the cortical plate (CP) and the marginal zone (MZ).

Fig. 2. Same area as Fig. 1. Nissl staining.

Fig. 3. DBH-like immunoreactivity (immunofluorescence technique). Note the presence of two plexuses of positive fibers: a superficial one, situated in the marginal zone, is highly fluorescent; a deep one is running in the inferior part of the intermediate zone.

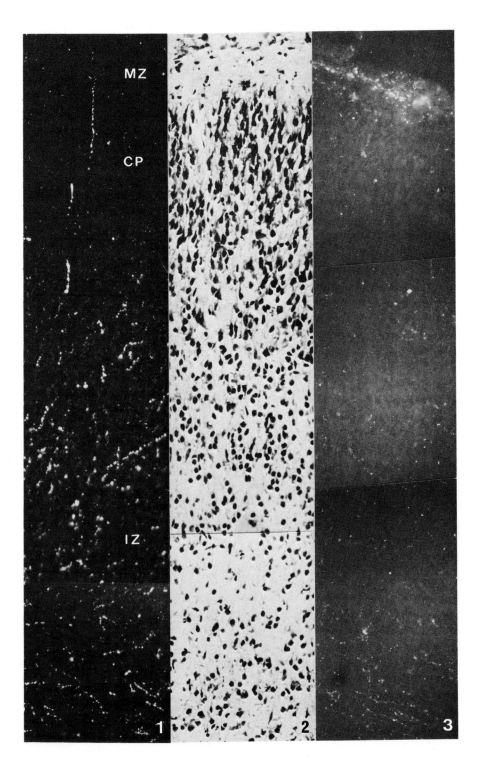

These two plexuses, parallel to the pial surface, invaded rapidly the whole neocortex following an antero-posterior gradient. Between them, perpendicular fibers first appeared at P0 in the medial frontal cortex. In the other cortical areas, all layers contained DBH reactive fibers at P5, but the adult pattern was reached at P14.

DISCUSSION

It appears that between embryonic day 16 and postnatal day 2, the distributions of DBH-like and TH-like immunoreactivity are strikingly different both from a cytoarchitectonic and a topographical point of view. DBH-like immunoreactive fibers appear in two strata, in the marginal and intermediate zone respectively, and progressively invade the other cortical layers at birth. These data are in agreement with the results obtained by Levitt and Moore (1979) and Schlumpf et al. (1980) using biochemical and fluorescence histochemical analysis of early noradrenergic innervation in the rat cerebral cortex. Interestingly enough, DBH immunoreactivity is higher in the marginal zone, like the endogenous content of norepinephrine visualized at P6 by Lidov et al. (1978) using fluorescence histochemistry. The distribution of TH-like positive fibers on the other hand follows an inside-out gradient: first located in the intermediate zone, they invade the cortical plate at birth and start to be visible in the molecular layer only at P1. Moreover, from E16 to P2, they are restricted to circumscribed areas which represent the regions of dopaminergic innervation in the adult. These results strongly suggest that during the early period of development in the cortex, TH was primarily visualized in dopaminergic terminals. This is in agreement with previous results (Hökfelt et al., 1977; Pickel et al., 1975) concerning the difficulty to visualize noradrenergic terminals in the cortex with TH-immunocytochemistry, but differ from recent data obtained by Specht et al. (1981). This discrepancy is possibly related to some technical difference.

When comparing the distribution in the early developing rat cerebral cortex of DBH-like immunoreactivity representing the noradrenergic system and TH-like immunoreactivity representing, under our experimental conditions, the dopaminergic system, it can be concluded that:

(1) the dopaminergic system contributes to the very early catecholaminergic innervation of the rat cerebral cortex recently emphasized by Schlumpf et al. (1980);

(2) from the beginning of the cortical differentiation, the distribution of the catecholaminergic innervation has the characteristics observed in the adult: a restricted distribution of the dopaminergic system to the frontal, supragenual, rhinal and suprarhinal and entorhinal cortex with a predominance in the deep cortical layers; a widespread projection of the noradrenergic system with a predominance in the molecular layer; and

(3) as already demonstrated for the noradrenergic system, the dopaminergic innervation first develops in one of the two cortical layers where the earliest differentiation during embryonic life, as well as the first synapses, have been observed (König et al., 1975). Whether dopaminergic terminals participate in the extensive monaminergic synaptogenesis identified in the rat cerebral cortex during the first postnatal week (Kristt, 1979) is currently under investigation.

REFERENCES

Berger, B., Tassin, J.P., Blanc, G., Moyne, M.A. and Thierry, A.M. (1974) Histochemical confirmation for dopaminergic innervation of the rat cerebral cortex after destruction of the noradrenergic ascending pathways. *Brain Res.*, 81: 332–337.

Berger, B., Di Porzio, U., Daguet, M.C., Gay, M., Vigny, A., Glowinski, J. and Prochiantz, A. (1982) Long-term development of mesencephalic dopaminergic neurons of mouse embryos in dissociated primary cultures. Morphological and histochemical characteristics. *Neuroscience*, 7: 193–205.

Brozoski, T.J., Brown, R.M., Rosvold, H.E. and Goldman, P.S. (1979) Cognitive deficit caused by regional depletion of dopamine in prefrontal cortex of rhesus monkey. *Science*, 205: 929–932.

Butler, I.J., O'Flynn, M.E., Seifert, W.E. and Howell, R.R. (1981) Neurotransmitter defects and treatment of disorders of hyperphenylalaninemia. *J. Pediat.*, 98: 729–733.

Dupin, J.C., Descarries, L. and de Champlain, J. (1976) Radioautographic visualization of central catecholamine neurons in newborn rat after intravenous administration of tritiated norepinephrine. *Brain Res.*, 103: 588–596.

Grzanna, R., Morrison, J.H., Coyle, J.T. and Molliver, M.E. (1977) The immunohistochemical demonstration of noradrenergic neurons in the rat brain: the use of homologous antiserum to dopamine-β-hydroxylase. *Neurosci. Lett.*, 4: 121–126.

Hamon, M. and Bourgoin, S. (1981) Ontogénèse des neurones monoaminergiques centraux chez les mammifères. In A. Minkowski (Ed.), *Biologie du Développement*, Flammarion Médecine Sciences, pp. 118–151.

Hökfelt, T., Johansson, O., Fuxe, K., Goldstein, M. and Park, D. (1977) Immunohistochemical studies on localization and distribution of monoamine neuron systems in rat brain. 2. Tyrosine hydroxylase in telencephalon. *Med. Biol.*, 55: 21–40.

König, N., Roch, G. and Marty, R. (1975) The onset of synaptogenesis in rat temporal cortex. *Anat. Embryol.*, 148: 73–88.

Kristt, D.A. (1979) Development of neocortical circuitry: quantitative ultrastructural analysis of putative monoaminergic synapses. *Brain Res.*, 178: 69–88.

Levitt, P. and Moore, R.Y. (1979) Development of the noradrenergic innervation of neocortex. *Brain Res.*, 162: 243–260.

Lidov, H.G.W., Molliver, M.E. and Zecevic, N.R. (1978) Characterization of the monoaminergic innervation of immature rat neocortex: a histofluorescence analysis. *J. comp. Neurol.*, 181: 663–680.

Lindvall, O., Björklund, A., Moore, R.Y. and Stenevi, U. (1974) Mesencephalic dopamine neurons projecting to neocortex. *Brain Res.*, 81: 325–331.

Loren, I., Björklund, A. and Lindvall, O. (1976) The catecholamine systems in the developing rat brain: improved visualization by a modified glyoxylic acid–paraformaldehyde method. *Brain Res.*, 117: 313–318.

Pickel, V.M., Joh, T.H., Field, P.M., Becker, C.G. and Reis, D.J. (1975) Cellular localization of tyrosine hydroxylase by immunohistochemistry. *J. Histochem. Cytochem.*, 23: 1–12.

Schlumpf, M., Shoemaker, W.J. and Bloom, F.E. (1980) Innervation of embryonic rat cerebral cortex by catecholamine-containing fibers. *J. comp. Neurol.*, 192: 361–377.

Seiger, A. and Olson, L. (1973) Late prenatal ontogeny of central monoamine neurons in the rat. Fluorescence histochemical observations. *Z. Anat. Entwickl.-Gesch.*, 140: 281–318.

Simon, H., Scatton, B. and Le Moal, M. (1980) Dopaminergic neurons are involved in cognitive functions. *Nature (Lond.)* 286: 150–151.

Specht, L.A., Pickel, V.M., Joh, T.H. and Reis, D.J. (1981) Light microscopic immunocytochemical localization of tyrosine hydroxylase in prenatal brain. II. Late ontogeny. *J. comp. Neurol.*, 199: 255–276.

Thierry, A.M., Blanc, G., Sobel, A., Stinus, L. and Glowinski, J. (1973) Dopaminergic terminals in the rat cortex. *Science*, 182: 499–501.

Verney, C., Molliver, M.E. and Grzanna R. (1982) Innervation noradrenergique du neocortex du rat au cours du développement: mise en évidence immunocytochimique à l'aide d'anticorps anti-dopamine-β-hydroxylase. *C.R. Acad. Sci. (Paris)*, 294: 35–38.

The Topographical Distribution of the Monoaminergic Innervation in the Basal Ganglia of the Human Brain

H. HÖRTNAGL, E. SCHLÖGL, G. SPERK and O. HORNYKIEWICZ

Institute of Biochemical Pharmacology, University of Vienna, A-1090 Vienna (Austria)

INTRODUCTION

Biochemical studies on post-mortem human brain material are fraught with many difficulties and limiting factors including age of the patient, disease state, immediate pre-mortem status and time elapsed between death and freezing of the brain. A largely neglected factor in human brain studies is the possible occurrence of a regionally uneven distribution of neurotransmitters within an individual brain nucleus. In the basal ganglia complex conspicuous changes in neurotransmitter levels have been observed in several neuropsychiatric diseases (e.g. Parkinson's disease, schizophrenia, Huntington's chorea) (Hornykiewicz, 1979; Bird et al., 1979; Crow et al., 1979; Farley et al., 1978b; Perry et al., 1973; Spokes, 1980). Within this complex the striatum comprises a large subcortical mass and receives its main afferents from the cerebral cortex, thalamus, substantia nigra and dorsal raphe nucleus (Graybiel and Ragsdale, 1979). There is increasing neurochemical evidence of inhomogeneities in the distribution of various neurotransmitter systems in the striatum of various species (Ternaux et al., 1977; Tassin et al., 1976; Fonnum and Walaas, 1979; Graybiel et al., 1981). However, little or no data are available on the distribution pattern of the monoaminergic systems within the human striatum.

It is obvious that the existence of larger differences in the intrastriatal neurotransmitter distribution may at least in part be responsible for the discrepancies found in the literature regarding normal values for striatal monoamines (e.g. dopamine; cf. Hornykiewicz, 1981). Difficulties in the anatomical classification of certain brain areas may further contribute to discrepancies of biochemical data in human brain studies. Thus, in the human basal ganglia complex the anatomically exact definition of the nucleus accumbens, situated within the rostro-ventral subdivision of the striatum (in the region of the junction between caudate nucleus and putamen) poses special difficulties. It is therefore not surprising that for this area large differences in monoamine levels (especially noradrenaline) have been reported from different laboratories (cf. Hornykiewicz, 1981).

The purpose of the present investigation was to determine, in the normal human brain, the biochemical distribution pattern of the known monoaminergic afferents (dopaminergic, noradrenergic, serotonergic) to the various nuclei of the basal ganglia complex. In doing so, we also hoped to obtain at least a biochemical characterization of the anatomically not yet clearly defined nucleus accumbens area.

[269]

MATERIAL AND METHODS

Human brain material

Post-mortem human brains were collected from 4 patients (3 females, 1 male; aged between 38 and 70 years) who died without any evidence of neurological or psychiatric disease. The interval from death to autopsy ranged from 3.4 to 23 hours (mean 12.6 ± 4.3).

All procedures involved in handling and freezing of human brains and the subsequent dissection of frozen brain material have been previously described (Lloyd et al., 1974; Farley and Hornykiewicz, 1977). Brain hemispheres separated from brainstem were kept frozen at –80 °C from 0.5 to 12 months until dissection. The topographical dissection was carried out on the basis of Riley's atlas of the human brainstem (Riley, 1960). Sixteen to 18 coronal sections (ca. 3 mm thickness) were cut beginning at the rostral pole of the caudate nucleus up to the caudal pole (cf. Hornykiewicz, 1981). The junction of the area between caudate and putamen in section 5 was further subdivided as indicated in Fig. 1. In the pallidum the internal and external segments were separated and analysed individually.

The right hemispheres were used for the estimation of dopamine (DA) and noradrenaline (NA), the left hemispheres for serotonin (5-HT) and 5-hydroxyindoleacetic acid (5-HIAA).

Biochemical analyses

Tissue samples were homogenized by ultrasonication in 20 vol. of 0.1 N perchloric acid containing 0.4 mM $NaHSO_3$. The homogenization was followed by centrifugation at 28,000 g for 10 min. For the determination of DA and NA the acidic metabolites were previously removed from the supernatant by extraction with ethylacetate (saturated with H_2O). The adsorption of the catecholamines to alumina oxide and their quantitative measurement by means of high performance liquid chromatography (HPLC) with electrochemical detection were performed as described recently (Sperk et al., 1981). For the determination of 5-HT and 5-HIAA an aliquot (100 μl) of the supernatant of the homogenate was directly applied to a HPLC system with electrochemical detection according to a recently developed method (Sperk, 1982).

Data analyses:

For the statistical analyses the paired Student's t-test was used. All data are given as means ± S.E.M., in μg/g wet tissue.

RESULTS

Rostro-caudal differences in the monoaminergic innervation of the basal ganglia

In Table I DA and NA levels in the rostral and caudal segments of caudate nucleus, putamen and globus pallidus are summarized. In the caudate nucleus, head and body were analysed separately. In the head of the caudate nucleus the DA level was significantly higher in the caudal portion (5.58 μg/g) as compared with the rostral part (2.42 μg/g). In contrast, in the body of the caudate the rostral part contained about 3 times more DA (6.01 μg/g) than the caudal part (2.21 μg/g; $P < 0.01$). There was also a significant decline of 5-HT in the whole caudate nucleus from rostral (0.47 μg/g) to caudal (0.23 μg/g; $P < 0.01$). In the putamen the concentration of DA tended to increase from rostral to caudal, although in our limited material this difference did not reach statistical significance. In respect to the noradrenergic innervation no rostro-caudal gradients could be observed in the caudate nucleus and putamen. In the globus pallidus, however, a very pronounced decrease of 5-HT from rostral to caudal could be detected in the internal as well as external segment (Table II).

TABLE I

Rostro-caudal differences in the levels of dopamine and noradrenaline in the caudate nucleus, putamen and pallidum

		Dopamine	Noradrenaline
		(μg/g wet tissue ± S.E.M.)	
Caudate nucleus head	rostral	2.42 ± 0.44	0.020 ± 0.004
	caudal	5.58 ± 0.84	0.034 ± 0.002
		$P < 0.02$	n.s.
Caudate nucleus corpus	rostral	6.01 ± 0.90	0.036 ± 0.002
	caudal	2.21 ± 0.48	0.033 ± 0.005
		$P < 0.01$	n.s.
Putamen	rostral	5.00 ± 0.50	0.064 ± 0.011
	caudal	7.21 ± 0.97	0.100 ± 0.022
		n.s.	n.s.
Globus pallidus internal segment	rostral	0.22 ± 0.11	0.085 ± 0.009
	caudal	0.13 ± 0.04	0.042 ± 0.007
		n.s.	$P < 0.01$
Globus pallidus external segment	rostral	1.19 ± 0.43	0.046 ± 0.008
	caudal	0.74 ± 0.34	0.052 ± 0.005
		n.s.	n.s.

Biochemical characterization of the junction between caudate nucleus and putamen (rostro-ventral striatum)

As can be seen in Fig. 1 our biochemical analyses in several subdivisions of the junction between caudate nucleus and putamen revealed very characteristic monoamine patterns. Thus, the junctional area 2a (cf. Fig. 1) – which in all probability includes parts of the nucleus accumbens (cf. Brockhaus, 1942; Riley, 1960) – contained 50-fold higher concentrations of NA than the adjacent portion of the caudate nucleus. A qualitatively similar pattern was observed for 5-HT; however, on a quantitative basis the difference in 5-HT level between the junction area 2a and the adjacent caudate was much smaller (2-fold) than that for NA. In contrast to NA and 5-HT, the DA level of the area 2a was significantly lower than that of the bordering caudate portion. Similar but less pronounced differences in monoamine levels were found between the area of the junction defined as 2b (cf. Fig. 1) and the adjacent portion of the putamen.

272

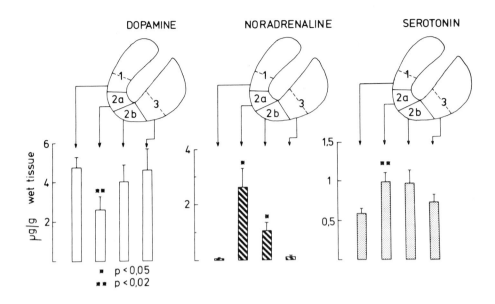

Fig. 1. Biochemical characterization of the junction between caudate nucleus and putamen (rostro-ventral striatum). 1, caudate nucleus; 2a, 2b, junction between caudate nucleus and putamen; 3, putamen. * $P < 0.05$ and ** $P < 0.02$ indicate the significance of the differences either between area 2a (including n.accumbens) and adjacent portion of caudate nucleus or between area 2b and adjacent portion of putamen.

Intra-nuclear differences in the turnover of 5-HT

As mentioned above, in both segments of the globus pallidus there was a rostro-caudal 5-HT gradient, with the rostral subdivision having markedly higher 5-HT levels than the caudal portion. In this respect, it appears intriguing that the gradient of the 5-HT turnover in this nucleus (as indicated by the molar ratio 5-HIAA to 5-HT) seemed to be in the opposite direction. This is suggested by the observation shown in Table II, that the ratio of 5-HIAA to 5-HT increased significantly from rostral to caudal.

TABLE II

Globus pallidus: Rostro-caudal differences in the levels of serotonin (5-HT), 5-hydroxyindoleacetic acid (5-HIAA) and the molar ratio 5-HIAA/5-HT

		5-HT	5-HIAA	Molar ratio
		($\mu g/g$ wet tissue $\pm$ S.E.M.)		5-HIAA/5-HT
Globus pallidus internal segment	rostral	0.79 ± 0.08	3.24 ± 0.72	3.82 ± 0.77
	caudal	0.20 ± 0.05	1.94 ± 0.37	9.64 ± 0.98
		$P < 0.01$	n.s.	$P < 0.02$
Globus pallidus external segment	rostral	0.66 ± 0.09	3.09 ± 0.83	4.19 ± 0.84
	caudal	0.29 ± 0.05	1.93 ± 0.44	6.27 ± 0.88
		$P < 0.02$	n.s.	$P < 0.05$

DISCUSSION

The present findings clearly demonstrate the existence of a marked diversity of the monoaminergic innervation within the various nuclei of the human basal ganglia complex. Such an inhomogeneity is not unexpected in view of the observations, obtained in various subhuman species, on the topographical distribution of various striatal neurotransmitters, neurotransmitter synthesizing or degrading enzymes as well as receptors. Besides inversely related rostro-caudal gradients of DA (Tassin et al., 1976) and 5-HT in the rat striatum (Ternaux et al., 1977), acetylcholinesterase and neuropeptides such as enkephalin and substance P are concentrated in discrete macroscopic patches, e.g. in the cat striatum (Graybiel et al., 1981). In the human striatum glutamate decarboxylase activity was found to be higher at the rostral level, whereas choline acetyltransferase was found to be higher at the caudal level (Gaspar et al., 1980).

Our observation of marked intra-regional gradients for DA, NA and 5-HT in the human basal ganglia have important implications for the interpretation of changes in neurotransmitter levels in pathological human brain material. Especially when the observed differences between values obtained from pathological and control material are comparatively small (as is often the case, e.g. in schizophrenic brain material; cf. Bird et al., 1979; Crow et al., 1979) special care seems to be essential in order to ensure that the control and pathological samples are taken from exactly the same subdivision of a given brain region.

Another noteworthy conclusion that can be drawn from our study is that in addition to intra-regional differences in steady-state levels, the turnover rate of monoamine transmitters may also show large variations in different parts of a given nucleus. Thus the molar ratio of 5-HIAA to 5-HT increased significantly from rostral to caudal in the internal as well as external segment of the globus pallidus. This may indicate that the serotoninergic neurons innervating the caudal part of the pallidum are characterized by a higher activity than those innervating the pallidum at the rostral level. The functional significance of this possibility is quite obvious. Some evidence for an uneven pattern in the ratio of dopamine to homovanillic acid has recently been reported for the human striatum (Adolfsson et al., 1979).

Finally, our results show that it is possible to define biochemically a subdivision of the junctional area of the rostro-ventral striatum which, in contradistinction to the immediately surrounding striatal tissues, contains significantly higher concentrations of NA and 5-HT, but lower DA levels, thus confirming, in principle, an earlier study using a different plane of dissection (Farley et al., 1978a). This characteristic distribution pattern of the three main brain monoamine neurotransmitters very likely represents a biochemical correlate of an anatomically distinct subdivision of the basal ganglia, possibly corresponding to the nucleus accumbens of subhuman species.

REFERENCES

Adolfsson, R., Gottfries, C.G., Roos, B.E. and Winblad, B. (1979) Post-mortem distribution of dopamine and homovanillic acid in human brain, variation related to age and a review of literature. *J. Neural Transm.*, 45: 81–105.

Bird, E.D., Crow, T.J., Iversen, L.L., Longden, A., Mackay, A.V.P., Riley, G.J. and Spokes, E.G. (1979) Dopamine and homovanillic acid concentrations in the post-mortem brain in schizophrenia. *J. Physiol. (Lond.)*, 293: 36–37P.

Brockhaus, H. (1942) Zur feineren Anatomie des Septum und des Striatum. *J. Physiol. Neurol.*, 51: 1–56.

Crow, T.J., Baker, H.F., Cross, A.J., Joseph, M.H., Lofthouse, R., Longden, A., Owen, F., Riley, G.J., Glover, V. and Killpack, W.S. (1979) Monoamine mechanisms in chronic schizophrenia: post-mortem neurochemical findings. *Brit. J. Psychiat.*, 134: 249–256.

Farley, I.J. and Hornykiewicz, O. (1977) Noradrenaline distribution in subcortical areas of the human brain. *Brain Res.*, 126: 53–62.

Farley, I.J., Price, K.S. and Hornykiewicz, O. (1978a) Monoaminergic systems in the human limbic brain. In K.E. Livingstone and O. Hornykiewicz (Eds.), *Limbic Mechanisms*, Plenum, New York, pp. 333–349.

Farley, I.J., Price, K.S., McCullough, E., Deck, J.H.N., Hordynski, W. and Hornykiewicz, O. (1978b) Norepinephrine in chronic paranoid schizophrenia: Above normal levels in limbic forebrain. *Science*, 200: 456–458.

Fonnum, F. and Walaas, I. (1979) Localization of neurotransmitter candidates in neostriatum. In I. Divac and R.G.E. Öberg (Eds.), *The Neostriatum*, Pergamon Press, Oxford, pp. 53–69.

Gaspar, P., Javoy-Agid, F., Ploska, A. and Agid, Y. (1980) Regional distribution of neurotransmitter synthesizing enzymes in the basal ganglia of human brain. *J. Neurochem.*, 34: 278–283.

Graybiel, A.M. and Ragsdale, C.W. (1979) Fiber connections in the basal ganglia. In M. Cuénod, G.W. Kreutzberg, and F.E. Bloom (Eds.), *Development and Chemical Specificity of Neurons, Progr. in Brain Res., Vol. 51*, Elsevier, Amsterdam, pp. 239–283.

Graybiel, A.M., Ragsdale, Jr., C.W., Yoneoka, E.S. and Elde, R.P. (1981) An immunohistochemical study of enkephalins and other neuropeptides in the striatum of the cat with evidence that the opiate peptides are arranged to form mosaic patterns in register with the striosomal compartments visible by acetylcholinesterase staining. *Neuroscience*, 6: 377–397.

Hornykiewicz, O. (1979) Brain dopamine in Parkinson's disease and other neurological disturbances. In A.S. Horn, J. Korf and B.H.C. Westerink (Eds.), *The Neurobiology of Dopamine*, Academic Press, New York, pp. 633–654.

Hornykiewicz, O. (1981) Importance of topographic neurochemistry in studying neurotransmitter systems in human brain: Critique and new data. In E. Usdin and P. Riederer (Eds.), *Transmitter Biochemistry of Human Brain Tissue*, Macmillan, London, pp. 9–24.

Lloyd, K.G., Farley, I.J., Deck, J.H.N. and Hornykiewicz, O. (1974) Serotonin and 5-hydroxyindoleacetic acid in discrete areas of the brainstem of suicide victims and control patients. *Advanc. Biochem. Psychopharmacol.*, 11: 387–397.

Perry, T.L., Hansen, S. and Kloster, M. (1973) Huntington's chorea: deficiency of gamma-aminobutyric acid in brain. *N. Engl. J. Med.*, 288: 337–342.

Riley, H.A. (1960) *An Atlas of the Basal Ganglia, Brainstem and Spinal Cord*, Hafner, New York.

Sperk, G. (1982) Simultaneous determination of serotonin, 5-hydroxyindoleacetic acid, 3,4-dihydroxyphenylacetic acid and homovanillic acid using high performance liquid chromatography with electrochemical detection. *J. Neurochem.*, 38: 840–843.

Sperk, G., Berger, M., Hörtnagl, H. and Hornykiewicz, O. (1981) Kainic acid induced changes of serotonin and dopamine metabolism in the striatum and substantia nigra of the rat. *Europ. J. Pharmacol.*, 74: 279–286.

Spokes, E.G.S. (1980) Neurochemical alterations in Huntington's chorea. A study of post-mortem brain tissue. *Brain*, 103: 179–210.

Tassin, J.P., Cheramy, A., Blanc, G., Thierry, A.M. and Glowinski, J. (1976) Topographical distribution of dopaminergic innervation and of dopaminergic receptors in the rat striatum. I. Microestimation of [^{3}H]dopamine uptake and dopamine contents in microdiscs. *Brain Res.*, 107: 291–301.

Ternaux, J.P., Héry, F., Bourgoin, S., Adrian, J., Glowinski, J. and Hamon, M. (1977) The topographical distribution of serotoninergic terminals in the neostriatum of the rat and the caudate nucleus of the cat. *Brain Res.*, 121: 311–326.

SECTION III

Rules of Development of the Central Nervous System

Cell Lineage in the Development of
the Leech Nervous System

DAVID A. WEISBLAT

Department of Molecular Biology, University of California, Berkeley, CA 94720 (U.S.A)

INTRODUCTION

Knowledge of the lines of descent of cells that compose the mature organism should help to discern basic mechanisms of development. The leech is well-suited for such cellular investigations of neurodevelopment because both the early embryo and the adult nervous system comprise identifiable cells accessible to experimental manipulation. In fact, the first studies of developmental cell lineage used leech embryos (Whitman, 1878, 1887). We have refined and extended such studies using intracellularly injected cell lineage tracers and ablatants with embryos of the leech *Helobdella triserialis.* A fuller account of the work presented here can be found elsewhere (Weisblat et al., 1978, 1980; Blair and Weisblat, 1982; Stent et al., 1982; Weisblat and Kim, 1982).

The yolky, 0.5 mm egg of *Helobdella* undergoes a series of stereotyped cleavages to produce an early embryo containing (among other blastomeres) four bilateral pairs of ectodermal precursors (the N, O, P and Q *teloblasts*) and one bilateral pair of mesodermal precursors (the M teloblasts). Individual teloblasts can be identified by their size and position within the embryo. Each teloblast undergoes several dozen highly unequal cleavages, producing a one cell wide column of *stem cells* called a *germinal bandlet.* The oldest stem cells (at the front of the bandlet) move away as new ones are produced by the parent teloblast. During gastrulation, the 10 bandlets of stem cells and their progeny come to lie parallel to the midline on the ventral side of the embryo, forming a structure known as the germinal plate. The leading ends of the bandlets are at the future head of the embryo; within each half-germinal plate the ectodermal bandlets are superficial and lie in the order n, o, p, q, from medial to lateral, and the m bandlet lies beneath them.

The situation of the left and right n bandlets (in direct apposition across the ventral midline) led Whitman to suggest that they give rise to the chain of segmental ganglia forming the ventral nerve cord. But the fates of individual stem cells and their progeny cannot be determined by the direct methods used to establish the lineage relations in the early leech embryo because they are small, numerous and lie in multiple layers in the germinal plate. We have pursued the question of the embryonic origins of the nervous system by labeling individual teloblasts early in development by intracellular injection of horseradish peroxidase (HRP), and then visualizing their progeny by histochemical staining later in embryogenesis, when the ganglia have already begun to approach their adult morphology.

[277]

RESULTS

Fig. 1a–e shows the pattern of HRP staining observed in late embryos after labeling specific teloblasts early in development. The labeled progeny of each

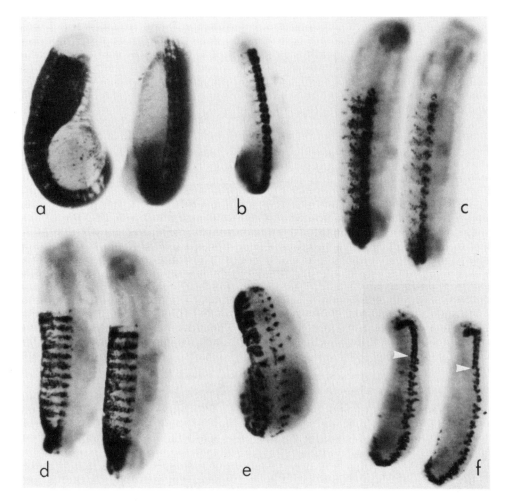

Fig. 1. Distribution of teloblast progeny revealed by HRP labeling. This figure shows embryos that were fixed and stained about six days after HRP had been injected into an identified teloblast. Except for those in panel a, a right hand teloblast in each embryo shown was labeled and, except for the embryos shown in panels e and f, teloblasts were labeled after the initiation of stem cell production, so that the anterior segments, which contain progeny of unlabeled stem cells, are unstained. All views are ventral unless otherwise indicated; anterior is up. a: lateral (left) and ventral (right) view of embryos in which the left hand M teloblast was labeled. Stain extends from the ventral midline to the lateral edge of the germinal plate. b: an N-labeled embryo. c: two O-labeled embryos. d: two P-labeled embryos. e: a Q-labeled embryo. This embryo bent during fixation so that the head is not visible in this photograph. f: two embryos, in each of which the right N teloblast was labeled with HRP soon after formation and the left N teloblast was ablated by DNAase injection after stem cell production was underway. Above the arrows are anterior ganglia formed from the full complement of stem cells; the stain pattern resembles that seen in panel b. Below the arrows are posterior ganglia lacking progeny of the left N teloblast; the normal pattern is disrupted and stain is seen on both sides of the ventral midline.

teloblast form a unique, segmentally repeating pattern within the germinal plate. In each case, the progeny are confined to the same side of the embryo as the labeled teloblast. Furthermore, in embryos in which the teloblast was injected after stem cell production had begun, there is a sharp anterior-posterior boundary to the stain pattern. This boundary corresponds to the boundary between anterior tissue produced from stem cells made prior to HRP injection and posterior tissue derived from stem cells made subsequently. Thus, there appears to be little or no migration of cell bodies across the midline or in the posterior to anterior direction within the germinal plate during normal development.

As predicted from the relative positions of the germinal bandlets within the germinal plate, the progeny of the N teloblast are largely confined to the medial

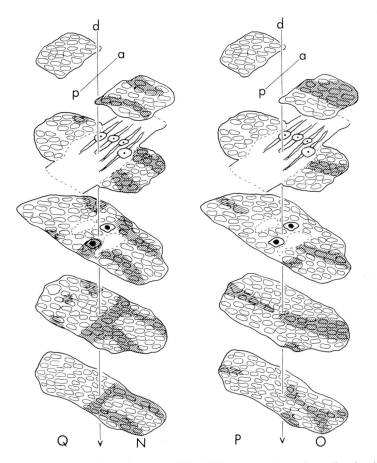

Fig. 2. Embryonic origins of the cells of the *Helobdella* segmental ganglion. The drawing shows 5 horizontal sections through a midbody segmental ganglion of the embryo at mid stage 10. (Dorsal aspect at the top; front edge facing away from the viewer.) The two pairs of dark, elongated contours in the center of the second section from the top represent identifiable muscle cells in the longitudinal nerve tract. They are descendants of the M teloblast pair. The two dark, circular contours in the center of the middle section represent two identifiable glial cells, each of which is a descendant of one N teloblast. The faint contours do not correspond to actual cells but are shown to indicate the approximate size, disposition and number of neurons in the ganglion. In each half-ganglion, cross-hatched domains contain descendants of the teloblast designated at the bottom of the figure.

portion of the germinal plate, in the vicinity of the ventral nerve cord. Although the shape of the repeating pattern of N-teloblast progeny conforms roughly to that of the segmental hemiganglion, there are unstained regions within each hemiganglion. The bulk of the O, P and Q teloblast progeny are progressively more laterally distributed, but there are clear exceptions to this rule. In particular, some progeny from each teloblast can be seen near the ventral midline; the distribution of these cells appears to complement that of the N teloblast progeny within the ganglionic borders.

These observations on intact embryos suggested that the segmental ganglia may have a more complex embryonic origin than was originally supposed. In fact, when labeled embryos were examined in section, it was found that each teloblast contributes a stereotyped, topographically distinct subpopulation of cells to the ipsilateral hemiganglia of the nerve cord. The major groups of cells arising from the ectoteloblasts are distributed as shown schematically in Fig. 2 (Weisblat and Kim, 1982). The N and O teloblasts each contribute many more cells to the ganglion than

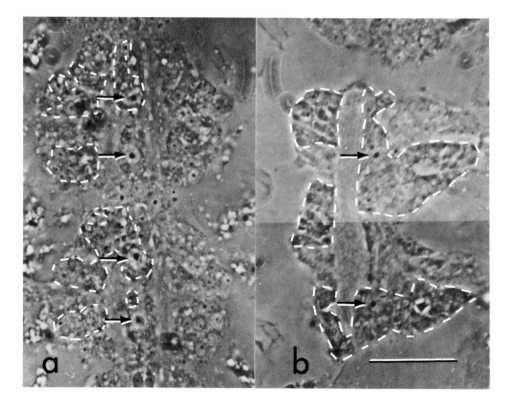

Fig. 3. Effects of N teloblast ablation. a: horizontal section through two normal ganglia of an embryo in which an N teloblast was labeled with HRP (cf. Fig. 1b). Dotted outlines indicate the regions of HRP stain visible in the original section. Arrows indicate the nuclei of the two giant neuropil glia in each ganglion. b: a similar section through two ganglia of an embryo in which one N teloblast was labeled with HRP and the other was ablated by DNAase injection. Note that, as in Fig. 1f, the HRP stain is on both sides of the midline. Also, only one neuropil glia can be seen in each ganglion. No other neuropil glia could be found in other sections through these ganglia. Anterior is up; scale bar = 25 μm.

do P and Q. A small number of additional cells in the ganglion arise from the M teloblast. Some of these are known to be nonneuronal (Weisblat et al., 1980); but some others are (Weisblat and Kim, 1982).

The sterotyped position of each teloblast's progeny in the embryonic ganglion, taken with the fixed position of identified neurons in the adult ganglion (cf. Nicholls and Baylor, 1968; Stuart, 1970), suggests that identified neurons may arise from specific teloblasts during normal development. Of the cells identifiable in the adult nervous system, only three, nonneuronal ones can be identified morphologically at the intermediate stage of development reached in these experiments. These are the two pairs of longitudinal muscle cells in the interganglionic connective nerve, which derive from the M teloblast, and the pair of giant glia associated with the ganglionic neuropil, each of which derives from one N teloblast (Fig. 3a). To probe the limits of the developmental determinacy indicated by these results, further experiments were done in which the right N teloblast was labeled with HRP and the left N teloblast was ablated by DNAase injection (Blair and Weisblat, 1982). Examination of such embryos, fixed, stained and sectioned, revealed that ganglia missing the progeny of one N teloblast also lack one neuropil glia (Fig. 3b). This deficit is seen even when progeny of the surviving N teloblast have aberrantly crossed the ventral midline and are present on both sides of the ganglion (Fig. 1f) (Blair and Weisblat, 1982).

DISCUSSION

The experiments reported here reveal that each teloblast of the early leech embryo, not just the pair of N teloblasts, contributes progeny to the segmental ganglia. There appears to be little or no migration of cell bodies across the midline or from posterior to anterior within the nerve cord during normal development. This implies that neuronal pathways within the leech central nervous system are established by process growth rather than by migration of cell bodies. There is movement of cell bodies during neurogenesis into the ventral nerve cord from laterally situated germinal bandlets, especially the q bandlet, but there is no evidence that any cell processes are left behind during this movement.

The significance of the distinct neuronal kinship groups from each of four ectoteloblast pairs, or why there are four pairs of ectodermal precursors and just one pair of mesodermal precursors, is not clear. Early cleavages in the leech embryo seem to result in the segregation of specific developmental fates. But the possibility implicit in Whitman's analysis, that different ectoteloblasts give rise to different tissue types, has been ruled out by the work reported here. Indeed, each ectoteloblast seems to give rise to both neural and body wall cells (Weisblat and Kim, 1982). A second hypothesis is that the teloblasts are developmentally equipotent, and are replicated to guarantee the production of a complete set of ectodermal structures. But the failure of the *Helobdella* embryo to generate a complete set of neuropil glia after N teloblast ablation argues against this interpretation, too. Alternatives include the segregation of identified neurons among the kinship groups on the basis of branching pattern, biochemical or biophysical traits, or spatial distribution of targets in the periphery. Further analysis of the lineage relations of identified cells in the leech nervous system, using techniques already at hand, should permit us to test these possibilities.

ACKNOWLEDGMENTS

I thank Gunther Stent, in whose laboratory this work was done, for his support and for many stimulating discussions, and Barbara Kellogg for assistance in the preparation of this manuscript. This work was supported by NIH Research Grant NS12818 and NSF BN577-19181.

REFERENCES

Blair, S.S. and Weisblat, D.A. (1982) Ectodermal interactions during neurogenesis in the glossiphoniid leech *Helobdella triserialis. Develop. Biol.*, 91: 64–72.

Nicholls, J.G. and Baylor, D.A. (1968) Specific modalities and receptive fields of sensory neurons in CNS of the leech. *J. Neurophysiol.*, 31: 740–756.

Stent, G.S., Weisblat, D.A., Blair, S.S. and Zackson, S.L. (1982) Cell lineage in the development of the leech nervous system. In N. Spitzer (Ed.), *Neuronal Development*, Plenum, New York, pp. 1–44.

Stuart, A.E. (1970) Physiological and morphological properties of motoneurones in the central nervous system of the leech. *J. Physiol. (Lond.)*, 209: 627–646.

Weisblat, D.A. and Kim (1982) in preparation.

Weisblat, D.A., Sawyer, R.T. and Stent, G.S. (1978) Cell lineage analysis by intracellular injection of a tracer enzyme. *Science*, 202: 1295–1298.

Weisblat, D.A., Harper, G., Stent, G.S. and Sawyer, R.T. (1980) Embryonic cell lineages in the nervous system of the glossiphoniid leech *Helobdella triserialis. Develop. Biol.*, 76: 58–78.

Whitman, C.O. (1878) The embryology of Clepsine. *Quart. J. Microscop. Sci.*, 18: 215–315.

Whitman, C.O. (1887). A contribution to the history of germ layers in Clepsine. *J. Morph.*, 1: 105–182.

Grasshopper Growth Cones:
Divergent Choices and Labeled Pathways

COREY S. GOODMAN, JONATHAN A. RAPER, SUSANNAH CHANG and ROBERT HO

Department of Biological Sciences, Stanford University, Stanford, CA 94305 (U.S.A.)

INTRODUCTION

The growth cones of individual neurons traverse long distances during embryogenesis, yet they find their correct targets and make their appropriate synaptic connections. We would like to understand how growth cones know where to go (pathway selection) and in particular, how the growth cones of different cells, confronted with the same environment, are determined to make different and stereotyped choices of which way to go.

Our results demonstrate that growth cones find their correct targets not by random growth, but rather by an active process of precise pathfinding. In this paper we will show that the growth cones of pioneer neurons in the central nervous system (CNS) establish stereotyped axonal pathways (see p. 290). In this section we will emphasize the divergent choices made by the growth cones of two sibling pioneer neurons. Then we will show that the growth cones of later cells follow specific axonal pathways laid down by pioneers, and when confronted with several available pathways, make specific choices of which one to follow (see p. 295). Here we will emphasize the divergent choices made by the growth cones of two sibling interneurons. Neuronal specificity results in large part from the ability of each individual growth cone to make a sequential series of pathway choices that take it to its correct target. These results lead us to propose the 'labeled pathways' hypothesis whereby axonal pathways are differentially labeled, probably by cell surface markers, and growth cones use these labels for guidance. One way to search for these 'labels' is to make monoclonal antibodies, and we will discuss our progress thus far using this approach (see p. 302).

We have been able to study the specific choices made by growth cones during embryogenesis by examining how a grasshopper makes its nervous system. The grasshopper embryo is a very favorable preparation because its nervous system is relatively simple, highly accessible, and well described. The questions of cell determination and pathway selection, common to all nervous systems, appear particularly solvable in the grasshopper embryo because of the precision and clarity with which they can be approached. In the living grasshopper embryo, individual neurons are large, accessible, and can be viewed with Nomarski interference contrast optics (Goodman and Spitzer, 1979; Goodman et al., 1979). The neuronal precursor cells are well described (Bate, 1976a; Bate and Grunewald, 1981). Individual identified neurons of known lineage can be studied from their birth to their maturation (Goodman and Spitzer, 1979; Goodman et al., 1979, 1981; Goodman, 1981); this is the only embryonic preparation in which this approach is possible. Pioneer neurons have been described which establish early axonal pathways in the peripheral and central nervous system (Bate, 1976b; Keshishian, 1980; Bate and Grunewald, 1981; Ho et al., 1981). Embryos can be cultured outside of the egg case for experimental manipulations (Goodman and Ridge, 1980; Whitington et al., 1981; Shankland et al., 1981). Thus, we can examine and manipulate the early events of cell interactions and cell determination during the proliferation and axonal outgrowth of individual neurons.

We have been studying the question of pathfinding by neuronal growth cones in grasshopper embryos by: (i) injecting the cells via their cell bodies, axons, or growth cones with a variety of intracellular dyes; and (ii) by selectively staining some of the cells with a monoclonal antibody called I-5. In this paper, we will discuss what we have learned about pathfinding in the CNS using both of these techniques, examining how pioneer growth cones make stereotyped axonal pathways, and how later growth cones make stereotyped choices of which pathway to follow. In particular, we will examine two divergent choices made by the growth cones of sibling cells, one by a pair of sibling pioneers establishing divergent pathways, and the other by a pair of sibling neurons following divergent pathways. In the end, we will suggest the 'labeled pathways' hypothesis based on these results.

GRASSHOPPER EMBRYOS

Like most metazoan animals, the grasshopper is a metameric animal with a basic repeating segmental body plan with regional specializations. The grasshopper's nervous system is segmentally arranged and corresponds to the metameric body plan of cephalic, thoracic, and abdominal segments (Fig. 1). Interneuron and motorneuron cell bodies lie in the CNS; sensory neurons are derived from body ectoderm and have their cell bodies in the periphery and their axons extending into the CNS. Within the CNS, there are several hundred thousand neurons, most of which are located in the brain and optic lobes. Fortunately, the chain of segmental ganglia is much simpler and contains at most only a few thousand neurons per segment. Early in embryogenesis each body segment has a segmental ganglion, but as development proceeds, some fusion of ganglia takes place leading to the final adult form. Each thoracic ganglion (T1–T3) contains about 3000 neurons; each abdominal ganglion (A1–A11) contains about 500 neurons. A growing list of neurons within the segmental ganglia can be described as individual unique cells (identified neurons) on the basis of their characteristic morphology, physiology, and biochemistry. Examples of two identified interneurons, called the 'G' and 'C' neurons, are shown in Fig. 2. These two identified neurons represent some of the variety of cell shapes found in a single segment. Interestingly, these two neurons are siblings that arise from a single cell division, and they are particularly accessible throughout their development. Thus, they have been ideal cells with which to study the specific and divergent choices made by the growth cones of sibling neurons (Raper and Goodman, 1981; Raper, Bastiani and Goodman, in preparation), a topic we will return to later (p. 295).

In the grasshopper embryo, as in all animals, the nervous system forms from the ectoderm. The ectodermal epithelium that generates the nervous system runs down the middle of the embryo from head to tail as a strip of contiguous plates of cells

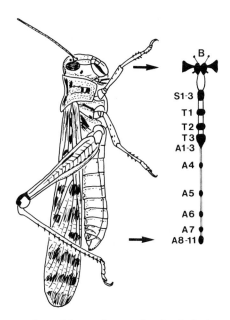

Fig. 1. Left: schematic diagram of an adult grasshopper showing its basic segmental body plan consisting of a head (including an unknown number of brain segments and segments S1–S3 which control the mouth parts), thorax (segments T1–T3, with 3 pairs of legs and 2 pairs of wings), and abdomen (segments Al–All). Right: schematic diagram of the grasshopper CNS showing the brain (B) and optic lobes, and the chain of unfused and fused segmental ganglia (S1–S3, T1–T3, Al–All). (Ganglia are a bit larger than in animal.) Each thoracic ganglion contains about 3000 neurons; each abdominal ganglion contains about 500 neurons.

(Fig. 3). The dorsal surface of this neural epithelium is covered by a conspicuous non-cellular basement membrane which separates it from the mesoderm; this basement membrane is probably secreted by the ectoderm at an early stage. Within the neural epithelium, certain cells specialize as neuronal precursors, rounding up and generally enlarging relative to the cells around them. There are two types of neuronal precursors from the segmental ganglia (Fig. 3): neuroblasts (NBs) (Bate, 1976a) and midline precursors (MPs) (Bate and Grunewald, 1981). A remarkable observation is that the number and pattern of precursor cells are repeatable from segment to segment from embryo to embryo (with minor changes at the anterior and posterior ends of the chain). In each segment there are two bilaterally symmetric plates containing 30 NBs each and an additional unpaired median NB (MNB). Individual NBs can be uniquely identified by their distinctive positions within the NB plates. There are also seven MPs arranged in a stereotyped pattern along the dorsal midline just anterior to the MNB.

Each MP divides only once to produce two neuronal progeny. Each NB maintains its large size as a stem cell while it divides repeatedly to give rise to a chain of smaller cells (ganglion mother cells, GMC) each of which divides once more to generate a chain of doublets (ganglion cells, GC), which then differentiate into neurons. Thus, each NB contributes a clone of neuronal progeny to the developing nervous system. Eventually, the NBs die and degenerate, with some having produced as few as 10 neuronal progeny and others as many as 100.

It is quite feasible to trace the ancestry of individual identified neurons and show

286

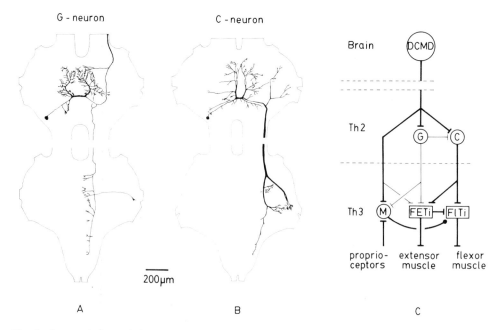

Fig. 2. A: morphology of G neuron in adult grasshopper. Cell body is in mesothoracic (T2) segment; major axon extends anteriorly up to brain (not shown). B: morphology of C neuron in adult grasshopper. Cell body is next to G's in T2 segment; major axon extends posteriorly down to metathoracic (T3) segment. C: identified monosynaptic connections onto and from G and C interneurons. The descending contralateral movement detector (DCMD) neuron from the brain synapses on both G and C (as well as onto interneuron M and onto the extensor motorneuron). The G neuron synapses onto C, M, and FETi (the fast extensor tibiae motorneuron). The C neuron synapses onto FETi and FlTi (the flexor tibiae motorneurons). Thick lines denote stronger synaptic connections. (This figure was kindly provided by Keir Pearson; data come from Pearson et al., 1980; and Pearson and Robertson, 1981, with permission.)

that they are produced during embryogenesis at specific points in the family tree of individual neuroblasts or MPs. The best documented examples are the first twelve progeny of the median neuroblast (MNB) (Goodman and Spitzer, 1979; Bate and Goodman, 1983a, b); the two progeny each of midline precursors 1, 2 and 3 (MP1, MP2, MP3) (Goodman et al., 1981; Bate and Grunewald, 1981; Ho, Raper and Goodman, in preparation); the first six progeny of neuroblast 7-4 (Raper, Bastiani, and Goodman, in preparation); and the first six progeny of neuroblast 4-4 (Taghert, Bate, and Goodman, in preparation). Two of these lineages, the first twelve progeny of the MNB and the first six progeny of NB 7-4, are shown schematically in Fig. 4. Fig. 5 shows Nomarski photographs of some of the progeny of the MNB (5A) and the two progeny of MP3 (5B). We are continuing to expand our maps of neuronal cell lineages to include many other large interneurons and motorneurons (Bate and Goodman, unpublished results). From these cell lineages we have learned that uniquely identified neurons arise from specific cell divisions of particular NBs or MPs, but we do not yet know the mechanisms underlying this cell-specific determination. Cells arising from the same final cell division can be quite similar, yet at the same time have individually distinctive characteristics (e.g. the dMP2 and vMP2 cells in the section on p. 295, and the G and C cells in the section on p. 300). Successive groups of cells can have certain features in common; their growth cones

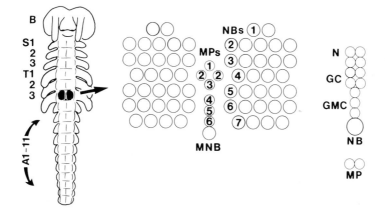

Fig. 3. Left: schematic diagram of a 30% embryo showing the segmental structure of the ectoderm (embryo is about 3 mm long). The middle of the ectoderm is a longitudinal strip of neuroepithelium which gives rise to the CNS. The location of the neuronal precursors for a single segment (T3) is drawn in black. Middle: pattern of neuronal precursors for a single segment (T3) includes two plates of 30 neuroblasts (NBs) arranged in a precise pattern of 7 rows, and 1 median NB (MNB) making a total of 61 NBs. Anterior to the MNB along the dorsal midline are seven other cells called midline precursors (MPs). Right: pattern of cell divisions of the neuronal precursors. The MPs divide only once and give rise to two progeny. The NBs maintain their large size as stem cells and divide repeatedly to give rise to a chain of ganglion mother cells (GMC). As each GMC gets about 3 cells away from the NB, it divides one final time into two ganglion cells (GC) making a chain of doublets, which then differentiate into neurons (N). NBs generate from 10 to 100 progeny in a reproducible pattern; all NBs finally die and degenerate.

often follow the same pathway initially (and only later diverge) and they often become secondarily dye coupled as groups of cells. In the end, each cell becomes a unique individual, its identity unfolding during embryogenesis as its growth cone makes specific choices of which axonal pathway(s) to follow. How a cell's growth cone chooses its

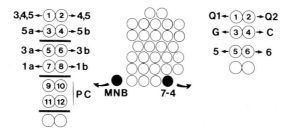

Fig. 4. Cell lineages of the MNB and NB 7-4. Schematic diagram of the right plate of neuroblasts (NBs) and the median neuroblast (MNB) from a single segment, showing the identities of the first twelve progeny of the MNB and the first six progeny of NB 7-4. From the first cell division of the MNB arises DUM 3, 4, 5 and DUM 4, 5, their names based on which of the 5 peripheral nerves they send axons out (3, 4, 5 is marked '1' because its growth cone comes out first); from its second cell division arises DUM 5a (DUMETi) and DUM 5b. Groups of 4 cells are separated by heavy lines because the growth cones from these 'quartets' of cells initially follow the same pathway. Of the second quartet of 4 cells, two send axons out nerve 3 and the next two send axons out nerve 1. The third quartet of cells all bifurcate in the posterior commissure (PC) (the ones before them bifurcate in the anterior commissure) and do not send axons out the peripheral nerves. From the first cell division of NB 7-4 arises Q1 and Q2, from its second cell division the G and C neurons, and from its third division cells '5' and '6'. See text for descriptions of these cells.

288

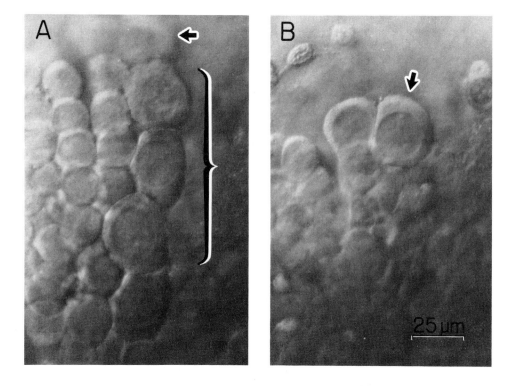

Fig. 5. Photomicrographs of the dorsal surface (desheathed) of the metathoracic (T3) ganglion of a 90% embryo visualized with Nomarski interference contrast optics, showing some of the progeny of the MNB (A) and the two progeny of MP3 (B). The plane of focus in A is dorsal to that in B. In A, the three oldest progeny of the MNB (from top to bottom: DUM 3, 4, 5, DUM 4, 5, and DUM 5a) are indicated by the bracket. The MP3 progeny lie deep to the focal plane (arrow) and anterior to the NMB progeny. In B, the H cell is indicated by the arrow. For further details, see Goodman et al. (1981).

appropriate pathway(s) appears to be the key factor in understanding the development of neuronal specificity.

METHODS FOR STUDYING PATHFINDING

Studies on grasshopper embryos make it clear that the key to understanding the development of neuronal specificity is unlocking the mystery of pathfinding. We have a three-fold strategy for studying pathfinding. First, we would like to describe the complete cellular environment in which particular growth cones make their cell-specific choices. Second, we would like to uncover the cellular rules underlying this specific pathfinding by manipulating the cellular environment around individual growth cones. Third, we would like to identify the biochemical guidance cues which are the molecular correlates of these pathfinding rules.

In order to study pathfinding by pioneer and follower growth cones, we have used and developed two different approaches (and are currently developing a third approach involving embryo culture and cellular manipulations). First, we inject the embryonic cells via their cell bodies, axons, or growth cones with a variety of intracellular dyes including Lucifer Yellow, cobalt dye, and horseradish peroxidase (HRP). The cells are then viewed with both the light and electron microscopes. In this way we can describe the behavior of individual growth cones and the cellular environment around them. Second, we have been making monoclonal antibodies against grasshopper neurons in the hope of uncovering developmentally important molecules involved in cell determination and pathway selection. One of the anti-bodies we have produced, called I-5, may be recognizing an antigen that is important during embryogenesis (Chang et al., 1981; Chang, Ho and Goodman, in pre-paration). Quite fortunately, the I-5 monoclonal antibody also serves as an excellent histological stain for our studies on pathfinding. We can selectively stain some of the embryonic cells with the I-5 antibody and then view them with an HRP-labeled second antibody as seen in the light microscope.

During the first half of embryonic development, the grasshopper embryo is very thin and sits on a bed of yolk. For our experiments, the embryo is removed from the egg case, separated from the yolk, and the embryonic membranes are removed from the ventral surface. The dorsal membrane of the embryo is opened, and the embryo is flattened and pinned out on a glass slide in a coffin surrounded by Sylgard. The dorsal surface of the neuroepithelium is then viewed with a Leitz 50X salt water immersion lens and Zeiss Nomarski interference contrast optics. The developing embryonic nervous system is only about 100 microns thick and can thus be viewed with excellent clarity and detail through the dorsal membrane. The early axonal pathways are formed on this dorsal basement membrane. The pioneer growth cones for each of the early pathways in the CNS use the membrane as the substrate on which to grow. Cell bodies in these young embryos are about 12–15 μm in diameter, axons about 1–2 μm in diameter, and growth cones about 2–5 μm in diameter; all are clearly visible and identifiable in the living preparation. Cell bodies, axons, or growth cones of early embryonic neurons can be routinely impaled with microelectrodes and a variety of dyes injected into them.

Our second methodological approach has been to make monoclonal antibodies against grasshopper neurons. Our goal is to find developmentally important mole-cules involved in cell determination and pathway selection. The great advantage of the monoclonal approach is that antibodies specific to individual antigens can be obtained from molecularly heterogeneous cells or tissues. The monoclonal anti-bodies were produced following standard procedures. Mice were injected with homogenized adult grasshopper ganglia (T2, T3, A1–A3), and the mouse spleen cells were fused with NS-1 myeloma cells using PEG 1540. Because we are interested in selecting for antibodies that recognize molecules expressed early in development, we screened the hybridomas for antibody specificity on 40% grasshopper embryos which were lightly fixed with 2% paraformaldehyde. We are currently injecting mice with 40% embryonic nervous systems and with membrane fractions of adult nervous systems to obtain additional monoclonal antibodies (Kotrla, in progress).

One of the monoclonal antibodies we have produced, called I-5, shows interesting patterns of cellular specificity and may be recognizing an antigen of developmental importance (Chang et al., 1981; Chang, Ho, and Goodman, in preparation). For example, the I-5 antibody selectively stains the peripheral pioneer neurons in the appendages and body wall (Fig. 6), as well as many central pioneers (Fig. 7A) and other neurons. Later in this paper (p. 302) we will describe in detail the selective staining by the I-5 antibody. However, in the next section we will use our data from

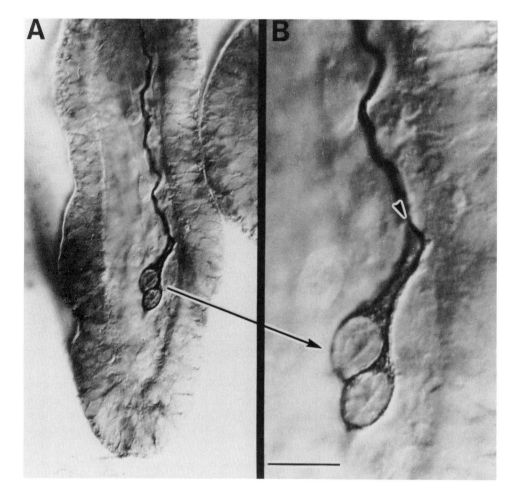

Fig. 6. A: photograph of antennae showing a pair of distal pioneer neurons as stained by the I-5 monoclonal antibody in a whole-mount embryo. B: enlarged view of same pair of pioneer neurons, showing two axons (arrow) fasciculating. Calibration bars = 50 μm in A and 20 μm in B.

the I-5 antibody in conjunction with our data from dye injections and microscopy to describe the divergent choices made by the growth cones of two sibling pioneer neurons.

DIVERGENT CHOICES BY PIONEER GROWTH CONES

Ross Harrison (1910) was the first to coin the word 'pioneer'. He noticed that during the development of the frog, the peripheral nerves are laid down early in embryonic life by "but a few fibers" which he termed the pathfinders or pioneers. "The fibers which develop later follow, in the main, the paths laid down by the pioneers". Thus, according to Harrison's definition, pioneers are cells whose growth cones navigate without having an existing nerve or axon to follow.

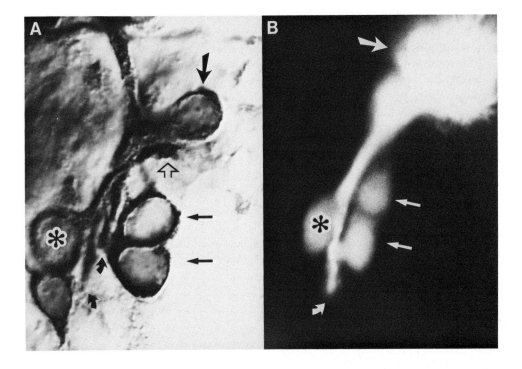

Fig. 7. A: photomicrograph of the dorsal surface of embryonic central nervous system showing a few of the central pioneer neurons as stained by the I-5 monoclonal antibody. Cell bodies shown include the MP1, aCC, pCC, Q1, and one additional cell body posterior to Q1. The two axons of the dMP2 and MP1 are shown running posteriorly, the one axon of the vMP2 running anteriorly, and the one axon of Q1 running towards the midline (note the growth cone of the Q1 cell just posterior to the MP1 cell body). The growth cones of the dMP2 and MP1 always extend along the basement membrane just lateral to the aCC and pCC cell bodies and just medial to the Q1 cell body. Large black arrow indicates the MP1 cell body, small black arrows the aCC and pCC cell bodies, and the asterisk the Q1 cell body. Small curved black arrows indicate the dMP2 (lateral) and MP1 (medial) growth cones extending posteriorly, and the short open arrow indicates the Q1 growth cone heading towards the midline. B: dye coupling (Lucifer Yellow, 450 MW) from the MP1 cell body via its axon to the cell bodies of the aCC, pCC, and Q1. The MP1 cell body appears enormous because of the intense fluorescence. Large white arrow indicates MP1 cell body, small white arrows the aCC and pCC cell bodies, and the asterisk the Q1 cell body. Small curved arrow indicates the MP1 growth cone extending posteriorly. In A and B cell body diameters are approximately 15 μm.

In the grasshopper, the cells subserving this pioneering role are typically large and conspicuous in both the peripheral (e.g. Fig. 6) (Bate, 1976b; Keshishian, 1980; Ho et al., 1981; Ho and Goodman, 1982) and central nervous system (e.g. Fig. 7A) (Bate and Grunewald, 1981; Ho et al., in preparation). Bate and Grunewald (1981) used serial electron and light micrographs and Nomarski optics to trace the first axons within the interganglionic connectives back to the progeny of midline precursors 1 and 2 (MP1 and MP2). Each MP2 divides once to give rise to a ventral daughter (vMP2) and a dorsal daughter cell (dMP2). The single MP1 gives rise to a pair of bilaterally symmetric daughters, each of which comes to lie dorsal to the two MP2 progeny (forming a trio of cells on each side of the midline of each segment). All three cells on each side send growth cones up to the basement membrane. The growth cone of the vMP2 turns and extends anteriorly; the growth cones of the dMP2 and the MP1 turn and extend posteriorly. In this way, the first longitudinal axonal pathways are generated on either side of the midline.

In this section, we will focus on our recent studies involving the divergent choices made by the growth cones of these three pioneer neurons on each side of the segment: the two sibling MP2 progeny and one of the two MP1 progeny. These are the very first growth cones to appear in the CNS. Three other cells are intimately associated with the posterior choice of the dMP2 and MP1 growth cones, namely the anterior corner cell (aCC), its sibling the posterior corner cell (pCC), and the Q1 cell. (The sibling aCC and pCC cells arise from the first division of NB 1-1; the Q1 and its sibling Q2 cell arise from the first division of NB 7-4.) We have observed the behavior of the vMP2, dMP2, and MP1 growth cones, and their relationship to the aCC, pCC, and Q1 cells, by using intracellular dye injections, Nomarski optics, and the I-5 antibody.

The growth cones of the two sibling progeny of the MP2, the dMP2 and vMP2, make divergent and stereotyped choices once they reach the dorsal basement membrane (Fig. 8B). Interestingly, their growth cones reach the basement membrane at about the same time in a variety of orientations relative to each other and to the growth cone of the MP1 (Fig. 8A). In some cases the vMP2 is the most anterior of the two siblings and in other cases the dMP2 is the most anterior; similarly, either growth cone can be the most lateral of the two. Within several hours, irrespective of how they reach the membrane, their growth cones begin to make their divergent choices as the vMP2 turns anteriorly and the dMP2 turns

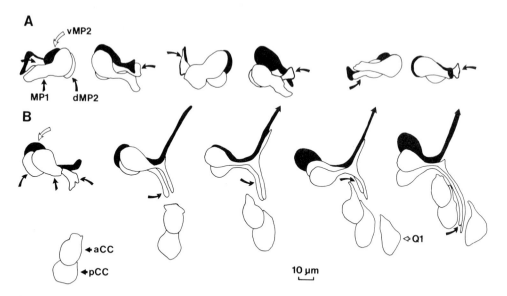

Fig. 8. Camera lucida drawings of vMP2, dMP2, and MP1 cells as growth cones reach the basement membrane (A), and later as they make their divergent and cell-specific choices of which way to grow. Drawings are from preparations stained with the I-5 antibody. Note that the vMP2 and dMP2 growth cones reach the basement membrane in a variety of orientations (A), yet grow off in specific directions (B). The dMP2 and MP1 growth cones extend in specific relationship to the aCC, pCC, and Q1 cell bodies.

posteriorly. The MP1 growth cone turns posteriorly and also sends a short anterior process whereas the dMP2 does not. These results support the idea that there is 'information' in the environment of these growth cones, and that they may be individually determined to respond to it.

All three of these central pioneer neurons stain with the I-5 monoclonal antibody. Furthermore, they show differential staining that is cell-specific. After their final cell division but before axonogenesis, the vMP2 stains darkly while its sibling, the dMP2, stains lightly (the MP1 also stains lightly). This differential staining is also expressed on their growth cones as they reach the basement membrane, and continues to be expressed on their growth cones and axons as they establish divergent axonal pathways (Fig. 9A). This result of cell-specific staining before axonogenesis between the two sibling cells shows that they have acquired a cell-specific determinant by this time. Interestingly, the cell-specific determinant correlates with the divergent choices made by their growth cones: the darkly stained vMP2 turning anteriorly and the lightly stained dMP2 and MP1 turning posteriorly. It is likely that the dMP2 and vMP2 acquire their cell-specific determinant either from their mitotic ancestry or from the position of their cell bodies immediately after their division (since they stain shortly thereafter). Nature has done an interesting experiment for us once thus far, in that on one side of one segment in an embryo that otherwise appeared totally normal, the MP2 division was in the horizontal rather than dorsal/ventral plane. In this case, one of the cells stained darkly and the other lightly, suggesting that their dorsal/ventral position may not be the important factor for their determination. In the future, we plan to manipulate and ablate these cells in order to understand how they become uniquely determined.

The growth cones of the dMP2 and vMP2 reach the basement membrane in a variety of orientations, yet within several hours make divergent and stereotyped choices of which way to go. What information in their environment provides guidance for their divergent choices? In looking for information in their environment, it is important to understand just how large their environment is. Each of

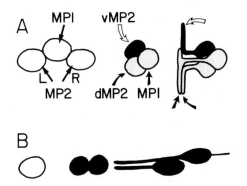

Fig. 9. Schematic diagram of staining pattern of I-5 monoclonal antibody on some central (A) and peripheral (B) pioneer neurons. A: three midline precursors (MP1 and MP2 on the left and right) each divide once and give rise to a trio of cells on each side of the midline, with from dorsal to ventral, the MP1, dMP2, and vMP2. After the cell division and before axonogenesis, the vMP2 stains darkly while the dMP2 and MP1 stain lightly with the antibody. This differential staining pattern persists on the growth cone and axons. B: the distal pioneer neurons in the appendages stain darkly with the I-5 monoclonal antibody after their final cell division and before axonogenesis; their axons also stain darkly.

these growth cones has many long, thin filopodia extending radially in many directions. The filopodia can be as long as 50 μm, and thus a growth cone can contact cells and other substrates within a diameter of 100 μm. One possible source of information available to them is polarity (anterior vs. posterior); the most likely source of such information would be the basement membrane. Alternatively, they may be orienting on 'landmark' cells that reside in opposite directions. In the posterior direction, there are three conspicuous cell bodies that are intimately involved in the formation of the early axonal pathways, and that are candidates for potential 'landmark' cells for the dMP2 and MP1 growth cones. These cells are the sibling anterior and posterior corner cells (aCC and pCC) and the Q1 cell, as shown in Figs. 7A and 8B.

As the growth cones of the dMP2, MP1, and vMP2 make their cell-specific choices, the aCC and pCC migrate anteriorly toward their characteristic position. The aCC and pCC are sibling cells that arise from the first cell division of NB 1-1 in the next posterior segment. They stain with the I-5 antibody once they are postmitotic and thus we can easily observe their migration in the fixed preparation with the antibody or in the living preparation with Nomarski optics. The aCC and pCC migrate anteriorly at about 5 μm per hour just under the basement membrane; they have flat lamellipodia and long thin filopodia extending from their anterior edges. As the aCC and pCC cell bodies migrate anteriorly, they and the growth cones of the dMP2 and MP1 appear to point towards one another and their filopodia overlap with each other. As the aCC and pCC finish their migration and assume their characteristic location just posterior to the MP1 cell body, the two growth cones of the dMP2 and the MP1 pass just lateral to them and between them and the Q1 cell body. Thus, if the aCC and pCC cell bodies are indeed important 'landmarks' for the guidance of the posteriorly extending dMP2 and MP1 growth cones, then we should be able to test this by ablating them before they have migrated anteriorly into the next segment. This is the type of experiment we plan for the future to uncover the guidance cues for the divergent choices of the vMP2 vs the dMP2 and MP1 growth cones.

The dMP2 and MP1 growth cones extend posteriorly and fasciculate on one another. Interestingly, either growth cone can be the leader; in some embryos MP1 is out in front, in others the dMP2 is the leader, and in still others they are running neck and neck. Whatever the guidance cue, either cell can respond to it. When the anteriorly extending vMP2 growth cone meets the posteriorly extending dMP2 and MP1 growth cones (from the next most anterior segment) near the segmental border, they do not fasciculate. Rather, the vMP2 growth cone passes on the medial side of the other two growth cones and all three continue growing in two parallel pathways along the basement membrane. Their growth cones do fasciculate, however, as they meet their segmental homologues from the next segment. It appears, then, that just as the vMP2 and dMP2 differentially stain with the I-5 antibody, so each of their growth cones can distinguish between the two sibling cells when it meets them in the next segment; it fasciculates on the axon of its homologue but not on the axon of its homologue's sibling.

One final point about the divergent choices of the sibling pioneers, the dMP2 and vMP2, concerns their dye coupling to other cells. (By dye coupling we mean the spread of the fluorescent dye Lucifer Yellow (450 MW) from the interior of one cell to another.) We have noticed distinctive patterns of dye coupling between the interiors of individually identified neurons at early stages of their differentiation (e.g. Fig. 7B) (Goodman and Spitzer, 1979; Bate and Grunewald, 1981; Raper and Goodman, 1981a). Dye coupling between related neurons (common lineage) appears to be common to many embryonic neurons whereas dye coupling to unrelated neurons is most common between the early pioneer neurons and specific other neurons in their environment. These specific patterns of intercellular coupling between pioneers and unrelated cells may be involved in pathfinding by pioneer growth cones. Here we will briefly describe the dye coupling from the dMP2 and MP1 growth cones to other cells in their environment.

When either the MP1 or dMP2 cells are filled with dye, the dye spreads into a reproducible and distinctive pattern of other cells according to the age of the embryo. Once their growth cones reach the basement membrane and extend filopodia in many directions (about the time they are making their posterior choice), dye spreads into the vMP2 and into the aCC, pCC, and Q1 cells (Fig. 7B). These last three cells (aCC, pCC, and Q1) are the cell bodies that the MP1 and dMP2 navigate between as they extend posteriorly. The coupling begins to occur before the growth cones contact the cell bodies of the aCC and pCC; this coupling is likely to be mediated by the filopodia since these are the only dye containing structures seen to span the gap between these cells. When the dMP2 and MP1 growth cones extend into the next posterior segment, they run parallel to the vMP2 axon from that segment but then fasciculate with the posteriorly extending axons of their homologues. Dye coupling occurs from the dMP2 or MP1 growth cones to their posterior ipsilateral homologues, but not to the vMP2 (even though the growth cones and later their axonal processes lie within a few microns of each other and their filopodia overlap). Thus it should be stressed that the dMP2 and MP1 growth cones do not become dye coupled to every cell in their vicinity; there are many growth cones, axons, and cell bodies around the injected cell's growth cone and axon well within the reach of its filopodia to which the dMP2 or MP1 are not coupled.

Whereas pioneer neurons tend to couple to specific patterns of unrelated as well as related cells as they establish the early axonal pathways, later neurons whose growth cones follow pioneer pathways (e.g. the G and C neurons, as described in the next section) tend to couple predominantly to specific groups of related neurons. Whether or not the coupling by the pioneers is involved in pathfinding, it strongly suggests a specific process of cell-to-cell recognition; growth cones and their filopodia contact many cells in their environment, but only become coupled to a specific subset of them.

DIVERGENT CHOICES BY FOLLOWER GROWTH CONES

In this paper we describe two types of pathfinding: that done by pioneer growth cones while establishing axonal pathways and that done by later growth cones while following axonal pathways. To study the second, we set out to find a group of related cells that started following the same pathway, were confronted with a choice of pathways, and then made cell-specific choices and differentiated into morphologically distinct identified neurons. Because of their high degree of accessibility from birth to maturation, we chose the first six progeny of NB 7-4 (Fig. 4), and in particular the two identified neurons G and C (Raper and Goodman, 1981b; Raper, Bastiani and Goodman, 1983a, b). Neuroblast 7-4 gives rise to about 100 progeny. From its first cell division arises a ganglion mother cell that divides into two neurons, Q1 and Q2. Q1 pioneers the first axonal pathway across the posterior commissure, and Q2 follows on its pathway. From the second division of NB 7-4 arises a ganglion mother cell that divides into two cells, one of which becomes interneuron G and the other interneuron C as shown in Fig. 2. Fortunately, these two identified neurons have been studied in Keir Pearson's laboratory (Pearson et al., 1980; Pearson and Robertson, 1981) and thus much is known about their morphology and synaptic connections in the adult grasshopper. The differences between these two neurons are of utmost behavioral importance; for example, the C neuron (of the mesothoracic or T2 segment) is involved in initiating the jump behavior and makes very strong synaptic connections onto extensor (FETi) and flexor (FlTi) motorneurons of the metathoracic (T3) jumping leg (Fig. 2C). The G neuron on the other hand makes only a weak synaptic connection onto the extensor motorneuron. The G neuron also synapses on the C neuron, but not vice versa. The morphologies of the two sibling cells have certain similarities, yet striking differences as well. The large axon of the G neuron runs anteriorly to the brain in the lateral portion of the ventral nerve cord; its small axon runs posteriorly to the next segment in a more medial portion of the nerve cord. The large axon of the C neuron runs posteriorly to the T3 segment in the lateral portion of the ventral nerve cord. The G neuron's dendrites are lateral and omega-shaped whereas the C neuron's dendrites are more medial and antler-shaped.

How do these cell-specific differences between the G and C neurons arise? The morphological development of both neurons results from a sequential series of specific choices made by their growth cones. Both sibling neurons send growth cones across the midline in the posterior commissure along the pathway pioneered by their earlier siblings Q1 and Q2. The first difference between the two pairs of cells, G and C vs. Q1 and Q2, is when the G and C growth cones extend across the medial longitudinal pathway on which the Q1 and Q2 growth cones got off. The first difference between the two sibling cells G and C is when they make divergent choices along a lateral axonal pathway on the contralateral side. The growth cone of the G neuron turns anteriorly while the growth cone of the C neuron turns posteriorly (the small posterior axon of the G neuron arises several days later from a secondary growth cone). The growth cones of both cells continue to make cell-specific choices as the cells develop their distinctive axonal and dendritic branching patterns and synaptic connections. Interestingly, the next pair of progeny from NB 7-4, cells '5' and '6', also follow the same pathway across the posterior commissure. When they reach the other side, they turn anteriorly on yet a different longitudinal pathway than that followed by Q1 and Q2 or by G and C. Our working hypothesis is that the entire sequence of choices made by the G and C growth cones, from their initial outgrowth to their final synaptic connections, is likely to involve similar cellular and molecular mechanisms. We have studied the first divergent choices because they are the most accessible. They occur early in development when the cellular enviroment and axonal pathways can be characterized and manipulated with relative ease.

G's growth cone reaches the contralateral side about 39% of development and C's reaches the same location about 40% (Fig. 10). On both the ipsilateral and con-tralateral sides of the ganglion, the G growth cone is confronted with several different longitudinal pathways. It grows past the ipsilateral and contralateral medial pathways (pioneered by the dMP2 and MP1) on which the Q1 and Q2 got off and

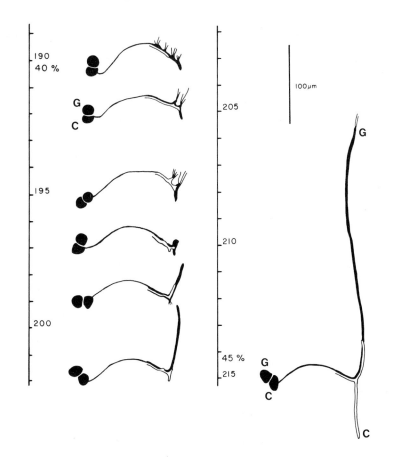

Fig. 10. Camera lucida drawings of G and C growth cones based on Lucifer Yellow injections at different times of development. Time line shows G growth cone making choice and extending anteriorly, and C growth cone just beginning to extend posteriorly.

extended posteriorly; it grows laterally to a different group of longitudinal pathways. In Nomarski optics we see at least three different longitudinal pathways in the vicinity of the G growth cone. The G growth cone often stops at this choice point for 6–10 h, and then elongates anteriorly along the most lateral longitudinal pathway (Fig. 10). While the G growth cone is at the choice point, it extends profuse tufts of filopodia (from 'active sites') in both the anterior and posterior directions radiating over several longitudinal pathways and many other axons. Before it begins to elongate anteriorly from one active site along its chosen pathway, other active sites often become quiescent and lose their tufts of filopodia.

The C growth cone arrives at the choice point several hours after the G growth cone and often assumes a very similar shape and position to G's with one major exception; G's growth cone is just ventral to the longitudinal axonal pathways while C's growth cone is immediately ventral to G's. For about 10 hours, C's growth cone waits at the choice point. For the next 10 hours, C's growth cone slowly elongates both anteriorly and posteriorly along the same axonal pathway that G chose to grow anteriorly on. Finally C's growth cone stops growing anteriorly and rapidly grows posteriorly.

298

This lateral pathway (called longitudinal pathway 3 or LP 3) upon which G and C make their divergent choices is formed by the axons of four cells (Fig. 11): A1, A2, P1, and P2. About the time that the G growth cone reaches the contralateral side of the ganglion, this lateral pathway is formed just under the basement membrane by the single growth cone of Al extending anteriorly, and the single growth cone of P1 extending posteriorly; their siblings follow closely behind them. These two pairs of cells grow in opposite directions along the basement membrane and meet at about the midpoint of the segment (Fig. 11); A1 appears to grow faster than P1 in this area. They continue growing past each other while fasciculating and forming a discrete axon bundle. By penetrating these growth cones and axons with microelectrodes and injecting them with Lucifer Yellow, we have revealed the identities of these cells and the time course of their growth. The A1 and A2 cells (which appear to be siblings) have their cell bodies in the next posterior segment on the contralateral side to the pathway they establish. The P1 and P2 cells (which also appear to be siblings) have their cell bodies in the same segment and on the same side as the lateral pathway they help to pioneer (Fig. 11). Thus, the lateral axonal pathway (LP 3) is initially formed by the axons of these four neurons originating in different segments and on different sides of the midline.

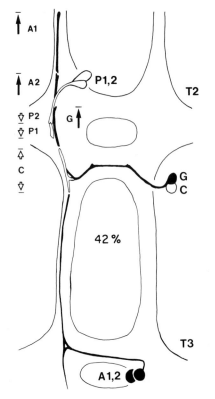

Fig. 11. Camera lucida drawings of cells in longitudinal pathway 3 (LP 3) based on intracellular injections of their axons (A1, A2, P1, and P2) and cell bodies (G, C) with Lucifer Yellow. The cell bodies of A1 and A2 are contralateral to the pathway in the next most posterior segment; the cell bodies of P1 and P2 are ipsilateral in the same segment as the pathway they help establish. Arrows mark direction of growth cone and lines in front of arrows mark extent of growth cone.

As the G and C growth cones make their divergent choices, they always fasciculate within the axon bundle formed by A1, A2, P1, and P2. There is a striking correlation concerning the G and C growth cones and the A and P axons. The arrival and departure times precisely correlate, in that the G growth cone turns anteriorly just behind the A1 and A2 axons, and the C growth cone waits and finally turns posteriorly just behind the P1 and P2 axons (Figs. 12 and 13). The G growth cone appears to follow A1 and A2 (Fig. 12), and the C growth cone appears to follow P1 and P2 (Fig. 13).

We have filled the G neuron with HRP and identified its axon and growth cone within this lateral bundle in electron micrographs (Raper, Bastiani and Goodman, 1983a, b). These cross sections confirm our data from Nomarski observations and dye injections, namely, that there are only four other axons in the bundle (A1, A2, P1, and P2) when G and C make their cell-specific choices. In time, many other axons will join this bundle.

These results lead us to suggest that the A1, A2, P1 and P2 axons are the 'guide fibers' for the G and C growth cones. We thus suggest the 'labeled pathways' hypothesis whereby individual bundles or subsets of axons with a bundle are labeled, and individual growth cones are determined to make cell-specific choices of which label to follow (this hypothesis is described in detail in the next section). We can test this hypothesis with G and C by determining if G and C make their appropriate choices in the absence of these identified axonal processes (A1, A2, P1, and P2).

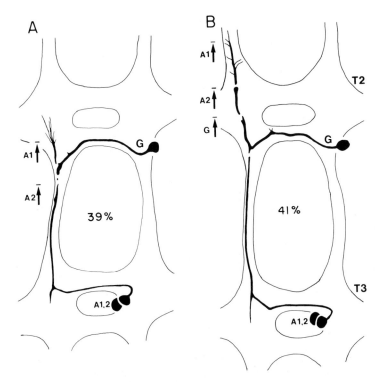

Fig. 12. Camera lucida drawings of A1, A2, and G cells showing G growth cone following A1 and A2 anteriorly in longitudinal pathway 3.

300

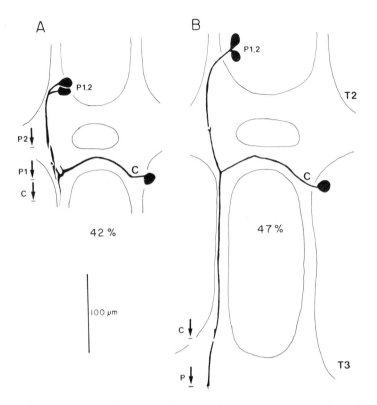

Fig. 13. Camera lucida drawings of P1, P2, and C cells showing C growth cone following P1 and P2 posteriorly in longitudinal pathway 3.

We would like to know when G and C become individually determined, that is, when they become committed to their cell-specific fates. One possibility is that their cell division is unequal such that they receive different determinants according to their mitotic ancestry. Alternatively, they may be equivalent cells at birth that achieve their neuronal specificity by some form of cellular interaction at a later time. For example, the cell that ultimately becomes G always sends out its growth cone first. This event might result from, or cause, some cellular interaction that uniquely determines the cells. On the other hand, the cells may remain equivalent until they reach the choice point. Here G's growth cone might win some competitive interaction because it arrives first and acquires a more desired position. We plan to test when G and C become individually determined by killing either cell at various times after their birth but before their divergent choices, or by delaying or impairing G's growth cone and thus allowing C to reach the choice point first.

THE 'LABELED PATHWAYS' HYPOTHESIS

No matter when G and C become individually determined, it is clear that they ultimately are confronted with several possible axonal pathways and invariably make divergent and specific choices. The G and C growth cones spread out over several pathways and extend filopodia over their surfaces. The 'labeled pathways' hypothesis suggests that they are sampling the pathways in search of guidance cues; these cues are likely to be specific cell surface molecules that label the pathways. The behavior of the growth cones suggests that the different pathways must be differentially labeled.

Thus, our observations on pathfinding by neuronal growth cones in the grasshopper embryo lead us to suggest the 'labeled pathways' hypothesis. This notion is not particularly new, in that it is compatible with previous results and in agreement with previous theories. Rather, it shifts the emphasis from passive guidance mechanisms to active guidance mechanisms and suggests specific experimental tests.

Previous studies on vertebrate motorneurons (Lance-Jones and Landmesser, 1980a, b), optic axons (Constantine-Paton and Capranica, 1975, 1976; Katz and Lasek, 1979), and Mauthner axons (Katz and Lasek, 1981), and on insect sensory axons (Ghysen and Janson, 1980; Anderson, in preparation), all conclude that surgically or genetically transplanted axons find and grow in their appropriate axon pathway. Singer et al. (1979) write:

"In addition to providing specific highways . . . the blueprint hypothesis implies that individual axons 'recognize' and follow particular itineraries even when challenged by multiple highways."

Katz and Lasek (1981), noting that the transplanted Mauthner axons bypass target areas where their neighboring host axons stop and synapse specifically, suggest that different axons can have different responses to the same environment and thus show ". . . differential recognition of specific environmental cues".

In *Drosophila*, Ghysen and Janson (1980) have used genetically transplanted axons to suggest the presence of labeled guides. Normally, the mesothoracic segment has a pair of wings and the metathoracic segment a pair of halteres. Distal campaniform sensilla from the wild type wing enter the mesothoracic segment and take specific pathways throughout the CNS. When the metathoracic halteres are transformed into wings in the mutant *bx pbx* (bithorax postbithorax), homeotic campaniform sensilla differentiate in the transformed segment. The axonal projection established by the homeotic axons, which enter the CNS in the metathoracic segment, is essentially identical to the normal projection from the mesothoracic wing neurons. The authors note that the homeotic axons grow along the appropriate pathway and display the normal branching and suggest that the growing axons recognize "a specific trail" which preexisted in the central nervous system.

Thus, the previous studies on vertebrate and invertebrate neurons lead to the notion that growth cones specifically search for and follow labeled axon tracts. Our studies on pathfinding by neuronal growth cones in grasshopper embryos has led to this same notion, that of 'labeled pathways'.

The 'labeled pathways' hypothesis states:

(i) that pioneer neurons establish stereotyped axonal pathways;

(ii) that these axonal pathways are differentially marked, most likely on their cell surfaces; and

(iii) that later growth cones are differentially determined in their ability to make specific choices of which labeled pathway to follow.

This hypothesis includes the notion that filopodia are actively involved in sampling the environment. The hypothesis does not address the issue of how pioneer growth cones navigate in an axonless environment. Here we speculate that surface interactions and/or intercellular coupling to 'landmark' cells may be important, as may polarity information on the basement membrane or elsewhere in their environment.

What appeals to us about the 'labeled pathways' hypothesis is that it is explicit. And what appeals to us about the grasshopper embryo as an experimental system is that this hypothesis can be tested and refined at the level of individually identified neurons, their growth cones, the axonal pathways they choose amongst, and the molecules that label their surfaces.

THE I-5 MONOCLONAL ANTIBODY

One of our goals in making monoclonal antibodies to grasshopper neurons, is to find developmentally important molecules involved in pathway selection by growth cones. Ideally, we would like to uncover the 'labels', be they associated with or secreted by the cell surface, or intracellular. This goal is actually part of our overall attempt to produce cell determination markers and cell interaction markers. By cell determination markers, we mean antibodies which specifically recognize neuronal precursor cells, subsets or individual precursor cells, or all of the members or specific subsets of individual neuroblast families. Here we would like to determine if there are cell lineage markers, if subsets of progeny share certain determinants, and if and when individual precursor cells and individual identified neurons acquire their cell-specific determinants. By cell interaction markers, we mean antibodies which specifically recognize molecules of potential developmental importance in cell inter-actions before axonogenesis, as guidance information for specific cell migrations, and as guidance information for growth cone navigation. Here we would like to deter-mine if there are cell-surface or intracellular markers indicative of the specific and divergent choices made by pioneer and follower growth cones.

One of the monoclonal antibodies we have produced thus far, called I-5, shows interesting patterns of cellular specificity early in neurogenesis and may be recogniz-ing an antigen of developmental importance (Chang et al., 1981; Chang, Ho, and Goodman, in preparation). At the very least, it is a powerful cell determination marker and histological tool. Staining of the embryo by the I-5 antibody first appears on many of the central (Fig. 7A) and peripheral (Fig. 6) pioneer neurons. The pioneer cell bodies in the periphery stain shortly after their final cell division; subsequently their growth cones and axonal processes stain (Fig. 6). With time, the cell body staining declines whereas the processes remain darkly stained. The antibody stains many other neurons in the CNS in addition to the pioneers. However, it does not stain all neurons, nor do all neurons that stain appear equally as dark (using an HRP-labeled second antibody). Rather, the antibody shows striking specificity. Of the central pioneers, for example, certain ones consistently stain darker than others. We have already mentioned that the vMP2 stains darkly while the dMP2 and MP1 stain lightly from embryo to embryo and segment to segment. The cell-specific difference in staining between the vMP2 and dMP2 appears before their growth cones emerge and continues to be expressed in their growth cones and axons. Many later developing neurons do not stain at all. Particular bundles of axons stain darkly. For example, in each abdominal segment there are two peripheral nerves: the dorsal nerve and the ventral nerve. Many axons in the dorsal nerve stain darkly whereas very few axons in the ventral nerve stain at all. The antibody also selectively stains some non-neuronal cells. For example, certain large mesodermal cells and a thin muscle over the segmental ganglia stain with the antibody, whereas mesodermal cells in general do not.

We are presently investigating both the molecular nature of the I-5 antigen and its subcellular localization. We are also pursuing the antibody in embryo culture to ascertain the functional importance of the antigen. Because it stains a selective subset of neurons, and in particular, a selective subset of axons and bundles in the embryo, it is of potential developmental importance. We are producing more monoclonal antibodies in the hope of finding more molecules of potential developmental importance. We already have several other antibodies which show interesting patterns of specificity in early embryos.

Our hope is that in grasshopper embryos we will be able to describe the complete cellular environment in which particular growth cones make their cell-specific choices, uncover the cellular rules underlying this specific pathfinding by manipulating the cellular environment, and identify the biochemical cues which are the molecular correlates of these pathfinding rules. The monoclonal antibody approach is one way for us to identify these biochemical cues.

ACKNOWLEDGEMENTS

We thank Michael Bastiani for help with the electron microscopy of the 'G' growth cone and its axonal pathway, and Paul Taghert for help with the characterization of the I-5 antibody in the adult nervous system. This work was supported by grants from the NSF, McKnight Foundation, and Sloan Foundation to C.S.G., and by a NIH Postdoctoral Fellowship to J.A.R. Support was also provided by institutional grants from the American Cancer Society and the NIH.

REFERENCES

Bate, C.M. (1976a) Embryogenesis of an insect nervous system. I. A map of the thoracic and abdominal neuroblasts in *Locusta migratoria. J. Embryol. exp. Morph.* 35: 107–123.

Bate, C.M. (1976b) Pioneer neurones in an insect embryo. *Nature (Lond.)*, 260: 54–56.

Bate, C.M. and Grunewald, E.B. (1981) Embryogenesis of an insect nervous system. II. A second class of neuron precursor cells and the origin of the intersegmental connectives. *J. Embryol. exp. Morph.*, 61: 317–330.

Chang, S., Ho, R., Raper, J.A. and Goodman, C.S. (1981) A monoclonal antibody which stains pioneer neurons and early axonal pathways in grasshopper embryos. *Soc. Neurosci. Abstr.*, 7: 347.

Constantine-Paton, M. and Capranica, R.P. (1975) Central projection of optic tract from translocated eyes in the leopard frog (*Rana pipiens*). *Science*, 189: 480–482.

Constantine-Paton, M. and Capranica, R.P. (1976) Axonal guidance of developing optic nerves in the frog. I. Anatomy of the projection from transplanted eye primordia. *J. comp. Neurol.*, 170: 17–32.

Ghysen, A. and Janson, R. (1980) Sensory pathways in Drosophila central nervous system. In O. Siddiqi, P. Babu, L.M. Hall and J.C. Hall (Eds.), *Development and Neurobiology of Drosophila*, Plenum Press, New York.

Goodman, C.S. (1981) Embryonic development of identified neurons in the grasshopper, In N.C. Spitzer (Ed.), *Neuronal Development*. Plenum Press, New York.

Goodman, C.S. and Ridge, K.A. (1980) Development of an identified neuron after removal of its peripheral targets in grasshopper embryos cultured in vitro. *Soc. Neurosci. Abstr.*, 6: 495.

304

Goodman, C.S. and Spitzer, N.C. (1979) Embryonic development of identified neurones: differentiation from neuroblast to neurone. *Nature (Lond.)*, 280: 208–214.

Goodman, C.S., O'Shea, M., McCaman, R.E. and Spitzer, N.C. (1979) Embryonic development of identified neurons: temporal pattern of morphological and biochemical differentiation. *Science*, 204: 1219–1222.

Goodman, C.S., Bate, M. and Spitzer, N.C. (1981) Embryonic development of identified neurons: origin and transformation of the H cell. *J. Neurosci.*, 1: 94–102.

Harrison, R.G. (1910) The outgrowth of the nerve fiber as a mode of protoplasmic movement. *J. exp. Zool.*, 9: 787–846.

Ho, R.K. and Goodman, C.S. (1982) Peripheral pathways are pioneered by an array of central and peripheral neurones in grasshopper embryos. *Nature (Lond.)*, 297: 404–406.

Ho, R., Chang, S. and Goodman, C.S. (1981) Monoclonal antibodies reveal the development of peripheral pioneer neurons and axonal pathways in grasshopper embryos. *Soc. Neurosci. Abstr.*, 7: 348.

Katz, M.J. and Lasek, R.J. (1979) Substrate pathways which guide growing axons in *Xenopus embryos. J. comp. Neurol.*, 183: 817–832.

Katz, M.J. and Lasek, R.J. (1981) Substrate pathways demonstrated by transplanted Mauthner axons. *J. comp. Neurol.*, 195: 627–641.

Keshishian, H. (1980) The origin and morphogenesis of pioneer neurons in the grasshopper metathoracic leg. *Develop. Biol.*, 80: 388–397.

Lance-Jones, C. and Landmesser, L. (1980a) Motoneurone projection patterns in embryonic chick limbs following partial deletions of the spinal cord. *J. Physiol. (Lond.)*, 302: 559–580.

Lance-Jones, C. and Landmesser, L. (1980b) Motoneurone projection patterns in the chick hind limb following early partial reversals of the spinal cord. *J. Physiol. (Lond.)*, 302: 581–602.

Pearson, K.G. and Robertson, M. (1981) Interneurons coactivating hindleg flexor and extensor motoneurons in the locust: their role in the jump. *J. Neurophysiol.*, in press.

Pearson, K.G., Heitler, W.J. and Steeves, J.D. (1980) Triggering of locust jump by multimodal inhibitory interneurons. *J. Neurophysiol.*, 43: 257–278.

Raper, J.A. and Goodman, C.S. (1981a) Transient dye coupling between developing neurons reveals patterns of intercellular communication during embryogenesis. In *Proc. 6th Symp. Ocular Vis. Dev.*, in press.

Raper, J.A. and Goodman, C.S. (1981b) The growth cones of two identified sibling neurons diverge at a particular choice point during grasshopper embryogenesis. *Soc. Neurosci. Abstr.*, 7: 347.

Raper, J.A., Bastiani, M.J. and Goodman, C.S. (1983a and b) Pathfinding by neuronal growth cones in grasshopper embryos. I. Divergent choices made by the growth cones of sibling neurons. *J. Neurosci.*, in press. II. Selective fasciculation onto specific axonal pathways. *J. Neurosci.*, in press.

Shankland, M., Goodman, C.S. and Bentley, D. (1981) An insect interneuron deprived of sensory innervation during its embryogenesis does not form the normal complement of dendritic branches. *Soc. Neurosci. Abstr.*, 7: 3.

Singer, M., Nordlander, R.H. and Egar, M. (1979) Axonal guidance during embryogenesis and regeneration in the spinal cord of the newt: the blueprint hypothesis of neuronal pathway patterning. *J. comp. Neurol.*, 185: 1–22.

Whitington, P., Bate, M., Seifert, E., Ridge, K.A. and Goodman, C.S. (1982) Survival and differentiation of identified embryonic neurones in the absence of their target muscles. *Science*, 215: 973–975.

Two Mechanisms for the Establishment of Sensory Projections in *Drosophila*

ERIC TEUGELS and ALAIN GHYSEN

Laboratoire de Génétique, Université Libre de Bruxelles, 67, rue des Chevaux,
1640 Rhode-St-Genèse (Belgium)

INTRODUCTION

The function of the nervous system relies on the establishment of specific connections between neurons. In order for the system to achieve a precise pattern of connections, each axon must be able to seek and find its own target, however distant this target may be. The mechanisms which guide axons towards their targets have been investigated in various ways. The approach we follow is to analyse the behavior of ectopic neurons, i.e. neurons which develop at abnormal locations.

We have chosen to examine this problem in insects, which present several distinctive advantages for this study. First, their sensory neurons derive from epidermal cells and remain located at the periphery, right under the epidermis. In the case of sensory bristles, it is therefore relatively easy to fill the underlying neuron simply by pulling the bristle and applying a solution of horseradish peroxidase to the exposed dendrite. Second, the exact arrangement of many sensory structures is strictly determined, and therefore each of these structures, as well as the associated neuron, can be uniquely recognized in all individuals of the same species. The third advantage, which is critical for our purpose, is the existence in various insects (and most notably in *Drosophila*) of a special class of mutations: the homoeotic mutations.

The homoeotic mutations affect the process of development in such a way that one segment, or part of it, is transformed into another segment. Contrary to most developmental mutations, the homoeotic do not seem to be simply disruptive: rather they appear to affect the basic regulatory mechanisms that underly the process of segmental determination. Besides their immense interest for the causal analysis of development, the homoeotic mutations provide us a unique opportunity to manipulate the sensory input to the central nervous system. This is illustrated by the first experiments along that line, which made use of mutants of *Drosophila* that transform the antenna into a leg (Deak, 1976; Stocker et al., 1976). In an elegant study, Deak showed that the chemosensory neurons of this ectopic leg succeed in establishing the connections appropriate for leg neurons, even though their axons enter the central nervous system at a place most unusual for leg neurons (i.e. the brain). Further progress with these mutants required that the course of the axons be visualized within the central nervous system; this has been complicated by the fact that most leg neurons and essentially all antennal neurons are difficult or impossible to fill individually. It is therefore impossible to single out given types of sensory structures for the analysis, and one has to examine the complete projection which includes many hundreds of axons from many types of sensory structures. An extensive study of this projection in normal and transformed antennae has shown that some components of the complex projection are modified when the antenna is replaced by a leg, while others are not (Stocker and Lawrence, 1981). It may be that the components which are not modified come from those neurons which are homologous in antenna and leg, while the new components observed in the mutant come from neurons which develop only on legs. However this important point cannot be settled until we can identify which type of sensory neuron is responsible for each component of the projection.

The other major set of homoeotic mutations in *Drosophila* transform the thoracic and abdominal segments one into another. These mutations are tightly clustered in the genome, where they define a complex locus: the bithorax complex (Lewis, 1978). Mutations in this locus are perfectly suited for our analysis because they yield transformations where the ectopic neurons are relatively easy to fill singly or in small groups. Further, the genetic analysis of the whole complex, as well as of its regulation, is much more advanced than in the case of any other developmental system (Lewis, 1978; Garcia-Bellido and Capdevila, 1979). Much work so far has been devoted to two of the mutations in this complex: bithorax (*bx*) and post-bithorax (*pbx*).

THE *bx pbx* MUTANT: REVIEW

The mutations *bx* and *pbx* transform respectively the anterior and posterior compartments (Garcia-Bellido et al., 1973) of the third thoracic segment (meta-thorax) into their counterpart of the second thoracic segment (mesothorax). In normal flies, the wing, the notum (dorsal part of the thorax) and most of the thoracic box are mesothoracic derivatives, while the metathorax is reduced to a narrow strip of epidermis which carries dorsally small appendages called halteres, and ventrally the pair of third legs. In flies homozygous for the double mutation *bx pbx*, the normal metathorax is extensively transformed into a second mesothorax: these flies have two thoracic boxes and two pairs of wings. Since the adult sensory neurons send their axons towards the central nervous system along pre-existing larval segmental nerves, all axons from the second (homoeotic) mesothorax still enter the central ganglion along the metathoracic nerve, posterior to the mesothoracic nerve which comprises the axons from the first (normal) mesothorax. We will now summarize the conclusions which have been reached by the analysis of the central projection of various normal and homoeotic sensory neurons (Ghysen, 1978, 1980; Palka et al., 1979).

(1) Sensory neurons innervating different types of sensory structures (e.g. mechanosensory bristles and campaniform sensilla) follow very different pathways in the central nervous system even though they enter it as a single bundle.

(2) Sensory neurons that innervate the same type of sense organ in the same region of the mesothorax follow the same pathway.

(3) We can therefore define four classes of mesothoracic sensory neurons, which follow four different pathways in the central nervous system: (A) the bristles on the

notum, (B) the bristles on the wing, (C) the campaniform sensilla on the proximal part of the wing blade, and (D) the campaniform sensilla on the distal part of the wing blade. The difference between A and B, and between C and D, corresponds both to differences in the structural details of the sense organs, and to differences in the developmental compartment in which they arise. We favor the hypothesis that the difference in compartmental identity is responsible for the choice of different δ pathways by neurons innervating similar sense organs (bristles for class A and B neurons, campaniform sensilla for class C and D neurons).

(4) In the mutant, we will call ectopic neurons those that develop on the second (homoeotic) mesothorax. The most remarkable feature of the projection from the ectopic neurons is that it is highly organized and reproducible. Furthermore, for at least two classes (A and D) the ectopic axons establish a projection which overlaps rather exactly the normal projection. This striking behavior led to the hypothesis (Ghysen, 1978) that sensory axons of a given class recognize one among various pre-existing pathways, and are guided along this pathway up to their targets.

It was conceivable that the normal axons, coming from the normal notum and wing, would be used as guides by the ectopic axons (Palka et al., 1979). However in experimental animals where the normal wing is absent, ectopic neurons of class D were still able to establish a normal projection (Ghysen and Janson, 1980). This indicates that the ectopic axons do not merely follow their normal counterparts, but rather both follow a common pre-existing pathway.

These results suggest that, at least for some sensory neurons of *Drosophila*, the recognition of the appropriate pathway plays an essential role in the development of the connectivity; they also show that the choice of which pathway to follow is strictly determined, and depends on the developmental history of the neuron. Similar results based on grafting experiments have since been obtained in the locust (Anderson and Bacon, 1979).

Contrary to neurons of class A and D, class B and C neurons are present not only on the wing but also on the normal metathoracic appendage, the haltere. It appears that, at least in the case of class C, the neurons tend to retain their metathoracic behavior, even though the epidermis surrounding them is extensively transformed to mesothoracic. This may reflect the fact that the mutations do not completely suppress the activity of the genes (Palka and Schubiger, 1980), or the possibility that different genes control the segmental identity of epidermis and of neurons. Support for the latter will be given elsewhere (Ghysen et al., 1983). Whatever the explanation, this resistance of metathoracic neurons to the homoeotic transformation makes them unsuitable for our analysis. However, misrouting experiments involving metathoracic class C neurons (Palka and Schubiger, 1980), as well as another class of metathoracic neurons not present in wings (Ghysen, 1978), suggest that these neurons too are guided within the central nervous system along a pathway that they specifically recognize.

THE *bxd* MUTANT: RESULTS

All neurons examined so far grow long distances within the central nervous system. We will now report the behavior of ectopic neurons which establish short projections. The thoracic ganglion of *Drosophila* comprises all the thoracic and abdominal segmental ganglia fused in a single mass. Dorsally, no sign of seg-

308

mentation remains; ventrally, three pairs of bulgings reveal the presence of the leg association centers, or leg neuromeres (Fig. 1a and b). Most of the leg sensory neurons project into the corresponding neuromere (Fig. 1c). Each leg is covered by about 375 mechanosensory bristles (M-bristles) arranged in proximo-distal or in transverse rows. In addition, each leg bears about 25 thinner, curved bristles. It seems possible that these are chemosensory bristles, and for the sake of nomenclature we will call them C-bristles. We restricted our analysis to the bristles on the tibia (about 150 M-bristles and 10 C-bristles). The projection from the M-bristles usually appears as a string of dots, and extends laterally on both sides of the neuromere so as to form a ring; on the contrary, the axon(s) from each C-bristle is clearly seen as a continuous line which extends ventrally under the neuromere and eventually sends ramifications which bend dorsalwards and enter the mass of the neuromere. The general organisation of M- and C-projections is very similar for the first, second and third legs (Figs. 1d and 2a–e).

The behavior of ectopic leg bristles was studied in the case of a mutant in the bithorax complex, bithoraxoid (*bxd*) (Lewis, 1963). In this mutant, the first abdominal segment is transformed into a metathorax, so that an extra pair of halteres and an extra pair of legs are formed. The halteres remain almost always invaginated inside the body; on the contrary the legs are often everted. We used the mutation in the hemizygous condition (*bxd/Df bx⁻*) so as to enhance the mutant phenotype. In

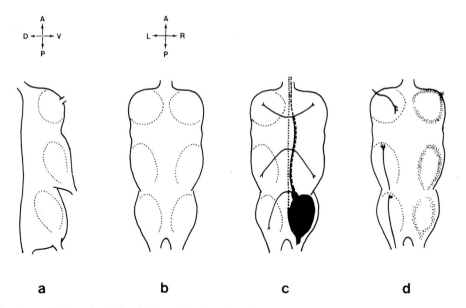

a   **b**   **c**   **d**

Fig. 1. a and b: lateral and dorsal views of the thoracico-abdominal ganglion of *Drosophila*. The dotted lines represent the outlines of the leg neuromeres. A and P, anterior and posterior; D and V, dorsal and ventral; L and R, left and right. c schematic drawing of the sensory projection from the right metathoracic leg. Most of the axons terminate in the corresponding neuromere; only three groups of axons extend to other regions of the central nervous system. One (dots) extends ventrally up to the brain, the second (dashed line) extends along the "ventral ellipse" where it sends medial branches (not shown) and up to the brain, the third (continuous line) send branches in the five other leg neuromeres as well as in the small wing neuromeres (not shown). d: schematic drawing of the projection from the C-bristles (left) and M-bristles (right) of the pro-, meso- and metathoracic legs. In c and d, the outlines of the leg neuromeres are shown on the left half of the ganglion (dotted lines).

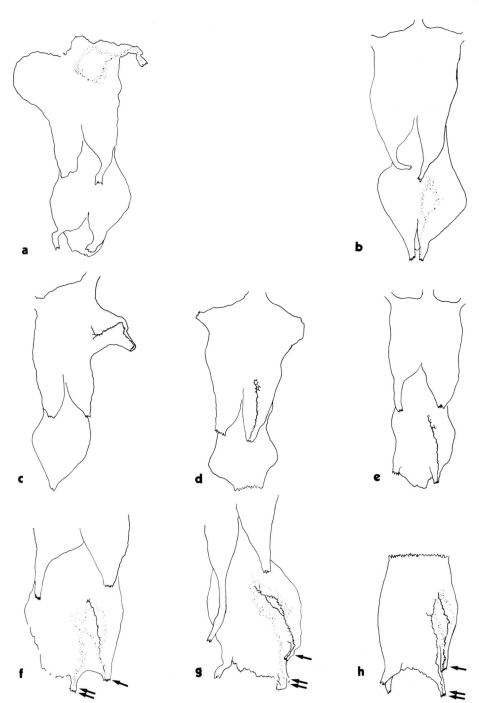

Fig. 2. Projection from leg sensory neurons. a and b: M-neurons on the pro- and metathoracic left legs. c, d and e: C-neurons from pro-, meso- and metathoracic left legs. f, g and h: projection from sensory neurons on the metathoracic and on the homoeotic (abdominal) legs in *bxd* mutants. See text for details. In all cases, the root of the normal metathoracic leg nerve is marked by an arrow, the root of the homoeotic leg nerve is marked by a double arrow.

this combination, the "abdominal" legs are often well developed and may even be very similar to the normal metathoracic legs in size. The nerve from the homoeotic leg enters the central nervous system at the position appropriate for the first abdominal nerve or slightly more ventrally, but in all cases posterior to the root of the normal metathoracic leg nerve (Ghysen and Deak, 1978). We filled M- and C-neurons of the homoeotic leg. Typical results are shown in Fig. 2f–h. In Fig. 2f, we pulled a few M-bristles on the homoeotic leg, as well as M- and C-bristles on the normal metathoracic leg. The homoeotic axons follow a course which is distinct from that of the normal axons, more medial and more dorsal, yet they end up in the same region of the metathoracic leg neuromere. In normal legs, the ring-like projection of the M-bristles actually contains two components: one which extends along the lateral and anterior side of the neuromere, and which originates from bristles of the anterior region of the leg, and the other extending along the posterior and medial sides of the neuromere, which originates from bristles of the posterior region of the leg (Vandervorst and Ghysen, in preparation). In Fig. 2g, we pulled anterior bristles of the normal leg, so that only the lateral and anterior component of the projection is marked. The homoeotic axons again follow a course that is different from the normal one, and they eventually project to the periphery of the meta-thoracic leg neuromere. In Fig. 2h, we pulled a single C-bristle on the homoeotic leg, as well as C- and M-bristles on the normal leg. The course of the homoeotic axon is completely different from the normal path: it proceeds along the dorsal side of the metathoracic leg neuromere, while the normal C-axon extends along the ventral side of the same neuromere; eventually however both normal and homoeotic C-axons terminate in the same region of the neuromere.

DISCUSSION

The results on homoeotic leg neurons clearly suggest that ectopic axons may reach their target by following an abnormal course. The results of the fillings do not prove that the homoeotic axons establish appropriate connections; however this can be tested by using a behavioral assay described elsewhere (Vandervorst and Ghysen, 1980). All seven bxd individuals which have been tested behaviorally gave responses to the stimulation of the M-bristles of the homoeotic leg; in all cases the response was qualitatively the same as that observed when stimulating M-bristles of normal metathoracic legs (P. Vandervorst, pers. commun.). Thus the homoeotic axons not only reach the appropriate region of the metathoracic neuromere, but in addition they make connections with the appropriate interneurons.

The observation that sensory axons may follow alternative pathways and yet end up in the same region of the central nervous system has already been reported in another homoeotic system, where neurons also project to nearby association centers (Stocker, 1982). These results are in striking contrast with the earlier results summarized above. We propose that this difference is related to the fact that leg neurons project locally, while the neurons examined earlier all extend over long distances within the central nervous system. In the case of the M- and C-neurons of the legs, the specification of the target would be enough to develop the appropriate pattern of connectivity: randomly growing growth processes would ensure that a contact with the nearby target be made. More likely, part of the course may be along paths of lesser resistance, or a preferred orientation of growth may be imposed by the layout of previous fibers. Thus the apparent reproducibility of the projection in normal flies would result from the general reproducibility of the development, without need for specific pathway recognition. On the other hand, neurons that have to reach distant targets seem to rely on a specific guidance system. Following the appropriate pathway will allow axons to be guided close enough to their targets, so that target recognition can take place. In the homoeotic mutants, the behavior of the ectopic neurons will depend on whether the neuron projects to local or to distant targets. In the first case the axons are not endowed with the ability to recognize a specific pathway; as long as they enter the central nervous system close enough to a target they may follow any course to reach that target. In the second case the axons will recognize and follow precisely the same pathway as normal axons, irrespective of where they make their first contact with their guide. This proposal is schematized in Fig. 3.

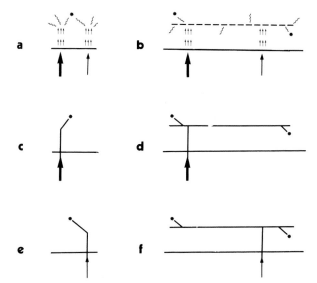

Fig. 3. A possible mechanism for the establishment of sensory projections. In all cases, the horizontal line represents the boundary of the central nervous system (above). The left column describes the situation of neurons that project to nearby targets, the right column corresponds to neurons that project to distant targets. a and b indicate the hypothetical elements used to establish a sensory projection in the central nervous system; c and d show how those elements give rise to the normal projection; and e and f show how the same elements give rise to the ectopic projection. For locally projecting neurons, the normal and ectopic axons follow different paths but end up on the same target (c and e), while for far-reaching neurons, normal and ectopic axons follow precisely the same path (d and f). Symbols: heavy arrow, normal sensory axon joining the ganglion; light arrow, ectopic sensory axon joining the ganglion; group of arrows, path of lesser resistance or preferred orientation; dashed line, specifically recognized pre-existing pathway; wavy lines, exploratory neurites; asterisks, targets.

SUMMARY

In the mutant *bithoraxoid* of *Drosophila*, an extra pair of metathoracic legs develop on the first abdominal segment. We describe the projection of two types of leg sensory neurons in normal and in mutant flies. The neurons of the extra legs do not follow the same path as those of the normal legs, yet they end up in the same region of the central nervous system. This is in contrast with earlier studies which showed that normal and ecotopic axons recognize and follow the same pathway. We propose that this difference is related to the fact that the neurons examined earlier have to travel long distances in the central nervous system, while the leg neurons analyzed in this report project locally.

ACKNOWLEDGEMENTS

This work was carried on under a contract between the Belgian government and the University of Brussels. A.G. is "Chercheur Qualifié" of the Fonds National de la Recherche Scientifique, Belgium. E.T. is a fellow of the IRSIA, Belgium.

REFERENCES

Anderson, H. and Bacon, J. (1979) Developmental determination of neuronal projection patterns from wind sensitive hairs in the locust, *Schistocerca gregaria*. *Develop. Biol.*, 72: 364–373.

Deak, I.I. (1976) Demonstration of sensory neurons in the ecotopic cuticle of *spineless-aristapedia*, a homoeotic mutant of *Drosophila*. *Nature (Lond.)*, 260: 252–254.

Garcia-Bellido, A. and Capdevila, M.P. (1979) Initiation and maintenance of gene activity in a developmental pathway of *Drosophila*. In S. Sobtenly and I. Sussex (Eds.), *The Clonal Analysis of Development*, Academic Press, New York, pp. 3–21.

Garcia-Bellido, A., Ripoll, P. and Morata, G. (1973) Developmental compartmentalization of the wing disc of *Drosophila*. *Nature New Biol.*, 245: 251–253.

Ghysen, A., (1978) Sensory neurons recognize defined pathways in *Drosophila* central nervous system. *Nature (Lond.)*, 274: 869–872.

Ghysen, A. (1980) The projection of sensory neurons in the central nervous system of *Drosophila*: choice of the appropriate pathway. *Develop. Biol.*, 78: 521–541.

Ghysen, A. and Deak, I.I. (1978) Experimental analysis of sensory pathways in *Drosophila*. *Wilhelm Roux' Arch.*, 184: 273–283.

Ghysen, A. and Janson, R. (1980) Sensory pathways in *Drosophila* central nervous system. In O. Siddiqi, P. Babu, L. Hall and J. Hall (Eds.), *Development and Neurobiology of Drosophila*, Plenum Press, New York, pp. 247–261.

Ghysen, A., Janson, R. and Santamaria, P. (1982) Genetic control of sensory pathways in *Drosophila*. Submitted.

Lewis, E.B. (1963) Genes and developmental pathways. *Amer. Zool.*, 3: 33–56.

Lewis, E.B. (1978) A gene complex controlling segmentation in *Drosophila*. *Nature (Lond.)*, 276: 565–570.

Palka, J. and Schubiger, M. (1980) Formation of central patterns by receptor cell axons in *Drosophila*. In O. Siddiqi, P. Babu, L. Hall and J. Hall (Eds.), *Development and Neurobiology of Drosophila*, Plenum Press, New York, pp. 223–246.

Palka, J., Lawrence, P.A. and Hart, H.S. (1979) Neural projection patterns from homoeotic tissue of *Drosophila* studied in *bithorax* mutants and mosaics. *Develop. Biol.*, 69: 549–575.

Stocker, R.F. (1982) Homeotically displaced sensory neurons in the proboscis and antenna of *Drosophilia* project into the same identified brain regions by different pathways. In preparation.

Stocker, R.F. and Lawrence, P.A. (1981) Sensory projections from normal and homoeotically transformed antennae in *Drosophila*. *Develop. Biol.*, 82: 224–237.

Stocker, R.F., Edwards, J.S., Palka, J. and Schubiger, G. (1976) Projection of sensory neurons from a homeotic mutant appendage, *Antennapedia*, in *Drosophila*. *Develop. Biol.*, 52: 210–220.

Vandervorst, P. and Ghysen, A. (1980) Genetic control of sensory connections in *Drosophila*. *Nature (Lond.)*, 286: 65–67.

Structural Analysis of Fiber Organization During Development

GÜNTER RAGER

*Institut für Anatomie und spezielle Embryologie I, rue Gockel,
CH-1700 Fribourg (Switzerland)*

INTRODUCTION

There is a great variety of topographically organized projections or maps in the nervous system of vertebrates both on the afferent and on the efferent side. These projections vary considerably in the degree of their precision from system to system; none of them has an absolute point-to-point connectivity. There may be some variation even from individual to individual in the same system; this is suggested, for example, by the occurrence of squint in children which varies in its degree and probably reflects same variation of the connectivity. Thus, it may be appropriate to use terms like order, precision, retinotopy and topography as fuzzy concepts and to deal with the problem of ordered mapping in a probabilistic way.

The variability of fiber projections will better be understood if the development of these projections is studied and factors are analyzed which may influence or determine the precision of a given map. The information content of the genome is probably not sufficient to determine the formation of these maps directly and in every detail; environmental or epigenetic factors may also contribute to a great extent. Up to now only very little is known about the environmental factors in terms of molecular biology, but our presently available scientific tools enable us to analyze these factors in terms of structure and time or in terms of morphogenesis. The development of an ordered map and the structural and temporal factors contributing to the organization of growing fibers are studied here using the retinotectal projection of the chick as a paradigm.

RESULTS AND DISCUSSION

Fiber organization in the retina

Ganglion cells are first generated in the posterior pole of the eye cup which roughly corresponds to the central area (Kahn, 1974; Rager, 1980a; Fig. 1). From there, generation of cells spreads to the retinal periphery with time. By this pattern of generation each cell is labeled in space and time. This is of importance since it determines the position of each axon in the optic fiber layer if all axons follow the same rules of growth.

[313]

314

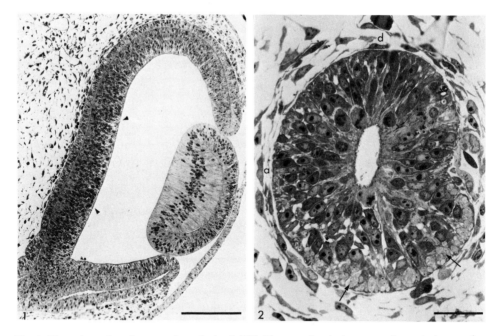

Fig. 1. The embryonic retina on embryonic day 3 (E3). The arrowheads demarcate the central zone where ganglion cells are first generated. Bar = 150 μm.

Fig. 2. Cross-section of the optic stalk on E4. The by far greatest part of the cross-sectional area is filled by neuroepithelial cells. Fiber bundles can be seen only in the ventral and posterior rim (arrows). d, dorsal; v, ventral. Bar = 25 μm.

Although ganglion cells are generated in a continuous and overlapping fashion, zones of newly formed ganglion cells can be distinguished at each developmental day. These zones of incremental growth can be designated as rings in a topological sense.

In the retina and in the optic stalk degenerating profiles of neuroepithelial cells can be seen before fibers arrive (Rager, 1981). Thereafter, like in the mouse (Silver, 1978; Silver and Robb, 1979), intercellular spaces appear which turned out to be oriented in the retina (Krayanek and Goldberg, 1981) and in the optic stalk (Silver and Sidman, 1980). Ganglion cell axons apparently use these intercellular spaces as an opportunity to grow towards the visual centers.

In the retina growing fibers show a regular pattern as observed in Golgi impregnated whole mounts (Rager, 1980a). They grow towards the optic fissure by the shortest possible route. By this pattern of growth neighborhood relations of ganglion cells are maintained in the fiber layer. Initially fibers are less well organized than at later stages of development. This phenomenon is correlated with the extension of the retina away from the optic fissure where the retina is firmly anchored. Thus, it is conceivable that oriented structures are formed by the radial extension of the retina.

The organization of fibers in the plane perpendicular to the optic fiber layer has been investigated with the electron microscope (Rager, 1980a). Sections were made near the central retinal area. The presence and the position of growth cones were used to determine whether later generated ganglion cells which are located more peripherally than central ones are represented in a special sublamina of the optic fiber layer or randomly distributed. We found that growth cones are located preferentially near to the inner limiting membrane. Thus, we concluded that the rings of incremental growth are always next to this membrane. However, it cannot yet be answered whether or not the surface of the inner limiting membrane is a necessary prerequisite for fiber guidance. By the radial growth and by the apposition of new sheets of fibers on the inner limiting membrane retinotopy is maintained in the optic fiber layer of the retina. These rules are valid for all retinal fibers with the exception of the circumferential fibers described by Goldberg and Coulombre (1972).

Fiber organization in the optic nerve

We have analyzed the position and distribution of retinal axons and growth cones in the optic stalk from the time on when fibers begin to invade the optic stalk. A cross-section on embryonic day 4 (E4) shows that the optic stalk is filled with neuroepithelial cells nearly exclusively. Fiber bundles are present only in the ventral and ventro-posterior rim near the pial surface (Fig. 2). Thus, the central retinal area, which is presumably circular, is transformed into a crescent in the optic stalk. One day later (E5) neuroepithelial cells are confined to the dorsal half of the stalk and degenerate to a great extent. The fiber compartment is considerably increased in size. It consists of bundles of thin axons which are located centrally and of small bundles containing mainly growth cones which are located close to the pial surface (Fig. 3). The presence and position of growth cones indicates that the next ring of incremental growth in the retina is transformed into a crescent of fibers which is added peripherally in the nerve. This pattern of innervation is continued during the next few days until the whole nerve is filled with fibers.

It is important to know the final organization of retinal fibers in the optic nerve, when all retinal fibers have grown through the optic nerve and formed synaptic contacts with their target neurons. We, therefore, have analyzed the organization of

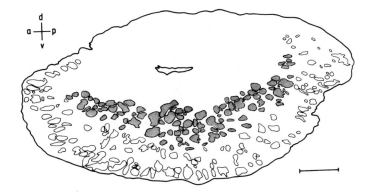

Fig. 3. Cross-section of the optic stalk on E5. The circumference of each fiber bundle was traced on a montage of electron micrographs. Each bundle was analyzed with respect to the presence of growth cones at a higher magnification. The stippled fields represent bundles which nearly exclusively consist of thin axons, the empty fields represent bundles which predominantly consist of growth cones. a, anterior; p, posterior; d, dorsal; v, ventral. Bar = 20 μm.

316

fibers in the middle third of the optic nerve using various morphometric parameters (Rager, 1980a). It turned out that the optic nerve is retinotopically organized thus being similar to the primate and human optic nerve as described by Polyak (1957) and different from the fish optic nerve as described by Scholes (1979). However, no data are yet available on the precision of retinotopy in the chick optic nerve. It has now to be understood, how retinotopy can be reestablished in the nerve when retinal rings have been transformed into crescents in the optic nerve head.

Transformation of the fiber pattern at the optic nerve head

The transformation of retinal rings into crescents in the nerve has to take place in the region of the optic fissure. This raises several problems. (1) By the pattern of intraretinal growth fibers originating in the periphery of the retina are located centrally in the optic fissure. How can this be reconciled with retinotopy in the optic nerve? (2) How are the rings transformed into crescents? (3) Where are the retinal quadrants represented in the crescents of the optic stalk?

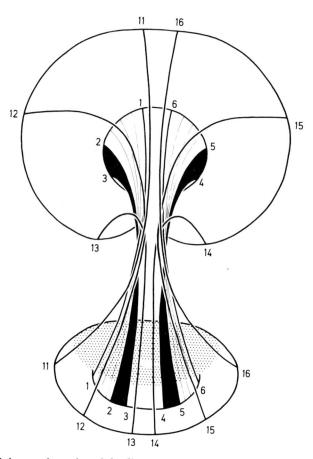

Fig. 4. A model of the transformation of the fiber organization at the optic fissure on E4 and E5. The upper half of the figure shows the central retinal area on E4 and the ring of incremental growth on E5. The lower half shows the corresponding crescents in the optic stalk on E4 and E5. The dorsal part of the optic stalk is filled with neuroepithelial cells (strippled area). The numbers indicate the position of ganglion cells which project to the respective fiber positions in the optic stalk.

In order to solve these problems I should like to propose a model which takes into consideration the following properties of fiber growth: (1) the growth velocity of fibers is constant which means that first fibers arriving at the optic fissure take the best available position which is ventral in the optic stalk and next to the optic fissure according to the local geometry at the transition from the eye cup to the optic stalk (3 and 4 in Fig. 4). Later arriving fibers (1 and 6 in Fig. 4) are positioned more anteriorly and posteriorly, thus forming a crescent; (2) fibers originating from more peripheral regions (11 through 16 in Fig. 4) are located more vitreally in the optic fiber layer of the retina and, therefore, more ventrally in the optic stalk than central retinal fibers, thus forming additional crescents; (3) the loss of neighborhood relations should be minimal; (4) the transformation of the fiber pattern should be as simple and regular as possible; (5) since retinotopy is found in the middle of the optic nerve (Rager, 1980a), the transformation from rings to crescents should allow that retinotopy is reestablished in a simple way in the optic nerve.

These five conditions are fulfilled in the model shown in Fig. 4. All neighborhood relations are eventually maintained except for fibers 1, 6 and 11, 16 which means that the retinal rings are split somewhere dorsally. The dorsally located neuroepithelial cells of the optic nerve degenerate or are transformed into glial cells with time. Thus, the split ends can again become adjacent and the topographical organization of fibers can match that of their perikarya in the retina. The fiber course shown in the model is consistent with our Golgi material (Rager, 1980b). Nevertheless it has to be tested further.

The course of fibers in the visual pathway

Except for the transformation at the optic nerve head and another transformation behind the chiasm, which is not yet fully understood, fibers are running parallel in the whole visual pathway. This ordered course of fibers is not disrupted by fibers coming from the other eye. At the chiasm both tracts penetrate each other forming alternating sheets (Rager, 1980a). The degree of order is very high already at early stages of development.

It is now interesting to know, what is the final outcome when fibers have travelled for such a long distance and passed through several transformations? Is there still order or are fibers widely scattered through the optic nerve so that retinotopic order is essentially lacking (Horton et al., 1979)? To answer this question we injected horseradish peroxidase (HRP) into various tectal sites and followed the retrograde transport. One example of these injections is shown in Fig. 5a and 5b, where the injection site together with the whole fiber tract can be seen on the same section. Although the injection site is large, fibers containing HRP stay together throughout the whole visual pathway and form a clearly confined bundle. In addition, this bundle is in the right position in terms of retinotopy. Thus, it would be perfectly adequate to state that retinal fibers are well ordered in the visual pathway. It is emphasized, however, that order is here understood in a probabilistic sense which allows some variation for any given fiber due to the many local factors influencing its growth. Thus, it can be concluded that the organization of fibers contributes in a high degree to the formation and to the precision of the retinotectal map. Recently there is increasing evidence that retinal projections in other visual systems are also

318

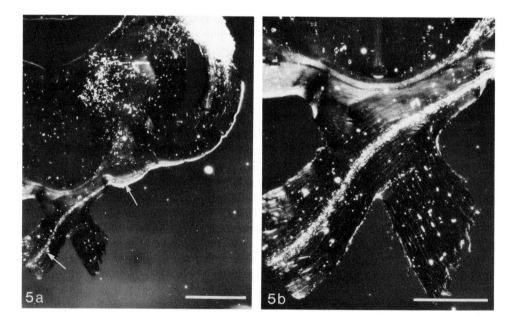

Fig. 5. Retrograde transport of horseradish peroxidase (HRP) injected into the optic tectum on postnatal day 11. Although the injection site is large, a confined bundle of fibers (arrows in a) can be traced back to the retina (low magnification in a, higher magnification of the same section in b). This bundle remains in the right retinotopic position and shows a high degree of order in the visual pathway of the chick. Bars = 2 mm (a) and 1 mm (b).

orderly organized (Aebersold et al., 1981; Scholes, 1979; Rusoff and Easter, 1980; Bunt and Horder, 1981).

CONCLUSION

We have analyzed the development of the retinotectal projection in the chick from the time when first ganglion cells are generated to the developmental stage when fibers start to invade the optic tectum. The invasion of the optic tectum itself has been studied earlier (Rager and Oeynhausen, 1979). From the developmental events in time and space we can infer a number of rules which are followed by growing fibers thus establishing a highly organized and ordered projection. I have to admit, however, that this analysis has to be pursued much further in order to obtain a complete set of developmental rules as far as they can be inferred from structural and temporal phenomena. Three points, however, can certainly be made: (1) epigenetic or environmental factors contribute considerably to the formation of a topographically organized map. Thus, the amount of genetic information necessary for the development of these maps is drastically reduced; (2) the environmental factors influence the formation of the map at every given site of the pathway, not only where pre- and postsynaptic cells interact; (3) it is not only one factor, but a multiplicity of factors each of which can be simple and rather unspecific per se. The complexity of the final map may be built up in the multidimensional space of developmental processes.

REFERENCES

Aebersold, H., Creutzfeldt, O.D., Kuhnt, U. and Sanides, D. (1981) Representation of the visual field in the optic tract and optic chiasma of the cat. *Exp. Brain Res.*, 42: 127–145.

Bunt, S.M. and Horder, T.J. (1981) Evidence for an orderly arrangement of optic axons within the optic nerves of the major non-mammalian vertebrate classes. *J. comp. Neurol.*, in press.

Goldberg, S. and Coulombre, A.J. (1972) Topographical development of the ganglion cell fiber layer in the chick retina. A whole mount study. *J. comp. Neurol.*, 146: 507–518.

Horton, J.C., Greenwood, M.M. and Hubel, D.H. (1979) Non-retinotopic arrangement of fibers in cat optic nerve. *Nature (Lond.)*, 282: 720–722.

Kahn, A.J. (1974) An autoradiographic analysis of the time of appearance of neurons in the developing chick neural retina. *Develop. Biol.*, 38: 30–40.

Krayanek, S. and Goldberg, S. (1981) Oriented extracellular channels and axonal guidance in the embryonic chick retina. *Develop. Biol.*, 84: 41–50.

Polyak, S.L. (1957) *The Vertebrate Visual System*, University of Chicago Press, Chicago.

Rager, G. (1980a) The development of the retinotectal projection in the chicken. *Advanc. Anat. Embryol. Cell Biol.*, 63.

Rager, G. (1980b) Die Ontogenese der retinotopen Projektion. Beobachtung und Reflexion. *Naturwissenschaften*, 67: 280–287.

Rager, G. (1981) The significance of neuronal cell death during the development of the nervous system. In H. Flohr and W. Precht (Eds.), *Lesion Induced Neuronal Plasticity in Sensorimotor Systems*, Springer, Berlin, pp. 3–12.

Rager, G. and Oeynhausen, B. von. (1979) Ingrowth and ramification of retinal fibers in the developing optic tectum of the chick embryo. *Exp. Brain Res.*, 35: 213–227.

Rusoff, A.C. and Easter, S.S. (1980) Order in the optic nerve of goldfish. *Science*, 208: 311–312.

Scholes, J.H. (1979) Nerve fiber topography in the retinal projection to the tectum. *Nature (Lond.)*, 278: 620–624.

Silver, J. (1978) Cell death during development of the nervous system. In M. Jacobson (Ed.), *Development of Sensory Systems, Handbook of Sensory Physiology, Vol 9*. pp. 419–436.

Silver, J. and Robb, R.M. (1979) Studies on the development of the eye cup and optic nerve in normal mice and in mutants with congenital optic aplasia. *Develop. Biol.*, 68: 175–190.

Silver, J. and Sidman, R.L. (1980) A mechanism for the guidance and topographic patterning of retinal ganglion cell axons. *J. comp. Neurol.*, 189: 101–111.

The Role of Fiber Ordering and Axon Collateralization in the Formation of Topographic Projections

KEVAN A.C. MARTIN and V. HUGH PERRY

Department of Experimental Psychology, South Parks Road, Oxford, OX1 3UD (U.K.)

INTRODUCTION

One of the most prominent features of the brain and spinal cord is the ubiquity of topographically ordered projections. The investigation and demonstration of these ordered projections has been a preoccupation of much of the physiological and anatomical investigations of the last three decades. This work has been primarily concerned with sensory projections, because of their relative ease of analysis, although recently progress has been made with the demonstration that motor outputs are also mapped (Murphy et al., 1978). Most of this work has been concerned to demonstrate the existence of topographically ordered projections with a view to delineating the existence of different subdivisions of nuclei or of the neocortex, each division of which may be concerned with some unique functional analysis. The actual investigation of the functional role of these multiple topographic projections has lagged behind the demonstration of their existence, although there has been no shortage of speculation as to their significance (Allman, 1977; Cowey, 1981; Merzenich and Kaas, 1980; Zeki, 1978). It is not our intention here to add further to this speculation, but rather to attempt to examine the factors which could lead to the formation of ordered projections.

The experimental investigation of the rules governing the formation of ordered projections or 'maps' has almost exclusively been the province of those working on the retinotectal system, of lower vertebrates in particular. We will briefly review the data on some major systems in mammals where the relationship between the ordering of the fibers in various nerves and tracts and the ordering of their terminals has been investigated. Unfortunately much of the evidence relies on observations made in the adult whereas ideally one would like to know the relationship existing during development. However, there are reasons which we will discuss, which makes the argument from the adult situation to the developmental one more tenable. The factors responsible for the formation of the peripheral motor system have recently been discussed by Horder (1978) and Landmesser (1980) and will not be considered here. We will thus concentrate specifically on sensory projections.

[321]

SOMATIC AFFERENT PATHS

Although there are variations between species in the organization of the spinal cord the ascending tracts can be divided into three main systems, the anterolateral quadrant pathways, the dorsolateral quadrant pathways and the dorsal funiculi. It is the last named of these which has been most studied with regard to the topography of its fibers and their connections. Most of the fibers in the dorsal funiculi are collaterals of the cells of the dorsal root ganglia, but only 25% of these fibers terminate in the gracile and cuneate nuclei, the remainder entering the gray matter of the cord above and below their entry points (Rethelyi and Szentagothai, 1973). The organization of the fasciculus gracilis has been studied anatomically and electrophysiologically by Whitsel et al. (1970), using cats and new world monkeys. The anatomical studies reveal that at the lumbar levels of the cord the fibers from individual roots, i.e. those supplying a single dermatome, remain segregated, but at cervical levels fibers of neighboring dermatomes overlap extensively. Similar findings have been reported for the old world monkey (Walker and Weaver, 1942; Carpenter et al., 1968).

Fibers are added laterally from successive dorsal roots as they ascend the cord. Within each dorsal root is contained a somatotopic map of the skin surface innervated by that root (Wall, 1960; Werner and Whitsel, 1967). Thus if a single root is partially transected, a degeneration free zone can be traced from the lumbar to the cervical regions of the cord (Whitsel et al., 1970). The neighborhood relations of the fibers within each root are therefore preserved. The progressive termination of fibers conveying deep sensation and the slowly adapting cutaneous fibers as one ascends from the lumbar to the cervical levels may in part be responsible for the increased overlap of the dermatomal projection. The net result of these fiber rearrangements is that cutaneous fibers which remain in the cervical levels of the cord are arranged in the same topographical order as that found in the nuclei of the dorsal funiculi (Walker and Weaver, 1942, Ferraro and Barrera, 1935, Hand, 1966; Gordon and Paine, 1960; Kruger et al., 1961). This same ordering appears to be preserved in the fiber projection from the dorsal column nuclei which form the medial lemniscus (Ferraro and Barrera, 1935; Walker, 1937; Werner and Whitsel, 1967). Most fibers in the medial lemniscus cross the midline at the level of the medulla. As they ascend further to their termination sites in nucleus ventralis posterior lateralis, the fibers rotate so that those which were originally placed ventrolaterally come to occupy a lateral position while the fibers which were dorsolateral come to occupy medial positions. They terminate in this order in the nucleus (Poggio and Mountcastle, 1963).

Although the fiber paths of the other main ascending spinal cord tracts have not been examined in such detail, the presence of somatotopic maps for the spinocervical tract neurons (Brown et al., 1980) and for the spinothalamic tract (Walker, 1942; Walker and Weaver, 1943; Morin et al., 1951) suggests that similar principles may be responsible for the organization of all three major somatosensory paths.

SPECIAL SOMATIC AFFERENTS: THE COCHLEAR NERVE

The cells which give rise to the cochlear nerve are positioned along the bony spiral lamina and collectively form the spiral ganglion. From the base to the apex of the Organ of Corti the ganglion cells become optimally stimulated by tones of progressively lower frequency. This tonotopic organization is also reflected in the nerve such that if small lesions are made in the cochlea, a restricted patch of degeneration can be traced along the nerve to restricted terminal locations in the cochlear nuclei (Sando, 1965). The studies of Lorenté de No (1933) show that the fibers of the cochlear nerve bifurcate to distribute their terminals in a highly orderly manner to the anteroventral and posteroventral portions of the cochlear nuclei. This regularity of termination is confirmed by the electrophysiological demonstration of tonotopically organized maps in the nuclei (Rose et al., 1959). Tonotopically organized maps have now been demonstrated at all levels of the auditory pathway (see review by Merzenich and Kaas, 1980).

During the formation of the cochlear spiral the first third of the basal spiral does not show any twisting. The fibers projecting from this portion of the spiral ganglion enter the cochlear nerve laterally and inferiorly and maintain this inferior position to their terminations in the cochlear nuclei and so form the axis of the cochlear nerve (Sando, 1965). Fibers from more apical positions in the ganglion spiral about this axis so that those from the most apical portion of the ganglion make about $1\frac{3}{4}$ turns about the axis formed by the basal fibers. These fiber arrangements are probably brought about during the morphogenesis of the cochlea, although little is known about the outgrowth of the cochlear fibers (see Rubel, 1978 for refs.).

TOPOGRAPHICAL RELATIONS OF THE OLFACTORY BULB EFFERENTS PROJECTING THROUGH THE LATERAL OLFACTORY TRACT (LOT)

In the central projections of the olfactory bulb, most of the mitral cell axons gather in a compact bundle called the lateral olfactory tract (LOT) which then fans out and terminates in the pyriform lobe. Anatomical analysis of the olfactory bulb projections using degeneration methods gave little indication of a topographic organization of the terminal distribution (White, 1965; Powell et al., 1965; Price and Powell, 1971). Shepherd and Haberly (1970) were, however, able to demonstrate a topographical ordering of the projection of the bulb into the LOT by stimulating at various sites in the tract and recording the antidromic evoked potentials in the bulb of the oppossum. Dorsal, ventral and lateral aspects of the bulb were found to project in strips of fibers lying in the dorsal, middle and ventral portions of the LOT. The medial portion of the bulb projected both ventrally and medially. In a later anatomical study Devor (1976) found in the hamster that this organization only applied to the initial portion of the LOT where Shepherd and Haberly (1970) had been stimulating. Fibers within the tract maintained their order for only about 1.5 mm distal to a partial transection of the tract. Lesions placed medially, centrally or laterally resulted in diffuse and homogeneous degeneration through all of the olfactory projection cortex. During development the fibers are seen to grow diffusely from the tract into the olfactory cortex (Schwob and Price, 1978). These findings thus demonstrate a lack of topographical organization of the fiber paths and their final terminations.

324

THE OPTIC NERVE

The visual system has been a focal point of studies of topographic mapping of sensory surfaces for many years. The early studies (reviewed by Horder and Martin, 1978) were content to examine only the relationship between fibers of the optic nerve and their origins in the retina. Of these early studies that of Pick (1896) is the most comprehensive. He found that after examining the cat, rabbit, rat and mouse only the mouse nerve did not show a localized patch of degeneration after a localized retinal lesion. These early studies were later extended to show that the optic fibers terminated in a topographic projection in the lateral geniculate nucleus (LGN; Brouwer and Zeeman, 1926). However, further work showed some disagreement on the ordering of the optic nerve. Lashley (1934) in the rat, Maturana (1960) and Fawcett (1980) in the frog, Hubel and Wiesel (1960) in the squirrel monkey and Horton et al. (1979) in the cat have provided evidence that the nerve is not well ordered. The question of the order in non-mammalian vertebrates has recently been reexamined in teleosts, anurans, urodeles, reptiles and birds by Bunt and Horder (1982). By tracing the course of horseradish peroxidase (HRP) filled fibers after local tectal or retinal applications of HRP they were able to demonstrate a high degree of order in all the species examined. In the frog Bunt and Horder (1982) found a small population of myelinated fibers which were only roughly organized in the nerve and

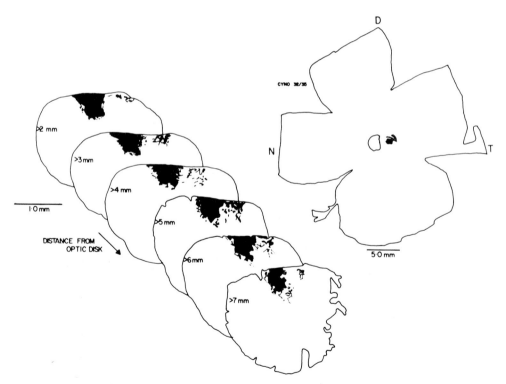

Fig. 1. The results of applying HRP to cut nerve fibers of the macular bundle in the optic nerve of the cynomologous monkey. One main patch and two subsidiary patches of HRP-labeled fibers (shown in black) can be distinguished in the nerve and three corresponding patches of labeled ganglion cells appear in the retina grouped around the foveal pit. D, dorsal; N, nasal; T, temporal.

which may have left the nerve to enter the basal optic nucleus and deep tectal layers (Herrick, 1942).

We have recently completed a similar study of a number of mammalian species. The animals, selected on the basis of different ganglion cell topographies, were old world monkey, sheep, cat, rock hyrax, rabbit and rat. Several methods were used to examine the nerve order. Most commonly the nerve was partially transected some distance from the eye and HRP was applied to the cut ends. Orthograde transport of the HRP revealed the centralwards relationships while the retrograde transport and filling of the retinal ganglion cell bodies revealed the retinal source of the cut fibers (see Figs. 1 and 2).

In other experiments a small cut was made in the nerve behind the eye and the eye was injected with HRP or [³H]proline. The cut fibers remained unfilled and could be traced centralwards to their termination sites. As the fibers approached the chiasm a small amount of local mixing was observed between the labeled and

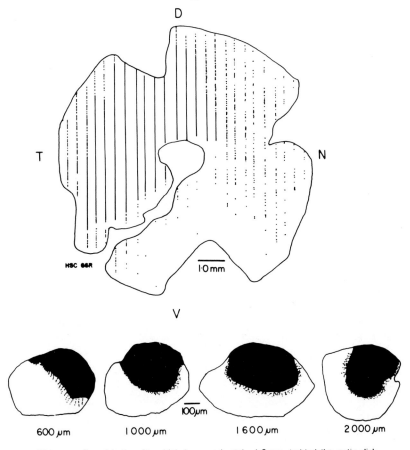

Fig. 2. A scale drawing showing the distribution of ganglion cells in the retina of the rat after an application of HRP to a partial cut in the optic nerve. Using an X–Y plotter, the flat mounted retina was scanned with a bar 250 μm in length and at each point where the bar passed over a cell a dot was placed. The continuous lines thus represent densely labeled regions while a single dot represents a single cell. The labeled bundle of fibers is shown in black on the drawings of coronal sections of the nerve.

unlabeled fibers. All methods showed that in all species neighboring retinal ganglion cells have neighboring axons in the nerve. Electrophysiological recording through the nerve in the monkey, sheep and cat revealed a similar topographic organization. Using similar methods Aebersold et al. (1981) have shown that the cat optic tract is topographically organized and Horder et al. (1979) have shown the mouse optic nerve to be well ordered.

In an attempt to obtain further details on the anatomical precision of the fiber terminations we have made minute iontophoretic injections of HRP into the most superficial layer of the rat tectum. This avoids damage to fibers of passage and the results of one such injection are shown in Fig. 3. The labeled cells are projecting to approximately the correct region of the tectum but there is clearly no 'point-to-point' projection of these small cells.

The main source of discrepancy between these results and those of previous investigators is probably technical. We have traced groups of fibers rather than individual fibers and have shown that although there may be a small proportion of fibers which do not travel in organized arrangements in the nerve, the vast majority of fibers *are* topographically organized.

The projection from the LGN to the primary visual cortex is also arranged in an orderly topographic fashion (Polyak, 1957; Spalding, 1952; Fig. 4). The highly orderly arrangement of the geniculocortical terminations has been well documented (e.g. Polyak, 1933; Daniel and Whitteridge, 1961).

DISCUSSION

The number of studies in which the topography of the projection and the ordering of the fibers has been examined are unfortunately few in number, although the relevant information must have existed in the material which was prepared. We have reviewed only the small number of topographic projections where the data are sufficiently detailed for some conclusion to be drawn. There is some evidence that other topographic projections, for example the projection from the septal nucleus (Mitchell et al., 1981) to the hippocampus and from Deiters nucleus to the spinal cord (Pompeiano and Brodal, 1957) are also innervated by orderly fiber arrangements. The evidence for non-topographic mapping is far more scarce and the olfactory bulb is the only example available where the fiber ordering has been examined in sufficient detail.

When reviewing the literature we had expected to find instances of an orderly termination pattern which was formed from disorderly arrangements of fibers. Some authors have suggested that this might be the situation in the optic nerve (Sperry, 1943; Horton et al., 1979) but our own data and that of others (Aebersold et al., 1981; Horder et al., 1979; Bunt and Horder, 1981) favor the existence of an orderly optic nerve throughout the phyla.

There are difficulties in extrapolating these findings back to the situation in development. However, we feel justified in assuming that if an ordered nerve is found in the adult then this is strongly indicative of orderly outgrowth of the fibers during development. It is possible to imagine mechanisms whereby an initially orderly arrangement of axons could be disrupted after the axons had terminated, by vascularization, glial movement towing fibers and by growth of perineural sheaths.

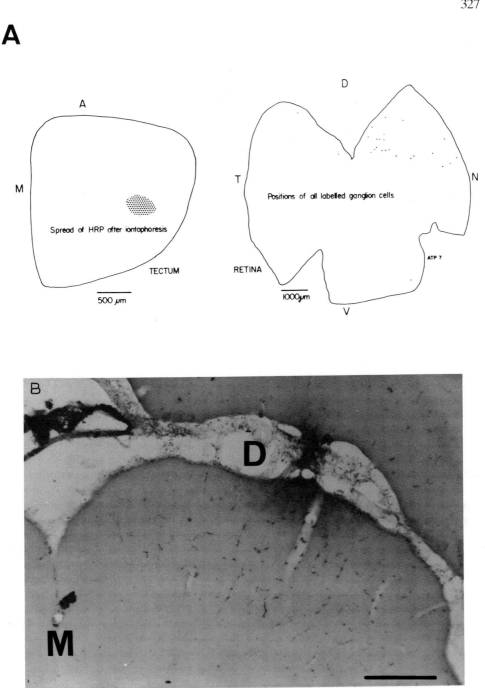

Fig. 3. A: the distribution of 24 retinal ganglion cells labeled after an iontophoretic injection of HRP into the upper one-third of the stratum griseum superficiale of the tectum. The size and position of the injection sites is shown in a dorsal view reconstruction of the tectum. The labeled ganglion cells cover about five times larger area of retina as would have been predicted from electrophysiological recordings. On tectal drawing, A is anterior and M medial. B: a coronal section of the injection site in the tectum. Bar = 500 μm, D, dorsal; M, medial.

328

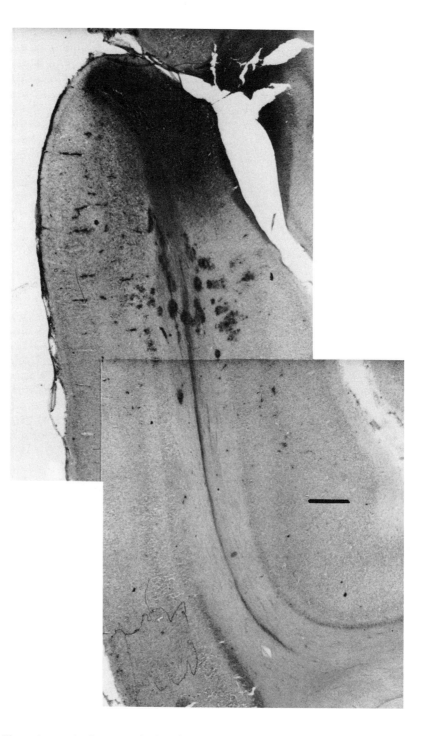

Fig. 4. Photomicrograph of a parasagittal section of the baboon visual cortex in which HRP had been injected into a localized region at the lip of the lunate sulcus. A discrete bundle of fibers can be traced running in the white matter. Bar = 1.0 mm (Unpublished study by K.A.C.M. and H. Kennedy).

Also some of the rotations of the fibers in the tracts (Polyak, 1957; Aebersold et al., 1981) may be accounted for by the morphogenetic movements of the terminal structure after the fibers have grown into it (Rakic, 1977a, b; Kalil, 1978). On the other hand it is difficult to imagine how an initially disorderly outgrowth of fibers could result in an orderly nerve in the adult.

Pathway specificity

If the relationship between the orderliness of the fiber projection and the orderliness of their terminations does turn out to be a consistent one in the light of further work, then it is appropriate to ask what underlying factors may determine this relationship. The orderliness of the fibers paths may indicate the existence of chemoaffinity pathway cues which are followed by the growing fibers (Attardi and Sperry, 1963). Alternatively this orderliness may merely be the reflection of a physical contact guidance (Weiss, 1941; Horder and Martin, 1978) of the growing fibers.

Against the chemoaffinity hypothesis is the evidence that whenever the developing system is perturbed, by for example exchanging eyes (Beazley, 1975), a significant number of fibers are misrouted and often terminate in the 'wrong' hemisphere. Many other examples of aberrant growth during development and regeneration have been reviewed by Horder and Martin (1978).

The problem of aberrant fibers is a serious one for chemospecific guidance since it is difficult to explain how events totally unrelated to the hypothesized specification of the cells can have such a profound effect on the guidance of fibers. If the guidance is largely mechanical in nature then the problem is less severe since the morphogenetic circumstances controlling fiber growth may alter with time or with the experimental manipulations of the kind described. Each fiber will be subject to slightly different mechanical conditions which may result in the misrouting of a small fraction of fibers even during normal development. With the demonstration that in the embryo there exist physical channels (Katz and Lasek, 1981; Nordlander and Singer, 1978; Nordlander et al., 1981; Silver, 1979, 1980; Silver and Sidman, 1980; Singer et al., 1979) which could act a mechanical guides to direct fibers to their termination sites, the argument for a largely mechanical guidance of fibers becomes even more compelling. There may also be an initial outgrowth of fibers analogous to the 'pioneer' fibers seen in arthropods (see Anderson et al., 1980; Bate, 1978) which could direct the growth of later formed axons (Silver, 1980). Thus the topographic organization or lack of it among the fibers in the pathways may simply be the result of the physical constraints on the direction of fiber growth during development.

Chemospecificity models also have difficulty in accounting for the presence of projections in the infant which are far more widely ramified than those found in the adult (Brown et al., 1976; Innocenti et al., 1977; Land and Lund, 1979; Perry and Cowey, 1981), In some systems these so-called 'exuberant' connections (Innocenti et al., 1977) are withdrawn (O'Leary et al., 1981) partially through functional influences (Lund et al., 1978). In other systems (see Cowan, 1973; Clarke and Cowan, 1976) cell death is responsible for increasing the specificity of the innervation. Functional mechanisms may also be responsible for the rearrangement of existing connections throughout development (Keating, 1974).

Target specificity

There is evidence to suggest that target specificity may also be of only a low order in that under conditions where fibers are unable to innervate their normal structures they will readily innervate other available termination sites (Frost, 1980; Lent and Schneider, 1980). This lack of strong target specificity may increase the significance of the mechanisms delivering fibers to the appropriate termination sites since any aberrant routing would result in inappropriate innervation. It may be of significance to note that even when fibers are terminating in completely inappropriate nuclei they still form topographic maps (Frost, 1980; Lent and Schneider, 1980; Sharma, 1981). Unless one assumes that chemospecific cues organizing maps are identical in different terminal regions (in which case the cues are not very specific), it is difficult to account for this form of observation in chemospecific terms.

In regeneration and development the polarity of the map can be experimentally altered (Bunt et al., 1979; Horder and Martin, 1977; Thompson, 1979) which strongly suggests that it is fiber self-ordering which is controlling the map development rather than a lock and key form of specificity. Whether the self-ordering needs to be an active process of recognition between fibers (Cook and Horder, 1977) or whether the existing ordering in the fibers is sufficient cannot yet be determined, although there is some evidence that fibers may terminate on a first-come-first-served basis (Bunt et al., 1978). There is also evidence to show that the time of outgrowth of fibers can determine the form of the fiber order in the nerve (Dawnay, 1979), the spatial arrangement of the terminals (Rager, 1981) and the position of the synapses from different projections on the same neuron (Gottlieb and Cowan, 1972).

The question as to whether the ordering in the fiber tracts is sufficient to account for the precision of the terminal ordering is a difficult one to answer for several reasons. One is that the data one needs are not available because the relationship between the fiber ordering and the ordering of the *terminations* has seldom been examined with sufficient precision. Usually the anatomical order of the fibers is compared with the map obtained by recording from the *post-synaptic* elements onto which the fibers synapse. This could give a deceptive impression of the precision of the terminal order because of functional interactions increasing the precision. For example, the large arbor size of the alpha retinal ganglion cell in the cat (Bowling and Michael, 1980) is not reflected in the map recorded post-synaptically (Sanderson, 1971). Our iontophoretic injection of HRP into the superficial layers of the tectum gave a scatter of retinal ganglion cells five times larger than that expected from the projection determined physiologically (Siminoff et al., 1966).

One of the few studies which has attempted to quantify the relationship between fiber order and order in the terminal field is that of Aebersold et al. (1981) who found that the scatter of receptive fields of fibers recorded in the tract was 2–5 times that found by post-synaptic recording in the LGN (Sanderson, 1975). As they point out, however, this may be an overestimate because of the pick-up range of the electrode, the mechanical displacement of fibers by the electrode, the method of analysing the variance and because the adult order may not be an accurate reflection of the actual order during development. Clearly one requires more precise anatomical analysis of the developmental relationships, perhaps along the lines of the iontophoretic study reported above.

Collaterals

The factors responsible for collateral formation are not well understood. It is possible that neurons have some specific genetic instruction to form a certain number of collaterals. Alternatively the formation of collateral branches and even the individual shapes of the arbors (Brown et al., 1981) may largely be the result of a response to the environment through which the axons are growing. There is evidence from adult studies that one stimulus to form collaterals is the presence of neighboring denervated areas (Liu and Chambers, 1958; Raisman and Field, 1973; Speidel, 1941). Similar stimuli may be present in the embryo where there are initially large uninnervated areas and where multiple innervation through collaterals is common in some systems (Crepel et al., 1976; Schwob and Price, 1978; Brown et al., 1976). One might therefore expect the cells which send their fibers out first to form the most collaterals. These cells may be the large neurons which in many places in the nervous system commence their final divisions before those of smaller neurons (e.g. Lawson et al., 1974: Rakic, 1977b; Forbes and Welt, 1981). Differential outgrowth may account for the differences in laminar termination found between larger and smaller fibers (Ferster and LeVay, 1978; Light and Perl, 1979).

Increasing collateralization is correlated with a decrease in the topographic precision of the terminal map, as for example in the olfactory bulb projection (Devor, 1976), the locus coeruleus projection (Gatter and Powell, 1977) and the projection of the median raphe nucleus (Azmitia and Segal, 1978). In these projections extensive collateralization of the initial fibers may result in the creation of many alternative contact guidance routes for the later growing fibers and so promote the lack of order in the projection. If this is the case then one might expect the ordering of collateralizing projections to be less precise. Whether the paths taken by other fiber groups are affected by the presence of collaterals may depend on the timing of the outgrowth, the number of fibers involved and the extent to which fiber sub-populations remain separate. There is evidence to suggest that different fiber subpopulations traveling in the same tract do tend to segregate (e.g. Aebersold et al., 1981; Light and Perl, 1978), and thus may grow relatively independently in the same gross pathway.

The formation of extensive collateral systems is not a feature of fibers growing along major tracts (Ramón y Cajal, 1960), which may account for the relative precision of the fiber ordering. However, work on the developing visual system has shown that as the optic fibers grow into the diencephalon they send out branchlets into possible termination sites, even if these sites (the medial geniculate nucleus, ventrobasal nucleus and inferior colliculus) do not receive optic projections in the adult (Perry and Cowey, 1981; unpublished observations). The final specificity may be determined by a complex set of competitive interactions between different fiber types and by various functional interactions, perhaps of a kind suggested by Changeux and Danchin (1976).

Mirror image maps

One puzzling feature of multiple topographic projections is that adjacent maps are often mirror symmetrically arranged (Scalia and Fite, 1974; Sanderson, 1975).

332

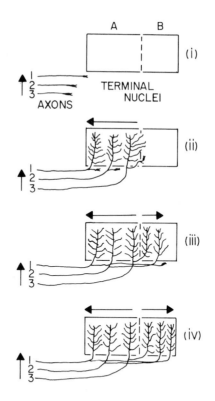

Fig. 5. An hypothetical schema whereby mirror-image maps could be formed in adjacent nuclei by collateralization. In (i), the axons 1, 2, and 3 grow into nucleus A and terminate (ii) on a first-come-first-served basis (iii). Note that fiber 3 can spread into the adjacent nucleus B which it then innervates by collateralization (iii). The remaining fibers 1 and 2 also give off collaterals and innervate nucleus B on a first-come-first-served basis (iv). The arrows show the polarity of the resultant projections. Such a schema may apply to the maps in the LGN and MIN of the cat, for example (see text).

There is evidence to suggest that this mirror imaging is not brought about by specific chemoaffinity cues (Horder and Martin, 1977; Bunt et al., 1978, 1979), but by the pattern of ingrowth of fibers and their interaction with other fiber subpopulations. Collateral growth could account for the mirror image arrangement found in adjacent visual nuclei like the LGN and medial interlaminal nucleus (MIN; Sanderson, 1971). The MIN projection is formed by collaterals of the alpha retinal ganglion cells (Bowling and Michael, 1980).

This could be simply accounted for by supposing that alpha cells grow initially into the LGN in an orderly fashion. The most medial fibers in the LGN would then be adjacent to an uninnervated MIN to which they would send a collateral branch as shown in Fig. 5. Successive orderly addition of collaterals would result in a mirror image collateral projection across the mediolateral dimension of the nucleus, but both maps would have the same anteroposterior ordering. Similar considerations could be applied to mirror image reversals along the rostrocaudal axis (Scalia and Fite, 1974).

CONCLUSIONS

In this paper we have reviewed the evidence showing a relationship between the orderliness of the fiber arrangement in nerves and tracts and the precision of their terminal map. This relationship is what would be expected if the formation of topographic projection is under the control of contact guidance mechanisms rather than chemospecific cues. We have thus emphasized the possible role of physical factors controlling nerve growth and the formation of topographic maps. This is not to deny the existence of any 'active' guidance mechanisms (Bunt et al., 1979) but to suggest that their role is subsidiary. Other mechanisms like cell death, collateral retraction, fiber-fiber interactions and function may have an important role in refining the topography and increasing the specificity of the system.

Our purpose in highlighting the contact guidance aspect of nerve growth is to draw attention to the many gaps in our knowledge about the timing and pattern of fiber growth and the morphogenetic changes which can influence the formation of specific connections. In this regard the study of the adult can be a hindrance rather than a help when attempting to account for the projections formed because one is only looking at the end-product of a complex chain of developmental interactions. However, if it is assumed that all connections are formed through chemoaffinity associations then all other mechanisms are irrelevant. The evidence presented above suggests the opposite.

It is only recently that techniques have become available to demonstrate unequivocally the presence of collateral branches among populations of neurons. The role of collateral development in the formation of topographic projections has been largely unexplored. We have suggested that they may account for the polarity of projections in some nuclei and that they may influence the degree of topographic precision of the system.

The morphogenetic interpretation of the development of topographic projections has many advantages as an explanatory model, as we have tried to indicate. Its principle advantage however, is to generate hypotheses which, when tested, will lead to a greater understanding of the factors controlling neural development.

ACKNOWLEDGEMENTS

Research supported by the M.R.C. Financial assistance from the Dale Fund is gratefully acknowledged by K.A.C.M.

REFERENCES

Aerbersold, H., Creutzfeldt, O.D., Kuhnt, U. and Sanides, D. (1981) Representation of the visual field in the optic tract and the optic chiasma of the cat. *Exp. Brain Res.*, 42: 127–145.

Albus, K. (1975) A quantitative study of the projection area of central visual field in area 17 of the cat 1: precision of the topography. *Exp. Brain Res.*, 24: 159–179.

Allman, J.M. (1977) Evolution of the visual system in early primates. In J.M. Sprague and A.N. Epstein (Eds.), *Progress in Psychobiology and Physiological Psychology, Vol. 7*, Academic Press, New York, pp. 1–53.

334

Anderson, H., Edwards, J.S. and Palka, J. (1980) Developmental neurobiology of invertebrates. *Ann. Rev. Neurosci.*, 3: 97–139.

Attardi, D.G. and Sperry, R.W. (1963) Preferential selection of central pathways by regenerating optic fibers. *Exp. Neurol.*, 7: 46–64.

Azmitia, E.L. and Segal, M. (1978) An autoradiographic analysis of the differential ascending projections of the dorsal and median raphe nuclei in the rat. *J. comp. Neurol.*, 179: 641–668.

Bate, C.M. (1978) Development of sensory systems in Arthropods. In M. Jacobson (Ed.), *Handbook of Sensory Physiology*, Springer, Berlin, pp. 1–53.

Beazley, L.D. (1975) Factors determining decussation at the optic chiasm by developing retinotectal fibers in *Xenopus*. *Exp. Brain Res.*, 23: 491–504.

Bowling, B. and Michael, C.R. (1980) Projection patterns of single physiologically characterized optic tract fibers in cat. *Nature (Lond.)*, 286: 899–902.

Brouwer, B. and Zeeman, W.P.C. (1926) The projection of the retina in the primary optic neuron in the monkey. *Brain*, 49: 1–35.

Brown, A.G., Fyffe, R.E.W., Noble, R., Rose, P.K. and Snow, P.J. (1980) The density distribution and topographical organization of spinocervical tract neurones in the cat. *J. Physiol. (Lond.).*, 300: 409–428.

Brown, A.G., Fyffe, R.E.W., Rose, P.K. and Snow, P.J. (1981) Spinal cord collaterals from axons of type II slowly adapting units in the cat. *J. Physiol. (Lond.)*, 316: 469–480.

Brown, M.C., Jansen, J.K.S. and Van Essen, D. (1976) Polyneuronal innervation of skeletal muscle in new-born rats and its elimination during maturation. *J. Physiol. (Lond.)*, 251: 387–422.

Bunt, S.M. and Horder, T.J. (1982) Evidence for an orderly arrangement of optic axons within the optic nerve of the major non-mammalian vertebrate classes. *J. comp. Neurol.*, in press.

Bunt, S.M., Horder, T.J. and Martin, K.A.C. (1978) Evidence that optic fibers regenerating across the goldfish optic tectum may be assigned termination sites on a "first-come-first-served basis". *J. Physiol. (Lond.)*, 276: 45–46P.

Bunt, S.M., Horder, T.J. and Martin, K.A.C. (1979) The nature of the nerve fibre guidance mechanism responsible for the formation of an orderly central visual projection. In R. Freeman (Ed.), *Development Neurobiology of Vision*, Plenum Press, New York, pp. 331–343.

Carpenter, M.B., Stein, B.M. and Shriver, J.R. (1968) Central projections of spinal dorsal roots in the monkey. II. Lower thoracic, lumbosacral and coccygeal dorsal roots. *Amer. J. Anat.*, 123: 75–118.

Changeux, J.P. and Danchin, A. (1976) The selective stabilization of developing synapses as a mechanism for the specification of neuronal networks. *Nature (Lond.)*, 264: 705–712.

Clarke, P.G.H. and Cowan, W.M. (1976) The development of the isthmo-optic tract in the chick, with special reference to the occurrence and correction of developmental errors in the location and connections of isthmo-optic neurones. *J. comp. Neurol.*, 167: 143–164.

Cowan, W.M. (1973) Neuronal death as a regulative mechanism in the control of cell number in the nervous system. In M. Rockstein (Ed.), *Development and Aging in the Nervous System*, Academic Press, New York, pp. 19–41.

Cook, J.E. and Horder, T.J. (1977) The multiple factors determining retinotopic order in the growth of optic fibers into the optic tectum. *Phil. Trans. roy. Soc. B.*, 278: 261–276.

Cowey, A. (1981) Why are there so many visual areas? In F.O. Schmidt, F.G. Worden, G. Adelman and S.G. Dennis (Eds.), *The Organization of the Cerebral Cortex*, M.I.T. Press, Cambridge, MA, pp. 395–413.

Crepel, F., Mariani, J. and Delhaye-Bouchard, N. (1976) Evidence of a multiple innervation of Purkinje cells by climbing fibers in the immature rat cerebellum. *J. Neurobiol.*, 7: 567–578.

Daniel, P.M. and Whitteridge, D. (1961) The representation of the visual field on the cerebral cortex in monkeys. *J. Physiol. (Lond.)*, 159: 203–221.

Dawnay, N.A.H. (1979) Chronotopic organization of the goldfish optic pathway. *J. Physiol. (Lond.)*, 290: 13–14P.

Devor, M. (1976) Fiber trajectories of olfactory bulb efferents in the hamster. *J. comp. Neurol.*, 166: 31–48.

Fawcett, I. (1980) Fibre organization in the optic nerve of *Xenopus laevis*. *J. Physiol. (Lond.)*, 306: 32P.

Ferraro, A. and Barrera, S.E. (1935) Posterior column fibers and their terminations in Macacus rhesus. *J. comp. Neurol.*, 62: 507–530.

Ferster, D. and LeVay, S. (1978) The axonal arborizations of lateral geniculate neurones in the striate cortex of the cat. *J. comp. Neurol.*, 182: 923–944.

Forbes, D.J. and Welt, C. (1981) Neurogenesis in the trigeminal ganglion of the albino rat: A quantitative autoradiographic study. *J. comp. Neurol.*, 199: 133–147.

Frost, D.O. (1980) Ordered anomalous retinal projections to the medial geniculate ventrobasal and lateral posterior nuclei. *Soc. Neurosci. Abstr.*, 6: 663.

Gatter, K.C. and Powell, T.P.S. (1977) The projection of the locus coeruleus upon the neocortex in the macaque monkey. *Neuroscience*, 2: 441–445.

Gordon, G. and Paine, C.H. (1960) Functional organization in the nucleus gracilis of the cat. *J. Physiol. (Lond.)*, 153: 331–349.

Gottlieb, D.I. and Cowan, W.M. (1972) Evidence for a temporal factor in the occupation of available synapse during development of the dentate gyrus. *Brain Res.*, 41: 452–456.

Hand, P.J. (1966) Lumbosacral dorsal root terminations in the nucleus gracilis of the cat. Some observations on terminal degeneration in other medullary sensory nuclei. *J. comp. Neurol.*, 126: 137–156.

Herrick, C.J. (1942) Optic and postoptic systems of fibers in the brain of *Necturus*. *J. comp. Neurol.*, 75: 487–544.

Horder, T.J. (1978) Functional adaptability and morphogenetic opportunism, the only rules for limb development? *Zoon*, 6: 181–192.

Horder, T.J. and Martin, K.A.C. (1977) Translocation of optic fibers in the tectum may be determined by their stability relative to surrounding fiber terminals. *J. Physiol. (Lond.)*, 271: 23–24P.

Horder, T.J. and Martin, K.A.C. (1978) Morphogenetics as an alternative to chemospecificity in the formation of nerve connections. In A.S.G. Curtis (Ed.), *Cell–Cell Recognition. Soc. Exp. Biol. Symp. XXII*, Cambridge Univ. Press, Cambridge, pp. 275–358.

Horder, T.J. and Martin, K.A.C. (1981) Some determinants of optic terminal localization and retinotopic polarity within fiber populations in the tectum of goldfish. Submitted for publication.

Horder, T.J., Mashkas, A. and Pilgrim, A.J. (1979) A method for the determination of fiber organization within the visual pathways of higher vertebrates. *J. Physiol. (Lond.)*, 296: 8–9P.

Horton, J.C., Greenwood, M.M. and Hubel, D.H. (1979) Non-retinotopic arrangement of fibers in the cat optic nerve. *Nature (Lond.)*, 282: 720–722.

Hubel, D.H. and Wiesel, T.N. (1960) Receptive fields of optic nerve fibers in the spider monkey. *J. Physiol. (Lond.)*, 155: 385–398.

Hubel, D.H. and Wiesel, T.N. (1972) Laminar and columnar distribution of geniculocortical fibers in the macaque monkey. *J. comp. Neurol.*, 140: 421–450.

Innocenti, G.M., Fiore, L. and Caminiti, R. (1977) Exurberant projections into the corpus callosum from the visual cortex of newborn cats. *Neurosci. Lett.*, 4: 237–242.

Jeffrey, G. and Perry, V.H. (1981) Evidence for ganglion cell death during development of the ipsilateral retinal projection in the rat. *Develop. Brain Res.*, 2: 176–180.

Kalil, R. (1978) Development of the dorsal lateral geniculate nucleus in the cat. *J. comp. Neurol.*, 182: 265–292.

Katz, M.J. and Lasek, R.J. (1981) Substrate pathways demonstrated by transplanted Mauthner axons. *J. comp. Neurol.*, 195: 627–641.

Keating, M.J. (1974) The role of visual function in the patterning of binocular visual connexions. *Brit. med. Bull.*, 30: 145–151.

Kruger, L.R., Siminoff, R. and Witkovsky, P. (1961) Single neuron analysis of dorsal column nuclei and spinal nucleus of trigeminal in cat. *J. Neurophysiol.*, 24: 333–349.

Land, P.W. and Lund, R.D. (1979) Development of the rat's uncrossed retino-tectal pathway and its relation to plasticity studies. *Science*, 205: 698–700.

Landmesser, L.T. (1980) The generation of neuromuscular specificity. *Ann Rev. Neurosci.*, 3: 279–302.

Lashley, K.S. (1934) The mechanism of vision. VII. The projection of the retina upon the primary optic centers in the rat. *J. comp. Neurol.*, 59: 341–373.

Lawson, S.N., Caddy, K.W.T. and Biscoe, T.J. (1974) Development of rat dorsal root ganglion neurones: Studies of cell birthdays and changes in mean cell diameter. *Cell Tiss. Res.*, 153: 399–413.

Lent, R. and Schneider, G.E. (1980) Order and disorder in the aberrant retinothalamic projection in hamsters with early tectal ablations. *Soc. Neurosci. Abstr.*, 6: 648.

Levinthal, F. and Levinthal, C. (1980) Development of retinotectal connections. *Soc. Neurosci. Abstr.*, 6: 293.

Light, A.R. and Perl, E.R. (1979) Re-examination of the dorsal root projection to the spinal dorsal horn including observations on the differential termination of coarse and fine fibers. *J. comp. Neurol.*, 186: 117–132.

Liu, C.-N. and Chambers, W.W. (1958) Intraspinal sprouting of dorsal root axons. *Arch. Neurol. Psychiat.*, 79: 46–61.

Lorente de No (1933) Anatomy of the eighth nerve. I. The central projection of the nerve endings of the internal ear. *Laryngoscope*, 43: 327–350.

Lund, R.D., Mitchell, D.E. and Henry, G.H. (1978) Squint-induced modification of callosal connections in cats. *Brain Res.*, 144: 169–172.

Mason, C.A., Polley, E.H. and Guillery, R.W. (1979) Retinotopic organization of axons in the optic nerve and tract of normal and Siamese cats. *Soc. Neurosci. Abstr.*, 5: 795.

Maturana, H.R. (1960) The fine anatomy of the optic nerve of anurans. An electron microscope study. *J. Biophys. Biochem. Cytol.*, 7: 107–120.

Merzenich, M.M. and Kaas, J.H. (1980) Principles of organization of sensory perceptual systems in mammals. In J.M. Sprague and A.N. Epstein (Eds.), *Progress in Psychobiology and Physiological Psychology, Vol. 9*, Academic Press, New York, pp. 1–42.

Mitchell, S.J., Rawlins, J.N.P., Steward, O. and Olton, D.S. (1982) Medial septal area lesions disrupt theta rhythm and cholinergic staining in medial entorhinal cortex and produce impaired radial arm maze behaviour in rats. *J. Neurosci.*, 2: 292–302.

Morin, F., Schwartz, H.G. and O'Leary, J.L. (1951) Experimental study of the spinothalamic and related tracts. *Acta psychiat. neurol scand.*, 26: 371–396.

Murphy, J.T., Kwan, H.C., MacKay, W.A. and Wong, Y.C. (1978) Spatial organization of precentral cortex in awake primates. III. Input–output coupling. *J. Neurophysiol.*, 41: 1132–1140.

Nordlander, R.H. and Singer, M. (1978) The role of the ependyma in regeneration of the spinal cord in the urodele amphibian tail. *J. comp. Neurol.*, 180: 349–374.

Nordlander, R.H., Singer, J.F., Beck, R. and Singer, M. (1981) An ultrastructural examination of early ventral root formation in amphibia. *J. comp. Neurol.*, 199: 535–551.

O'Leary, D.D.M., Stanfield, B.B. and Cowan, W.M. (1981) Evidence that the early postnatal restriction of the cells of origin of the callosal projection is due to the elimination of axonal collaterals rather than to the death of neurones. *Develop. Brain Res.*, 227: 607–617.

Perry, V.H. and Cowey, A. (1981) A sensitive period for ganglion cell degeneration and the formation of aberrant retino-fugal connections following tectal lesions in rats. *Neuroscience*, 7: 583–594.

Pick, A. (1896) Untersuchungen uber die topographischen Beziehungen zwischen Retina, Opticus und gekreutztem Tractus opticus beim Kaninchen. *Nova acta acad. Caes. Leop.-Car. Germ. nat. cur.*, 66: 1–24.

Poggio, G.F. and Mountcastle, V.B. (1963) The functional properties of ventrobasal thalamic neurons studied in unanaesthetized monkeys. *J. Neurophysiol.*, 26: 775–806.

Polyak, S. (1933) A contribution to the cerebral representation of the retina. *J. comp. Neurol.*, 57: 541–617.

Polyak, S. (1957) *The Vertebrate Visual System*, Univ. Chic. Press, Chicago.

Pompeiano, O. and Brodal, A. (1957) The origin of the vestibulospinal fibers in the cat. An experimental study with comments on the descending medial longitudinal fasciculus. *Arch. ital. Biol.*, 166–195.

Powell, T.P.S., Cowan, W.M. and Raisman, G. (1965) The central olfactory connexions. *J. Anat. (Lond.)*, 99: 791–813.

Price, J.L. and Powell, T.P.S. (1971) Certain observations on the olfactory pathway. *J. Anat. (Lond.)*, 110: 105–126.

Rager, G. (1981) The development of the retinotectal projection in the chicken. In A. Brodal et al. (Eds.), *Advanc. Anat. Embryol. Cell Biol., Vol. 63*, Springer, New York, pp. 1–92.

Raisman, G. and Field, P.M. (1973) A quantitative investigation of the development of collateral reinnervation after partial deafferentation of the septal nuclei. *Brain Res.*, 50: 241–264.

Rakic, P. (1977a) Prenatal development of the visual system in the rhesus monkey. *Phil. Trans. Roy. Soc. B*, 278: 245–260.

Rakic, P. (1977b) Genesis of the dorsal lateral geniculate nucleus in the rhesus monkey: Site and time of origin, kinetics of proliferation, routes of migration and pattern of distribution of neurons. *J. comp. Neurol.*, 176: 23–52.

Ramon y Cajal, S. (1960) *Studies in Vertebrate Neurogenesis*. Transl. L. Guth. Charles C. Thomas, Springfield, IL.

Rethelyi, M. and Szentagothai, J. (1973) Distribution and connections of afferent fibres in the spinal cord. In A. Iggo (Ed.), *Handbook of Sensory Physiology. II. Somatosensory system*, Springer, Berlin, pp. 207–252.

Rose, J.E., Galambos, R. and Hughes, J.R. (1959) Microelectrode studies of the cochlear nuclei of the cat. *Bull. Johns Hopk. Hosp.*, 104: 211–251.

Rubel, E.W. (1978) Ontogeny of structure and function in the vertebrate auditory system. In M. Jacobson (Ed.), *Handbook of Sensory Physiology, Vol. IX: Development of Sensory Systems*, Springer, New York, pp. 135–237.

Sanderson, K.J. (1971) The projection of the visual field to the lateral geniculate and medial interlaminar nuclei in the cat. *J. comp. Neurol.*, 143: 101–115.

Sando, I. (1965) The anatomical interrelationships of the cochlear nerve fibers. *Acto oto-laryng.*, 59: 417–436.

Sapiro, J.A., Silver, J. and Singer, M. (1980) Orderly fasciculation in the early optic nerve of *Xenopus laevis*. *Soc. Neurosci. Abstr.*, 6: 296.

Scalia, F. and Fite, K. (1974) A retinotopic analysis of the central connections of the optic nerve in the frog. *J. comp. Neurol.*, 158: 455–478.

Schwob, F.E. and Price, J.L. (1978) The cortical projection of the olfactory bulb: development in fetal and neonatal rats correlated with quantitative variations in adult rats. *Brain Res.*, 151: 369–374.

Schatz, C.J. and Rakic, P. (1981) The genesis of efferent connections from the visual cortex of the fetal rhesus monkey. *J. comp. Neurol.*, 196: 287–307.

Sharma, S.C. (1981) Retinal projection in a non-visual area after bilateral tectal ablation in the goldfish. *Nature (Lond.)*, 291: 66–67.

Shepherd, G.M. and Haberly, L.B. (1970) Partial activation of olfactory bulb: analysis of field potentials and topographical relation between bulb and lateral olfactory tract. *J. Neurophysiol.*, 33: 643–653.

Silver, J. (1979) Guidance and topographic patterning of retinal ganglion cell axons. *Soc. Neurosci. Abstr.*, 5: 179.

Silver, J. (1980) Mechanisms of axonal guidance during the formation of central nervous system commissures. *Soc. Neurosci. Abstr.*, 6: 487.

Silver, J. and Sidman, R.L. (1980) A mechanism for the guidance and topographic patterning of retinal ganglion cell axons. *J. comp. Neurol.*, 189: 101–111.

Siminoff, R., Schwassmann, H.O. and Kruger, L. (1966) An electrophysiological study of the visual projection to the superior colliculus in the rat. *J. comp. Neurol.*, 127: 435–444.

Singer, M., Nordlander, R.H. and Eghar, M. (1979) Axonal guidance during embryogenesis and regeneration in the spinal cord of the newt: the blueprint hypothesis of neuronal pathway patterning. *J. comp. Neurol.*, 185: 1–22.

Spalding, J.M.K. (1952) Wounds of the visual pathway. Part 1. The visual radiation. *J. Neurol. Neurosurg. Psychiat.*, 15: 99–109.

Speidel, C.C. (1941) Adjustments of nerve endings. *Harvey Lect.*, 36: 126–158.

Sperry, R.W. (1943) Visuomotor coordination in the newt (*Triturus viridescens*) after regeneration of the optic nerve. *J. comp. Neurol.*, 79: 33–55.

Thompson, I.D. (1979) Changes in the uncrossed retinotectal projection after removal of the other eye at birth. *Nature (Lond.)*, 279: 63–66.

Walker, A.E. (1937) Experimental studies of topical localization within the thalamus of the chimpanzee. *Proc. kon. ned. Akad. Wet.*, 40: 198–206.

Walker, A.E. (1942) Somatotopic localization of spinothalamic and secondary trigeminal tracts in mesencephalon. *Arch. Neurol Psychiat.*, 48: 884–889.

Walker, A.E. (1943) Central representation of pain. *Res. Publ. Assoc. nerv. ment. Dis.*, 23: 63–85.

Walker, A.E. and Weaver, T.A. (1942) The topical organization and termination of the posterior columns in Macca mulatta. *J. comp. Neurol.*, 76: 145–158.

Wall, P.D. (1960) Cord cells responding to touch, damage and temperature of skin. *J. Neurophysiol.*, 23: 197–210.

Wässle, H. and Illing, R.B. (1980) The retinal projection to the superior colliculus in the cat. A quantitative study with HRP. *J. comp. Neurol.*, 190: 333–356.

Weiss, P. (1941) *Nerve Patterns: The Mechanics of Nerve Growth. Third Growth Symp., Vol. 5*, pp. 163–203.

Werner, G. and Whitsel, B.L. (1967) The topology of the dermatomal projections in the medial lemniscal system. *J. Physiol. (Lond.)*, 192: 123–144.

White, L.E. Jr. (1965) Olfactory bulb projections in the rat. *Anat. Rec.*, 152: 465–479.

Whitsel, B.L., Petrucelli, L.M., Sapiro, G. and Ha, H. (1970) Fiber sorting in the fasciculus gracilis of squirrel monkeys. *Exp. Neurol.*, 29: 227–242.

Zeki, S.M. (1978) Functional specialization in the visual cortex of the rhesus monkey. *Nature (Lond.)*, 274: 423–428.

The Topography of the Initial Retinotectal Projection

C.E. HOLT

MRC Biophysics Unit, King's College, London University, 26–29 Drury Lane, London WC2B 5RL (U.K.)

INTRODUCTION

One of the striking features of the nervous system is the precise and ordered way in which separate populations of neurons become connected. In sensory systems where spatial resolution of input is important, afferent nerve fibers project from the receptor structure to targets centrally where their synaptic terminals are arranged in a pattern which is topologically equivalent to their cells of origin in the periphery. Thus, the visual field is mapped topographically in the tectum of the midbrain in lower vertebrates, where the distribution of optic terminals reflects the arrangement of ganglion cells in the eye (Gaze, 1959, 1970; Maturana et al., 1959).

Many studies have been directed at how this neurological map forms and an important finding to emerge recently is that optic axons are also topographically ordered en route to the tectum (Scalia and Fite, 1974; Bunt and Horder, 1978; Scholes, 1979; Rusoff and Easter, 1980; Fujisawa et al., 1981). A consequence of this pathway organization during development and growth is that optic nerve fibers are delivered to the tectum in correspondence with their final destinations and supports theories of map formation based on mechanical growth constraints, such as those proposed by Horder and Martin (1978).

On the other hand, in lower vertebrates, retinal afferents regenerate after they are severed and form a normal map in the tectum (Sperry, 1943) despite being dis-ordered along their pathways (Meyer, 1980; Fujisawa, 1981). Order in the regenerated tectal map does not emerge immediately but follows an initial phase of disorder (Gaze and Jacobson, 1963; Meyer, 1980). Anatomical observations (Meyer, 1980) show that ordered pathway topography is not essential for orderly map formation, at least in regeneration, and suggests that highly selective recognition processes are at work between afferents and their post-synaptic contacts, such as those invoked by Sperry (1943, 1944, 1963).

A question of fundamental interest is how the retinal projection is arranged during early development. Are optic fibers ordered retinotopically during the initial stages of tectal innervation or, as in regeneration, are the first population of fibers disordered becoming progressively less so at subsequent stages of development? Electrophysiological studies on the developing frog visual system are consistent with the latter since they show an initial period of disorder (Gaze et al., 1972, 1974). In contrast, however, the anatomical studies described here, show that the topography of the retinal projection in *Xenopus laevis* is ordered from the beginning of tectal innervation.

[339]

METHOD FOR LABELING DEVELOPING POPULATIONS OF NERVE FIBERS

To determine the topography of the growing retinotectal projection, different parts were labeled by exposing groups of precursor retinal cells to [³H]amino acid. The label becomes incorporated into structural proteins during neuronal differentiation so that growing axons can be identified autoradiographically.

Before and at the beginning of retinal differentiation, *Xenopus* embryos stages 24–31 (Nieuwkoop and Faber, 1956) were lightly anesthetized in 1:10,000 tricaine methane sulphonate (MS 222, Sandoz) in two-thirds strength Niu Twitty solution (Rugh, 1962) at pH 7.6, dejellied and placed in operating wells in a wax coated petri dish. Whole eye primordia or dorsal and ventral halves and less were dissected out with fine tungsten needles and transferred with a pipette to a droplet of operating medium containing [³H]proline (specific activity 117 Ci/mmol) at a concentration of 400 µCi/ml in which they were incubated for 15–20 min. Care was taken in ventral eye surgery to include the optic stalk region to ensure labeling the entire presumptive retina (Holt, 1980). The [³H]proline incubated eye tissue was then washed repeatedly in fresh medium and replaced orthotopically in its original orientation. Animals were reared at 20 °C postoperatively, fixed 1–10 days later (stage 40–48) in 2.5% glutaraldehyde in 0.2 M phosphate buffer (pH 7.4), embedded in paraffin wax and serially sectioned at 6 µm and 12 µm. Sections were mounted on gelatin coated slides, dehydrated, dewaxed and dipped in K5 photographic emulsion (Ilford) for light microscope autoradiography. Autoradiographs were developed 2–8 weeks later.

THE INITIAL RETINAL PROJECTION

The first ganglion cell axons differentiate around stage 28/9 (approximately 1.5 days postfertilization; Grant and Rubin, 1980) and are first observed in the tectum approximately 24 h later around stage 38/9 (Chung et al., 1975; Grant et al., 1980). In this study the retinal projection was examined a few hours after the arrival of the first fibers at the tectum (stage 40 onwards) and is referred to as the initial projection. There are approximately 1000 optic fibers at stage 40 (Wilson, 1971).

In experiments on 51 embryos, 27 were successful in that the eye appeared normal and the central projection was labeled. The major findings are briefly described here. Fig. 1a shows an example of an autoradiograph from a stage 43 eye whose dorsal half was exposed to [³H]proline at stage 27/8. Silver grains are confined to cells in the dorsal half of the retina where they are fairly uniformly distributed. The boundary dividing labeled and unlabeled regions is only violated in the dendritic and ganglion cell axon layers. Labeled axons (arrow) can be seen coursing ventrally towards the optic nerve head; grains seen extending 30 µm ventrally in the inner plexiform layer reflect the spread of amacrine and ganglion cell dendritic arborization. Transverse sections through the optic nerve head (Fig. 1b) frequently show label confined to the dorsal half indicating that axons exit from the eye preserving their retinotopic order as in older animals (Fawcett, 1981). Although the cross-section of the optic nerve (15 µm) approaches the limit of resolution, order can be seen close to the eye but cannot be detected nearer the chiasm which is consistent with recent observations in the mature optic nerve (Fawcett, 1981).

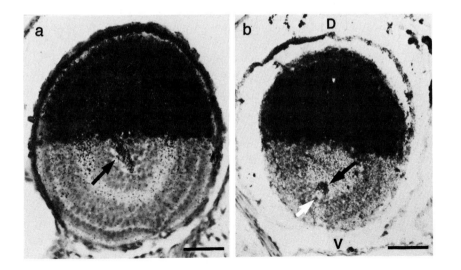

Fig. 1. Autoradiographs of a stage 43 (a) and 45 (b) eye in transverse section; the dorsal half of each was incubated in [³H]proline at stage 26/7. a: the autoradiographic grains (black) are confined to the dorsal half of the eye and are only found ventral to the labeled boundary in the inner plexiform layer (lightly stained region), indicating the extent of ganglion cell and amacrine cell dendrites, and in the ganglion cell axon layer where axons are seen coursing ventrally (arrow) towards the optic nerve head. b: the optic nerve head (arrows) shows grains confined to its dorsal half as well as to the dorsal half of the retina; the black arrow indicates the labeled half and the white arrow the unlabeled half. Dorsal and ventral axes of a and b are the same; the nasal and temporal axes are reversed (a) right eye, (b) left eye. D, dorsal; V, ventral. Bar = 100 μm.

Fig. 2a shows the retinal projection labeled in the midbrain. This is an autoradiograph of a section taken parasagittally through the optic tract and tectum of a stage 40 individual (approximately 3 days postfertilization) whose contralateral eye (ventral half) was incubated in [³H]proline at stage 26. Here, optic fibers are labeled in the optic tract, thalamic centers and in the tectal neuropil. Label is slightly more dense in the tectal neuropil which indicates that terminals are arborizing. Tectal layering is not yet apparent although a few cells found rostral to the central mass indicate its beginnings. A few labeled fibers can also be seen running caudally from the tract towards the accessory optic system, the basal optic neuropil, which appears not to form until later (stage 45/6) when characteristic laminations appear. This difference in timing between the initial innervation of the tectum and the basal optic neuropil may reflect a corresponding difference in the sequence of differentiation of ganglion cell types subserving different functions. For instance, in the pigeon the basal optic neuropil is served exclusively by afferents from a distinct population of displaced ganglion cells in the retina (Fite et al., 1981).

In the adult frog, optic fibers are segregated in the optic tract and thalamic centers so that dorsal fibers run ventrally and ventral ones dorsally; the lateral and medial regions of the tectum are occupied by fibers from dorsal and ventral parts of the retina respectively (Scalia and Fite, 1974). Localization of label in the mediolateral dimension of the tectum was compared between individuals with labeled dorsal and ventral eye halves or fragments. Fig. 2b and c shows sections drawn from different levels of tectum and diencephalon. The medial and lateral extremes of the tectal neuropil are shown plus two sections at intermediate levels, one passing through the

342

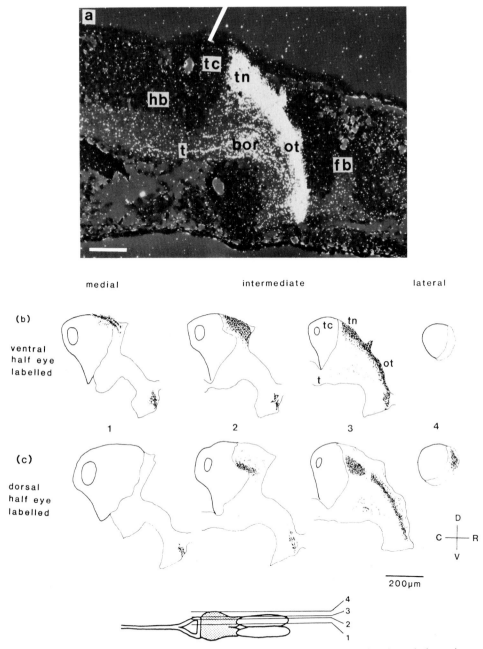

Fig. 2. a: a combined bright- and dark-field autoradiograph of a parasagittal section through the optic tract and tectum of a stage 40 animal. The ventral half of the contralateral eye was incubated in [³H]proline at stage 26. Autoradiographic grains (white) are seen in the optic tract (ot) and tectal neuropil (tn); grains caudal to the ot show fibers of the basal optic root (bor). Bar = 100 μm. b and c: camera lucida drawings made from autoradiographs through the tectum and optic tract in the parasagittal plane. Both a and b are from stage 40 animals where: a, the ventral half of the contralateral eye was labeled at stage 26 and, b, the dorsal half was labeled at stage 25. Drawing b3 corresponds with Fig. 2a. The numbers refer to the level through the midbrain and correspond to those indicated in the whole brain outline. Medial, intermediate and lateral are levels through the tectal neuropil. Grains are represented with black dots. D, dorsal; V, ventral; R, rostral; C, caudal; tc, tectal central cell mass; fb, forebrain; hb, hindbrain; t, tegmentum.

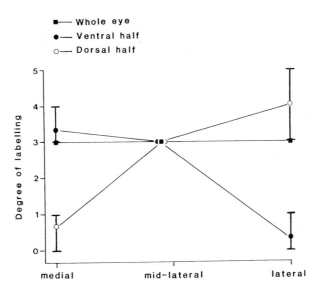

Fig. 3. A summary graph of the data taken from 11 animals (early stage 40s) where either the whole eye or dorsal and ventral halves and fragments were labeled with [³H]proline at mid-stage 20s. The grain density in the tectal neuropil from serial reconstructions was scored subjectively on a relative scale of 0–5 by comparison with the standard. The section through the optic tract was taken as the standard (as in Fig. 2a) and given the value 3 against which labeling in the medial and lateral extremes were compared. The distribution of values obtained by this procedure from different animals is indicated by the vertical bar and the points from which the lines have been drawn (open and filled circles: squares) are the averaged values.

optic tract. The projections from dorsally and ventrally labeled eyes are consistently different each showing a characteristic distribution of label. Labeling in the tectal neuropil from dorsally labeled eyes (Fig. 2c) is most dense laterally becoming less so medially, whereas projections from ventrally labeled eyes (Fig. 2b) show the reverse, with label most dense medially becoming less so laterally. The degree of labeling with respect to the position in the midbrain is shown in Fig. 3 where results from 11 animals have been pooled. These results clearly show that the dorsal half of the eye projects laterally and ventral half medially in the tectal neuropil. The width of the tectal neuropil at stage 40/1 is ~60 μm and label from half the projection spreads ~45 μm which indicates that arborizations are not extensive, probably less than 30 μm. The position of the label in the optic tract also differs (Fig. 2b and c) with dorsal fibers located ventrally (~30 μm ventral to diencephalic border) and ventral fibers located dorsally along the edge of the diencephalon.

CONCLUSIONS

These results show that the initial optic fiber projection is retinotopically arranged both en route to and in the neuropil of the immature tectum. This agrees with studies on chick where embryonic retinal ablations were used to show that the adult pattern of innervation is present in the early projection (De Long and Coulombre, 1965; Crossland et al., 1974). It is unclear why the anatomical findings here should differ from the functional studies of Gaze et al. (1972, 1974) which indicate that an ordered retinotectal map does not emerge until later in development (stage 47). However, in a recent series of tectal recordings (Holt and Harris, 1983) functional ordering was found at corresponding stages of development (stage 41 onwards).

A major conclusion from these studies is that during development a disordered pattern of axonal growth and tectal innervation does not precede the emergence of an ordered retinotectal map. In contrast, it has been shown anatomically that during regeneration the pattern of retinal axon terminals is at first disordered but becomes progressively ordered over the following months (Meyer, 1980). The implication which arises from this is that the processes of map formation during regeneration differ from those in development. However, if one considers that terminals have to modify their synaptic contacts to allow for changes in geometry occurring in normal development and growth (Gaze et al., 1974; Keating, 1974), then the sorting out of grossly misplaced terminals in regeneration can be seen as the result of a mechanism that exists normally only to produce much smaller modifications.

ACKNOWLEDGEMENTS

I thank John Scholes for his help and guidance throughout and Helen Saibil for helpful comments on the manuscript. This work was supported by a Science Research Council studentship.

REFERENCES

Bunt, S.M. and Horder, T.J. (1978) Evidence for an orderly arrangement of optic axons in the central pathways of vertebrates and its implications for the formation and regeneration of optic projections. Soc. Neurosci. Abstr., 4: 468.

Chung, S.H., Stirling, R.V. and Gaze, R.M. (1975) The structural and functional development of the retina in larval Xenopus. J. Embryol. exp. Morph., 33: 915–940.

Crossland, W.J., Cowan, W.M., Rogers, L.A. and Kelly, J.P. (1974) The specification of the retinotectal projection in the chick. J. comp. Neurol., 155: 127–164.

De Long, G.R. and Coulombre, A.J. (1965) Development of the retinotectal topographic projection in the chick embryo. Exp. Neurol., 13: 351–363.

Fawcett, J. (1981) How axons grow down the Xenopus optic nerve. J. Embryol. exp. Morph., 65: 219–233.

Fite, K.V., Brecha, N., Karten, H.J. and Hunt, S.P. (1981) Displaced ganglion cells and the accessory optic system of pigeon. J. comp. Neurol., 195: 279–288.

Fujisawa, H., Watanabe, K., Noboru, T. and Ibata, Y. (1981) Retinotopic analysis of fibre pathways in amphibians. I. The adult newt Cynops pyrrhogaster. Brain Res., 206: 9–10. II. The frog Rana nigromaculata. Brain Res., 206: 21–26.

Fujisawa, H. (1981) Retinotopic analysis in the regenerating retinotectal system of the adult newt Cynops pyrrhogaster. Brain Res., 206: 27–37.

Gaze, R.M. (1959) Regeneration of the optic nerve in Xenopus laevis. Quant. J. exp. Physiol., 44: 290–308.

Gaze, R.M. (1970) Formation of Nerve Connections, Academic Press, New York.

Gaze, R.M. and Jacobson, M. (1963) A study of the retinotectal projection during regeneration of the optic nerve in the frog. Proc. roy. Soc. B, 157: 420–448.

Gaze, R.M., Chung, S.H. and Keating, M.J. (1972) Development of the retinotectal projections in Xenopus. Nature New Biol., 236: 133–135.

Gaze, R.M., Keating, M.J. and Chung, S.-H. (1974) The evolution of the retinotectal map during development in Xenopus. Proc. roy. Soc. B., 185: 301–330.

Grant, P., Rubin, E. and Cima, C. (1980) Ontogeny of the retina and optic nerve in Xenopus laevis. I. stages in the early development of the retina. J. comp. Neurol., 189: 593–613.

Grant, P. and Rubin, E. (1980) Ontogeny of the retina and optic nerve in *Xenopus laevis*. II Ontogeny of the optic fibre pattern in the retina. *J. comp. Neurol.*, 189: 671–698.

Holt, C. (1980) Cell movements in *Xenopus* eye development. *Nature (Lond.)*, 287: 850–852.

Holt, C.E. and Harris, W.A. (1983) Order in the initial retinotectal map in *Xenopus*: a new technique for labelling growing nerve fibres. In press.

Keating, M.J. (1974) The role of visual functioning in the patterning of binocular visual connections. *Brit. med. Bull.*, 30: 145–151.

Maturana, H.R., Lettvin, J.Y., McCulloch, W.S. and Pitts, W.H. (1959) Physiological evidence that cut optic nerve fibres in the frog regenerate to their proper places in the tectum. *Science*, 130: 1709–1710.

Meyer, R.L. (1980) Mapping the normal and regenerating retinotectal projection of goldfish with autoradiographic methods. *J. comp. Neurol.*, 189: 273–289.

Nieuwkoop, P.D. and Faber, J. (1956) *Normal Tables of Xenopus laevis*, North-Holland, Amsterdam.

Rugh, R. (1962) *Experimental Embryology*, 3rd edn., Burgess Publ., Minneapolis, MN.

Rusoff, A.C. and Easter, S.S. (1980) Order in the optic nerve of goldfish. *Science*, 208: 311–312.

Scalia, R. and Fite, K. (1974) A retinotopic analysis of the central connections of the optic nerve in the frog. *J. comp. Neurol.*, 158: 445–478.

Scholes, J.H. (1979) Nerve fibre topography in retinal projection to the tectum. *Nature (Lond.)*, 278: 620–624.

Sperry, R.W. (1943) Visuomotor coordination in the newt (*Triturus viridescens*) after regeneration of the optic nerve. *J. comp. Neurol.*, 79: 33–55.

Sperry, R.W. (1944) Optic nerve regeneration within return of vision in anurans. *J. Neurophysiol.*, 7: 57–69.

Sperry, R.W. (1963) Chemoaffinity in the orderly growth of nerve fibres patterns and connections. *Proc. nat. Acad. Sci. U.S.A.*, 50: 703–710.

Wilson, M.A. (1971) Optic nerve fibre counts and retinal ganglion cell counts during development of *Xenopus laevis* (Daudin). *J. exp. Physiol.*, 56: 83–91.

Genomic and Non-Genomic Actions of Nerve Growth Factor in Development

LLOYD A. GREENE, PAULETTE BERND*, MARK M. BLACK**, DAVID E. BURSTEIN, JAMES L. CONNOLLY, ADRIANA RUKENSTEIN and P. JOHN SEELEY

Departments of Pharmacology and (D.E.B.) Pathology, NYU School of Medicine, 550 First Avenue, New York, NY 10016, and (J.L.C.) Department of Pathology, Harvard Medical School, Boston, MA 02215 (U.S.A.)

INTRODUCTION

Chemical signals appear to play important roles in development of neural tissue. For example, they may function to spatially and temporally coordinate the differentiation of specific cell groups, to provide tropic signalling and guidance, and to mediate cell–cell communication and feedback. Moreover, because of their potential to function extracellularly, chemical signals could work either in restricted local environments, or, more diffusely, over long distances.

Within the last thirty years, a number of macromolecular factors have been identified that can influence the development and differentiation of the nervous system (for reviews see Greene, 1981; Sensenbrenner, 1981; Varon and Adler, 1977). The nerve growth factor protein (NGF) is the first discovered of such macromolecules (Levi-Montalcini and Angeletti, 1968) and is well familiar to most neuroscientists. Because NGF can be easily obtained and purified, it has been exceptionally well characterized with respect to its biochemistry and biology (Bradshaw, 1978; Greene and Shooter, 1980; Levi-Montalcini and Angeletti, 1968; Thoenen and Barde, 1980). Consequently, NGF is presently the most useful model available for studying the actions of chemical factors that regulate neural development.

The particular aim of the present essay is to explore the role of the genome in the action of nerve growth factor. The major conclusions supported here will be (a) that NGF has two separable classes of actions on its target cells; (b) that one class of actions involves specific regulation of gene transcription; (c) that another class of actions involves short-latency, local events that are independent of gene transcription; (d) that full expression of either class of action is dependent on expression of the other class; and (e) that both classes of action play important roles in regulating neuronal development: the transcription-dependent class may bring about long-term regulation of overall neuronal differentiation while the transcription-independent class may permit rapid, local control of neurite outgrowth. While the experimental basis for these conclusions specifically relates to NGF, it is hypothesized that other growth factors possess similar classes of action on the nervous system.

*Present address: Department of Anatomy, University School of Medicine, Philadelphia, PA 19140, U.S.A.
**Present address: Department of Anatomy, Mt. Sinai Medical Center, New York, NY 10029, U.S.A.

GENERAL CONSIDERATIONS OF NGF AND ITS ACTIVITY

A material that promoted neurite outgrowth from sensory and sympathetic ganglia was first identified in sarcoma tumors (Levi-Montalcini and Angeletti, 1968). Large quantities of this material, named nerve growth factor (NGF), were subsequently discovered in snake venom and in adult male mouse submaxillary glands (Levi-Montalcini and Angeletti, 1968). While the latter is the major source of NGF for experimentation, proteins with similar biological activity and related structure appear to be present in all vertebrates. The biologically active species of mouse NGF is a protein of mol. wt. $\simeq 27,000$ that is composed of two identical non-covalently bound chains whose sequence has been determined (Bradshaw, 1978; Greene and Shooter, 1980). The major target cells for NGF are sympathetic and sensory neurons (Levi-Montalcini and Angeletti, 1968; Thoenen and Barde, 1980). Most other types of neurons do not exhibit detectable responses to the molecule. The effects of NGF are most pronounced during development but, at least for sympathetic neurons, responses may also be noted in the adult. Major biological actions of NGF include (see Bradshaw, 1978; Greene and Shooter, 1980; Levi-Montalcini and Angeletti; 1968; Thoenen and Barde, 1980, for reviews): (1) maintenance of survival, (2) promotion of neurite outgrowth and regeneration, (3) directional guidance of neurite outgrowth, (4) stimulation of anabolic activity and (5) regulation of enzymes involved in the synthesis of neurotransmitters. As noted above, the aim of this essay is to review the evidence that NGF promotes these and other actions via both genomic and non-genomic mechanisms.

EXPERIMENTAL MODELS

Evaluation of the role of the genome in NGF's mechanism requires an appropriate experimental system. In vivo and in vitro preparations of sympathetic and sensory neurons have been quite useful in this regard. These preparations do, however, possess certain drawbacks. In particular, since these neurons require NGF for survival, it is difficult to compare their behaviors with and without NGF treatment, especially over times greater than a few hours. Moreover, since these neurons are unavoidably exposed to NGF in vivo before their use for experiments, it is possible to observe only ongoing, rather than initial responses to the factor. A more recently introduced system without such problems is the PC12 line of rat pheochromocytoma cells (Dichter et al., 1977; Greene and Rein; 1977; Greene and Tischler, 1976, 1982). These cells do not require NGF for survival in serum-containing medium. In the absence of exogenous NGF, PC12 cells strongly resemble their non-neoplastic counterparts, adrenal chromaffin cells: they contain chromaffin granules and synthesize and store large amounts of catecholamines, but do not possess neurites. When PC12 cells are treated for several days with physiological levels of NGF, they cease proliferation and acquire many neuronal properties such as long, branching neurites, electrical excitability, and synaptic-like vesicles. The PC12 system provides the important advantages that it may be used to examine initial responses of cells previously unexposed to NGF and that the cells can be compared before and after exposure to the factor. These properties of the PC12 system have made it particularly useful for uncovering both transcriptional and non-transcriptional actions of NGF.

TRANSCRIPTIONAL ACTIONS OF NGF

Experiments with PC12 cells have revealed a number of responses to NGF that are apparent only after latencies of days. In instances in which testing has been possible, these responses are blocked by specific inhibitors of RNA synthesis and thus appear to require gene transcription. Some of these are reviewed below.

Neurite outgrowth

Initiation of neurite outgrowth in PC12 cultures by NGF is sensitive to treatment with the RNA synthesis inhibitors actinomycin-D, cordycepin and camptothecin (Burstein and Greene, 1978). As discussed below, these compounds do not block neurite outgrowth by cells pre-exposed to NGF and hence their inhibition of neurite initiation appears to be due to their anti-transcriptional activities rather than to less specific direct blockade of neurite growth. These and other observations have led to the "priming" model for the mechanism by which NGF promotes neurite outgrowth (Burstein and Greene, 1978; Greene et al., 1980). According to this model, NGF causes target cells, via a selective stimulation of gene transcription, to synthesize and accumulate material which is required for production of neurites.

Neurotransmitter metabolism

As noted above, NGF regulates the activities of several enzymes involved in the metabolism of neurotransmitters including tyrosine hydroxylase, dopamine-β-hydroxylase, choline acetyltransferase and acetylcholinesterase. Consistent with a transcriptional mechanism, enhancement of the levels of these enzymes in ganglia or cultured cells by NGF occurs with a latency of at least 24 h. For the case of regulation of acetylcholinesterase activity in PC12 cells, this action of NGF is specifically blocked by low concentrations of inhibitors of transcription (Greene and Rukenstein, 1981). There is also evidence that regulation of tyrosine hydroxylase activity in sympathetic ganglia by NGF has a transcriptional basis (MacDonnell et al., 1977).

Protein synthesis

Comparison by means of 1- and 2-dimensional polyacrylamide gel electrophoresis of PC12 cultures before and after exposure to NGF has revealed no qualitative changes in the composition of the 1000 or so most abundant peptides present in the cells (Garrels and Schubert; 1979; McGuire et al; 1978). On the other hand, a few quantitative changes in composition have been detected that appear over time courses of days (Garrels and Schubert, 1979; McGuire and Greene, 1980; McGuire et al., 1978), and there is evidence that at least several of these have a transcriptional basis. These include increases in the levels of an 80,000 mol. wt. protein (McGuire and Greene, 1980), and of glycoproteins of apparent mol. wt. 25,000–30,000 and 230,000 (McGuire et al., 1978). The latter is a surface component named NILE (NGF-inducible large external) glycoprotein that is also present in sympathetic ganglia and brain (Lee et al., 1981) and which present findings indicate is a specific marker for neurons (S.R.M. Salton et al.). It is not presently known whether any of these proteins play a causal role in priming.

Other long-latency responses

Several additional responses of PC12 cells to NGF occur with time courses of days and, although not yet tested for sensitivity to inhibitors of RNA synthesis, could have transcriptional bases. One example is acquisition of electrical excitability. Prior to NGF

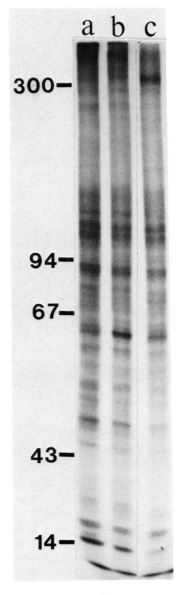

Fig. 1. SDS polyacrylamide gel (6.5–13%) pattern of ^{32}P-labeled proteins in PC12 pheochromocytoma cultures exposed to NGF for (a) 0 h, (b) 2 h or (c) 9 days. Numbers at left denote apparent molecular weight $\times 10^{-3}$. Note the long-term relative increase in labeling of a band at ~300,000 mol. wt. This component corresponds to authentic MAP-1 protein. Note also the transient increase in relative labeling of a band at apparent mol. wt. 60,000 that is evident at 2 h, but not at 9 days of NGF treatment.

exposure, PC12 cells are not electrically excitable. After a latency of 3–5 days of NGF treatment, the cultures show a progressive increase in the proportion of cells in which action potentials may be evoked (Dichter et al., 1977). Recent studies (Rudy et al., 1982) indicate that this change might in part be due to an increase in number and density of surface membrane sodium channels. A second example is the possible regulation of NGF of its own receptors. Preliminary binding and autoradiographic experiments (P. Bernd, unpublished) suggest that PC12 cells exposed to NGF for more than 2–3 days have a several-fold higher density of surface NGF receptors than do cells without NGF pretreatment. A third example is the finding (Black and Greene, 1982) that the microtubules in PC12 cultures treated with NGF for 3 weeks appear to be considerably more resistant to colchicine than do microtubules in NGF-untreated PC12 cultures. This resistance to colchicine is not present after only 24 h of NGF treatment and hence NGF may bring about a long-term shift in the equilibrium between monomeric and polymeric tubulin. This effect could in turn play an important role in the formation and/or maintenance of neurites. A final example concerns recent observations of the pattern of proteins that become labeled during exposure of PC12 cultures to [^{32}P]orthophosphate. Such experiments reveal that as a function of time of pre-exposure to NGF, there occurs, with a latency of several days, a progressive increase in the relative labeling of a high ($\geq$300,000) mol. wt. material as well as of a band of apparent mol. wt. 65,000–70,000 (Fig. 1). The former material corresponds to type 1 of the high molecular weight microtubule associated proteins (MAP-1) while the latter is in the region of the tau MAPs. Both materials appear to be associated with the cell cytoskeleton. Since MAPs may play significant roles in promoting the formation and stabilization of microtubules as well as in linking these structures to other elements of the cell (Lasek and Shelanski, 1981), the possible relationship between such findings and neurite outgrowth is particularly intriguing.

SHORT-LATENCY, NON-TRANSCRIPTIONAL ACTIONS OF NGF

Experiments with PC12 cells and cultured neurons have uncovered a class of responses to NGF that occur with latencies of seconds to hours and that are not sensitive to inhibitors of transcription. In considering such responses it is particularly important to distinguish between those that merely play causal links in the chain of NGF's mechanism of action and those that in themselves modify the phenotypic behavior of target cells. Often, this distinction is difficult to make, but, in the present discussion, it is the latter type of responses that will be the focus of interest. Several examples follow.

Promotion of neurite outgrowth and regeneration by primed cells

Stimulation of neurite outgrowth from freshly dissected cultured sensory and sympathetic neurons is apparent within several hours of NGF treatment (Levi-Montalcini and Angeletti, 1968). Partlow and Larrabee (1971) reported that this behavior occurs even when transcription is blocked by high concentrations of actinomycin-D. Similarly, regrowth of neurites by PC12 cells pre-treated or "primed" with NGF for at least several days and then divested of their processes by mechanical shearing: (a) requires the presence of NGF, (b) begins within several hours, and (c) is insensitive to inhibitors of transcription (Burstein and Greene, 1978). This behavior of neurons and of "primed" PC12 cells contrasts with that of "unprimed" PC12 cells (i.e. those without prior exposure to NGF). That is, as noted above, in unprimed cultures, initiation of neurite outgrowth by NGF: (a) has a latency of about 18 h, (b) has a slow time course prolonged over days, and (c) requires RNA synthesis (Burstein and Greene, 1978). One mechanism consistent with these observations is that neurite outgrowth requires not only a transcriptional pathway, but also a rapidly activated, non-transcriptional pathway. It has been hypothesized (Burstein and Greene, 1978) that the transcriptional pathway leads to accumulation of material required for neurite production. Even when such material is present, however, it appears that promotion of outgrowth cannot occur unless the non-transcriptional pathway is also activated. In this light, the ability of NGF to promote rapid neurite growth by primed cells even when RNA synthesis is blocked would be due to the presence of specific material accumulated during pre-exposure to NGF as well as to activation of the non-transcriptional pathway. Moreover, it has been suggested that the rapid, actinomycin-resistant response of neurons to NGF in vitro is a consequence of prior exposure to NGF (or priming) in vivo (Burstein and Greene, 1978; Greene et al., 1980).

While it is of course not certain that all aspects of the priming model will eventually be confirmed, the major point to be stressed here is that stimulation of process outgrowth and regeneration by NGF includes a separable, rapidly activated component that is independent of gene transcription.

Local actions of NGF at growth cones

Several different experiments have revealed short-latency, local effects of NGF on the movement and structure of growth cones. Using a chamber device that permitted the cell bodies of cultured sympathetic neurons to be exposed to medium different from that bathing the distal ends of their processes, Campenot (1977) demonstrated that neurites would only remain or grow into local environments containing NGF. Griffin and Letourneau (1980) reported that increasing the concentration of NGF in cultures of sensory neurons resulted in a rapid, reversible partial withdrawal of growth cones. In another study, Gundersen and Barrett (1980) used micropipets to expose the growth cones of cultured neurons to concentration gradients of NGF. Within 20 min of such exposure, the growing tips of the neurites turned toward the direction of higher NGF concentration. These types of findings suggest that NGF exerts rapidly initiated, local actions on the maintenance and direction of movement of growth cones. Furthermore, while the RNA synthesis requirements of such actions were not tested in the above studies, their short latencies are strongly consistent with a non-transcriptional mechanism.

Recent time-lapse videography experiments in our own laboratory with PC12 cells and sympathetic neurons have revealed further evidence for actions of NGF on growth cones (Seeley and Greene, 1983). In NGF-treated cultures, the recordings confirm previous findings that growth cones are often flattened structures which both translate along the substrate as a whole and which show continuous movement of labile, finger-like projections which probe the culture substrate and medium. Withdrawal of NGF from such cultures results within several hours in a progressive arrest of growth cone translation and motility and often, in rounding up of the growth cone into a "beaded" structure. Readdition of NGF rapidly elicits a dramatic change in growth cone behavior. With a latency of no more than several minutes, the growth cones re-flatten and highly motile projections reappear. After a latency of about half an hour, forward translational movement of the neurite tip is once again apparent. These rapid responses to NGF readdition occur even when the growth cone is separated from the cell body by neurite transection and hence are independent of transcription.

In summary, NGF appears rapidly able to regulate the maintenance, structure, motility, elongation and direction of growth cone movement by a mechanism that is independent of gene transcription. As will be discussed below, these actions could provide for local regulation of neurite outgrowth.

Rapid regulation of cell surface NGF receptors

There is abundant evidence that target cells for NGF possess specific surface receptors for the factor (see Bradshaw, 1978; Greene and Shooter, 1980, for review). Experiments with PC12 cells have revealed, as has been previously noted to occur for many other peptide receptors (Anderson et al., 1977), rapid regulation of the number of NGF receptors in response to NGF itself. That is, within several hours after PC12 cells are initially exposed to NGF, there occurs a 50–90% drop in the capacity of the cells to bind NGF (Calissano and Shelanski, 1980). Moreover, recovery of receptor binding capacity takes place within 12–24 h of NGF exposure. This phenomenon of "down-regulation" is distinct from the longer-term effect described above in which NGF appears to cause a long-latency increase in the number and cell surface density of NGF receptors. Suggestions have been made that ligand-mediated down-regulation of receptors could play an important role in regulating responsiveness of cells to peptide hormones (Anderson et al., 1977). Conceivably, increases in NGF concentration could elicit rapid responses followed shortly thereafter by decreased sensitivity to the factor. Recovery would occur only over a longer time. The effect of this would be to "sharpen" the time-course of responses to increases in NGF concentration. Such a mechanism might be particularly effective on a local scale.

Cell surface architecture

Observations by scanning and transmission electron microscopy have revealed a rapidly initiated (within 30 sec) sequence of changes in cell surface architecture that occurs in response to NGF and which is not affected by the presence of RNA synthesis inhibitors (Connolly et al., 1979, 1981). Among these changes are alterations in microvillus number, the transitory appearance and disappearance of surface ruffles, the formation of blebs and an increase in the cell surface density of coated pits. Fig. 2 shows examples of some of these effects. It has been hypothesized that such responses might in part relate to internalization of NGF and to the down-regulation of NGF receptors. Short-term alterations of cell surface in response to NGF have been observed on neurites and growth cones as well as on the cell body (J. Connolly et al., unpublished). Hence these changes might also conceivably play a role in the above described actions of NGF on growth cone motility and translation.

Cell survival

A major action of NGF is to maintain the survival of developing sympathetic and

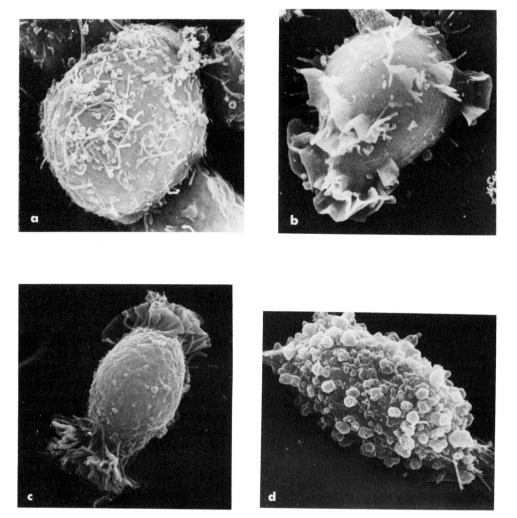

Fig. 2. Short-latency actions of NGF on PC12 cell surface architecture. a: scanning electron micrograph (SEM) of PC12 cell not treated with NGF. The surface has numerous small blebs and microvilli. × 4600. b: SEM of a PC12 cell after 3 min NGF treatment. Microvilli at this time are markedly decreased. Large ruffles become prominent on the dorsal surface of the cell and then at the periphery. × 4200. c: SEM of a PC12 cell 15 min after NGF treatment. The dorsal surface is quite smooth and some ruffling activity is seen at the periphery. × 4500. d: SEM of a PC12 cell 90 min after NGF treatment. The large blebs become prominent on the cells between one and four hours. × 4900.

sensory neurons (Levi-Montalcini and Angeletti, 1968). For example, if these neurons are deprived of NGF in vitro, irreversible changes may be detected within 4–6 h and by 12–18 h, the cells are dead. Inhibitor experiments such as those first described by Partlow and Larrabee (1971) show that NGF can maintain cell viability even when RNA synthesis is almost completely blocked. Hence, the effects of NGF on survival appear to be not only rapidly occurring, but are at least in part independent of transcription.

CONCLUSIONS AND CLOSING REMARKS

This paper has reviewed evidence for two separable classes of NGF's action on target cells. One class is observable within latencies of seconds to hours and is independent of de novo RNA synthesis. The other class is evident after latencies of hours to days and requires de novo synthesis of RNA. There are several points of interest which follow from these observations.

While the classes of NGF's action can be experimentally dissected from one another, they also exhibit a high degree of interdependence. For instance, in a permissive sense, long-term transcriptional actions of NGF can be expressed only if cell viability is maintained by the factor; as noted above, maintenance of viability is at least in part short latency and independent of transcription. Also, initiation of neurite outgrowth in PC12 cultures appears to require both transcriptional and non-transcriptional actions of NGF. Expression of other long-term genome-regulated effects of NGF may similarly require short-latency actions of the factor. Conversely, full expression of certain rapid responses to NGF may depend on long-term actions at the level of the genome. One clear example is embodied in the phenomenon of "priming" in which rapid transcription-independent stimulation of neurite regeneration in PC12 cultures occurs only if the cells have undergone prior transcriptional responses to NGF. The actions of NGF at growth cones also appear to be dependent on priming. A possible mechanism for such priming is that NGF transcriptionally regulates the synthesis of molecules which in turn mediate short-latency actions of the factor.

While both classes of NGF's action may be interdependent, each may also play a different type of role in directing neuronal development. Selective actions of NGF on the genome may provide for long-term, overall regulation of differentiation. For example, transcriptional mechanisms may elicit qualitative alterations in the cell phenotype, such as induction of neuronal differentiation of immature neuroblasts. Genomic actions may also quantitatively modulate cell phenotype as, for instance, by altering the level of neurotransmitter synthesis or by promoting global increases in neurite production. On the other hand, non-transcriptional actions of NGF could provide for rapid, local responses to the factor. An example might be regulation of the extent and direction of growth cone movement in response to changes in local concentration of NGF. Such types of responses could be restricted to a localized portion of the neuron and would not necessitate the time lag required for synthesis of macromolecules in the cell body and their transport to remote areas of processes. It has been suggested that NGF can be synthesized by target cells and there is evidence that NGF can be taken up by sympathetic and sensory nerve endings and retrogradely transported to cell bodies (see Thoenen and Barde, 1980, for review). In this light, NGF reaching cell bodies either locally, by humoral means, or by retrograde transport could bring about long-term, transcriptional responses that regulate the general differentiated state of the cell. Locally released NGF, on the other hand, could elicit short-latency, direct influences of targets on nearby growth cones.

A final point to be made is that although this discussion has necessarily focused on NGF, it is not unlikely that other neuronal "growth factors" possess either or both of the presently described classes of action. Perhaps the principles expressed here will be of use in functionally characterizing the roles of these factors as well.

ACKNOWLEDGEMENTS

We thank Ms. Margaret DiPiazza for her expert technical assistance and Ms. Yvel Calderon for aid in preparation of this manuscript. The experiments described here were supported by grants from the USPHS (NS 16036 and 17888) and March of Dimes Birth Defects Foundation. Mark Black was supported by a USPHS Postdoctoral Fellowship from NINCDS; Paulette Bernd was a Postdoctoral Fellow of the Pharmaceutical Manufacturers Association and P. John Seeley was a NATO Postdoctoral Fellow.

REFERENCES

Anderson, R.G.W., Brown, M.S. and Goldstein, J.L. (1977) Role of the coated endocytotic vesicle in the uptake of receptor-bound low density lipoprotein in human fibroblasts. *Cell*, 10: 351–364.

Black, M.M. and Greene, L.A. (1982) Changes in the colchicine susceptibility of microtubules associated with neutrite outgrowth: studies with nerve growth factor-responsive PC12 pheochromocytoma cells. *J. Cell Biol.*, 95: 379–386.

Burstein, D.E. and Greene, L.A. (1978) Evidence for both RNA-synthesis-dependent and -independent pathways in stimulation of neurite outgrowth by nerve growth factor. *Proc. nat. Acad. Sci. U.S.A.*, 75: 6059–6063.

Bradshaw, R.A. (1978) Nerve growth factor. *Ann. Rev. Biochem.*, 47: 191–216.

Calissano, P. and Shelanski, M.L. (1980) Interaction of nerve growth factor with pheochromocytoma cells. Evidence for tight binding and sequestration. *Neuroscience*, 5: 1033–1039.

Campenot, R.B. (1977) Local control of neurite development by nerve growth factor. *Proc. nat. Acad. Sci. U.S.A.*, 74: 4516–4519.

Connolly, J.L., Greene, L.A., Viscarello, R.R. and Riley, W.D. (1979) Rapid, sequential changes in surface morphology of PC12 pheochromocytoma cells in response to nerve growth factor. *J. Cell Biol.*, 82: 820–827.

Connolly, J.L., Green, S. and Greene, L.A. (1981) Pit formation and rapid changes in surface morphology of sympathetic neurons in response to nerve growth factor. *J. Cell Biol.*, 90: 176–180.

Dichter, M.A., Tischler, A.S. and Greene, L.A. (1977) Nerve growth factor-induced increase in electrical excitability and acetylcholine sensitivity in a rat pheochromocytoma cell line. *Nature (Lond.)*, 268: 501–504.

Garrels, J.I. and Schubert, D. (1979) Modulation of protein synthesis by nerve growth factor. *J. biol. Chem.*, 254: 7978–7985.

Greene, L.A. (1981) Chemical factors influencing neuronal development. In T.A. Sears (Ed.), *Neuronal-Glial Cell Interrelationships*, Springer-Verlag, Berlin, pp. 303–320.

Greene, L.A. and Rein, G. (1977) Release, storage and uptake of catecholamines by a clonal cell line of nerve growth factor (NGF) responsive pheochromocytoma cells. *Brain Res.*, 129: 247–263.

Greene, L.A. and Rukenstein, A. (1981) Regulation of acetylcholinesterase activity by nerve growth factor: Role of transcription and dissociation from effects on proliferation and neurite outgrowth. *J. biol. Chem.*, 256: 6363–6367.

Greene, L.A. and Shooter, E.M. (1980) The nerve growth factor: Biochemistry, synthesis, and mechanism of action. *Ann. Rev. Neurosci.*, 3: 353–402.

Greene, L.A. and Tischler, A.S. (1976) Establishment of a noradrenergic clonal line of rat adrenal pheochromocytoma cells which respond to nerve growth factor. *Proc. nat. Acad. Sci. U.S.A.*, 73: 2424–2428.

Greene, L.A. and Tischler, A.S. (1982) PC12 pheochromocytoma cultures in neurobiological research. *Advanc. Cell. Neurobiol.*, 3: 373–414.

Greene, L.A., Burstein, D.E. and Black, M.M. (1980) The priming model for the mechanism of action of nerve growth factor: Evidence derived from clonal PC12 pheochromocytoma cells. In E. Giacobini, A. Vernadakis and A. Shahar (Eds.), *Tissue Culture in Neurobiology*, Raven Press, New York, pp. 313–319.

Griffin, C.G. and Letourneau, P.C. (1980) Rapid retraction of neurites by sensory neurons in response to increased concentrations of nerve growth factor. *J. Cell Biol.*, 86: 156–161.

Gundersen, R.W. and Barrett, J.N. (1980) Characterization of the turning response of dorsal root neurites toward nerve growth factor. *J. Cell Biol.*, 87: 546–554.

Lasek, R.J. and Shelanski, M.L. (1981) Cytoskeletons and the architecture of nervous systems. *Neurosci. Res. Prog.*, 19: 1–153.

Lee, V., Greene, L.A. and Shelanski, M.L. (1981) Identification of neural and adrenal medullary surface membrane glycoproteins recognized by antisera to cultured rat sympathetic neurons and PC12 pheochromocytoma cells. *Neuroscience*, 6: 2773–2786.

Levi-Montalcini, R. and Angeletti, P.U. (1968) The nerve growth factor. *Physiol. Rev.*, 48: 534–569.

MacDonnell, P.C., Tolson, N. and Guroff, G. (1977) Selective de novo synthesis of tyrosine hydroxylase in organ cultures of rat superior cervical ganglia after in vivo administration of nerve growth factor. *J. biol. Chem.*, 252: 5859–5863.

McGuire, J.C. and Greene, L.A. (1980) Nerve growth factor stimulation of specific protein synthesis by rat PC12 pheochromocytoma cells. *Neuroscience*, 5: 179–180.

McGuire, J.C., Greene, L.A. and Furano, A.V. (1978) NGF stimulates incorporation of glucose or glucosamine into an external glycoprotein in cultured rat PC12 pheochromocytoma cells. *Cell*, 15: 357–365.

Partlow, L.M. and Larrabee, M.G. (1971) Effects of a nerve growth factor, embryo age, and metabolic inhibitors on growth of fibers and on synthesis of ribonucleic acid and protein in embryonic sympathetic ganglia. *J. Neurochem.*, 18: 2101–2118.

Rudy, B., Kirschenbaum, B. and Greene, L.A. (1982) Nerve growth factor-induced increase in saxitoxin binding to rat PC12 pheochromocytoma cells. *J. Neurosci.*, 2: 1405–1411.

Salton, S.R.J., Richter-Landsberg, C., Greene, L.A. and Shelanski, M.L. (1983) Nerve growth factor inducible large external (NILE) glycoprotein: Studies of a central and peripheral neuronal marker. *J. Neurosci.*, in press.

Seeley, P.J. and Greene, L.A. (1983) Short-latency, local actions of nerve growth factor on growth cones. *Proc. nat. Acad. Sci. U.S.A.*, in press.

Sensenbrenner, M. (1977) Dissociated brain cells in primary cultures. In S. Federoff and L. Hertz (Eds.), *Cell, Tissue and Organ Cultures in Neurobiology*, Academic Press, New York, pp. 191–213.

Thoenen, H. and Barde, Y.-A. (1980) Physiology of nerve growth factor. *Physiol. Rev.*, 60: 1284–1335.

Varon, S. and Adler, R. (1981) Trophic and specifying factors directed to neuronal cells. *Advanc. Cell. Neurobiol.*, 2: 115–163.

Inhibition of Protease Activity Can
Lead to Neurite Extension in
Neuroblastoma Cells

DENIS MONARD, EVELYN NIDAY, ALAIN LIMAT and FRANK SOLOMON

Friedrich Miescher-Institut, P.O. Box 2534, CH-4002 Basel (Switzerland) and (F.S.) Department of Biology and Center for Cancer Research, MIT, Cambridge, MA 02139 (U.S.A.)

INTRODUCTION

Neurite extension is one of the first morphological steps in neuronal differentiation. A study on the nature and the regulation of the biochemical events involved in this phenomenon requires an appropriate experimental model. The extension of neurites in neuroblastoma cells offers a number of experimental advantages for such an approach (Haffke and Seeds, 1975).

Glial cells, including gliomas, release a macromolecular factor which induces a dose-dependent neurite outgrowth in neuroblastoma cells (Monard et al., 1973). This change in neuronal cellular morphology is also promoted by the medium conditioned by certain primary cultures of rat brain. There is a correlation between the presence of glial factor activity in such media and the age of the animal from which the primary culture was derived (Schürch-Rathgeb and Monard, 1978). These results suggest the importance of exogenous signals for the regulation of neurite outgrowth. They also imply that this phenomenon can be modulated by glial–neuronal interactions.

In the nervous system, neuroblast migration precedes neurite extension and further neuronal differentiation. The role of cell surface protease activity in cell migration has been stressed in many developmental systems (Sherman et al., 1976; Topp et al., 1976). Migrating cells, including cells transformed by oncogenic viruses, have more cell surface proteolytic activity than stationary, differentiated cells (Unkeless et al., 1973; Ossowski et al., 1974). Cell surface proteolytic activity is usually measured by the activity of cell derived plasminogen activators (Unkeless et al., 1974). Plasminogen activators or urokinase are serine proteases converting plasminogen to plasmin which is then able to degrade fibrin (Williams, 1951). Plasminogen activator production has been detected in cerebellar cultured cells dissociated at the time of active granule cell migration (Krystosek and Seeds, 1978). Recently a marginal increase in neurite outgrowth has been reported when human neuroblastoma cells are incubated in a medium supplemented with plasminogen depleted serum (Becherer and Wachsman, 1980). We found that the medium conditioned by glioma cells is strongly inhibitory in the plasminogen activator assay. We therefore started to explore the possibility that inhibition of cell surface associated proteases is involved in the glia induced neurite extension in neuroblastoma cells.

[359]

INHIBITION OF PLASMINOGEN ACTIVATION BY PURIFIED PREPARATION OF GLIAL FACTOR

Serum-free glia conditioned medium (SFCM) is produced on a roller auto-harvester system, centrifuged and concentrated about 20–25-fold with an Amicon hollow fiber DC-2 apparatus. A dose of about 1100 ng of protein of this concentrate is required to induce optimal neurite extension in the neuroblastoma assay we have developed (Schürch-Rathgeb and Monard, 1978). After high speed centrifugation, glial factor activity can be purified using anion exchange, Affi-Blue and car-boxymethyl (CM)-Sepharose chromatography (Limat et al., in preparation). About 1 ng protein of this purified material is then required to obtain optimal neurite extension. Thus about a 1000-fold increase in specific activity is achieved by this procedure.

Such purified preparations of glial factor inhibit the activation of plasminogen by urokinase, as measured with a very sensitive assay using [^{125}I]fibrin as substrate (Table I). Although we have not yet been able to demonstrate that such CM-Sepharose purified glial factor preparations are also able to inhibit other serine proteases like trypsin, chymotrypsin or thrombin, these results are not conclusive. The assays for these proteases are not as sensitive as the urokinase test. Therefore the amount of protein available in our preparations (at the most 0.5 µg/ml) could be insufficient to detect inhibitory activity in these assays.

EFFECT OF PROTEASE INHIBITORS ON NEURITE EXTENSION

Since a serine protease inhibitory activity might be involved in glial factor activity, we asked whether well known serine protease inhibitors could promote neurite extension. The results in Table II demonstrate that among the different protease inhibitors tested, only leupeptin and hirudin can efficiently induce neurite outgrowth,

TABLE I

Inhibition of plasminogen activation by purified glial factor activity

Glial factor activity was purified by the procedure mentioned in the text. Urokinase was measured by monitoring the degradation of [^{125}I]fibrin as described by Unkeless et al. (1973). 0.2 µl of the CM-Sepharose pool tested here promoted neurite extension in 49.4% of the neuroblastoma cells under the conditions des-cribed earlier (Schürch-Rathgeb and Monard, 1978).

	cpm [^{125}I]fibrin released in 17 h
Urokinase 1 mU	3116 ± 22
+2 µl glycine buffer	4130 ± 23
+2 µl CM-Sepharose pool	542 ± 125
+5 µl glycine buffer	3062 ± 81
+5 µl CM-Sepharose pool	138 ± 13

TABLE II

Effect of protease inhibitors on neurite outgrowth

The different inhibitors were dissolved in medium and added during the 4 h bioassay described earlier (Schürch-Rathgeb and Monard, 1978).

Inhibitor	Concentration	% cells with neurites
None	–	18.7 ± 1.7
Hirudin	0.5 ng/ml	53.2 ± 3.9
	2.5 ng/ml	62.3 ± 5.4
Leupeptin	10^{-4} M	61.7 ± 2.7
Soya bean trypsin inhibitor	10 ng/ml	23.8 ± 2.2
	2 μg/ml	46.5 ± 2.9
	10 μg/ml	31.6 ± 6.4
Aprotinin	0.14 TIU*/ml	26.6 ± 2.4
Ovomucoid	5 μg/ml	25.4 ± 1.0
Benzamidine	10^{-3} M	23.7 ± 1.7
TLCK (N-α-tosyl-L-lysyl chloromethyl ketone)	10^{-4} M	24.9 ± 7.5

*One trypsin inhibitor unit (TIU) will inhibit 2 trypsin units by 50% where one trypsin unit will hydrolyze 1.0 μmol of α-N-benzoyl-DL-arginine-*p*-nitroanilide per minute at pH 7.8 at 25°C.

thus mimicking glial factor activity. It is important to stress the high potency of hirudin which already shows neurite promoting activity at a concentration as low as 0.5 ng/ml. The fact that the other inhibitors tested do not promote neurite extension at such low concentration suggests a fairly high specificity for the type of cell surface protease involved.

INHIBITION OF GLIAL FACTOR ACTIVITY BY THROMBIN

Since hirudin is an inhibitor highly specific for thrombin (Markwardt, 1955; Markwardt and Walsmann, 1958), we therefore tested the effect of thrombin on glial factor activity. Extremely low concentrations of thrombin are able to antagonize the neurite extension promoted by concentrated serum-free glia conditioned medium (Fig. 1). It is interesting that this antagonism is also specific since urokinase and trypsin, other serine proteases, are not able to abolish glial factor activity when tested at such low concentrations. In fact, trypsin will inhibit only at 250 ng/ml and urokinase does not

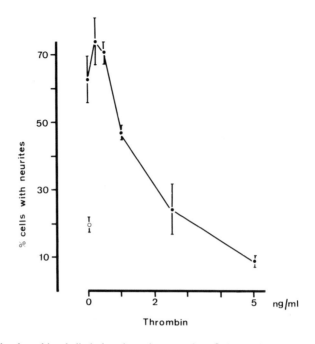

Fig. 1. Inhibition by thrombin of glia-induced neurite extension. ●, increasing concentrations of thrombin were added to 10 μl of SFCM in the 4 h bioassay (Schürch-Rathgeb and Monard, 1978). ○, control culture incubated without SFCM.

show any inhibition when tested at 20 Plough units/ml or about 4 μg/ml (Results not shown).

COMMENTS

The fact that an inhibitor of urokinase activity, present in the concentrated glia conditioned medium, copurifies with glial factor activity in our procedure could still be coincidental. At this stage we are trying to determine whether both activities are due to the same protein. Such studies should also indicate if glial factor activity is solely due to inhibition of proteolytic activity. The stimulation of neurite extension by extremely low concentrations of hirudin argues against a pure coincidence. We have already stressed the specificity of both the proteases and the inhibitors which show an inhibitory or a stimulatory effect on neurite extension. It is therefore difficult to explain why purified glial factor inhibits urokinase, but that the reverse is not true. This could indicate that the neuroblastoma cell surface protease involved is distinct from urokinase and preferentially interacts with the inhibitor present in purified preparations of glial factor activity. In fact, the extremely low concentration of hirudin necessary to promote neurite extension would rather support a "thrombin-like" character for the protease activity associated with the neuroblastoma cells. This argument is further supported by the very low concentration of thrombin required to antagonize glial factor activity. Here it is important to stress that the biological effects triggered by thrombin in platelets or fibroblasts require higher concentrations (10 μg/ml or 1 μg/ml, respectively) (Lapetina and Cuatrecasas, 1979; Chen and Buchanan, 1975; Carney et al., 1978). As mentioned earlier, the failure to demonstrate thrombin inhibitory activity in purified preparation of glial factor activity could simply be due to the very sensitive assays required for the small amount of inhibitory protein available. A strong species specificity for urokinase could also explain the lack of inhibition of glial factor activity by the human urokinase tested in the present experiments.

Again, the possibility that protease inhibitory activity and glial factor activity are distinct entities has not yet been ruled out. Nevertheless, the promotion of neurite extension by low concentrations of hirudin clearly indicates that inhibition of a cell surface associated proteolytic enzyme can play a key role in neuronal morphological differentiation. It is very tempting to speculate that this phenomenon makes biological sense: neuronal neurite outgrowth does take place at the time neuroblast migration has stopped. Surrounding glial cells could therefore release protease inhibitory substances which would modulate this cellular neuronal event.

ACKNOWLEDGEMENTS

We would like to thank M. Rentsch for technical assistance, Dr. H. Fritz for the gift of hirudin and Drs. J.D. Vassalli and E. Reich for their help in setting up the urokinase assay.

REFERENCES

Becherer, P.R. and Wachsman, J.T. (1980) Increased neurite development and plasminogen activator expression by exposure of human neuroblastoma cells to a plasminogen-deficient growth medium. *J. cell. Physiol.*, 104: 47–52.

Carney, D.H., Glenn, K.C. and Cunningham, D.D. (1978) Conditions which affect initiation of animal cell division by trypsin and thrombin. *J. cell. Physiol.*, 95: 13–22.

Chen, L.B. and Buchanan, J.M. (1975) Mitogenic activity of blood components. I Thrombin and prothrombin. *Proc. nat. Acad. Sci. U.S.A.*, 72: 131–135.

Haffke, S.C. and Seeds, N.W. (1975) Neuroblastoma: the *E. coli* of neurobiology? *Life Sci.*, 16: 1649–1658.

Krystosek, A. and Seeds, N.W. (1978) Plasminogen activator production by cultures of developing cerebellum. *Fed. Proc.*, 37: 1702.

Lapetina, E.G. and Cuatrecasas, P. (1979) Stimulation of phosphatidic acid production in platelets precedes the formation of arachidonate and parallels the release of serotonin. *Biochim. biophys. Acta*, 573: 394–402.

Markwardt, F. (1955) Untersuchungen über Hirudin. *Naturwissenschaften*, 42: 537–538.

Markwardt, F. and Walsmann, P. (1958) Die Reaktion zwischen Hirudin und Thrombin. *Hoppe-Seylers Z. Physiol. Chem.*, 312: 85–98.

Monard, D., Solomon, F., Rentsch, M. and Gysin, R. (1973). Glia-induced morphological differentiation in neuroblastoma cells. *Proc. nat. Acad. Sci. U.S.A.*, 70: 1894–1897.

Ossowski, L., Quigley, J.P. and Reich, E. (1974). Fibrinolysis associated with oncogenic transformation. *J. biol. Chem.*, 249: 4312–4320.

Schürch-Rathgeb, Y. and Monard, D. (1978) Brain development influences the appearance of glial factor-like activity in rat brain primary cultures. *Nature (Lond.)*, 273: 308–309.

Sherman, M.I., Strickland, S. and Reich, E. (1976) Differentiation of early mouse embryonic and teratocarcinoma cells in vitro: plasminogen activator production. *Cancer Res.*, 36: 4208–4216.

Topp, W., Hall, J.D., Marsden, M., Teresky, A.K., Rifkin, D., Levine, A.J. and Pollack, R. (1976). In vitro differentiation of teratomas and the distribution of creatine phosphokinase and plasminogen activator in teratocarcinoma-derived cells. *Cancer Res.*, 36: 4217–4223.

Unkeless, J.C., Tobia, A., Ossowski, L., Quigley, J.P., Rifkin, D.B. and Reich, E. (1973) An enzymatic function associated with transformation of fibroblasts by oncogenic viruses. *J. exp. Med.*, 137: 85–111.

Williams, J.R.B. (1951) The fibrinolytic activity of urine. *Brit. J. exp. Pathol.*, 32: 530–537.

In Vitro Studies on Central Dopaminergic Neurons' Development

A. PROCHIANTZ, M.-C. DAGUET, U. DI PORZIO, A. HERBET and J. GLOWINSKI

INSERM U 114, Collège de France, 11, place Marcelin Berthelot, 75231 Paris Cedex 05 (France) and (U. di P.) Laboratorio Embriologia Molecolare, Via Toiano 2, Arco Felice, Napoli (Italy)

INTRODUCTION

The pattern of development of nerve fibers, both at the periphery and in the central nervous system (CNS) seems to be dictated through specific interactions between the growing tip of the neuron and its environment. Growth of the neurites is asymmetric and seems to be directed by the ability of the growth cones to follow specific pathways or to recognize specific diffusible signals. In a similar fashion the terminal arborizations will only develop inside precise territories, as if the neurite was able to descriminate between target and non-target structures.

It is long ago that Levi-Montalcini and Hamburger have demonstrated the existence of diffusible proteic factors able to stimulate nerve growth (1951). Indeed, due to their pioneering work and to that of many other contributors it was possible to show that the noradrenergic sympathetic neurons and some sensory neurons needed the presence of a nerve growth factor (NGF) for their survival and growth (Bradshaw, 1978). It was also suggested that NGF may exert some sort of chemotactic guidance on the growing sympathetic and sensory cells (Levi-Montalcini, 1976; Letourneau, 1978; Campenot, 1977). More recently, a factor having growth stimulating properties for the parasympathetic cholinergic neurons from the chick ciliary ganglion has been characterized (Adler et al., 1979). It is noteworthy that in both cases the factors can be synthesized by the cells located in the target area (Landa et al., 1980; Ebendal et al., 1980). However, at least in the case of the NGF, important amounts of the factor can be detected in non-target territories.

In contrast with the results accumulated concerning the peripheral neurons the existence of specific growth factors (target specific and nerve type specific) in the brain is still questioned. In the last few years we have addressed this question using the following experimental model: dissociated dopaminergic (DA) mesencephalic neurons from the embryonic mouse were grown in the presence or in the absence of their striatal target cells and the development of these DA neurons was compared in both experimental conditions. The use of the DA nigrostriatal system was mainly dictated by two considerations: (1) DA neurons are not very numerous and their localization in the brain is well known, and (2) the innervation of their target territory (the striatum) is massive and convergent. These points allow us to stress the similarity between the DA nigrostriatal pathway and any system constituted by an homogenous cell population within a ganglion and its target territory.

[365]

RESULTS

Growth of central DA neurons

Central DA neurons were localized in 13-day-old embryo brain sections by immunocytochemistry using an antibody against tyrosine hydroxylase (TH). The region of the brain containing these DA cells was dissected, and the cells were dissociated and plated as already described (Prochiantz et al., 1979). The morphological development of the DA neurons was followed biochemically and morphologically (Berger et al., 1982). It was shown that they can develop for very long periods of time (over six weeks) during which they extend long varicose processes. The ability of the cells to specifically take up exogenous tritiated dopamine ([³H]DA) and to synthesize the neuromediator from its tritiated tyrosine precursor was also demonstrated and shown to increase with time. Loaded or synthesized [³H]DA could be released by the cells into the medium when they were incubated in the presence of veratridine. This release is calcium dependent and is blocked in the presence of tetrodotoxin (TTX), indicating the presence on the DA cells of fast sodium channels (Daguet et al., 1980).

Influence of striatal target cells

When 13-day-old mesencephalic cells were grown in the presence of striatal target cells from 15-day-old embryos (cocultures), it was shown that the ability of the cells to take up exogenous [³H]DA and to synthesize it from [³H]tyrosine was increased by at least two-fold, either after 8 days or after 15 days in vitro (Prochiantz et al., 1979). The absolute number of DA neurons was not modified in coculture and it was concluded that this effect reflected an enhanced maturation of the DA cells in the presence of their target cells. Indeed, since these experiments had been done with cells grown in the presence of serum, the presence of glial elements was inevitable and it was not established whether these elements were important in the observed enhancement of DA cells maturation. In order to elucidate this point we repeated these experiments in a serum-free chemically defined medium complemented with proteins, hormones and salts (CDM) as described by different authors (Bottenstein et al., 1980). In these conditions the number of non neuronal cells was very much reduced (95% at least) as estimated by the number of flat cells able to incorporate tritiated thymidine during the first two days in culture. In spite of this net decrease in the number of non-neuronal cells the ability of DA cells to take up and synthesize [³H]DA was still enhanced in the presence of their striatal target cells. From this it was concluded that this effect was due to direct or indirect interactions between neuronal cells exclusively (Di Porzio et al., 1980).

In the course of this study on the development of central DA neurons in CDM we found out that the survival of these cells was very much reduced (less than 10 days) when compared to that observed in the presence of serum. The survival time could be increased again (up to three weeks) by conditioning the CDM on a layer of either glial or neuronal cells. In these conditions the cell population was still composed of neurons (95% at least), as demonstrated by the number of cells stained with an antibody against neurofilaments versus that of cells stained with an antibody against vimentine and/or glial fibrillary acidic protein (Prochiantz et al., 1982). Again it was demonstrated that in these conditions after eight and fifteen days in coculture the ability of DA cells to take up and synthesize [³H]DA was increased, without changes in the total number of DA neurons (Di Porzio et al., 1980).

Research of molecular clues

The results briefly described above suggested that the presence of striatal neurons was beneficial to the development in vitro of DA neurons. Such an interaction could be indirect (synthesis of diffusible factors) or direct (cell–cell interactions). A series of experiments was performed in order to test the hypothesis that striatal membranes may bear molecular signals able to stimulate DA maturation. Crude striatal membranes were prepared from mice of different ages. These membranes were added to the mesencephalic neurons in vitro and the ability of the cells to take up [³H]DA after three days in culture was measured. We found out that coculturing mesencephalic cells with striatal membranes from two- and three-week-old mice resulted in an increased [³H]DA uptake capacity of the DA neurons. This effect was not observed when younger (one-week-old) or adult membranes were used. Crude membrane preparations from other parts of the brain such as parietal cortex, mesencephalon, cerebellum or hippocampus had no effect on the [³H]DA uptake capacity of the DA neurons. It was also found that the striatal membranes had no effect on the ability of mesencephalic GABAergic neurons to take up exogenous tritiated GABA (Prochiantz et al., 1981). One possible interpretation of these results is that at the period of maximal synaptogenesis, molecular clues exist at the surface of striatal target cells which stimulate DA fibers growth, this stimulation being reflected in vitro by an increase uptake of [³H]DA per DA neuron.

CONCLUSION

The target cells can influence afferent neurons development through the synthesis of diffusible factors and/or through direct neuron-neuron contacts. In our experimental model we were able to cultivate central mesencephalic DA neurons and to show that their development was increased in the presence of their striatal target neurons. At the moment we have not been able to monitor in conditioned medium from striatal cells the presence of a diffusible factor that would stimulate DA cells maturation. This does not preclude the existence of such factors that in our conditions might be too diluted, or unstable. We therefore focused our attention on a possible role of membrane interactions. If membrane interactions exist in vivo between DA mesencephalic neurons and striatal neurons, they can only concern the DA terminals and the striatal cells. It was not unlikely that striatal membranes may therefore provide a substrate on which a DA terminal would find specific molecular clues enhancing their growth. Such a possibility is stressed by the work of Bonhoeffer and Huf (1980) who showed that growth cones of retina ganglion cells have a marked preference for their tectal target cells. Our results suggest that a similar phenomenon may also be true for DA terminals and striatal membranes at the time of maximal synaptogenesis. Interestingly enough non target structures do not seem to bear the signals enhancing DA neurons maturation. In view of these results and of our interpretation it is noteworthy, that it has been recently demonstrated that membrane preparations from the tectum are able to bind to retina ganglion cell neurites and that this property is not shared by membranes prepared from other parts of the brain (Halfter et al., 1980).

REFERENCES

Adler, R., Landa, K.B., Manthorpe, M. and Varon, S. (1979) Cholinergic neuronotrophic factors: intraocular distribution of trophic activity for ciliary neurons. *Science*, 204: 1434–1436.

Berger, B., Di Porzio, U., Daguet, M.-C., Gay, M., Vigny, A., Glowinski, J. and Prochiantz, A. (1982) Long-term development of mesencephalic dopaminergic neurons of mouse embryos in dissociated primary cultures: morphological and histochemical characteristics. *Neuroscience*, 7: 193–205.

Bonhoeffer, F. and Huf, J. (1980) Recognition of cell types by axonal growth cones in vitro. *Nature (Lond.)*, 288: 162–164.

Bottenstein, J.E., Skaper, S.D., Varon, S.S. and Sato, G. (1980) Selective survival of neurons from chick embryo sensory ganglionic dissociates utilizing serum-free medium. *Exp. Cell. Res.*, 125: 183–190.

Bradshaw, R.A. (1978) Nerve growth factor. *Ann. Rev. Biochem.*, 47: 191–216.

Campenot, R.B. (1978) Local control of neurite development by nerve growth factor. *Proc. nat. Acad. Sci. U.S.A.*, 74: 4516–4519.

Daguet, M.-C., Di Porzio, U., Prochiantz, A., Kato, A. and Glowinski, J. (1980) Release of dopamine from dissociated mesencephalic dopaminergic neurons in primary cultures in absence or presence of striatal target cells. *Brain Res.*, 191: 564–568.

Di Porzio, U., Daguet, M.-C., Glowinski, J. and Prochiantz, A. (1980) Effect of striatal target cells on in vitro maturation of mesencephalic dopaminergic neurones grown in serum-free conditions. *Nature (Lond.)*, 288: 370–373.

Ebendal, T., Olson, L., Sieger, A. and Hedlund, K.-O. (1980) Nerve growth factor in the rat iris. *Nature (Lond.)*, 286: 25–28.

Halfter, W., Clavicz, M. and Schwarz, U. (1980) *Nature*, 292, 67.

Landa, K.B., Adler, R., Manthorpe, M. and Varon, S. (1980) Cholinergic neuronotrophic factors III. Developmental increase of trophic activity for chick embryo ciliary ganglion neurons in their intraocular target tissues. *Develop. Biol.*, 74: 401–408.

Letourneau, P.C. (1978) Chemotactic response of nerve fiber elongation to nerve growth factor. *Develop. Biol.*, 66: 183–196.

Levi-Montalcini, R. (1976) The nerve growth factor: its role in growth, differentiation and function of the sympathetic adrenergic neuron. In M.A. Corner and D.F. Swaab (Eds.), *Perspective in Brain Research, Progr. Brain Res., Vol. 45*, Elsevier/North-Holland, Amsterdam, pp. 235–258.

Levi-Montalcini, R. and Hamburger, V. (1951) Selective growth stimulating effect of mouse sarcoma on the sensory and sympathetic nervous system of the chick embryo. *J. exp. Zool.*, 116: 321–362.

Prochiantz, A., Di Porzio, U., Kato, A. and Glowinski, J. (1979) In vitro maturation of mesencephalic dopaminergic neurons from mouse embryos is enhanced in presence of their striatal target cells. *Proc. nat. Acad. Sci. U.S.A.*, 76: 5387–5381.

Prochiantz, A., Daguet, M.-C., Herbet, A. and Glowinski, J. (1981) Specific stimulation of in vitro maturation of mesencephalic dopaminergic neurones by striatal membranes. *Nature (Lond.)*, 293: 570–573.

Prochiantz, A., Delacourte, A., Daguet, M.-C. and Paulin, D. (1982) Intermediate filament proteins in mouse brain cells cultured in the presence or absence of fetal calf serum. *Exp. Cell Res.*, 139: 404–410.

Roles for Retrograde Factors in Synapse Formation at the Nerve–Muscle Junction

C.E. HENDERSON

Institut Pasteur, Neurobiologie Moléculaire, 25 Rue du Docteur Roux, 75015 Paris (France)

At the molecular level, the rules of synapse formation in the peripheral nervous system are poorly understood. Nevertheless, some of the molecular interactions between the developing nerve cell and its potential target have proved amenable to experimental study, mainly by the methods of in vitro cell culture. These interactions may be classed either as "anterograde", such as the effect of the nerve on the specialization of what is to become the postsynaptic membrane, or, conversely, as "retrograde" (Changeux, 1979). It has been proposed for many systems that soluble or membrane-bound "retrograde factors" derived from the target cell affect three major parameters of nerve cell development: (i) cell survival; (ii) synthesis of enzymes involved in neurotransmitter metabolism; and (iii) neurite outgrowth and stabilization.

The nerve growth factor (NGF) has been much studied as a candidate for the role of physiological retrograde factor (Thoenen and Barde, 1980). Its action in the periphery, however, is restricted to sensory and sympathetic neurons. Several observations suggest that motor neurons too are dependent for their normal development upon the presence of their target tissues. In the chick embryo, early extirpation of the target muscle leads to an enhancement of naturally-occurring cell death. This is true for spinal motoneurons after limb bud extirpation (Hollyday and Hamburger, 1976) and for the ciliary neurons of the cholinergic ciliary ganglion after removal of the eye (Landmesser and Pilar, 1974). Neurons destined normally to die can be "rescued" by increasing the volume of available target tissue. In the light of these results, much effort has been devoted to the identification of retrograde factors involved in these two systems.

In the case of the ciliary ganglion, several putative factors have been detected. One of them, ciliary neuronotrophic factor (CNTF), is required for the survival in culture of dissociated ganglionic neurons (Adler et al., 1979). It is found at high specific activities in the intraocular target tissues at the time when neuronal death occurs in the ciliary ganglion (Landa et al., 1980) and has been partially purified (Manthorpe et al., 1980; Bonyhady et al., 1980). A second factor, polyornithine-attachable neurite-promoting factor (PNPF) which promotes neurite outgrowth from CNTF-supported neurons, is found in media conditioned by a wide variety of cells (Adler et al., 1981) and is only active when bound to a positively-charged culture substratum (Collins, 1978). Separable activities have been found in eye extract that stimulate, respectively, neuronal growth and choline acetyltransferase activity in cultures of ciliary ganglionic neurons (Nishi and Berg, 1981). Other workers report a macromolecular factor from chick gizzard that stimulates synapse formation in cocultures of chick ciliary ganglion neurons and rat myotubes (Miki et al., 1981).

[369]

Our understanding of factors affecting the development of spinal motoneurons is less advanced. High molecular weight fractions of medium conditioned by skeletal myotubes have been reported to increase levels of choline acetyltransferase in cultures of dissociated spinal neurons (Giller et al., 1977; Brookes et al., 1980; Godfrey et al., 1980), and to support the survival in such cultures of motoneurons putatively identified by their choline acetyltransferase (CAT) content (Schnaar and Schaffner, 1980) or by their ability to transport horseradish peroxidase (HRP) retrogradely from the limb muscles (Bennett et al., 1980). Neurite outgrowth from rat spinal cord explants was enhanced by media conditioned by primary cultures of skeletal muscle, fibroblasts, or lung cells (Dribin and Barrett, 1980). The active factor(s) was of high molecular weight but did not appear to be βNGF or fibronectin. Mesenchymal embryonic limb target tissue exerted a neurite-promoting effect upon spinal cord explants from *Rana pipiens* (Pollack et al., 1981).

We have used dissociated chicken spinal neurons cultured in serum-free medium to study the effects of skeletal muscle-derived factors on neurite outgrowth (Henderson et al., 1981). When neurons from 4.5-day (stage 25) embryos were cultured for 20 h in minimum essential medium ("non-conditioned medium"), less than 10% of the living cells bore one or more neurites (Fig. 1a, c). Parallel cultures performed in minimal essential medium that had been exposed for 2 days to fused skeletal myotubes ("conditioned medium") developed levels of neurite ourgrowth of >30% cells with neurite (Fig. 1b, c), and this response varied in a dose-dependent manner with conditioned medium concentration, allowing the units of neurite-promoting activity in a given sample to be measured.

This rapid quantitative assay defined in vitro an activity that affects a process closely related to that of neurite outgrowth in vitro. Using this assay, the active factor(s) in muscle-conditioned medium was shown to be trypsin-sensitive and to be associated with species of molecular weights 40,000, 500,000 and >10⁶. Conditioned medium (protein concentration 50 μg/ml) was active either in the presence or

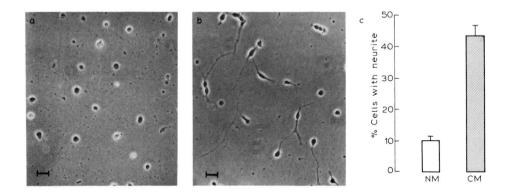

Fig. 1. Effect of muscle-conditioned medium on neurite outgrowth from spinal cord cells. a and b: phase-contrast micrographs (scale = 20 μm) of dissociated spinal cord cells after 22 h of culture in non-conditioned (a) and conditioned (b) serum-free medium. c: quantitative assay of neurite extension after 20 h in non-conditioned (NM) and conditioned (CM) medium. Vertical bars represent the S.E.M. of results from four dishes from each medium. These cultures contained 23 ± 1 living cells per microscopic field in non-conditioned medium and 26 ± 2 per field in conditioned medium. (From Henderson et al., 1981, with permission.)

absence of 10% serum. Neither NGF, insulin, BSA or media conditioned by cultures of lung, heart or C6 glioma showed any activity in this bioassay; although media conditioned by skin fibroblasts or liver did enhance neurite outgrowth, their specific activities were lower than that of muscle-conditioned medium. Under conditions in which they were responsive to NGF, conditioned medium only slightly enhanced neurite outgrowth from explanted dorsal root ganglia. Thus the neurite-promoting activity shows some specificity as regards both its source and its target.

Two possible explanations of the effect of conditioned medium were considered: (a) all healthy neurons were intrinsically capable of neurite outgrowth but only in conditioned medium did they receive sufficient metabolic support for this to occur; or (b) conditioned medium had a direct action on the initiation of neurite outgrowth from healthy, responsive but morphologically undifferentiated neurons. In a recent study (Henderson et al., 1983), it was shown that although neurons cultured in the absence of conditioned medium developed only low levels of neurite outgrowth, they survived and were capable of responding to conditioned medium added after up to one day in culture. The growth factor(s) in muscle-conditioned medium therefore acts as a specifying factor for neurite outgrowth rather than simply as a metabolic support. Nevertheless, persistence of neurites once the cells have responded to the growth factor was shown to require the continued presence of conditioned medium.

Neurite-promoting factors from other sources are considered to act in vitro either by binding direct to responsive neurons (Sutter et al., 1979) or by "coating" the culture substratum so as to create a favorable terrain for neurite development (Collins, 1978). We showed that the present factor binds to polyornithine but not to tissue culture plastic under cell culture conditions. Nevertheless, spinal neurons responded to conditioned medium equally well on both substrata, suggesting that the partition of growth factor between supernatant and substratum is not important for its activity. It most probably interacts directly with the spinal neurons.

It is interesting to compare the mode of action in vitro of this factor with those of known neurite-promoting factors for other chicken neurons. Like NGF, it can act in soluble form (Frazier et al., 1973) and is required to be continuously present. At least in culture, however, it has no comparable effect on the survival of responsive neurons. The PNPF of ciliary neurons is only active when bound to the culture substratum. This was not true for the active factor in our muscle-conditioned medium, as shown both by its different affinities for polyornithine and plastic substrata and by the observation that there was an almost complete loss of neurites after removal of conditioned medium from cells cultured on tissue culture plastic. It seems likely therefore that the muscle-derived factor(s) in our system differs in its mode of action from both NGF and PNPF.

One important question remains to be answered before the possible importance of such a factor in the ontogenesis of the neuromuscular junction can be assessed. Are the responsive cells in these cultures motoneurons? In 4.5-day chicken embryos, most motoneurons are postmitotic while proliferation continues in other parts of the neural tube (Hamburger, 1948), and indeed in cultures of spinal cord from embryos of this age about 50% of the neurons are capable of forming functional synapses with skeletal myotubes (Berg and Fischbach, 1978). For comparison, the percentage of cells that responded to muscle-conditioned medium varied between 30% and 60% in different experiments. We calculated that, in our hands, 6×10^4 cells per spinal cord survived the plating step and put out neurites. The estimated number of

α-motoneurons in the 4-day cord is 5×10^4 (Barald and Berg, 1979). Nevertheless, we cannot be sure that the responsive cells in these culture were motoneurons.

It remains to be seen whether putative growth factors such as this one identified by their action in vitro will turn out to play the role proposed for them, or any role, in vivo. Does the present factor, for instance, stimulate de novo neurite outgrowth from postmitotic neurons or is it involved in later stages of synapse development, when the growth cone is only a short distance from the muscle? Two observations suggest that the very early stages of neurite outgrowth from motoneurons might not be completely dependent on the presence of the target muscle mass. First, although in chicken embryos whose limb bud has been extirpated all the corresponding motoneurons subsequently die, axons are nevertheless sent out as far as the wound, where they form a neuroma (Oppenheim et al., 1978). Secondly, in embryos that have been X-irradiated to destroy all muscle tissue, the principal nerve tracts are reported to develop normally although no subsequent branching occurs (Lewis et al., 1981). A possible explanation comes from the observation that under the right in vitro conditions spinal cord explants can develop significant levels of neurite outgrowth and CAT activity even in the absence of exogenous factors (Meyer et al., 1979; Norrgren and Ebendal, 1981). Although none of these observations completely eliminates the possibility that even at these early stages the muscle liberates a soluble "retrograde" factor upon which the motoneurons are dependent, and with which the spinal cord could be "impregnated" before target removal, it is perhaps easier to envisage a developmental programme whereby only at later stages are synapse formation and definition of the neural network regulated by an interplay of "anterograde" and "retrograde" factors acting over a relatively short distance. A crucial step in our understanding of these phenomena will be the production of specific antibodies to putative growth factors and a careful analysis of the processes that they disrupt in vivo during the development of the nervous system. With this aim in mind, assays based on differentiation in dissociated cell culture seem one of the more rapid and quantitative foundations to a purification procedure.

REFERENCES

Adler, R., Landa, K.B., Manthorpe, M. and Varon, S. (1979) Cholinergic neuronotrophic factors: intraocular distribution of trophic activity for ciliary neurons. Science, 204: 1434–1436.

Adler, R., Manthorpe, M., Skaper, S.D. and Varon, S. (1981) Polyornithine attached neurite-promoting factors (PNPFs). Culture sources and responsive neurons. Brain Res., 206: 129–144.

Barald, K.F. and Berg, D.K. (1979) Autoradiographic labeling of spinal cord neurons with high affinity choline uptake in cell culture. Develop. Biol., 72: 1–14.

Bennett, M.R., Lai, K. and Nurcombe, V. (1980) Identification of embryonic motoneurons in vitro: their survival is dependent on skeletal muscle. Brain Res., 190: 537–542.

Berg, D.K. and Fischbach, G.D. (1978) Enrichment of spinal cord cell cultures with motoneurons. J. Cell Biol., 77: 83–98.

Bonyhady, R.E., Hendry, I.A., Hill, C.E. and McLennan, I.S. (1980) Characterization of a cardiac muscle factor required for the survival of cultured parasympathetic neurons. Neurosci. Lett., 18: 197–202.

Brookes, N., Burt, D.R., Goldberg, A.M. and Bierkamper, G.G. (1980) The influence of muscle-conditioned medium on cholinergic maturation in spinal cord cell cultures. Brain Res., 186: 474–479.

Changeux, J.P. (1979) Molecular interactions in adult and developing neuromuscular junction. In The Neurosciences Fourth Study Program, MIT Press, Cambridge, MA, pp. 749–778.

Collins, F. (1978) Induction of neurite outgrowth by a conditioned medium factor bound to culture substratum. *Proc. nat. Acad. Sci. U.S.A.*, 75: 5210–5213.

Dribin, L.B. and Barrett, J.N. (1980) Conditioned medium enhances neuritic outgrowth from rat spinal cord explants. *Develop. Biol.*, 74: 184–195.

Giller, E.L., Neale, J.H., Bullock, P.N., Schrier, B.K. and Nelson, P.G. (1977) Choline acetyltransferase activity of spinal cord cell cultures increased by co-culture with muscle and by muscle-conditioned medium. *J. Cell Biol.*, 74: 16–29.

Godfrey, E.W., Schrier, B.K. and Nelson, P.G. (1980) Source and target cell specificities of a conditioned medium factor that increases choline acetyltransferase activity in cultured spinal cord cells. *Develop. Biol.*, 77: 403–418.

Hamburger, V. (1948) The mitotic patterns in the spinal cord of the chick embryo and their relation to histogenic processes. *J. comp. Neurol.*, 88: 221–283.

Henderson, C.E., Huchet, M. and Changeux, J.P. (1981) Neurite outgrowth from embryonic chicken spinal neurons is promoted by media conditioned by muscle cells. *Proc. nat. Acad. Sci. U.S.A.*, 78: 2625–2629.

Henderson, C.E., Huchet, M. and Changeux, J.P. (1983) Characterization of the neurite-promoting activity for spinal neurons in muscle-conditioned media. *Develop. Biol.*, submitted.

Hollyday, M. and Hamburger, V. (1976) Reduction of the naturally occurring motor neuron loss by enlargement of the periphery *J. comp. Neurol.*, 170: 311–320.

Landa, K.B., Adler, R., Manthorpe, M. and Varon, S. (1980) Cholinergic neuronotrophic factors III. Developmental increase of trophic activity of chick embryo ganglion neurons in their intraocular target tissues. *Develop. Biol.*, 74: 401–408.

Landmesser, L. and Pilar, G. (1976) Fate of ganglionic synapses and ganglion cell axons during normal and induced cell death. *J. Cell Biol.*, 68: 357–374.

Lewis, J., Chevallier, A., Kieny, M. and Wolpert, L. (1981) Muscle nerve branches do not develop in chick wings devoid of muscle. *J. Embryol. exp. Morph.*, 64: 211–232.

Manthorpe, M., Skaper, S., Adler, R., Landa, K. and Varon, S. (1980) Cholinergic neuronotrophic factors: fractionation properties of an extract from selected chick embryonic eye tissues. *J. Neurochem.*, 34: 69–75.

Meyer, T., Burkart, W. and Jockusch, H. (1979) Choline acetyltransferase induction in cultured neurons: dissociated spinal cord cells are dependent on muscle cells, organotypic explants are not. *Neurosci. Lett.*, 11: 59–62.

Miki, N., Hayashi, Y. and Higashida, H. (1981) Characterization of chick gizzard extract that promotes neurite outgrowth in cultured ciliary neurons. *J. Neurochem.*, 37: 627–633.

Nishi, R. and Berg, D.K. (1981) Two components from eye tissue that differentially stimulate the growth and development of ciliary ganglion neurons in cell culture. *J. Neurosci.*, 1: 505–513.

Norrgren, G. and Ebendal, T. (1980) Test of the possible action of trophic factors upon embryonic chick CNS neurons. *Neurosci. Lett.*, Suppl. 5: S124.

Oppenheim, R.W., Chu-Wang, I.-W. and Maderdrut, J.L. (1978) Cell death of motoneurons in the chick embryo spinal cord. The differentiation of motoneurons prior to their induced degeneration following limb-bud removal. *J. comp. Neurol.*, 177: 87–112.

Pollack, E.D., Muhlach, W.L. and Liebig, V. (1981) Neuronotrophic influence of mesenchymal limb target tissue on spinal cord neurite growth in vitro. *J. comp. Neurol.*, 200: 393–405.

Schnaar, R.L. and Schaffner, A.E. (1981) Separation of cell types from chicken and rat spinal cord: characterization of motoneuron enriched fractions. *J. Neurosci.*, 1: 204–217.

Sutter, A., Riopelle, R.J., Harris-Warrick, R.M. and Shooter, E.M. (1979) NGF receptors: characterization of two distinct classes of binding sites on chick embryo sensory ganglia cells. *J. biol. Chem.*, 249: 2188–2194.

Thoenen, H. and Barde, Y.-A. (1980) Physiology of nerve growth factor. *Physiol. Rev.*, 60: 1284–1335.

Monoclonal Antibodies Used to Study the Interaction of Nerve and Muscle Cell Lines

WILLIAM D. MATTHEW and LOUIS F. REICHARDT

Department of Physiology, University of California, San Francisco, CA 94143 (U.S.A.)

INTRODUCTION

The objective of our laboratory is to understand the biochemical mechanisms responsible for the formation, maintenance and modification of chemical synapses. We are trying to define the sequence of events which occurs during synapse formation and identify the molecules that are responsible for this interaction between defined neuronal and target types. We have chosen an immunological approach as one means of accomplishing our objective and intend to use antibodies to identify, localize and quantitate synaptic molecules.

In hopes of obtaining antibodies specific for synaptic molecules, monoclonal antibodies have been prepared from mice immunized with rat brain synaptic membranes. Since monoclonal antibodies recognize single determinants, they have the potential to identify individual molecules important in the development and function of the synapse. Such antibodies should be very useful for studying the molecular organization of the synapse. Furthermore, they should be capable of purifying relevant molecules and organelles (synapses and vesicles) for structural studies and also be useful for determining the function of these antigens. We have isolated several hundred cell lines which secrete antibodies that bind to neural antigens. Antibodies have been identified which distinguish the basic cell types of the brain and a variety of cellular organelles (Matthew et al., 1981b). We have characterized the antigens defined by many of these antibodies and have begun to use these antibodies to study synaptogenesis in culture.

As one model system of neuronal differentiation, we have studied the differentiation of a neuron-like cell line (PC-12) in response to nerve growth factor or in co-culture with a cell line derived from skeletal muscle. Rat pheochromocytoma cells (PC-12) are a tumor cell line derived from the adrenal (Greene and Tischler, 1976). In culture they appear as small round cells and divide mitotically. When the culture medium is supplemented with nerve growth factor (NGF), PC-12 cells stop dividing and extend processes (Greene and Tischler, 1976). This cell line synthesizes, stores and releases norepinephrine and acetylcholine (Greene and Tischler, 1976) and is capable of forming synapses in culture (Schubert et al., 1977). A co-culture system of pheochromocytoma cells and a muscle cell line, C2 (Yaffe and Saxel, 1977), has been developed in hopes of inducing differentiation of these cells. When C2 cells are maintained in serum-rich growth medium, they proliferate as myoblasts. When the serum concentration is reduced in these cultures, the cells fuse into myotubes. Using monoclonal antibodies and indirect immunofluorescense procedures, we have shown

[375]

that PC-12 cells and C2 myotubes in co-culture develop specialized contacts with each other.

The rationale for using two cell lines, rather than primary dissociated cells, is the potential for using somatic cell genetics to analyze the function of molecules defined by our monoclonal antibodies. Using antibodies and complement, we have selected PC-12 mutants which do not display a specific proteoglycan on their cell surface. Such procedures can be used to obtain mutants in a variety of surface molecules. Many of our monoclonal antibodies bind to the plasma membrane or cytoplasmic components of PC-12 cells. Differentiation will be monitored by localizing all these antigens in co-cultures and those that are localized to synaptic regions will be given priority for selecting mutants. Currently PC-12 cell differentiation has been monitored by localizing two different antigens – a synaptic vesicle associated protein and a cell surface proteoglycan.

NERVE GROWTH FACTOR INDUCES REDISTRIBUTION OF SYNAPTIC VESICLES IN PC-12 CELLS

A monoclonal antibody, #48, has been described which binds a 65 kdalton protein on the outer surface of synaptic vesicles (Matthew et al., 1981a). This protein is restricted to synaptic and neurosecretory vesicles in a variety of neuronal and neural tissues. Antibody 48 has been used to purify vesicles and transmitters from PC-12 cells (Matthew et al., 1981a) and can be used to localize vesicles in these cells using indirect immunofluorescense procedures. When PC-12 cells are grown mitotically in culture (without nerve growth factor) and stained with monoclonal antibody 48, the vesicle antigen is distributed uniformly in the cytoplasm. Fig. 1A shows the diffuse staining pattern seen in these cells. When PC-12 cells are differentiated in nerve growth factor and induced to extend processes, the vesicles are clustered in process varicosities (Fig. 1B). The cell body stains with approximately the same intensity as undifferentiated cells except the pattern is less diffuse and appears as tiny specks. This antibody provides a very sensitive, rapid and reliable method for localizing vesicle clusters and, therefore, potential synaptic contacts. The distribution of vesicles also serves to monitor PC-12 cell differentiation.

PC-12, C2 CO-CULTURE

Rat pheochromocytoma cells (PC-12) were plated on top of C2 muscle cells in C2 growth medium. After 24 h the cultures were fed with muscle fusion medium. Myotubes began forming within 48 h and cultures were stained with monoclonal antibodies after four to seven days in fusion medium. The myotubes and unfused C2 cells form a very thick carpet of cells. The PC-12 cell bodies are difficult to distinguish lying on top of the muscle cells and virtually none of the PC-12 processes can be visualized with phase optics.

Monoclonal antibodies to a neuronal surface proteoglycan have been described (Matthew, 1981). Indirect immunofluorescent labeling with any of the anti-proteoglycan antibodies (3, 15, 22, 31, 42) allows the PC-12 cells to be visualized in these cultures with great detail. The cell bodies stain very brightly as do all the axonal processes.

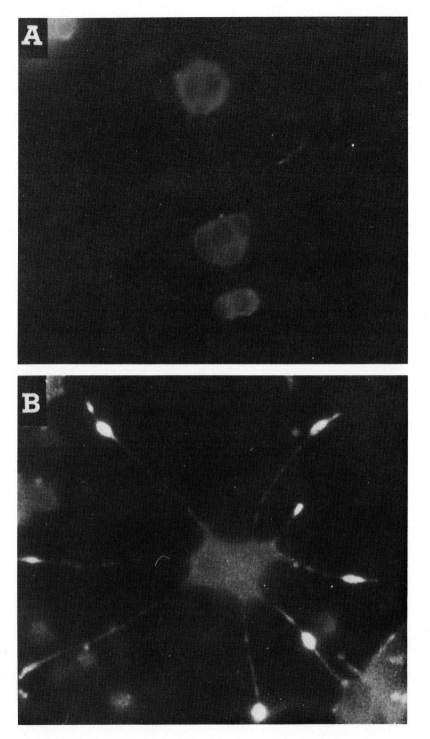

Fig. 1. Nerve growth factor induces localization of vesicles in PC-12 cells. PC-12 cells were grown on collagen-coated glass coverslips. Coverslips were removed from culture dishes, rinsed in phosphate buffer and fixed-permeabilized in absolute methanol at −20°C for 30 sec. The coverslips were immersed in PBS containing 5% calf serum and immunofluorescent staining was completed with antibody 48 + fluorescein coupled goat anti-mouse Ig serum. Photograph A shows undifferentiated PC-12 cells and photograph B shows cells grown in nerve growth factor.

Two types of processes are found in these cultures. As mentioned, the PC-12 cell bodies lie above the muscle cells. One set of processes lie in this focal plane and connect all the PC-12 cell bodies to each other. These processes are smooth, show no varicosities and tend to be bundled. An example of these processes is shown in Fig. 2A. Another type of PC-12 process is seen in these cultures. The PC-12 cells send a very large number of processes into the muscle cell layer. They tend to follow the length of myotubes and are highly varicose. An example of this is illustrated in Fig. 2B (the same field shown in Fig. 2A but focused on a lower plane). There appears to be a specific association between the PC-12 processes and the muscle cells.

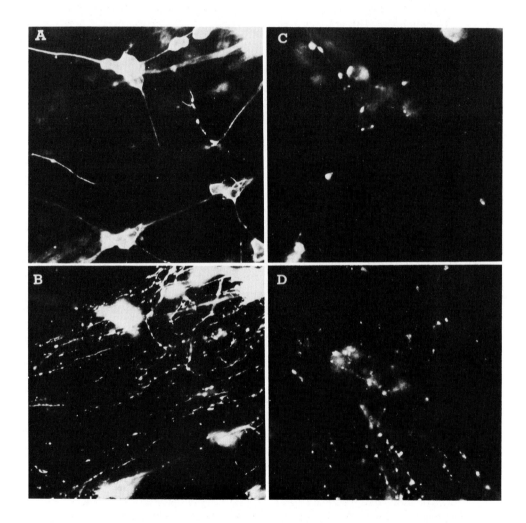

Fig. 2. Indirect immunofluorescense on PC-12, C2 co-cultures. The cells on the left were stained with monoclonal antibody #22 and fluorescein conjugated goat anti-mouse Ig serum. Photograph A is focused on a higher plane where the PC-12 cell bodies are located. Photograph B is on a lower plane where the myotubes are attached to the coverslip. The cells on the right were fixed in methanol at −20°C for 5 min, incubated with hybridoma #48 culture fluid and fluorescein coupled goat anti-mouse Ig antisera. Photograph C is focused on the upper plane where the PC-12 cell bodies lie, whereas D is focused on the myotube layer

VESICLE LOCALIZATION IN CO-CULTURES

Based on the distribution of varicosities (Fig. 2B), it is assumed that most of the transmitter-containing vesicles are associated with the processes on the muscle cells. To verify this, indirect immunofluorescense techniques were used with the anti-synaptic vesicle antibody in order to localize putative synapses. After examining hundreds of cells, it is clear that there are relatively few vesicles in the PC-12 cell bodies or the bundled processes linking the cell bodies. The only significant fluorescent staining in this focal plane is where the processes terminate on a PC-12 cell body or where a process crosses a myotube. A representative photograph focused on the PC-12 cell bodies is shown in Fig. 2C. When the camera is focused on the muscle cell layer, a large amount of localized fluorescense is seen (Fig. 2D). Hence, the large number of varicose processes which are associated with the myotubes are filled with synaptic vesicles.

C2 MYOTUBES INDUCE PC-12 DIFFERENTIATION IN THE ABSENCE OF NERVE GROWTH FACTOR

Cocultures were established in C2 fusion medium with and without the addition of purified nerve growth factor (NGF). When the PC-12 cells were examined by indirect immunofluorescence with anti-proteoglycan and anti-vesicle monoclonal antibodies they appeared identical (data not shown). Both cultures appeared as the photographs in Fig. 2. Therefore, C2 cells either synthesize NGF or are capable of inducing differentiation of PC-12 cells without NGF. To determine the mechanism, cocultures were established with and without anti-NGF serum. A high concentration of anti-NGF was maintained in these cultures in order to determine if C2 cells synthesize NGF. Cells grown without anti-NGF extend elaborate processes as previously described. When anti-NGF was included the PC-12 cells still differentiate and extend processes. Furthermore, PC-12 cells plated onto paraformaldehyde fixed C2 cultures in the presence of anti-NGF developed neurites and localized their synaptic vesicles. Apparently C2 myotubes synthesize a molecule(s), distinct from NGF, which is able to elicit the differentiation of PC-12 cells.

DISCUSSION

We have shown that nerve growth factor induces clustering and redistribution of synaptic vesicles in a neuron-like (PC-12) cell line (Fig. 1). A coculture system has been described which consists of PC-12 cells and a fusing muscle cell line (C2). Two different types of neuronal processes can be distinguished in cocultures. One is smooth, does not associate closely with myotubes and contains relatively few synaptic vesicles. The second type of process is highly varicose, contains a large number of vesicles and is closely associated with myotubes. It would appear that these two types of cells interact closely in culture and may actually form synapses analogous to the neuromuscular junction.

There are probably many signals which are used in this cell to cell interaction. One signal is able to mimic the effects of NGF since antiserum to NGF does not block neurite outgrowth. The signal which directs vesicles to the processes which contact myotubes has not been determined. It is possible this signal is a component of C2 extracellular matrix since primary sympathetic ganglion neurons will extend processes in the absence of NGF if they are plated on proteoglycan components from C2 cells (Lander et al., 1982). The exact nature and mechanism of this signal will be investigated.

This coculture system will be used to assay the distribution of all our monoclonal antibodies that recognize molecules synthesized by PC-12 cells. We have defined three distinct types of PC-12 membrane – cell bodies, smooth processes and varicose processes. These can be easily distinguished and provide a simple screen for synaptic molecules. The distribution of muscle surface molecules – acetylcholine receptors, acetylcholinesterase and basement membrane antigens (Sanes and Hall, 1979) will also be monitored. Once this system has been defined with respect to these molecules, antibodies will be used to disrupt differentiation. PC-12 mutants have been developed (Matthew, 1981) and will be used in this system to investigate the role of these surface molecules. This coculture system should be valuable in identifying putative synaptic antigens and for studying their roles in synaptogenesis.

SUMMARY

Using a monoclonal antibody which recognizes a protein restricted to synaptic vesicles, we have shown that a neuron-like cell line (PC-12) redistributes its vesicles in response to nerve growth factor (NGF). The interaction between PC-12 cells and a fusing skeletal muscle derived cell line (C2) has been characterized using monoclonal antibodies. When PC-12 cells are cocultured with C2 myotubes, the PC-12 cells differentiate, forming two distinct types of axonal processes on top of the myotubes. Both types of processes can be localized using an antibody to a surface proteoglycan. One type of process forms a network between the PC-12 cell bodies. These neurites appear smooth without any variocosities. The second type of process is much more plentiful, appears thin, highly varicose and makes contacts along the length of the myotubes. Immunofluorescent staining with the antibody to the vesicle antigen shows the majority of vesicles are contained in the processes which closely contact the myotubes. PC-12 cells maintain their processes in coculture in the presence of antiserum to nerve growth factor.

ACKNOWLEDGEMENTS

We thank our colleagues at UCSF, especially Drs. Zach Hall and Laura Silberstein, for advice and assistance. Research was supported by grants to L.F.R. from the National Science Foundation, Muscular Dystrophy Association, McKnight Foundation, March of Dimes Birth Defects Foundation, and Wills Foundation. L.F.R. is a Sloan Foundation Fellow.

REFERENCES

Greene, L. and Tishler, A. (1976) Establishment of a noradrenergic clonal line of rat adrenal pheochromocytoma cells which responds to nerve growth factor. *Proc. nat. Acad. Sci. U.S.A.*, 73: 2424–2428.

Lander, A.D., Fujii, D.K., Gospodarowicz, D. and Reichardt, L.F. (1982) Characterization of a factor that promotes neurite outgrowth: evidence linking activity to a heparan sulfate proteoglycan. *J. Cell Biol.*, 94: 574–585.

Matthew, W.D. (1981) *Biochemical Studies using Monoclonal Antibodies to Neural Antigens*, Ph.D. Thesis, University of California, San Francisco.

Matthew, W.D., Tsavaler, L. and Reichardt, L.F. (1981a) Identification of a synaptic vesicle specific membrane protein with a wide distribution in neuronal and neurosecretory tissue. *J. Cell Biol.*, 91: 257–269.

Matthew, W.D., Tsavaler, L. and Reichardt, L.F. (1981b) Monoclonal antibodies to synaptic membranes and vesicles. In R. McKay, M.C. Raff and L.F. Reichardt (Eds.), *Monoclonal Antibodies to Neural Antigens*, Cold Spring Harbor, pp. 163–180.

Sanes, J.R. and Hall, Z.W. (1979) Antibodies that bind specifically to synaptic sites on muscle fiber basal lamina. *J. Cell Biol.*, 83: 357–370.

Schubert, D., Heinemann, S. and Kidokoro, Y. (1977) Cholinergic metabolism and synapse formation by a rat pheochromocytoma cell line. *Proc. nat. Acad. Sci. U.S.A.*, 74: 2579–2583.

Yaffe, D. and Saxel, O. (1977) Serial passaging and differentiation of myogenic cells isolated from dystrophic mouse muscle. *Nature (Lond.)*, 270: 725–727.

Elimination of Synapses During the Development of the Central Nervous System

J. MARIANI

Département de Biologie Moléculaire, Institut Pasteur, Paris Cedex 15 (France)

During the development of the nervous system, after the setting out of neuronal somas, the growth of their processes (axons and dendrites) leads to the formation of a network of synaptic connections that in the adult exhibits both precision and diversity. Synaptic contacts are generally established between partners belonging to well-defined and homogeneous *categories* of cells (see Changeux, this book). These *classes* of synapses represent a first level of order within the system; the specificity of recognition between appropriate classes of cell is strict but probably not absolute: functional "heterologous synapses" might be formed between cells which under normal conditions never form synapses. For example, mossy fibers in the cerebellum synapse with Purkinje cell dendrites when their normal targets, the granule cells, are missing (see review in Mariani et al., 1977; Wilson et al., 1981).

The accuracy of synaptic connections *within* a given class of synapses represents another level of complexity. Without doubt the connections between subsets of neurons are very precisely established, although it is not clear to what extent the connections have to be precise to generate a given behavior (in other words a certain "degeneracy" might exist between connectivity and behavior, see Changeux et al., 1973; Edelman, 1978). At this level of resolution the problem becomes a quantitative one: to match the number of pre- and post-synaptic cells, and to regulate the number and the distribution of synaptic contacts within a population of target cells (Purves and Lichtman, 1980). Several mechanisms have been proposed for the creation of such order and diversity (see review in Changeux and Danchin, 1976; Changeux and Mikoshiba, 1978; Changeux, 1979); many of them are not in fact mutually exclusive, since the acquisition of such a synaptic accuracy is likely to be not a single step process but a progressive and sequential one. According to this view, a given nerve terminal could recognize and innervate transiently more partners than it will in the final stage; additional order is brought within this "limited redundancy" of connectivity by the selective elimination of some of the previously formed contacts (Changeux et al., 1973; Changeux and Danchin, 1976).

One example of elimination of functional synapses during normal development has been known for more than a decade (Redfern, 1970). This is the neuromuscular junction, where each muscle fiber is contacted by a single axon in the adult but by several during development. If such transient polyneuronal innervation were unique to the muscle, it could not be used as a general model of synapse formation. Thus it was essential to demonstrate that synapse elimination occurs also between developing neurons, and especially in the central nervous system.

The best experimental situation, at least from an electrophysiological point of view, for demonstrating synapse elimination is when it leads to the extreme case of only one fiber remaining on the target. Such one-to-one relationships are rather unfrequent in the central nervous system and in this respect, the synapse between climbing fibers (CF) and Purkinje cells (PC) in the cerebellar cortex of mammals is particularly interesting since each Purkinje cell is innervated by only one CF collateral in the adult (Ramón y Cajal, 1911; Eccles et al., 1966). Moreover, the development of the cerebellar network is mostly postnatal in the rat (Altman, 1972) and the response of Purkinje cells through climbing fiber activation is recognizable electrophysiologically in adult (Eccles et al., 1966) and in young animals (Crepel, 1971). Thus it was possible to investigate the formation of CF–PC contacts in developing rats by means of electrophysiological recordings and elucidate how the one-to-one relationship was established.

In a first series of experiments, unitary extracellular recordings and collision experiments were mainly used (Delhaye-Bouchaud et al., 1975; Crepel et al., 1976); evidence was obtained that in the cerebellum of 8–9-day-old rats more than 50% of Purkinje cells recorded were innervated by more than one climbing fiber, in contrast with the monoinnervation of the adult, established on postnatal day 15.

Recently, we have obtained more direct evidence by systematic intracellular recordings from Purkinje cells in developing rats aged from postnatal day 3 until adulthood (Mariani and Changeux, 1980b, 1981a, b). The climbing fiber pathway was stimulated electrically either in the region of the fastigial nucleus (JF stimulation) or in the inferior olivary nucleus (IO stimulation) whose axons constitute the climbing fibers. The criteria used to recognize the multiple innervation were the same at all the ages studied and are illustrated in Fig. 1.

The typical full-spike climbing fiber response (CFR) was evoked through JF stimulation (Fig. 1A). After disappearance of the spike-generating mechanism the typical underlying postsynaptic potential mediated through climbing fiber (CF-EPSP) was recorded, and fully reversed when a depolarizing DC current was applied through the microelectrode (Fig. $1B_2$) (Eccles, 1964; Llinas and Nicholson, 1976). Basically a PC was considered as innervated by a single CF collateral when the CF-EPSP evoked by stimulation of the CF pathway was all-or-none in amplitude (Fig. $1B_1$ and B_2). In the same cell, the CF-EPSPs occurring in the background discharge were also all-or-none in amplitude (Fig. $1B_3$). On the other hand, a PC was considered as innervated by several CF collaterals when the amplitude of the CF-EPSP was graded in a stepwise manner, either when the intensity of stimulation was slightly increased (Fig. $1C_1$ to C_5) or during the background spontaneous discharge (Fig. $1C_6$). A detailed discussion of the criteria used to demonstrate multiple innervation has been provided elsewhere (Mariani and Changeux, 1981a).

Two parameters were followed to describe more precisely the phenomenon of regression (Fig. 2): (a) the percentage of multiply-innervated cells remained more or less on a plateau from postnatal day 3 to 7 (around 90–95%) and subsequently decreased until postnatal day 15 (Fig. 2A); (b) the mean number of observed steps in the evoked CF-EPSPs was taken as a minimal estimate of the mean number of CF collaterals per PC. It increased from day 3 to 5 where it reached a peak value around 3.5 fibers per PC and then decreased regularly down to one step on day 15 indicating that the mono-innervation is established at this age. Similar results have been obtained

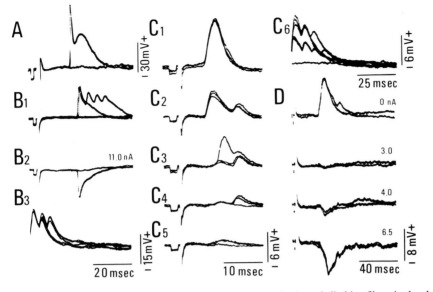

Fig. 1. Intracellular recordings of Purkinje cell responses to the activation of climbing fibers in developing rats. IO stimulation was used in A, B and D, and JF stimulation was used in C. Several sweeps are superimposed in all traces. A: full spike climbing fiber response evoked in a 10-day-old rat. The response was all-or-none in character. B_1–B_3: all-or-none CF-EPSP evoked from another PC in a 9-day-old animal. Reversal of the EPSP was obtained (B_2) with a DC depolarizing current of 11 nA. Resting potential of the cell was -42 mV. B_3: all-or-none CF-EPSP in the spontaneous discharge of the same PC as in B_1 and B_2. C_1–C_6: CF-EPSPs recorded in a PC of a 5-day-old rat. The intensity of stimulation was increased smoothly from C_5 to C_1 and several steps appeared in the amplitude of the response. D: reversal properties of CF-EPSP in a 4-day-old rat; The maximal response (0 nA) almost fully reversed with a depolarizing current of 6.5 nA. Resting potential of the cell was -37 mV. (From Mariani and Changeux, 1981a, with permission.)

independently by Crepel et al. (1981). Additional evidence for a transient multiple innervation of PCs by CFs was obtained by recording both the *spontaneous* discharge of the CF-mediated activity of PCs and the *spontaneous* activity of inferior olivary neurons (whose axons constitute the CFs) (Fig. 3A); the ratio of these two values provided another estimate of the mean number of CFs per PC (Fig. 3B) that fitted closely with the data obtained by the study of evoked CF-EPSPs.

To summarize, electrophysiological arguments strongly suggest that synapse elimination occurs during the formation of the synapses between climbing fibers and Purkinje cells in the developing cerebellum of rats. The anatomical counterparts of this demonstration have been provided recently at the electron microscope level (Triller and Sotelo, 1980; Sotelo and Triller, in preparation). It should be added that preliminary data indicate that in the cerebellum (as in the muscle) synapse elimination occurs probably by withdrawal of axon collaterals rather than by cell death of presynaptic neurons (i.e. inferior olivary neurons) (Delhaye-Bouchaud and Mariani, unpublished results).

The first question raised by such an example of synapse elimination is obviously the generality of the phenomenon.

In the peripheral nervous system, besides that of the neuromuscular junction, extensively studied in several species (Redfern, 1970; see review in Changeux, 1979; Jansen and Lomo, 1981), three other examples of synapse elimination have been added

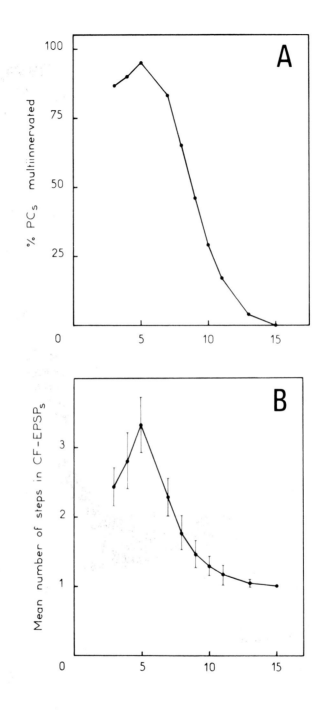

Fig. 2. Evolution with age of the multiple innervation of PCs by CFs in developing rats. A: evolution of the observed percentage of PCs multiply innervated by CFs. B: evolution of the mean number of steps in CF-EPSPs recorded from singly and multiply innervated PCs. Vertical bars represent the confidence limit interval of the mean at each age (at 95%). (From Mariani and Changeux, 1981a, with permission.)

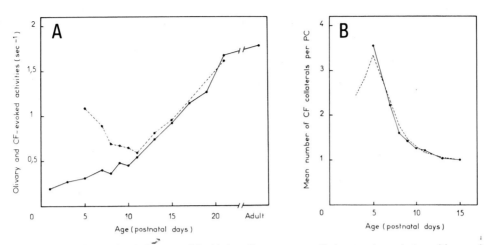

Fig. 3. Comparative study of olivary and Purkinje cell spontaneous discharges. A: evolution with age of spontaneous discharge of IO neurons (●——●) versus CF-mediated discharge (●– – – –●) of the global population of PCs. B: mean number of CF collaterals per PC estimated by the ratio between IO and PC discharges (●——●). Note the good agreement with the value determined using the mean number of steps in the evoked response (dashed line). (From Mariani and Changeux, 1981b, with permission.)

more recently: the submandibular ganglion of the rat (Litchtman, 1977), the superior cervical ganglion of the hamster (Lichtman and Purves, 1980) and the ciliary ganglion of the rabbit (Johnson and Purves, 1981). In the cervical ganglion of the hamster a feature was disclosed that might be relevant for the central nervous system: synapse elimination occurs also when the target cell remains innervated by more than one presynaptic fiber in the adult.

In the central nervous system, to our knowledge the only example of removal of functional synapses during normal development is the climbing fiber–Purkinje cell synapse. However, anatomical evidence for synapse elimination has been obtained for the axon hillock of spinal motor neurons (Ronnevi and Conradi, 1974; Conradi and Ronnevi, 1975) and for the sensory quadrant of the spinal cord of embryonic primates (Knyihar et al., 1978). Synapse elimination is also strongly suspected to occur in the developing visual cortex, particularly of cats and monkeys: cortical neurons in layer IV of the primary visual cortex are organized in columns of ocular dominance; in very young animals an overlap exists between adjacent columns that decreases gradually with maturation, possibly through the loss of some connections, but this has not yet been demonstrated in the years that have elapsed since the early work of Hubel and Wiesel (Hubel and Wiesel, 1963; for references see Rakic, 1977; Schatz and Stryker, 1978).

Thus, examples of synapse elimination during development remain relatively few. By way of contrast, however, there are increasingly numerous reports of the tendency of axons to undergo an exuberant growth during normal development, with subsequent partial retraction: this occurs in particular for connections between cortical areas, especially the transcallosal ones (Innocenti et al., 1977; Innocenti and Caminiti, 1979; Ivy et al., 1979; Goldman-Rakic, 1981), for the uncrossed retinal projections on several structures (lateral geniculate body, superior colliculus, visual cortex) and in different species (Rakic, 1976, 1977; Hubel et al., 1977; Land and Lund, 1979; Frost et al., 1979). It is also the case for the recurrent collateral plexus of Purkinje cell axons (Ramón y Cajal, 1911) and the rat olfactory cortex (Price et al., 1976). For all these cases, it would be necessary to search for possible elimination of synapses associated with retraction of axonal collaterals.

The second important question raised by the elimination of synapses is that of the mechanism involved.

At variance with what occurs in the periphery, synapse elimination in the cerebellum (and probably in the whole central nervous system) exhibits a peculiar feature: the regression occurs within a given category of afferences (i.e. the climbing fiber system) while other classes of afferences make synapses on the Purkinje cells, mainly the parallel fibers (the axons of the granule cells) and the inhibitory interneurons (Altman, 1972). It has been shown that the multiple innervation persists in the adult when Purkinje cells develop in a cellular milieu devoid of granule cells such as occurs in X-irradiated rats (Woodward et al., 1974; Puro and Woodward, 1978; Crepel and Delhaye-Bouchaud, 1979) or in *weaver* and *reeler* mutant mice (Crepel and Mariani, 1976; Siggins et al., 1976; Mariani et al., 1977; Puro and Woodward, 1977). The multiple-innervation persists also when parallel fibers are present but fail to form synaptic contacts with PCs as in *staggerer* mice (Mariani and Changeux, 1980a; Crepel et al., 1980). The extent of the remaining multiple innervation in the mutant mice is similar to its maximum extent in developing rats (Mariani, 1982). On the contrary, a certain degree of regression occurs in X-irradiated rats (Crepel et al., 1981).

As a whole these results suggest that the regression of supernumerary synapses depends on the formation of granule cells and their synapses with Purkinje cells; it is possible that the granule cells that take up their position during the first postnatal week play a more critical role than those formed later (Delhaye-Bouchaud et al., 1978). The underlying mechanism of the regression remains largely unknown in the cerebellum. In view of some results obtained in more simple systems such as neuromuscular junction, it is tempting to speculate that the activity of the olivocerebellar system might regulate directly or not the regression of the multiple innervation and that retrograde factors emitted by the target might play a role (Henderson, this volume). These mechanisms have been recently reviewed in detail (Changeux and Danchin, 1976; Changeux, 1979; Purves and Lichtman, 1980; Willshaw, 1981; see also Fishman and Nelson, 1981) and will not be considered here, since they are still largely hypothetical.

The third important feature of the development of CF–PC synapses concerns the number of contacts that CFs can make on a given PC and their location.

At early stages, CFs synapse on perisomatic processes of the Purkinje cells, and progressively shift towards their dendritic location as the perisomatic processes disappear (Ramón y Cajal, 1911; Altman, 1972). This (apparent) translocation occurs while the multiple innervation is regressing but the two phenomena are unlikely to be linked: the synaptic boutons belonging to different CFs can coexist in dendrites of PCs in developing rats (Sotelo and Triller, personal communication) and the comparison between the location and the multi- or mono-innervated character of CF–PC synapses in several mutant mice (see Table I) suggests that these two parameters are relatively independent.

While both the translocation and the elimination of some CF collaterals occur, the number of synaptic contacts made by a given CF on a Purkinje cell strikingly increases (although quantitative data are still lacking for this point). Thus, what is called "synapse elimination" is not necessarily associated with a reduction in the overall number of synaptic contacts. As already underlined by Purves and Lichtman (1980), during

TABLE I

Comparison between location and mono- or multiply-innervated character of CF–PC synapses in rodents.

		Synapses between climbing fibers and Purkinje cells	
		Location of Purkinje cells	Mono- or multi-innervation
Normal rats	Young	Somas	Multi-innervation
	Adult	Dendrites	Mono-innervation
Experimental adult animals	*Weaver* mice X-irradiated rats *Reeler* mice (ectopic PCs)	Dendrites	Multi-innervation
	Staggerer mice	Soma and base of dendrites	Multi-innervation
	Hyperspiny mice*	Soma and base of dendrites	Mono-innervation

*Guenet, Sotelo and Mariani (unpublished results).

synapse elimination in other systems, this means that a growing axon can make an increasing number of contacts on a decreasing number of target cells. However, the important phenomenon remains that the number of targets (Purkinje cells) innervated by the axon collaterals of one olivary neuron decreases during normal development (by a factor of about 4). In other words, the size of the "olivary unit" is reduced as it occurs for other neural units in the periphery (Johnson and Purves, 1981). A crucial but still unanswered question is to know if this reduction leads to the emergence of subsets of Purkinje cells defined by topological and functional criteria. During the development of the lobster single motoneurons innervate initially muscles of three segments with a subsequent restriction to a single segment probably by loss of functional synapses (Stephens and Govind, 1981). In mammalian muscles, however, the muscle fibers belonging to different motor units are randomly mixed (see review in Brown et al., 1976) and the study of peripheral fields of single motoneurons is difficult. On the contrary, in the adult cerebellar cortex, there is a precise somatotopic representation of the periphery through climbing fiber projection, at least for certain sensory modalities (see, for example, Rushmer et al., 1980). It is an attractive (and testable) hypothesis that the elimination of supernumerary CF–PC synapses leads to the formation or refinement of these maps during development. Selective elimination of synapses would then represent a fundamental (and maybe modulable) mechanism for progressively defining the repertoire of connections of a given subset of neurons, or in other words for creating both precision and complexity in the connections of the central nervous system.

ACKNOWLEDGMENTS

We wish to thank Drs P. Benoit, J.P. Changeux, C. Henderson and J.L. Popot for helpful discussions, and E. Couelle for typing the manuscript.

REFERENCES

Altman, J. (1972) Postnatal development of the cerebellar cortex in the rat. III. Maturation of the components of the granular layer. *J. comp. Neurol.*, 145: 465–514.

Brown, M.C., Jansen, J.K.S. and Van Essen, D. (1976) Polyneural innervation of skeletal muscle in newborn rats and its elimination during maturation. *J. Physiol. (Lond.)*, 261: 387–422.

Changeux, J.P. (1979) Molecular interactions in adult and developing neuromuscular junction. In *The Neurosciences. Fourth Study Program*, MIT Press, Cambridge, MA, pp. 749–778.

Changeux, J.P. and Danchin, A. (1976) Selective stabilization of developing synapses, a mechanism for the specification of neuronal networks. *Nature. (Lond.)*, 264: 705–712.

Changeux, J.P. and Mikoshiba, K. (1978) Genetic and "epigenetic" factors regulating synapse formation in vertebrate cerebellum and neuromuscular junction. In M.A. Corner et al. (Eds.), *Maturation of the Nervous System, Progress in Brain Research, Vol. 48*, Elsevier/North-Holland, Amsterdam, pp. 44–64.

Changeux, J.P., Courrège, P. and Danchin, A. (1973) A theory of the epigenesis of neuronal networks by selective stabilization of synapses. *Proc. nat. Acad. Sci. U.S.A.*, 70: 2974–2978.

Conradi, S. and Ronnevi, L.O. (1975) Spontaneous elimination of synapses on cat spinal motoneurons after birth: do half of the synapses on the cell bodies disappear? *Brain Res.*, 92: 505–510.

Crepel, F. (1971) Maturation of climbing fiber responses in the rat. *Brain Res.*, 35: 272–276.

Crepel, F. and Delhaye-Bouchaud, N. (1979) Distribution of climbing fibers on cerebellar Purkinje cells in X-irradiated rats. An electrophysiological study. *J. Physiol. (Lond.)*, 290: 97–112.

Crepel, F. and Mariani, J. (1976) Multiple innervation of Purkinje cells by climbing fibers in the cerebellum of the weaver mutant mouse. *J. Neurobiol.*, 7: 579–582.

Crepel, F., Mariani, J. and Delhaye-Bouchaud, N. (1976) Evidence for a multiple innervation of Purkinje cells by climbing fibers in the immature rat cerebellum. *J. Neurobiol.*, 7: 567–578.

Crepel, F., Delhaye-Bouchaud, N., Guastavino, J.M. and Sampaio, I. (1980) Multiple innervation of cerebellar Purkinje cells by climbing fibers in staggerer mutant mouse. *Nature (Lond.)*, 283: 483–484.

Crepel, F., Delhaye-Bouchaud, N. and Dupont, J.L. (1981) Fate of the multiple innervation of cerebellar Purkinje cells by climbing fibers in immature control, X-irradiated and hypothyroid rats. *Develop. Brain Res.*, 1: 59–71.

Delhaye-Bouchaud, N., Crepel, F. and Mariani, J. (1975) Mise en évidence d'une multiinnervation temporaire des cellules de Purkinje du cervelet par les fibres grimpantes au cours du développement chez le rat. *C.R. Acad. Sci. (Paris)*, 281: 909–912.

Delhaye-Bouchaud, N., Mory, G. and Crepel, F. (1978). Differential role of granule cells in the specification of synapses between climbing fibers and cerebellar Purkinje cells in the rat. *Neurosci. Lett.*, 9: 51–58.

Eccles, J.C. (1964) *The Physiology of Synapses*, Springer, New York.

Eccles, J.C., Ito, M. and Szentagothai, J. (1967). *The Cerebellum as a Neuronal Machine*. Springer, Berlin.

Eccles, J.C., Llinas, R. and Sasaki, K. (1966) The excitatory synaptic action of climbing fibers on the Purkinje cells of the cerebellum. *J. Physiol. (Lond)*, 182: 268–296.

Edelman, G. (1978) Group selection and phasic reentrant signaling: a theory of higher brain function. In *The Mindful Brain*, MIT Press, Cambridge, MA, pp. 51–100.

Fishman, M.C. and Nelson, P.G. (1981) Depolarization-induced synaptic plasticity at cholinergic synapses in tissue culture. *J. Neurosci.*, 1: 1043–1051.

Frost, D.O., So, K.F. and Schneider, G.E. (1979) Postnatal development of retinal projections in syrian hamsters: a study using autoradiographic and anterograde degeneration techniques. *Neuroscience*, 4: 1649–1677.

Goldman-Rakic, P. (1981) Prenatal formation of cortical input and development of cytoarchitectonic compartments in the neostriatum of the rhesus monkey. *J. Neurosci.*, 1: 721–735.

Hubel, D.H. and Wiesel, T.N. (1963) Receptive fields of cells in striate cortex of very young, visually inexperienced kittens. *J. Neurophysiol.*, 26: 994–1002.

Hubel, D.H., Wiesel, T.N. and LeVay, S. (1977) Plasticity of ocular dominance columns in monkey striate cortex. *Phil. Trans. roy. Soc. Lond. B*, 2: 377–409.

Innocenti, G.M. and Caminiti, R. (1979) Postnatal shaping of callosal connections from sensory areas. *Exp. Brain Res.*, 38: 381–394.

Innocenti, G.M., Fiore, L. and Caminiti, R. (1977) Exuberant projection into the corpus callosum from the visual cortex of newborn cats. *Neurosci. Lett.*, 4: 237–242.

Ivy, G.O., Akers, R.M. and Killackey, H.P. (1979) Differential distribution of callosal projection neurons in the neonatal and adult rat. *Brain Res.*, 173: 532–537.

Jansen, J.K.S. and Lomo, T. (1981) The development of neuromuscular connections. *Trends NeuroSci.*, 7: 178–181.

Johnson, D.A. and Purves, D. (1981) Postnatal reduction of neural unit size in the rabbit ciliary ganglion. *J. Physiol. (Lond.)*, 318: 143–159.

Knyihar, E., Csillik, B. and Rakic, P. (1978) Transient synapses in the embryonic primate spinal cord. *Science*, 202: 1206–1209.

Land, P.W. and Lund, R.D. (1979) Development of the rat's uncrossed retinotectal pathway and its relation to plasticity studies. *Science*, 205: 698–700.

Lichtman, J.W. (1977) The reorganization of synaptic connexions in the rat submandibular ganglion during post-natal development. *J. Physiol. (Lond.)*, 273: 155–177.

Lichtman, J.W. and Purves, D. (1980) The elimination of redundant preganglionic innervation to hamster sympathetic ganglion cells in early postnatal life. *J. Physiol. (Lond.)*, 301: 213–228.

Llinas, R. and Nicholson, C. (1976) Reversal properties of climbing fiber potential in cat Purkinje cells: an example of a distributed synapse. *J. Neurophysiol.*, 39: 311–323.

Mariani, J. (1982) Extent of multiple innervation of Purkinje cells by climbing fibers in the olivo-cerebellar system of *weaver*, *reeler* and *staggerer* mutant mice. *J. Neurobiol.*, 13: 119–126.

Mariani, J. and Changeux, J.P. (1980a) Multiple innervation of Purkinje cells by climbing fibers in the cerebellum of the adult staggerer mutant mouse. *J. Neurobiol.*, 11: 41–50.

Mariani, J. and Changeux, J.P. (1980b) Etude par enregistrements intracellulaires de l'innervation multiple des cellules de Purkinje par les fibres grimpantes dans le cervelet du rat en développement. *C.R. Acad. Sci. (Paris)*, 291: 97–100.

Mariani, J. and Changeux, J.P. (1981a) Ontogenesis of olivocerebellar relationships. I. Studies by intracellular recordings of the multiple innervation of Purkinje cells by climbing fibers in the developing rat cerebellum. *J. Neurosci.*, 1: 696–702.

Mariani, J. and Changeux, J.P. (1981b) Ontogenesis of olivocerebellar relationships. II. Spontaneous activity of inferior olivary neurons and climbing fiber-mediated activity of cerebellar Purkinje cells in developing rats. *J. Neurosci.*, 1: 703–709.

Mariani, J., Crepel, F., Mikoshiba, K., Changeux, J.P. and Sotelo, C. (1977) Anatomical, physiological and biochemical studies of the cerebellum from reeler mutant mouse. *Phil. Trans. B*, 281: 1–28.

Price, J.L., Moxkley, G.F. and Schwob, J.E. (1976) Development and plasticity of complementary afferent fiber systems to the olfactory cortex. *Exp. Brain Res.*, Suppl. 1: 148–154.

Puro, D.G. and Woodward, D.J. (1977) The climbing fiber system in the weaver mutant. *Brain Res.*, 129: 141–146.

Puro, D.G. and Woodward, D.J. (1978) Physiological properties of afferents and synaptic reorganization in the rat cerebellum degranulated by postnatal X-irradiation. *J. Neurobiol.*, 9: 195–215.

Purves, D. and Lichtman, J.W. (1980) Elimination of synapses in the developing nervous system. *Science*, 210: 153–157.

Rakic, P. (1976) Prenatal genesis of connections subserving ocular dominance in the rhesus monkey. *Nature (Lond.)*, 267: 467–471.

Rakic, P. (1977) Prenatal development of the visual system in rhesus monkey. *Phil. Trans. B*, 278: 245–260.

Ramón y Cajal, S. (1911) *Histologie du Système Nerveux de l'Homme et des Vertébrés. I et II*. Maloine, Paris.

Redfern, P.A. (1970) Neuromuscular transmission in new-born rats. *J. Physiol. (Lond.)*, 209: 701–709.

Ronnevi, L.O. and Conradi, S. (1974) Ultrastructural evidence for spontaneous elimination of synaptic terminals on spinal motoneuron in the kitten. *Brain Res.*, 80: 335–339.

Rushmer, D.S., Woollacott, M.H., Robertson, L.T. and Laxer, K. (1980) Somatotopic organization of climbing fiber projections from low threshold cutaneous afferents to pars intermedia of cerebellar cortex in the cat. *Brain Res.*, 181: 17–30.

Schatz, C.J. and Stryker, M.P. (1978) Ocular dominance in layer IV of the cat's visual cortex and the effects of monocular deprivation. *J. Physiol. (Lond.)*, 281: 267–283.

Siggins, G., Henriksen, J. and Landis, S. (1976) Electrophysiology of Purkinje neurons in the weaver mouse: iontophoresis of neurotransmitters and cyclic nucleotides, and stimulation of the nucleus locus coeruleus. *Brain Res.*, 94: 19–44.

Stephens, P.J. and Govind, C.K. (1981) Peripheral innervation fields of single lobster motoneurons defined by synapse elimination during development. *Brain Res.*, 212: 476–480.

Triller, A. and Sotelo, C. (1980) In *Proc. First Meet. Int. Soc. Develop. Neurosci.*, Strasbourg.

Willshaw, D.J. (1981) The establishment and subsequent elimination of polyneuronal innervation of developing muscle: theoretical considerations. *Proc. roy. Soc. B*, 212: 233–252.

Wilson, L., Sotelo, C. and Caviness, U.S. (1981) Heterologous synapses upon Purkinje cells in the cerebellum of the reeler mutant mouse: an experimental light and electron microscopic study. *Brain Res.*, 213: 63–75.

Woodward, D.J., Hoffer, B.J. and Altman, J. (1974) Physiological and pharmacological properties of Purkinje cells in rat cerebellum degranulated by postnatal X-irradiation. *J. Neurobiol.*, 5: 283–304.

Geniculo-Cortical Connections in Primates: Normal and Experimentally Altered Development

PASKO RAKIC

Section of Neuroanatomy, Yale University School of Medicine, 333 Cedar Street, New Haven, CT 06510
(U.S.A.)

INTRODUCTION

The emphasis in this communication is on the emergence of afferent connections from the dorsal lateral geniculate nucleus (LGd) of the thalamus to the primary visual cortex (area 17) in the cerebrum of fetal rhesus monkeys. I started this series of studies with the hope that it would enhance our understanding of normal and pathological development in the human visual system and perhaps elucidate indirectly the pathogenesis of various congenital disorders of the cerebral cortex. The developing visual cortex seems to be a reasonable experimental model for that purpose because its cellular organization and characteristics of binocular and color vision are remarkably similar in both monkeys and man (Polyak, 1957; Shkolnik-Jarros, 1971; Hubel and Wiesel, 1977; Hitchcock and Hickey, 1981).

It is essential for discussion of the present topic to underscore that all neurons that comprise the primate visual system are generated (have their last cell division) before birth (Rakic, 1974, 1977a, b). Furthermore, basic visual connections from the retina via the thalamus to the cortex and reciprocal cortico-thalamic fibers are also layed down before birth (Rakic, 1976, 1977b; Shatz and Rakic, 1981). It should be emphasized that pregancy lasts about five and a half months (165 days) in the rhesus monkey and nine months in the human and that all of the observed developmental events and structural changes during this protracted period in both primate species occur in the absence of visual experience. Therefore, functional validation explanation for these events that require trial and error mechanisms involving visual experience can be eliminated.

Background information on the precise time of origin of each class of visual cortical neurons is based on our extensive analysis of autoradiographic data obtained from postnatal rhesus monkeys that had been exposed to a pulse of [³H]thymidine at different embryonic (E) days, and early postnatal (P) days. Thus, we learned that neurons destined for the primary visual cortex are generated between the 43rd embryonic day (E43) and E102 with layer IV stellate cells – the major target of LGd axons terminals – being produced from E70 to E85 (Rakic, 1974). Following their last cell divisions, near the ventricular surface of the occipital lobe, these young neurons have to migrate to their final positions in the prospective cortical plate at a precisely specified time and rate in order to acquire appropriate input from various intrinsic and extrinsic sources (Rakic, 1975, 1977b). The mode and possible cellular mechanisms of this migration during these early developmental events are described elsewhere (Rakic, 1972, 1978, 1981a). Here, I will focus only on later stages of cortical differentiation that involve the formation of synapses with afferents that arrive at the cortical plate from the LGd via the optic radiation.

The first part of the chapter will be concerned with the basic anatomical organization of geniculo-cortical input in the adult monkey. The second part will deal with critical developmental events and prenatal mechanisms that may be at play during the genesis of the normal pattern of geniculo-cortical connections in primates. In the third part, the morphological consequences of selective prenatal destruction of eye(s) which affect secondarily the development of central visual pathways will be used as a criterion for determining the extent of capacity for synaptic reorganization within the primate visual cortex.

ADULT ORGANIZATION OF GENICULO-CORTICAL AFFERENTS

In order to provide a basis for the study of development and modifiability of thalamo-cortical afferents, it is essential to describe the organization of basic visual projections in adult rhesus monkeys. Primary visual cortex (area 17 of Brodmann) is perhaps among the best understood regions of the primate neocortex. In adult rhesus monkey, it occupies a surface area of about 900–1000 mm^2 and is on average a 1.8 mm thick sheet of gray matter consisting of nerve cells that are arranged in six well delineated layers (Fig. 1). Although our knowledge of the anatomy and physiology of the primary visual cortex in this species has accumulated for over 50 years (i.e. see Polyak, 1957, for review of early works), the meaning of these subdivisions has become reasonably clear only recently (Hubel and Wiesel, 1977; Lund, 1981; Gilbert and Wiesel, 1981). Perhaps the best understood component of visual cortex is the granular layer IV, which receives the major portion of the geniculate projection and can be further subdivided into four sublayers, each of which have specific input-output relationships (Fig. 1). As evident from Fig. 1C, a major output of layer IV is to the upper (supragranular) layers which in turn project heavily to the lower (infragranular) layers (Lund, 1981; Gilbert and Wiesel, 1981). It is possible that the development of synaptic connections within the visual cortex follows this synaptic hierarchy with input to layer IV emerging relatively early and input to the supragranular and the infragranular layers developing in succession at later stages.

For the purpose of this presentation, I will emphasize only two aspects of geniculo-cortical input to layer IV, both of which are anatomically segregated in the adult monkey: these are the binocular and X- and Y-like systems. The binocular system of connections subserves stereoscopic vision whereas the X- and Y-like systems, among their other functional properties, are in monkey presumably related mainly to color and contrast vision (Schiller and Malpeli, 1978; Shapley et al., 1981). The distinction between these sets of projections in the cortex is possible because geniculate terminals that subserve one or the other eye or belong to X- or Y-like neuronal categories project to separate cortical territories. Thus, they can be recognized in autoradiograms prepared from monkeys that had received an ocular injection of high doses of radioactive tracers. Since this research strategy and the

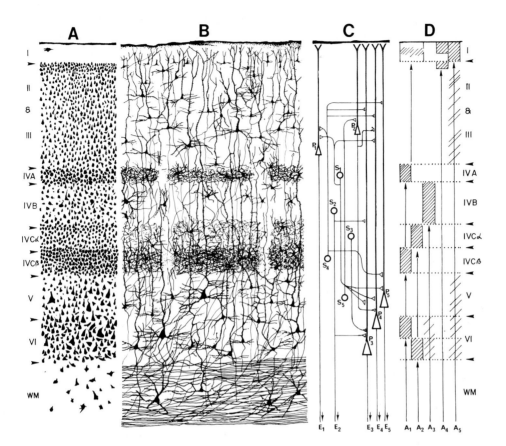

Fig. 1. Composite diagram of the laminar and columnar organization and input-output relationship of the primary visual cortex of the rhesus monkey which integrates observations derived by several investigators using a variety of techniques (for recent reviews see also Hubel and Wiesel, 1977; Lund, 1981; Gilbert and Wiesel, 1981). On the left (A) the cytoarchitectonic appearance of the visual cortex (area 17) in Nissl strain displays horizontal cell stratification into layers and sublayers. The adjacent diagram (B) shows the appearance of visual cortex in Golgi impregnated preparations superimposed with afferent axonal plexuses in sublayers IVA and IVC strained by a reduced silver method. As verified by the autoradiographic method, these afferents form 350–400 µm wide columns, only one of which (flanked by two half-columns) is illustrated. Column C displays a simplified diagram of local neuronal circuits. Thus layer IV cells, the main recipient of geniculo-cortical fibers, have differential projections: stellate cells of sublayers IVCβ (S_4) and IVCα (S_1) project predominantly to layer III, where they synapse either directly upon dendrites of efferent pyramidal cells (P_1 and $P_{3,4}$) or indirectly through another local circuit neuron (small pyramidal cell P_2). The majority of stellate cells of sublayer IVCα (e.g. S_3) probably contact efferent pyramids (P_3) within layer V. Some stellate cells of layer IVB (S_2) contact nearby neurons within the same layer but also project to adjacent visual association cortex (E_2). However, most visual efferents are formed by large pyramidal cells of layer V and VI ($P_{3,4,5}$) which project differentially to subcortical structures: P_3 to superior colliculus (E_3): P_4 to the parvocellular moiety of lateral geniculate nucleus (E_4) and P_5 to the magnocellular moiety (E_5). The right hand column (D) displays the relative position of terminal fields from five major afferent systems: A_1 (from parvocellular moiety of LGd); A_2 (from magnocellular moiety of LGd); A_3 (from superior temporal cortex); A_4 (from inferior pulvinar) and A_5 (from area 18).

same technical procedure is used also for the subsequent analysis of development of normal and experimentally altered visual connections, some elaboration of the technique and method of analysis is provided below.

When one eye of the monkey is injected with about 1 mCi of [³H]proline or its mixture with [³H]fucose, radioactivity is transported anterogradely to the LGd and only three out of the six LGd laminae become heavily labeled (Wiesel et al., 1974). Two of them are small-celled or parvocellular laminae and they are considered to receive basically X-like input (Dreher et al., 1976; Schiller and Malpeli, 1978), although some input from Y-like cells has also been recently recorded (Shapley et al., 1981). The single remaining labeled lamina is large-celled and it receives exclusively Y-like input. The parvocellular and magnocellular moieties of the monkey LGd project to different sublayers of the visual cortex (Hubel and Wiesel, 1972).

For present purposes, it is important that both binocular and X- and Y-like systems remain anatomically segregated from their point of origin in the retina all the way to the fourth cortical layer. This can be demonstrated anatomically because small, but autoradiographically detectable amounts of radioactivity are transported transneuronally through the geniculo-cortical system following injections of tritiated aminoacids and sugars into one eye (Grafstein, 1969). Using this approach one can

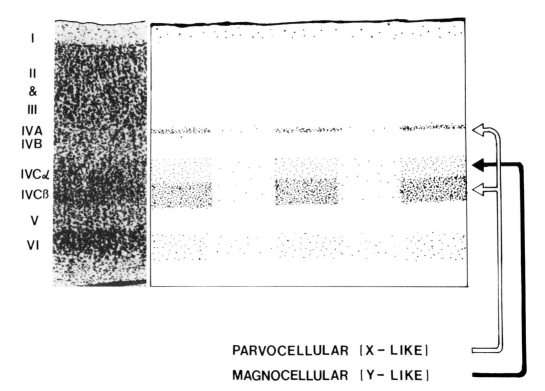

PARVOCELLULAR [X – LIKE]

MAGNOCELLULAR [Y – LIKE]

Fig. 2. Semidiagrammatic illustration of the distribution of geniculo-cortical terminals in the primary visual cortex (area 17) of a normal adult rhesus monkey. On the left is a photograph of a cresyl violet-stained section to indicate corresponding cortical layers. Drawings on the right illustrate ocular dominance columns exposed by alternating labeled and unlabeled territories and selective distribution over sublayers IVA, IVCα and IVCβ in animal injected with radioactive tracers into one eye. (Further explanation in text.)

analyze the cortical distribution of geniculate projections originating from each of the three labeled LGd laminae. Thus, as illustrated in Fig. 2, fibers from left and right eyes project mainly to layer IV in the form of alternating ocular dominance columns and the parvocellular and magnocellular moieties of LGd terminate in different sublayers within their columns (Hubel and Wiesel, 1972). As schematically illustrated in Fig. 1, layers IVA and IVCβ receive input from parvocellular layers; while layer IVCα receives input from magnocellular layers (see also Fig. 1). Thus, terminal fields of both binocular (belonging to one or the other eye) and X- and Y-like (presumably color and contrast vision) systems can be recognized in light microscopic autoradiograms.

Our research strategy was designed to determine the timing and manner in which these two afferent systems are normally established and then to try to manipulate their formation by removing one eye at appropriate developmental stages in monkey embryos. Some of the more obvious questions that could be answered by such experiments are: When do geniculo-cortical fibers enter the developing cortical plate? Do they enter it before or after their major target neurons in layer IV are generated and/or attain their final positions? Do geniculo-cortical axons enter exclusively the territory of the prospective cytoarchitectonic area 17 or are they initially more diffusely distributed? Are the geniculo-cortical fibers subserving the two eyes segregated at the time they enter the developing cortical plate? If not, do they sort out before or after birth? Is the development of the vertical distribution of X- and Y-like systems into separate sublayers of layer IV independent of the horizontal segregation of geniculo-cortical fibers into ocular dominance columns?

THE TIMETABLE AND MODE OF NORMAL DEVELOPMENT OF GENICULO-CORTICAL CONNECTIONS

Contrary to general understanding and our predictions of one decade ago (e.g. Sidman and Rakic, 1973), specific thalamic afferents from LGd enter the developing cortex only after the principal target cells in layer IV complete their migrations and attain appropriate positions within the developing cortical plate (Rakic, 1976). This sequence of developmental events was possible to demonstrate only after the advent of two types of autoradiographic methods: one that enables tagging DNA of migrating cells (described in Introduction) and the other that permits the use of the transneuronal transport method for tracing long neuronal connections. In addition, the refinement of procedures for prenatal surgery enabled us to remove fetal monkeys from the uterus, inject or enucleate an eye and replace the fetus in the uterus (Rakic, 1976). In this particular set of experiments, monkey fetuses were sacrificed two weeks after unilateral eye injection of radioactive tracers (mixture of [^{3}H]proline and [^{3}H]fucose) and subsequently processed for light microscopic autoradiography. The two week interval between the injection and sacrifice of the fetus was chosen to allow sufficient time transneuronally for the label to be transported transneurally and to fill geniculo-cortical axons.

As illustrated semidiagramatically in Fig. 3, the autoradiographic analysis indicated that geniculo-cortical axons enter the occipital lobe at relatively early stages but that they do not invade the developing cortical plate until the beginning of the second half of gestation (Rakic, 1976, 1979b). The same material clearly shows that

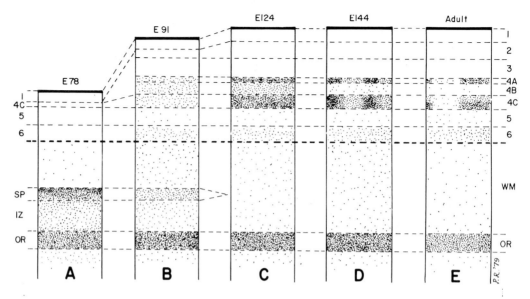

Fig. 3. Semidiagrammatic summary of development of geniculo-cortical connections and ocular-dominance columns in the occipital lobe of the rhesus monkey from the end of the first half of pregnancy to adulthood. The columns illustrate a portion of the lateral cerebral wall in the region of area 17 as seen in autoradiograms of animals that had received unilateral injection of a mixture of [³H]proline and [³H]fucose 14 days earlier. The age of animals at the moment of sacrifice is provided at the top of each column in embryonic (E) and postnatal (P) days. Note that at E78 the cortical plate consists of only layers 6, 5, and a small portion of 4C. Abbreviations: IZ, intermediate zone; OR, optic radiation; SP, deep portion of subplate layer; WM, white matter. (From Rakic, 1979b, with permission.)

in the monkey fetus LGd axons grow selectively towards prospective area 17, stopping rather abruptly at the border to area 18 (Fig. 4). Following arrival at the cortex around mid gestation (E91 specimen), geniculate axons carrying input from each eye first become distributed uniformly over the entire territory of layer IV (Rakic, 1976, 1977b). Three weeks before birth (E144), afferents begin to segregate vertically into sublayers IVA, IVCα and IVCβ, that receive separate input from parvo and magnocellular layers indicating the possible emergence of the X- and Y-like systems (Fig. 3). Furthermore, geniculate fibers begin also to sort out horizontally into alternating high and low grain density areas indicating emergence of ocular dominance columns (Rakic, 1976). These columns, initially 250–300 μm wide, subsequently expand and by the second postnatal month reach the normal adult width of 350–400 μm (Hubel et al., 1977).

Although there must be some spillover of radioactivity at the level of LGd, it does not alter the interpretation of our autoradiographic data. The strongest evidence that the intermixing of fibers subserving the left and right eye is real comes from our experiments with short and long survival following monocular eye injection at midgestational period. Thus, in a fetus injected at E78 and sacrificed one day later (E79) the entire LGd is labeled regardless of whether the injection is given to the left or right eye. However, in another fetus whose eye was injected at about the same time (E77) but which was sacrificed fourteen days later (E91) the distribution of retinal fibers shows territories of higher and lower grain densities. If the diffuse labeling of the first case is a result of a spillover of a radioactive molecule from one layer

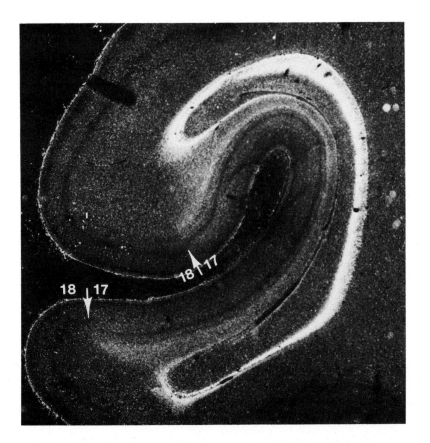

Fig. 4. Autoradiogram of a coronal section through the occipital lobe of a 124-day-old monkey fetus whose left eye was injected with a mixture of [³H]proline and [³H]fucose 14 days before sacrifice. Transneuronally transported radioactivity is most dense in the optic radiation but some fibers enter the developing cortical plate within area 17 in the depth of calcarine fissure. Note that geniculo-cortical fibers do not spread to adjacent area 18.

to the next, the pattern label in the LGd would not change fourteen days later. Therefore, we concluded that the uniform label at the early stage is not an artifact, but rather a result of intermixing of fibers originating from the two eyes. The interpretation of the cortical data is somewhat more complex. However, quantitative and electrophysiological analyses performed on developing kittens also supports the notion that the intermixing of geniculate fiber terminals at the cortical level is a real phenomenon (LeVay et al., 1978). Furthermore, since the boundary between radioactive territories and non-radioactive territories in both vertical and, at the later stages of development, also in the tangential direction, is rather sharp, spillover of radioactivity at the cortical level must be negligible. A final and most important point is that the label at the cortical level is still uniform in monkey fetuses near the term when the input from the left and right eye within the LGd is already well segregated. Thus, although detailed quantitative analysis of grain counts has not been done in the monkey cortex we can reaffirm our previous statement that development of the geniculo-cortical connections in primates proceeds through two broad phases (Rakic, 1976, 1981b). In the *first phase* LGd axons subserving input from each eye invade the cortical plate but their endings are distributed over the entire layer IV in an intermixed manner. In the *second phase* terminals subserving left and right eye sort out horizontally into ocular dominance stripes, while the axons belonging presumably to X- and Y-like system segregate vertically.

DEVELOPMENT OF GENICULO-CORTICAL CONNECTIONS IN THE ABSENCE OF ONE EYE

Analysis of the mode of normal development of geniculo-cortical projections provides new and intriguing information which raises several questions relevant to possible cellular mechanisms involved in formation of territorial distribution of axonal terminals within the cortex. For example, does competition between the two eyes play a role in formation of segregated input to the cortex? This issue can be resolved by removing one eye at a critical developmental period and then allowing the operated fetus to be delivered and to survive for a few months after birth. Here, I will limit my discussion to our recent autoradiographic findings in the visual cortex of such animals, although obviously structural changes occurring in the LGd are also intimately involved.

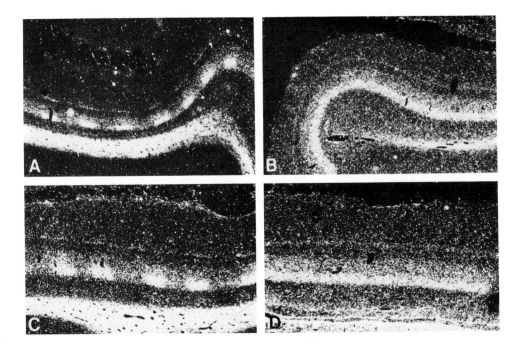

Fig. 5. Dark-field illumination photomicrograph of autoradiograms showing distribution of transneuronally transported radioactive tracers in primary visual cortex of normal adult monkeys (A and C) and in adult monkeys whose one eye has been enucleated during the first third of pregnancy (B and D). Note lack of alternating ocular dominance columns in the cortex of experimental animals. The distribution of silver grains over sublayers of layer IV remain similar to that in the control. See Fig. 6 for the diagrammatic illustration of differential grain distribution in enucleated monkeys.

The major finding relevant for the topic of this chapter is that the distribution of LGd terminals in the primary visual cortex of the mature monkey is abnormal if one eye is enucleated at critical periods of their fetal life (Rakic, 1981b). This phenomenon can be demonstrated by the transneuronally transported radioactive tracers injected into one eye of mature monkeys in which the contralateral eye was enucleated during the second fetal month (at E63). In such cases ocular dominance stripes fail to develop (Rakic, 1979a, 1981b). Rather, the LGd axon terminals within layer IV form two continuous and uniform horizontal lines confined to layers IVA and IVC (Figs. 5 and 6). Since, as described in the preceding section, LGd projections subserving two eyes initially overlap, these results can be explained, at least in part, by a failure of terminals subserving the remaining eye to retract from the territory that normally becomes occupied exclusively by terminals subserving the other (enucleated) eye. Although the results of these experiments clearly show that cortical neurons which normally receive input from the left eye, now receive input from the right eye, at present, we cannot determine which LGd neurons issue these projections. It is possible that this abnormal connectivity is established by genetically "proper" set of LGd neurons or by the selective elimination or rearrangement of geniculo-cortical connections. This is a challenging question for the future research

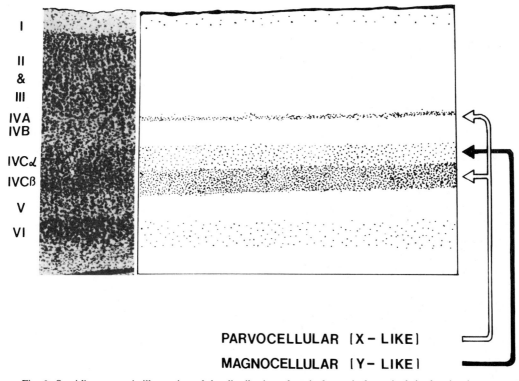

Fig. 6. Semidiagrammatic illustration of the distribution of geniculo-cortical terminals in the visual cortex of a two-month-old monkey in which one eye was enucleated during the first third of gestation and the remaining eye injected with radioactive tracers two weeks before sacrifice. The distribution of grains is aligned with photograph of cresyl violet-stained visual cortex to show relative positions of horizontal, uniform sheets of projections without any sign of ocular dominance columns. Note, however, that vertical segregation of input into sublayers IVA, IVCα and IVCβ is clearly indicated. (Based on Rakic, 1981b).

which should involve electrophysiological, histochemical or anatomical analyses in mature monkeys that were prenatally enucleated.

In contrast to the absence of visible horizontal segregation into ocular dominance stripes, the vertical segregation of the thalamic input into cortical sublayers IVA, IVCα and IVCβ as well as elimination of the transient projection to layers IVB appear to be achieved normally (compare Fig. 5A and B). Since the sublayers IVA, and IVCβ in the visual cortex receive input from the parvocellular moiety of the LGd while IVC receives input from magnocellular moieties of the LGd (Hubel and Wiesel, 1972), it seems reasonable to assume that segregation of X- and Y-like systems in cortex may have proceeded normally.

CONCLUSIONS

The present experiments show that geniculo-cortical fibers enter the territory of prospective area 17 only after their major target neurons have attained final positions in the cortical plate. Furthermore, it appears that the integrity of projections from the two eyes during prenatal development is a necessary condition for the establishment of the normal distribution of retino-geniculate and indirectly of geniculo-cortical terminals and for their proper synaptic organization within the primate visual cortex. More specifically, the process of competition between the retinal terminals from two eyes at the level of LGd appears to be essential for proper cortical development. The latter assumption is based on the finding that LGd neurons and their interconnections form abnormally although individual LGd neurons may receive morphologically normal synaptic input from a single eye (Rakic, 1981b). Thus, the very process of competition between terminals originating from two eyes provides essential conditions for the normal development of LGd. Information about the absence of this competition at the level of LGd must somehow be conveyed to the visual cortex via the optic radiation.

Our study of the mode of normal development of geniculocortical projection also indicates that binocular competition, critical for the initial formation of the normal visual cortex, does not involve visual experience per se since the described morphogenetic changes occur before birth. However, although visual experience does not play a role in these embryonic events, the spontaneous electrical activity from the two retinae may be of significance (Stryker, 1982). Present findings also do not exclude the possible influence of binocular vision on the final stages of cortical synaptogenesis. At these late stages of development vision may play a considerable role as indicated by the recent report of the organization of ocular dominance columns in dark-reared kittens (Swindale, 1981). Finally, our radioautographic analysis indicates further that the dependence of normal development upon prenatal binocular competition may be a selective one; segregation of the terminal distribution of axons from magnocellular and parvocellular moieties of LGd in the cerebral cortex appears to proceed normally in prenatally enucleated animals while ocular dominance stripes in these same cases fail to segregate.

Mechanisms underlying segregation of afferents in the primate visual cortex are not understood, although a combination of selective elimination of fibers and active retraction of terminals that may involve cell death and/or translocation of already formed synapses seem like reasonable working hypothesis. Anatomical study of the visual cortex of postnatal cats indicates that the emergence of stripes may depend upon selective retraction of portions of axon terminal arbors (LeVay and Stryker, 1979). At present, however, we cannot exclude the possibility that selective cell death in the LGd and/or late but massive ingrowth of "appropriate" fibers may also contribute to the emergence of the adult striped pattern. Similar cellular mechanisms have been postulated in other systems with multiple input such as the cerebellum (Changeux and Danchin, 1976), peripheral ganglia (Purves and Lichtman, 1980), and neostriatum (Goldman-Rakic, 1981). These sorting out phenomena could be achieved by axon-axon competition or by axon-target recognition. Although the cellular mechanisms are not solved, the present sets of experiments on embryonic visual cortex illustrate vividly how an error in development or a lesion of a single neural structure can alter development and functional connectivity of distant but transsynaptically related regions of the complex primate brain.

REFERENCES

Changeux, J.-P. and Danchin, A. (1976) Selective stabilization of developing synapses as a mechanism for the specification of neural networks. *Nature (Lond.)*, 264: 705–712.

Dreher, B., Fukuda, Y. and Rodieck, R.W. (1976) Identification, classification, and anatomical segregation of cells with X-like and Y-like properties in the lateral geniculate nucleus of old-world primates. *J. Physiol. (Lond.)*, 258: 433–452.

Gilbert, C.D. and Wiesel, T.N. (1981) Laminar specialization and intracortical connections in cat primary visual cortex. In F.O. Schmitt (Ed.), *The Organization of the Cerebral Cortex*, MIT Press, Cambridge, MA, pp. 163–191.

Goldman-Rakic, P.S. (1981) Prenatal formation of cortical input and development of cytoarchitectonic compartments in the neostriatum of the rhesus monkey. *J. Neurosci.*, 1: 721–735.

Grafstein, B. (1971) Transneuronal transfer of radioactivity in the central nervous system. *Science*, 172: 177–179.

Hitchcock, P.F. and Hickey, T.L. (1980) Ocular dominance columns: evidence for their presence in humans. *Brain Res.*, 182: 176–179.

Hubel, D.H. and Wiesel, T.N. (1972) Laminar and columnar distribution of geniculocortical fibers in the macaque monkey. *J. comp. Neurol.*, 146: 421–450.

Hubel, D.H. and Wiesel, T.N. (1977) Functional architecture of macaque monkey visual cortex. *Proc. roy. Soc. B*, 198: 1–59.

Hubel, D.H., Wiesel, T.N. and LeVay, S. (1977) Plasticity of ocular dominance columns in monkey striate cortex. *Phil. Trans. B*, 278: 131–163.

LeVay, S. and Stryker, M.P. (1979) The development of ocular dominance columns in the cat. In J.A. Fernondelli (Ed.), *Aspects of Developmental Neurobiology, Soc. Neurosci. Symposia*, 4: 83–98.

LeVay, S., Hubel, D.H. and Wiesel, T.N. (1975) The pattern of ocular dominance columns in macaque visual cortex revealed by a reduced silver stain. *J. comp. Neurol.*, 159: 559–576.

LeVay, S., Stryker, M.P. and Shatz, C.J. (1978) Ocular dominance columns and their development in layer IV of the cat's visual cortex: a quantitative study. *J. comp. Neurol.*, 179: 223–244.

Lund, J.S. (1981) Intrinsic organization of the primary visual cortex area 17, as seen in Golgi preparations. In F.O. Schmitt (Ed.), *The Organization of the Cerebral Cortex*, MIT Press, Cambridge, MA, pp. 106–124.

Polyak, S.L. (1975) *The Vertebrate Visual System*, Univ. of Chicago Press, Chicago.

Purves, D. and Lichtman, J.W. (1980) Elimination of synapses in the developing neuron system. *Science*, 261: 467–471.

Rakic, P. (1972) Mode of cell migration to the superficial layers of fetal monkey neocortex. *J. comp. Neurol.*, 145: 61–84.

Rakic, P. (1974) Neurons in rhesus monkey visual cortex: systematic relation between time of origin and eventual disposition. *Science*, 183: 425–427.

Rakic, P. (1975) Timing of major ontogenetic events in the visual cortex of the rhesus monkey. In N.A. Buchwald and M. Brazier (Eds.), *Brain Mechanisms in Mental Retardation*, Academic Press, New York, pp. 3–40.

Rakic, P. (1976) Prenatal genesis of connections subserving ocular dominance in the rhesus monkey. *Nature (Lond.)*, 261: 467–471.

Rakic, P. (1977a) Genesis of the dorsal lateral geniculate nucleus in the rhesus monkey: Site and time of origin, kinetics of proliferation, routes of migration and pattern of distribution of neurons. *J. comp. Neurol.*, 176: 23–52.

Rakic, P. (1977b) Prenatal development of the visual system in the rhesus monkey. *Phil. Trans. B*, 278: 245–260.

Rakic, P. (1978) Neuronal migration and contact guidance in primate telencephalon. *Postgrad. med. J.*, 54: 25–40.

Rakic, P. (1979a) Genetic and epigenetic determinants of local neuronal circuits in the mammalian central nervous system. In F.O. Schmitt and F.G. Worden (Eds.), *The Neurosciences. Fourth Study Program*, MIT Press, Cambridge, MA, pp. 109–127.

Rakic, P. (1979b) Genesis of visual connections in the rhesus monkey. In R. Freeman (Ed.), *Developmental Biology of Visual System*, Plenum, New York, pp. 249–260.

Rakic, P. (1981a) Developmental events leading to laminar and areal organization of the neocortex. In F.O. Schmitt (Ed.), *The Cerebral Cortex*, MIT Press, Cambridge, MA, pp. 34–71.

Rakic, P. (1981b) Development of visual centers in the primate brain depends on binocular competition before birth. *Science*, 214: 928–931.

Schiller, P.H. and Malpeli, J.G. (1978) Functional specificity of lateral geniculate nucleus laminae in the rhesus monkey. *J. Neurophysiol.*, 41: 788–797.

Shapley, R., Kaplan, E. and Soodak, R. (1981) Spatial summation and contrast sensitivity of X and Y cells in the lateral geniculate nucleus of the macaque. *Nature (Lond.)*, 292: 543–545.

Shatz, C. and Rakic, P. (1981) The genesis of efferent connections from the visual cortex of the fetal monkey. *J. comp. Neurol.*, 196: 287–307.

Shkolnik-Yarros, E.G. (1971) *Neurons and Interneuronal Connections of the Central Visual System*. Plenum, New York, 295 pp.

Sidman, R.L. and Rakic, P. (1973) Neuronal migration, with special reference to developing human brain: a review. *Brain Res.*, 62: 1–35.

Stryker, M.P. (1982) The role of visual afferent activity in the development of ocular dominance columns. *Neurosci. Res. Prog. Bull.*, in press.

Swindale, N.V. (1981) Absence of ocular dominance patches in dark-reared cats. *Nature (Lond.)*, 290: 332–333.

Wiesel, T.N., Hubel, D.H. and Lam, D.M.K. (1974) Autoradiographic demonstration of ocular dominance columns in the monkey striate cortex by means of transneuronal transport. *Brain Res.*, 79: 273–279.

The Corticostriatal Fiber System
in the Rhesus Monkey: Organization
and Development

PATRICIA S. GOLDMAN-RAKIC

Section of Neuroanatomy, Yale University School of Medicine, 333 Cedar Street, New Haven, CT 06510
(U.S.A.)

INTRODUCTION

Over the past decade, methods for defining the biochemical, physiological and morphological properties of neurons in the central nervous system have developed at an unprecedented pace. These developments have revolutionized our ideas and concepts about virtually every component structure of the nervous system. This "anatomic revolution" has had a particularly profound impact on our understanding of the two largest forebrain structures – the neocortex (for recent reviews, see Schmitt et al., 1981; Rakic and Goldman-Rakic, 1982) and the neostriatum (e.g. Chase et al., 1979). Perhaps recent advances in unraveling the anatomical complexities of these structures seems the more impressive because only a decade ago the telencephalon was so poorly understood.

Analysis of the neocortex and neostriatum in the frontal lobe of primates has been a preoccupation of my laboratory for many years. We have been especially interested in prefronto-striatal connections in large part because they play an important role in cognitive functions (Goldman and Rosvold, 1972). Our goal has been to use advanced neurobiological methods to penetrate the cellular and hodological organization of this complex system as an avenue toward understanding its functions in normal behavior and in mental disease. In this chapter I will report some recent findings that may be of particular relevance to the "higher brain functions" that constitute the focus of this conference.

ORGANIZATION OF CORTICOSTRIATAL PROJECTIONS IN ADULT MONKEY

Although one of the major efferent pathways of cerebral cortex terminates in the neostriatum, corticostriatal projections were denied for most of the present century. Only with the advent of silver methods for the impregnation of degenerating fibers was clear evidence obtained that such connections existed (e.g. Devito and Smith, 1964; Kemp and Powell, 1970). These earlier studies established that practically the entire neocortex projects to the neostriatum; and further that these projections are arranged topographically. For example, the frontal cortex projects to the head of the caudate nucleus while the more posterior cortical regions in the parietal, occipital and

406

temporal lobes project to progressively more caudal territories in the "body" and "tail" of the caudate nucleus.

More recently the use of axonal transport of radioactive tracers to study central nervous system connectivity has confirmed in major outline the existence of massive projections from the cerebral cortex to neostriatum and in addition has occasioned revision in our ideas about the size, topography and configuration of corticostriatal fibers particularly in a gyrencephalic brain such as that of the rhesus monkey. For example, analysis of the corticostriatal fibers by autoradiography indicates that the overlap among fiber terminals representing different cortical regions is much more extensive than previously realized. In the case of prefrontal-striatal connections, these project not only to the head of the caudate nucleus in the frontal lobe as previously described but also throughout the entire rostrocaudal length of the nucleus to its tail in the temporal lobe (Goldman and Nauta, 1977). Similarly, corticostriatal projections that originate in posterior cortical areas extend more anteriorly than previously reported on the basis of fiber degeneration analysis (Yeterian and Van Hoesen, 1978).

The autoradiographic studies not only showed that certain projections were more extensive than believed but also, conversely, that some projections to this structure had been overestimated. Thus, lesion studies had suggested a large input to the caudate nucleus from the primary motor cortex (Kemp and Powell, 1970) whereas the axonal transport studies indicate that motor areas project only sparsely to the

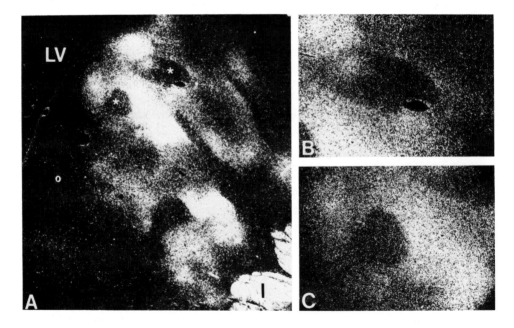

Fig. 1. Photograph of the caudate nucleus under dark-field illumination illustrating the fenestrated distribution of prefrontal axons in a rhesus monkey that received an injection of [³H]proline and [³H]leucine into the homolateral prefrontal cortex. A: low magnification photo in which the caudate nucleus is bounded by the lateral vertricle (LV) in the upper left hand corner and by the internal capsule (I) at the lower right. B and C: higher magnification photographs of the elliptical and rounded territories surrounded by prefrontal input marked by asterisks in A.

caudate nucleus and more prominently to the putamen (Goldman and Nauta, 1977; Künzle, 1975). Thus, although the caudate and putamen have long been regarded as a unitary structure, the anatomical arrangement of its cortical input is indicative instead of a possible division of labor between these two neostriatal components. On the basis of our present knowledge about the organization of corticostriatal connections, one may speculate that the caudate nucleus in primates is more closely functionally related to the association cortex while the putamen may be involved to a greater degree with sensorimotor functions.

From the point of view of cellular mechanisms, the most interesting and novel finding that has materialized from autoradiographic studies in the last five years is the discovery that cortical fiber termination within the caudate nucleus is neither uniform nor random but instead displays an intricate pattern in which terminals are concentrated in irregularly shaped patches that are partly confluent and partly separated by areas which are devoid of labeled prefrontal fibers (Goldman and Nauta, 1977). As illustrated in Fig. 1, many of the heavily labeled territories in the caudate nucleus contain unlabeled fenestrations that are circular or elliptical in shape. On the basis of the configuration of these afferent connections, it may be reasoned that prefrontal fibers spatially alternate in the caudate nucleus with other sources of striatal afferents. However, other hypotheses are equally plausible. For example, there is indirect evidence that neocortical regions having reciprocal corticocortical connections converge in the same region of the caudate nucleus (Yeterian and Van Hoesen, 1978). Thus terminals with divergent cortical origins may overlap in the neostriatum or alternatively they may interdigitate in regions of the nucleus around or even within the elliptical core territories.

CYTOARCHITECTONIC ORGANIZATION OF THE ADULT PRIMATE NEOSTRIATUM

The caudate nucleus is the major synaptic target of afferents from the frontal association cortex, and its cellular organization has considerable bearing on the terminal pattern of cortical input. It should be pointed out that in contrast to the cerebral cortex or dorsal thalamus, which are organized into cellular layers, cytoarchitectonic fields and/or nuclei, the neostriatum of primates has traditionally been regarded as a cytologically homogeneous structure composed mainly of medium sized neurons mixed with occasional large neurons scattered in an apparently irregular manner throughout a complex neuropil (e.g., Carpenter, 1976; Kemp and Powell, 1971a, b; Mettler, 1968). Such cytoarchitectonic uniformity of the neostriatum seemed puzzling in light of increasing evidence for heterogeneous organization of neostriatal connections and certain features of intrinsic cytochemistry. As mentioned, Nauta and I found that the distribution of frontal association afferents in the caudate nucleus exhibit marked discontinuities. Similar discontinuities have also been reported for projections from the motor and limbic cortex (Künzle, 1975; Yeterian and Van Hoesen, 1978) as well as for thalamostriatal connections (Kalil, 1978; Royce, 1978). Furthermore, there is increasing evidence for a "patchy" distribution of various putative neurotransmitters in the neostriatum, including dopamine (Olson et al., 1972; Tennyson et al., 1972) and enkephalin (Graybiel et al., 1981; Pickel, 1980), as well as for acetylcholinesterase (Butcher and Hodge, 1976;

408

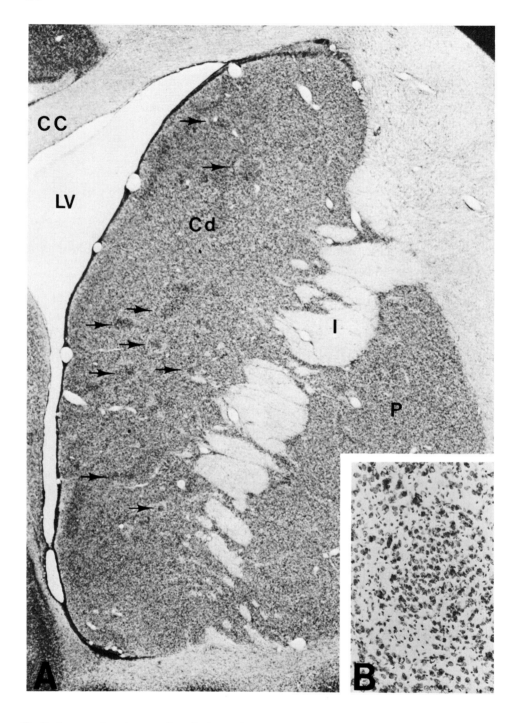

Fig. 2. A: coronal sections cut through the caudate nucleus (Cd) and putamen (P) of a rhesus monkey showing the distribution and shapes of cellular islands (arrows) surrounded by a homogeneous cellular matrix. B: higher magnification photograph of one of the cellular islands encircled by a cell-sparse capsule. I, internal capsule; LV, lateral ventricle; CC, corpus callosum.

Graybiel and Ragsdale, 1978; Kostovic-Knezevic et al., 1979) and opiate receptors (Atweh and Kuhar, 1977; Herkenham and Pert, 1981; Pert et al., 1976).

Various pieces of the "striatal puzzle" recently began to fit together with the discovery that different classes of neuronal somata in the primate neostriatum are not uniformly distributed but instead are arrayed in distinctive cellular compartments, distinguished by differences in cell size, density, and staining properties (Goldman-Rakic, 1981b, 1982). As illustrated in Fig. 2, two types of cellular compartments have been observed in standard Nissl stained sections: (1) islands of tightly packed darkly-staining cells encapsulated by a thin ring of fibers, embedded in; (2) a background or matrix of more loosely packed lighter staining neurons that are distributed more irregularly. These cell groupings are well defined in 35–40 μm celloidin-embedded tissue and they are also clearly visible in frozen sections providing the tissue is well fixed, devoid of cutting artifact and properly stained. Although cellular islands are occasionally observed in the putamen, they are much more prominent and prevalent in the head and body of the caudate nucleus.

These cellular islands in the primate neostriatum display a variety of sizes and shapes. Although they may assume elongated and irregular geometric forms, the most conspicuous and easily recognizable profiles in coronal sections are round or elliptical and their long-axis diameters range from 300 to 600 μm. In the sagittal plane, the shapes of islands are more variable. They may take the form of small or large cylindrical profiles or assume elongated vermiform configurations that extend for distances of 500–1500 μm in a given section. Although we have not reconstructed these cellular configurations, on the basis of their appearance in the three cardinal planes (Fig. 3), I have proposed that a three dimensional model of a

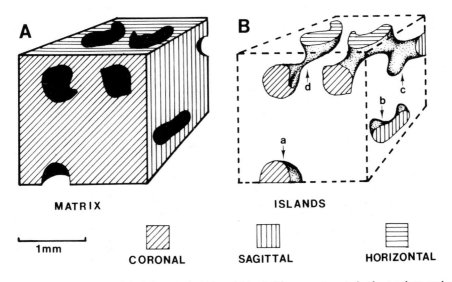

Fig. 3. Three-dimensional model of the matrix (A) and island (B) compartments in the caudate nucleus based on analysis of cytoarchitectonic areas as seen in coronal (slanted grid lines), sagittal (vertical grids) and horizontal (horizontal grids) sections. The islands occupy less than 10% of the tissue volume of the caudate nucleus and take on variable sizes and shapes that range from round (a) and elliptical (b) to considerably more complex (c, d). (From Goldman-Rakic, 1982, with permission.)

block of caudate tissue would probably take the form of a Swiss cheese in which the holes represent the space occupied by cellular islands. In this model, cellular islands represent a relatively small fraction of the total volume of the nucleus (Goldman-Rakic, 1981b). Summarizing, these recent observations indicate that the neostriatum in primates should be viewed as a cytoarchitectonically heterogeneous structure composed of at least two distinct cellular compartments which may now be related to the histochemical and functional diversity of the neostriatum.

RELATIONSHIP BETWEEN CORTICAL INPUT AND CELLULAR COMPARTMENTS

The similarity of the shape and distribution of cellular compartments in the caudate nucleus (Goldman-Rakic, 1982) to the fenestrated pattern of corticostriatal termination described earlier (Goldman and Nauta, 1977; Goldman, 1978; Goldman-Rakic, 1981a) raises the question of whether there is any correspondence between striatal cytoarchitecture and the distribution of corticostriatal afferents in this structure. The prefrontal cortex is highly suitable for examining this question because of the high density and patterning of its projections to the caudate nucleus (Goldman and Nauta, 1977a). In order to expose these possible spatial relationships, autoradiograms from monkeys that had received injections of [³H]proline and [³H]leucine in the prefrontal granular cortex were examined under both dark- and bright-field illumination, allowing simultaneous comparison of autoradiographic labeling and cytoarchitecture. As described previously, analysis of this material under dark-field illumination showed that prefrontal projections to the caudate nucleus terminate in discontinuous fields surrounding round or elliptically shaped territories which are devoid of prefrontostriatal input. Cytoarchitectonic analysis of these territories has now revealed that the "holes" in the terminal fields contain cellular islands (Goldman-Rakic, 1981b, 1982). Dense accumulations of radioactivity are present over both the fiber annuli that surround the islands as well as over the matrix compartment of the caudate nucleus but do not invade the territory of the cellular islands. The finding that cortical afferents project exclusively to the territory of the matrix compartment and cell poor capsule but not to the cellular islands suggests that cortical terminals have an explicit synaptic affinity for cells located in the matrix compartment and a corresponding lack of attraction to island cells. In order to further understand the nature of this selectivity in terminal patterning, we next examined the development of the corticostriatal pathway.

PRENATAL FORMATION OF CORTICAL INPUT AND CYTOARCHITECTONIC COMPARTMENTS

Since our initial autoradiographic studies demonstrated that the prefronto-striatal efferents in the rhesus monkey are already well developed in the neonatal period (Goldman and Nauta, 1977), it became necessary to study prenatal stages in order to obtain data on the timing, sequence and mode of development of these connections. Accordingly I injected microquantities of tritiated amino acids into the prospective prefrontal cortex in ten fetal rhesus monkeys of various gestational ages, allowed them to survive for 1–3 days and subsequently processed their brains for autoradiography (Goldman-Rakic, 1981b). The youngest fetus was injected on the 69th embryonic day, and sacrificed at E70 (E69–70) and the oldest was injected at E152 and sacrificed at E155 (E152–155).

A finding from this study of prenatal development that has particular relevance to the present chapter is that the genesis of the prefrontostriatal innervation involves a transformation from a diffuse pattern of distribution observed at early stages of gestation to one that becomes intricately patterned in the last third of pregnancy. Thus, as illustrated in Figs. 4 and 5, some prefrontal efferents reach their target in the homolateral neostriatum by E69. Thereafter, their number increases steadily throughout the gestational period, and possibly even into postnatal life (see Fig. 7 in Goldman-Rakic, 1981b). Early in gestation, between E69 and E95 the corticostriatal input is distributed diffusely within the neostriatum and there is no evidence of the type of fiber clustering that is characteristic of the fenestrated corticostriatal projection in the mature rhesus monkey (Goldman and Nauta, 1977). However, as the density of corticostriatal fibers increases, there is a progressive sorting out of fibers within the neostriatum such that by E105, autoradiograms contain some relatively ill-defined areas of lower grain density encircled by an otherwise homogeneous field of radioactivity. This process of segregation continues until E133 when the mature pattern of distribution of prefrontal axons surrounding sharply defined oval or elliptical territories that are devoid of prefrontal input is finally achieved (Goldman-Rakic, 1981b). Except for a possible increment in fiber density, and slight increase in the size of fenestrations, there is little change in configuration of corticostriatal input after this period. It should be emphasized that although the distribution of cortical fibers is arranged as in the adult a full month before birth, neither the cortical terminals nor the striatal neurons are fully mature at this age. In the monkey, synaptogenesis in the caudate nucleus begins as early as E65 (Brand and Rakic, 1979b) but additional synapses continue to form and differentiate through at least the first 16 weeks of postnatal life (DiFiglia et al., 1980). Our autoradiographic and cytoarchitectonic study in fetal monkeys demonstrates only that the basic pattern of ingrowth of fibers and their distribution in the neostriatum are well established at least one month before birth.

Another finding that may have considerable bearing on understanding the development of synaptic connectivity in the neostriatum is that segregation of corticostriatal input is paralleled by and temporally correlated with the development of cytoarchitectonic differentiation of the neostriatum. Before E100, when the corticostriatal fibers are distributed diffusely, the cellular organization of the neostriatum is also rather uniform and does not display cellular compartmentalization into island or matrix zones. However, after that period when fibers begin to disappear or retract from some territories, the cytological composition of the neostriatum also begins to change and island and matrix compartments begin to emerge. Although I have not followed the onset and development of these two cellular events in close temporal sequence, the dual processes of segregation of fiber input and cytoarchitectonic compartmentalization appear to occur at about the same time. A similar synchrony occurs in the establishment of lamina-specific connections from the two eyes and the emergence of separate ipsilateral and contralateral laminae in the lateral geniculate body of the fetal rhesus monkey (Rakic, 1976). The present results indicate that a biphasic transformation from diffuse to patterned input occurs in both non-sensory and sensory systems alike.

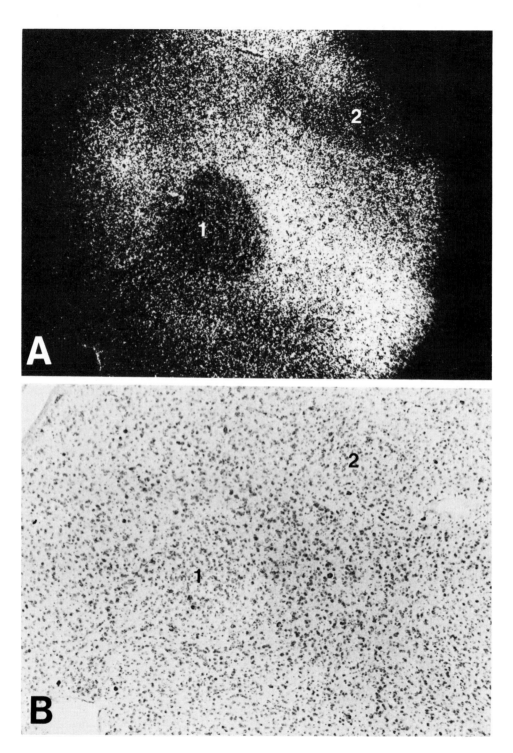

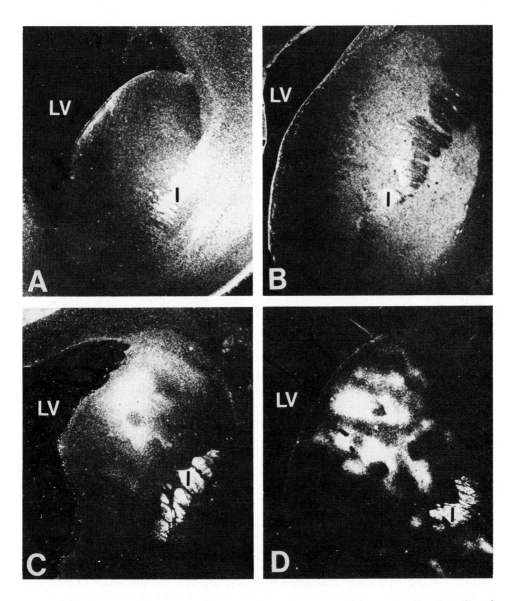

Fig. 5. Dark-field illumination photographs of autoradiograms prepared from coronal sections through the neostriatum of fetal and neonatal monkeys that were sacrificed at: embryonic day (E) 70 (A); E105 (B); E134 (C) and postnatal day (P) 11 (D). This figure displays the progressive compartmentalization of corticostriatal terminal fields from diffuse and uniform (A and B) to fenestrated (C and D). LV, lateral ventricle; I, internal capsule.

Fig. 4. Photographs displaying the relationship between the distribution of corticostriatal input (A) and neostriatal islands (B) as revealed in a rhesus monkey the prefrontal cortex of which was injected one week prior to sacrifice. A: photograph under dark-field illumination of prefrontostriatal projection to the head of the caudate nucleus with two label-free cores indicated by arabic numbers. B: the very same slide as in A photographed under bright-field illumination to expose the cellular islands within the label-free cores.

BIOCHEMICAL HETEROGENEITY OF FETAL STRIATUM

The biphasic development of discontinuous corticostriatal terminal fields and segregation of cellular compartments within the neostriatum is also reminiscent of other morphological and biochemical changes that have recently been described in this structure. One can only speculate about how the development of cell aggregates and cortical input may be related to the dopamine-fiber "islands" that originate in the substantia nigra (Olson et al., 1972; Tennyson et al., 1972) or to dense and light zones of acetylcholinesterase (AChE) activity observed within the neostriatum (Butcher and Hodge, 1976; Graybiel and Ragsdale, 1979; Kostovic et al., 1979). However, it might be suggested that the patches defined by dense AChE centers and pale AChE perimeters described in the neostriatum of human fetuses and neonates may correspond respectively to the cell clusters and fiber annuli described in the present study. This would imply that early in development island cells may be cholinergic or may receive cholinergic input whereas matrix cells presumably receive glutamatergic input from corticostriatal neurons (Kim et al., 1977). It should not be overlooked, however, that although both dopamine and acetylcholinesterase staining exhibit discontinuities in the neostriatum of immature rodents, carnivores and man, at maturity, the uneven distributions of these neurotransmitters is overshadowed by a more diffuse pattern of staining (Olson et al., 1972; Butcher and Hodge, 1976; Graybiel and Ragsdale, 1979). If this pattern of change is a progression from specific-to-diffuse, as it appears on the surface to be, it is opposite to the diffuse-to-patterned transformation that occurs in the corticostriatal terminal fields in monkey. Thus, many questions about the spatial and temporal relationships of the intrinsic and extrinsic fiber systems within the neostriatum still remain to be answered (for further discussion, see Goldman-Rakic, 1982).

MECHANISMS FOR SORTING OUT OF CORTICOSTRIATAL CONNECTIONS

Two basic types of cellular mechanisms can be proposed to account for how corticostriatal fibers are transformed from an initially diffuse to a fenestrated pattern in the mature brain. One possibility is a competition between cortical and other inputs for synaptic space in the various cellular compartments of the developing neostriatum. Such rivalry would imply that corticostriatal terminals are displaced to the periphery of neostriatal islands by an influx of competing fibers from another source such as the thalamus, the substantia nigra and/or the midbrain raphe complex, which may have higher affinities than corticostriatal input from the "island" cells. This readjustment of cortical terminals would undoubtedly be aided by translocations of target cells and dendrites upon which they terminate. Also, if the corticostriatal projections to the islands have already formed some synaptic junctions before E95, as seems likely (Brand and Rakic, 1979), the competition hypothesis would further require that these are later broken. This would not be unprecedented; indeed elimination of synapses seems to be the rule rather than the exception during development (for review, see Purves and Lichtman, 1980; Changeux and Danchin, 1976; also Crepel et al., 1976).

Unfortunately, very little is yet known about the synaptic terminations of corti-

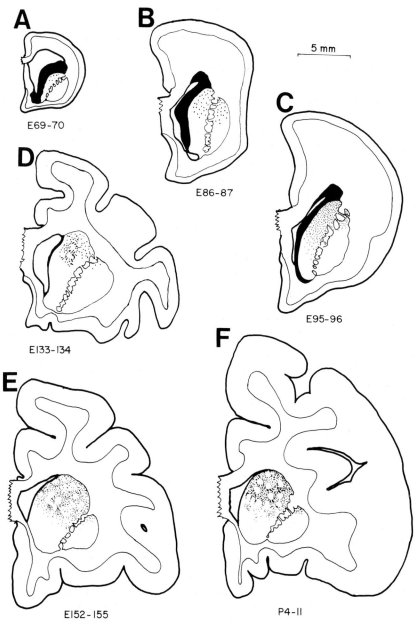

Fig. 6. Summary semidiagrammatic illustration of the time and mode of establishment of corticostriatal projections in the developing rhesus monkey. Following the convention used throughout this article, the first number under each drawing refers to the embryonic (E) or postnatal (P) day of [³H]proline and [³H]leucine injection into the superior bank of the developing principal sulcus; the second number indicates the day of sacrifice. Around E70, a small contingent of prefrontal fibers enter the territory of developing neostriatum which is still receiving neurons and glia from the proliferative zone of the ganglionic eminence (black area). Between E86 and E96 when all neostriatal neurons have been generated, many more cortical fibers enter the caudate nucleus and putamen. At these ages as at earlier fetal stages, the corticostriatal input is uniformly distributed throughout the neostriatum. Beginning around E105 (not shown) fenestrations begin to appear in the cortical terminal fields, a process which is completed by E133, one month before birth. The pattern of corticostriatal fiber distribution at E133 appears nearly identical to that observed in older fetuses (E152–155) and neonatal (P4–11) monkeys, though synaptogenesis in this structure is far from complete. (From Goldman-Rakic, 1981b, with permission.)

costriatal axons in fetal monkeys nor about their relationship to the timing and sequence of arrival of the various other neostriatal afferents during primate development. Based on present knowledge, it is likely that fibers of subcortical origin invade the neostriatum at least as early if not earlier than the corticostriatal input. Neurons of the brain stem (Levitt and Rakic, 1980) and thalamus (Dekker and Rakic, 1980) which project to the neostriatum are already generated in the monkey between E30 and E45 and between E38 and E43, respectively. However, these fibers may not innervate the neostriatum and differentiate their terminal fields until midgestation. Another likely source of fibers involved in competition for synaptic space may come from other nonfrontal cortical areas of the same hemisphere. Competition from homotopic neurons of the opposite hemisphere appears to be ruled out by our evidence of their paucity (Goldman-Rakic, 1981b). Whatever their source, other neostriatal inputs must either overlap the corticostriatal projection during the period of gestation when it is diffusely distributed or else develop later in gestation. The other possible explanation for the formation of the cortical terminal patterns in the neostriatum is the selective elimination of a subpopulation of cortical neurons that initially projected to the neostriatal islands. Cell death has been considered by many to be one of the principal mechanisms for shaping neural centers and establishing appropriate connections (e.g., Cowan, 1973; Clarke and Cowan, 1975; Knyihar et al., 1978). If this is applicable to the formation of corticostriatal terminal fields, cortical cell death must occur in a nonrandom fashion in order to produce "empty" elliptical areas within fiber clusters.

Any mechanism that may be responsible for the developmental transformation from a diffuse to a fenestrated distribution of corticostriatal axon terminals will also have to account for the formation of cellular islands in the neostriatum. This developmental interdependence of two classes of neurons that eventually become synaptically connected needs to be further elaborated to determine whether cytological changes in the target structure induce or are induced by compartmentalization of ingrowing axons. Since the neostriatum is becoming well characterized anatomically, histochemically and biochemically the formation of compartments in this structure may provide a valuable model for the analysis of mechanisms involved in neuronal specificity in complex systems. Its value as a model is further enhanced by the present evidence that a transformation of corticostriatal input from overlapping and diffuse to a segregated pattern appears to reflect a general rule governing the formation of central neuronal connections – one that applies not only to the ascending radiations of sensory afferent systems but also the major descending efferent projections of the association neocortex.

REFERENCES

Atweh, S.F. and Kuhar, M.J. (1977) Autoradiographic localization of opiate receptors in rat brain. III. The telencephalon. *Brain Res.*, 134: 393–405.

Brand, S. and Rakic, P. (1979) Synaptogenesis in the caudate nucleus of pre- and postnatal rhesus monkeys. *Anat. Rec.*, 193: 490.

Butcher, L.L. and Hodge, G.K. (1976) Postnatal development of acetylecholinesterase in the caudate-putamen nucleus and substantia nigra of rats. *Brain Res.*, 106: 223–240.

Carpenter, M. (1976) Anatomical organization of the corpus striatum and related nuclei. In M. Yahr (Ed.), *The Basal Ganglia*, Raven Press, New York, pp. 1–36.

Changeux, J.-P. and Danchin, A. (1976) Selective stabilization of developing synapses, a mechanism for the specification of neuronal networks. *Nature (Lond.)*, 264: 705–715.

Chase, T.N., Wexler, N.S. and Barbeau, A. (Eds.) (1979) *Advances in Neurology, Vol. 23*, Raven Press, New York.

Clarke, P.G.H. and Cowan, W.M. (1976) Ectopic neurons and aberrant connections during neuronal development. *Proc. nat. Acad. Sci. U.S.A.*, 72: 4455–4458.

Crepel, F., Delhaye-Bouchand, N. and Mariani, J. (1976) Evidence for a multiple innervation of Purkinje cells by climbing fibers in the immature rat cerebellum. *J. Neurobiol.*, 7: 567–578.

Cowan, W.M. (1973) Neuronal death as a regulative mechanism in the control of cell number in the nervous system. In M. Rockstein (Ed.), *Development and Aging in the Nervous System*, Academic Press, New York, pp. 59–86.

Dekker, J.J. and Rakic, P. (1980) Genesis of the neurons in the motor cortex and VA-VL thalamic complex in rhesus monkey. *Soc. Neurosci. Abstr.*, 6: 205.

DeVito, J.L. and Smith, Jr., O.A.S. (1964) Subcortical projections of the prefrontal lobe of the monkey. *J. comp. Neurol.*, 123: 413–424.

DiFiglia, M., Pasik, P. and Pasik, T. (1980) Early postnatal development of the monkey neostriatum: A Golgi and ultrastructural study. *J. comp. Neurol.*, 190: 303–331.

Goldman, P.S. (1978) Neuronal plasticity in primate telencephalon: anomalous crossed cortico-caudate projections induced by prenatal removal of frontal association cortex. *Science*, 202: 768–770.

Goldman, P.S. and Rosvold, H.E. (1972) The effects of selective caudate lesions in infant and juvenile rhesus monkeys. *Brain Res.*, 43: 53–66.

Goldman, P.S. and Nauta, W.J.H. (1977) An intricately patterned prefronto-caudate projection in rhesus monkey. *J. comp. Neurol.*, 171: 369–386.

Goldman-Rakic, P.S. (1981a) Development and plasticity of primate frontal cortex. In F.O. Schmitt, F.G. Worden, S.G. Dennis and G. Adelman (Eds.), *The Organization of the Cerebral Cortex*, MIT Press, Cambridge, MA, pp. 69–97.

Goldman-Rakic, P.S. (1981b) Prenatal formation of cortical input and development of cytoarchitectonic compartments in the neostriatum of the rhesus monkey. *J. Neurosci.*, 1: 721–735.

Goldman-Rakic, P.S. (1982) Cytoarchitectonic heterogeneity of the primate neostriatum: subdivision into island and matrix cellular compartments. *J. comp. Neurol.*, 205: 398–413.

Graybiel, A.M. and Ragsdale, C.W. (1979) Histochemically distinct compartments in the striatum of human being, monkey and cat demonstrated by the acetylthiocholinesterase staining method. *Proc. nat. Acad. Sci. U.S.A.*, 75: 5723–5726.

Graybiel, A.M., Ragsdale, Jr., C.W., Yoneoka, E.S. and Elde, R.P. (1981) An immunohistochemical study of enkephalin and other neuropeptides in the striatum of the cat with evidence that the opiate peptides are arranged to form mosaic patterns in register with the striosomal compartments visible by acetylcholinesterase staining. *Neuroscience*, 6: 377–397.

Herkenham, M. and Pert, C. (1981) Mosaic distribution of opiate receptors, parafascicular projections and acetylcholinesterase in rat striatum. *Nature (Lond.)*, 291: 415–417.

Kalil, K. (1978) Patch-like termination of thalamic fibers in the putamen of the rhesus monkey: an autoradiographic study. *Brain Res.*, 140: 333–339.

Kemp, J.M. and Powell, T.P.S. (1970) The cortico-striate projection in the monkey. *Brain*, 93: 525–546.

Kemp, J.M. and Powell, T.P.S. (1971a) The structure of the caudate nucleus of the cat: light and electron microscopy. *Phil. Trans. B*, 262: 383–401.

Kemp, J.M. and Powell, T.P.S. (1971b) The termination of fibers from the cerebral cortex and thalamus upon dendritic spines in the caudate nucleus: a study with the Golgi method. *Phil. Trans. B*, 262: 429–439.

Kim, J.-S., Hassler, R., Haug, P. and Paik, K.-S. (1977) Effect of frontal cortex ablation on striatal glutamic acid level in rat. *Brain Res.*, 132: 370–374.

Knyihar, E., Csillik, B. and Rakic, P. (1978) Transient synapses in the embryonic primate spinal cord. *Science*, 202: 1206–1209.

Kostovic-Knezevic, Lj., Kostovic, I., Krompotic-Nemanic, J. and Kelovic, Z. (1979) Acetylcholinesterase (AChE) staining in the growing telencephalic structures of the human fetus. *Verh. Anat. Ges.*, 73: 667–669.

Künzle, H. (1975) Bilateral projections from precentral motor cortex to the putamen and other parts of the basal ganglia. *Brain Res.*, 88: 195–210.

Levitt, P. and Rakic, P. (1979) Genesis of central monoamine neurons in the rhesus monkey. *Soc. Neurosci. Abstr.*, 5: 341.

418

Mettler, F.A. (1968) Anatomy of the basal ganglia, In P.J. Vinken and G.W. Bruyn (Eds.), *Handbook of Clinical Neurology, Vol. 6*, North-Holland, Amsterdam, pp. 1–55.

Olson, L., Seiger, A. and Fuxe, K. (1972) Heterogeneity of striatal and limbic dopamine innervation: Highly fluorescent islands in developing and adult rats. *Brain Res.*, 44: 283–288.

Pert, C.B., Kuhar, M.J. and Snyder, S.H. (1976) The opiate receptor: autoradiographic localization in rat brain. *Proc. nat. Acad. Sci. U.S.A.*, 73: 3729–3733.

Pickel, V.M., Sumal, K.K., Beckley, S.C., Miller, R.J. and Reis, D.J. (1980) Immunocytochemical localization of enkephalin in the neostriatum of rat brain: a light and electron microscopic study. *J. comp. Neurol.*, 189: 721–740.

Purves, D. and Lichtman, J.W. (1980) Elimination of synapses in the developing nervous system. *Science*, 210: 153–157.

Rakic, P. (1976) Prenatal genesis of connections subserving ocular dominance in the rhesus monkey. *Nature (Lond.)*, 261: 467–471.

Rakic, P. and Goldman-Rakic, P.S. (1982) Development and modifiability of the cerebral cortex. *Neurosci. Res. Prog. Bull.*, 20: 429–611.

Royce, J.G. (1978) Cells of origin of subcortical afferents to the caudate nucleus: a horseradish peroxidase study in the cat. *Brain Res.*, 153: 465–475.

Schmitt, F.O., Worden, F., Dennis, S.G. and Adelman, G. (Eds.) (1981) *The Organization of the Cerebral Cortex*, MIT Press, Cambridge, MA.

Tennyson, V.M., Barrett, R.E., Cohen, G., Cote, L., Heikkila, R. and Mytilineou, C. (1972) The developing neostriatum of the rabbit: correlation of fluorescence histochemistry, electron microscopy, endogenous dopamine levels, and [^{3}H]dopamine uptake. *Brain Res.*, 46: 251–285.

Yeterian, E.H. and Van Hoesen, G.W. (1978) Cortico-striate projections in the rhesus monkey: The organization of certain cortico-caudate connections. *Brain Res.*, 139: 43–63.

Possible Cellular Basis for Prolonged Changes of Synaptic Efficiency – A Simple Case of Learning

PER ANDERSEN

Institute of Neurophysiology, University of Oslo (Norway)

Learning is one of the fundamental properties of animals, reaching its highest form in man. The phenomenon is essential for the survival of the organism in that it provides the means to adapt to different environmental changes. Both in man and animals, the achievement and execution of various behaviors clearly depend heavily upon the ability to learn. With the increased degree and speed of adaptation provided by learning, the likelihood of survival increases greatly.

Whether an attempt to explain the nerve changes underlying learning follows a network or a connectionist approach, a definite physical change in the nerve cells and their connections seems necessary. Although the network explanation implies a change of the dynamic state of the participating neurons in the network, the time-locked changes in the network somehow must have a mechanistic explanation. With a connectionist approach, mechanical or chemical changes in or between the nerve elements are obvious necessities.

The most probable locus for such changes are the synaptic contacts. In this context, I shall use the term learning in a broad sense, describing a modification of behavior resulting from previous experience of one or several stimuli, also where these stimuli are associated with other stimuli or responses as well. Learning, thus defined, comprises several categories of changes including the simple non-associative forms habituation, dishabituation and sensitization, the more complex associative forms of classical and instrumental conditioning and more advanced forms (Kandel, 1978).

It is often assumed that the higher functions like learning are best looked for in the most complicated nervous systems and within these, in the most intricate areas, notably the cerebral cortex. However, the complexity which is called upon to explain phenomena of learning and memory does in itself hinder a thorough analysis of the phenomena. Nevertheless, a very large amount of work has been devoted to studies using cortical tissue as the substratum for studies on learning mechanisms in intact animals. In spite of the large amount of empirical data assembled in this way, showing that a number of learning paradigms can be mimicked, this approach has been somewhat disappointing. Although recordings from single units in various parts of the brain have shown that associative learning in the form of conditioning reflexes can be set up with sensory, direct stimulation and chemical mediation as the unconditioned stimulus (Bureš and Burešová, 1970), the mechanism by which the process operates has eluded the experimenters. The obvious reason is the lack of experimental control of all inputs to the system, and, particularly, to the detailed processes across the membrane of the participating cells and of their immediate environment. Similar comments can be raised towards studies with anodal polarization of cortex, which may give very long-lasting changes in firing to direct and sensory stimulation (Rusinov, 1953; Morrel, 1961; Lippold, 1970).

In search of preparations which lend themselves more easily to an experimental approach while still maintaining properties relevant to learning, interesting results were obtained by Spencer and his associates, studying the very long-lasting post-tetanic potentiation in motoneurons. However, the required tetanizing stimuli had frequencies in the upper range or above those seen in Ia fibers under physiological conditions, and the tetani had to last for several tens of minutes. However, when such high frequency long-lasting tetani were used, Spencer and April (1970) observed powerful potentiation which could last for several hours. The test reflex in question was the monosynaptic reflex of the cat hind limb. The long-lasting potentiation was curtailed, however, by an early and severe post-tetanic depression which probably is due to blockade of the impulses in the afferent fiber terminals, due to the associated hyperpolarization. However, as a case of relatively short-lasting plastic change, the phenomenon could well be of major importance in demonstrating definite changes in the connectivity in the spinal cord (Spencer and April, 1970).

Another example of activity-induced long-lasting changes in the mammalian spinal cord is the decrement of the flexor reflex following repeated cutaneous stimuli observed by Spencer and his associates (Spencer et al., 1966a, b, c).

At the other end of the spectrum, the use of simpler preparations, in which greater experimental control can be brought to bear, has proven remarkably successful. In particular, studies on the gastropod *Aplysia californica* have proven extremely successful (Kandel, 1978). Also, isolated brain slices have been useful for a study of plastic changes in cortical tissue. These preparations allow techniques which permit more direct analysis of the induced changes at a cellular level. In this short survey, I shall deal with some of the cellular changes which follow training periods in *Aplysia* and in hippocampal slices.

One of the plastic changes that can be successfully studied in *Aplysia* is the process of habituation. In order to study reflex habituation, Kandel (1978) and coworkers have chosen the defensive withdrawal reflex of the external organs of the mantle cavity in *Aplysia*. The respiratory organ, the gill, is found inside a chamber, which is covered by a protective sheet of the mantle shelf, which terminates in a soft tube, the siphon. When a weak, or moderately intense tactile stimulus is applied to the siphon or the mantle shelf, both the siphon and the gill contract and withdraw into the mantle cavity (Pinsker et al., 1970). This defensive reflex may undergo two elementary forms of learning: habituation and sensitization. When the same tactile stimulus is applied several times some minutes apart, the withdrawal reflex gradually diminishes, but reappears after a rest period. The Kandel group has defined the neuronal net which operates in the withdrawal reflex (Kandel, 1978). By recording from the motoneurons which control the gill withdrawal, Kupferman et al. (1970) were able to describe the neuronal correlates of the habituation as a reduced number of action potentials to a constant tactile stimulus. Furthermore, simplifying the system by stimulation of the appropriate sensory nerve and blocking interneuronal activity with high calcium/low magnesium, Castellucci and Kandel (1974) found a gradual depression of the EPSP as the most likely cause of the habituation. In this situation, they made a quantal analysis. The reduced EPSP amplitude during habituation was associated with a reduction in the quantal content (m) while the quantal size (q) remained unchanged. This result indicates that the locus of the short-term habituation at this identified synapse is presynaptic. Even more remarkable, by testing animals which had received a training regime composed by several brief sessions of habituation training of 10 trials each, Castellucci et al. (1978) found that reduced transmission remained as long as three weeks in a considerable fraction of the synapses in question. This is particularly important for our general discussion, since it shows that both short- and long-term habituation may be located at the same synaptic locus, at least in this preparation.

Another process which has been studied with great success is sensitization. This means an enhancement of a reflex produced by strong or noxious stimulus to the head or neck. The enhancement may last from minutes to weeks and depends upon the strength and duration of the priming stimulus. It resembles classical conditioning in that activity in one input system facilitates the reflex activity in another. However, the sensitizing and test stimuli need not be temporally associated. At the cellular levels the sensitization of the gill withdrawal reflex in *Aplysia* turned out to be caused by an increased number of discharges from the gill motoneuron due to increased synaptic potentials. A quantal analysis showed that the process was explained by an increased quantal content, while again the quantal size remained constant (Castellucci and Kandel, 1974).

The increased EPSP is also associated with an increased presence of cyclic AMP in the ganglion (Cedar et al., 1972). Brunelli et al. (1976) further showed that serotonin caused a similar facilitation of the EPSP. Finally, intracellular injection of cyclic AMP also produced facilitation, whereas cyclic GMP and 5'-AMP were ineffective. Kandel (1978) concluded that the effect of serotonin is mediated by way of cyclic AMP, which again modulates the intracellular calcium concentration presynaptically. Because of the duration of the effect the process is most likely due to an alteration of the calcium channels, either by changing their number or properties (Fig. 1), and not just due to an increased release due to increased intraterminal calcium.

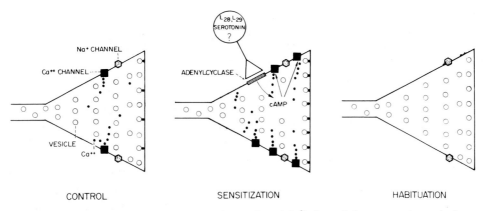

Fig. 1. Diagram to explain how modulation of the number of Ca^{2+}-channels in presynaptic terminals may explain the increased probability of release of transmitter during sensitization and reduced probability during habituation. (From Kandel, 1978, with permission.)

Another promising preparation for studying cellular attributes of simple learning processes has been the long-term potentiation (LTP) of synaptic transmission in hippocampal and dentate synapses (Lømo, 1966; Bliss and Lømo, 1973; Douglas and Goddard, 1975). Later, the same type of long-lasting facilitation has been shown to occur at several synapses in the hippocampal formation. The phenomenon requires that the receiving cells are driven by a short train of impulses within their physiological range of discharge, for example 10–15 Hz for 10 sec. In intact animals, such a train to the perforant path fibers which synapse on dentate granule cells may give rise to prominent synaptic facilitation, lasting for several weeks (Bliss and Gardner-Medwin, 1973). Even more effective is one or a few stimulus trains at high frequency, delivered with intervals of some seconds (Douglas, 1977). The process can also be seen in isolated brain slices (Schwartzkroin and Wester, 1975). The potentiation appears to be homosynaptic since other inputs to the same cell do not show the change (Andersen et al., 1977; Lynch et al., 1977), although claims have been made that heterosynaptic facilitation also exists (Misgeld et al., 1979). The process appears as an increase of the extracellular EPSP in response to a standard input. Furthermore, the population spike, signifying the nearly synchronous discharge of a great number of cells shows a prominent increase (Bliss and Lømo, 1973). An adequate measure of the number of afferent fibers is a prerequisite for claims of changes in synaptic transmission at the time courses in question. Usually, this has been achieved by stimulation with constant current pulses and by constructing input-output curves to demonstrate that the threshold is not changed. Small movements of either stimulation or recording electrodes as well as polarization, changes in anesthetic level, edema or other non-specific changes can easily imitate a facilitatory effect, however.

For a study of the LTP mechanism the advent of brain slices (Yamamoto and McIlwain, 1966; Richards and Sercombe, 1968; Skrede and Westgaard, 1971) has been a great advantage. In the transverse hippocampal formation, it is possible to monitor the size of the afferent volley (Andersen et al., 1978) and also perform long-lasting intra- or extracellular recordings from cells under study. Furthermore, the stratification of the afferent fibers to the pyramidal cells of the hippocampal formation allows the selective activation of two or more inputs to the same cell. Using two such separate inputs, Andersen et al. (1977) and Lynch et al. (1977) found that only the tetanized pathway showed a persistent increase of synaptic transmission. The facilitation occurs in two steps, an early fast phase followed by a more prolonged one (McNaughton, 1977). The first phase is probably a post-tetanic potentiation, following the same rules as found in other preparations. The long-lasting tail, lasting for up to 2 h in slice preparations, is the long-term potentiation proper. In most cells, it is preceded by a short period (3–6 min) of depression. The depression is heterosynaptic in that it affects all synaptic responses, excitatory as well as inhibitory, and also testing pulses across the soma membrane. By recording the field potential at the site of the activated synapses, it appears that the LTP process is due to an increased inward synaptic current. By recording from single units, there is a clear and long-lasting increase in the probability of discharge to a matched input compared with the situation before tetanization (Andersen et al., 1980). Recorded intracellularly, there is an increased size and rate of rise of the EPSP and the latency of the spike is reduced (Fig. 2).

When compared to an input/output curve taken before tetanization there is a

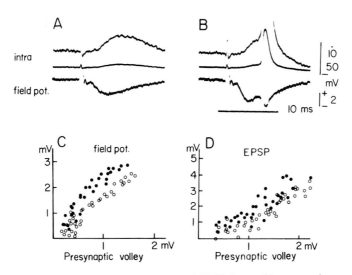

Fig. 2. A: upper two traces are intracellularly recorded EPSP from a hippocampal pyramid at high and low gain. Lower trace is extracellular record taken at the level of the activated synapses. B: as A, but 10 min after a 50 Hz, 5 sec tetanus was delivered to the afferent pathway. C: relation between the presynaptic volley size (abscissa) and the extracellular EPSP before (open circles) and after (filled circles) tetanization. D: as C, but ordinate gives size of intracellular EPSP.

clear increase in the probability of discharge as well as a reduced latency for a corresponding size of the input volley. By testing the excitability of the soma membrane with long hyperpolarizing pulses, there is no change in the membrane resistance nor in the membrane potential in well penetrated cells. Thus, the first, tentative conclusion is that there is an increased EPSP without changes in the input resistance of the cell, indicating an increase of liberated transmitter, similar to the facilitatory process in *Aplysia* (Kandel, 1978). The process does not depend upon the simultaneous discharge of the postsynaptic cell, since neither parallel antidromic nor weak synaptic activation is followed by the described change. Furthermore, tetanization during hyperpolarization of the cell recorded from is still followed by long-term potentiation (Wigström et al., 1982).

Since the EPSP is increased without a reduction of the total input resistance, an increased amount of liberated transmitter is part of the mechanism. However, there is a disturbing discrepancy between the relatively large change of the extracellular EPSP and the moderate increase of the intracellular EPSP. Furthermore, when the increased probability of discharge and the reduced spike latency are matched to a calibration curve produced by increasing input volleys, the post-tetanic changes are much larger than those that can be ascribed to the moderate EPSP increase. Therefore, an additional factor seems to be at play. Possibly this factor may be located on the postsynaptic side of the synapse. However, since the soma membrane did not show any changes of its passive electric properties, the change may occur locally. This local change may involve a change in ionic composition or changes in the spine membrane associated with the increased depolarizing synaptic current. In this context, it is interesting to note that the soma membrane often shows anomalous rectification (Hotson et al., 1979). Recent experiments with long-lasting depolarizing pulses suggest that the dendritic membrane may create regenerative activity in the

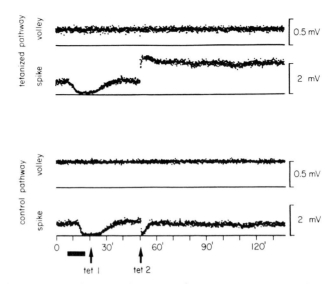

Fig. 3. Amplitude of presynaptic volley (upper trace) and population spike (lower trace) of CA1 hippocampal cells. Upper half gives data from tetanized pathway, lower half shows responses to a not tetanized input to another part of the dendritic tree of the same cell population. Thick bar indicates removal of calcium ions. tet 1 indicates a train of 50 Hz, 5 sec when synaptic transmission but not fiber action potentials were blocked; tet 2 is a similar train after re-admission of calcium. Only the last is followed by a potentiated population spike (LTP). The control side shows a short-lasting depression which is non-specific. (From Andersen et al., 1980, with permission.)

form of long-lasting potentials (Lanthorn et al., 1981). A possible explanation is that the long, intense depolarization caused by the tetanizing stimulation, causes a change in the postsynaptic membrane, possibly altering the calcium channels. Long-lasting depolarizing potentials in these cells have been ascribed to calcium currents (Schwartzkroin and Slawsky, 1977; Wong and Prince, 1978). This explanation resembles that given by Kandel (1978) for the presynaptic change in *Aplysia*.

The possibility that the presynaptic change is dependent upon the intracellular calcium level is suggested by substitution experiments in which tetanization was performed when the perfusion fluid was without calcium ions (Fig. 3). Calcium ions were readmitted just after the tetanization (tet 1), and normal synaptic transmission ensued, but no long-term potentiation appeared. LTP developed, however, when a new tetanizing period was delivered with a normal calcium level (tet 2). Although the experiment is open to alternative explanations, it is consistent with the view that presynaptic calcium concentration is an important mediator for the process. In this context it would be similar to the process already described in detail for *Aplysia* gill withdrawal reflex.

Recently, it has been claimed that noradrenaline (NA) is necessary for LTP to occur in dentate granule cells (Bliss et al., 1981). Interestingly, NA has been seen to block Ca^{2+}-mediated potentials in hippocampal neurons (Segal, 1981), probably by interference with calmodulin. These data do not yet give a coherent picture, but indicate an interesting area for future research.

Finally, it is of great importance to distinguish between the locus of enhancement discussed above and the locus of control (Goddard, 1980; Douglas et al., 1982). Because the tetanizing stimulus needs to be above a certain strength before the LTP phenomenon is seen, the simultaneous activation of a group of neighboring fibers seems a requirement for the process. This, however, does not mean that a given number of postsynaptic cells must be brought into action for the process to develop. By feeding in a commissural input, which gives inhibition of dentate granule cells, just before a tetanizing input, Douglas et al. (1982) were able to prevent the LTP altogether. This result suggests that the locus of enhancement is postsynaptic. This, however, is not necessarily the case. Unfortunately, no well controlled intracellular study of dentate EPSP enhancement is available. From the extracellular records, however, it appears likely that the LTP in the perforant path/granule cell synapse also is associated with an increased transmitter release. The absence of LTP following inhibition of the receiving cell during tetanization implies that postsynaptic modifications play a part in the change, but this does not by itself negate the presynaptic role.

In short, long-term potentiation of hippocampal and dentate neurons seems to have many of the properties one would like to ascribe to a simple learning process. The response apparently involves both presynaptic and postsynaptic processes, but the locus of control may be presynaptic only. Apparently, alteration of calcium channels may well prove of crucial importance both pre- and postsynaptically for the LTP process. Thus, although there is a long distance between the gastropod withdrawal reflex and mammalian hippocampal cortical neurons, they may well share fundamental properties associated with learning processes.

REFERENCES

Andersen, P., Sundberg, S.H., Sveen, O. and Wigström, H. (1977) Specific long-lasting potentiation of synaptic transmission in hippocampal slices. Nature (Lond.), 266: 736–737.

Andersen, P., Silfvenius, H., Sundberg, S.H., Sveen, O. and Wigström, H. (1978) Functional characteristics of unmyelinated fibers in the hippocampal cortex. Brain Res., 144: 11–18.

Andersen, P., Sundberg, S.H., Swann, J.N. and Wigström, H. (1980) Possible mechanisms for long-lasting potentiation of synaptic transmission in hippocampal slices from guinea pigs. J. Physiol. (Lond.), 302: 463–482.

Bliss, T.V.P. and Gardner-Medwin, A.R. (1973) Long-lasting potentiation of synaptic transmission in the dentate area of the unanaesthetized rabbit following stimulation of the perforant path. J. Physiol. (Lond.), 232: 357–374.

Bliss, T.V.P. and Lømo, T. (1973) Long-lasting potentiation of synaptic transmission in the dentate area of the anaesthetized rabbit following stimulation of the perforant path. J. Physiol. (Lond.), 232: 331–356.

Bliss, T.V.P., Goddard, G.V., Robertson, H.A. and Sutherland, R.J. (1981) Noradrenaline depletion reduces long-term potentiation in the rat hippocampus. In O. Feher and F. Joo (Eds.), Cellular Analogues of Conditioning and Neural Plasticity, Advanc. Physiol. Sci., Vol. 36, pp. 175–185.

Brunelli, M., Castellucci, V. and Kandel, R.R. (1976) Synaptic facilitation and behavioral sensitization in Aplysia: possible role of serotonin and cyclic AMP. Science, 194: 1178–1181.

Bureš, J. and Burešová, O. (1970) Plasticity in single neurons and neural populations. In G. Horn and R.A. Hinde (Eds.), Short-Term Changes in Neural Activity and Behavior, University Press, Cambridge, pp. 363–403.

Castellucci, V.F. and Kandel, E.R. (1974) A quantal analysis of the synaptic depression underlying habituation of the gill-withdrawal reflex in Aplysia. Proc. natl. Acad. Sci. U.S.A., 71: 5004–5008.

Castellucci, V.F., Carew, T.J. and Kandel, E.R. (1978) Cellular analysis of long-term habituation in the gill-withdrawal reflex of Aplysia californica. Science, 202: 1306–1308.

Cedar, H., Kandel, E.R. and Schwartz, J.H. (1972) Cyclic adenosine monophosphate in the nervous system of Aplysia californica. I. Increased synthesis in response to synaptic stimulation. J. gen. Physiol., 60: 558–569.

Douglas, R.M. (1977) Long-lasting synaptic potentiation in the rat dentate gyrus following brief high-frequency stimulation. Brain Res., 126: 361–365.

Douglas, R.M. and Goddard, G.V. (1975) Long-term potentiation of the perforant path-granule cell synapse in the rat hippocampus. *Brain Res.*, 86: 205–215.

Douglas, R.M., Goodard, G.V. and Riives, M. (1982) Inhibitory modulation of long-term potentiation: evidence for a postsynaptic locus of control. *Brain Res.*, 240: 259–272.

Goddard, G.V. (1980) Component properties of the memory machine: Hebb revisited. In P.W. Jusczyk and R.M. Klein (Eds.), *The Nature of Thought; Essays in Honour of D.O. Hebb*, Lawrence Erlbaum Assoc., New Jersey, pp. 231–247.

Hotson, J.R., Prince, D.A. and Schwartzkroin, P.A. (1979) Anomalous inward rectification in hippocampal neurons. *J. Neurophysiol.*, 42: 889–895.

Kandel, E.R. (1978) *A Cell-Biological Approach to Learning*, Soc. Neurosci., Bethesda, MD, p. 90.

Kupferman, I., Castellucci, V., Pinsker, H. and Kandel, E.R. (1970) Neuronal correlates of habituation and dis-habituation of the gill-withdrawal reflex in *Aplysia. Science*, 167: 1743–1745.

Lanthorn, T., Storm, J. and Andersen, P. (1981) Responses of hippocampal CA1 pyramidal neurones in vitro to depolarizing currents of long duration. *Neurosci. Lett.*, Suppl. 7: S383.

Lippold, O.C.J. (1970) Long-lasting changes in activity of cortical neurones. In G. Horn and R.A. Hinde (Eds.), *Short-Term Changes in Neural Activity and Behavior*, University Press, Cambridge, pp. 405–432.

Lømo, T. (1966) Frequency potentiation of excitatory synaptic activity in the dentate area of the hippocampal formation. *Acta physiol. scand.*, 68, Suppl. 277: 128.

Lynch, G.S., Dunwiddie, T. and Gribkoff, V. (1977) Heterosynaptic depression: a postsynaptic correlate of long-term potentiation. *Nature (Lond.)*, 266: 737–739.

McNaughton, B.L. (1977) Dissociation of short- and long-lasting modification of synaptic efficacy at the terminals of the perforant path. *Soc. Neurosci. Abstr.*, 3: 517.

Misgeld, U., Sarvey, J.M. and Klee, M.R. (1979) Heterosynaptic postactivation potentiation in hippocampal CA3 neurons: long-term changes of the postsynaptic potentials. *Exp. Brain Res.*, 37: 217–229.

Morrell, F. (1961) Electrical signs of sensory coding. In G.C. Quarton, T. Melnechuk and F.O. Schmitt (Eds.), *The Neurosciences*, Rockefeller University Press, New York, pp. 452–469.

Pinsker, H., Kupferman, I., Castellucci, V. and Kandel, E.R. (1970) Habituation and dishabituation of the gill-withdrawal reflex in *Aplysia. Science*, 167: 1740–1742.

Richards, C.D. and Sercombe, R. (1968) Electrical activity observed in guinea-pig olfactory cortex maintained in vitro. *J. Physiol. (Lond.)*, 197: 667–683.

Rusinov, V.S. (1953) An electrophysiological analysis of the connecting function in the cerebral cortex in the presence of a dominant area. In *Abstr., 19th Int. Congr. Physiol.*, Montreal, p. 719.

Schwartzkroin, P. and Slawsky, M. (1977) Probable calcium spikes in hippocampal neurons. *Brain Res.*, 135: 157–161.

Schwartzkroin, P. and Wester, K. (1975) Long-lasting facilitation of a synaptic potential following tetanization in the in vitro hippocampal slice. *Brain Res.*, 89: 107–119.

Segal, M. (1981) The action of norepinephrine in the rat hippocampus: intracellular studies in the slice preparation. *Brain Res.*, 206: 107–128.

Skrede, K.K. and Westgaard, R.H. (1971) The transverse hippocampal slice: a well-defined cortical structure maintained in vitro. *Brain Res.*, 35: 589–593.

Spencer, W.A. and April. R.S. (1970) Plastic properties of monosynaptic pathways in mammals. In G. Horn and R.A. Hinde (Eds.), *Short-Term Changes in Neural Activity and Behavior*, University Press, Cambridge, pp. 433–474.

Spencer, W.A., Thompson, R.F. and Neilson, D.R., Jr. (1966a) Response decrement of the flexion reflex in the acute spinal cat and transient restoration by strong stimuli. *J. Neurophysiol.*, 29: 221–239.

Spencer, W.A., Thompson, R.F. and Neilson, D.R., Jr. (1966b) Alterations in responsiveness of ascending and reflex pathways activated by iterated cutaneous afferent volleys. *J. Neurophysiol.*, 29: 240–252.

Spencer, W.A., Thompson, R.F. and Neilson, D.R., Jr (1966c) Decrement of ventral root electrotonus and intracellularly recorded PSPs produced by iterated cutaneous afferent volleys. *J. Neurophysiol.*, 29: 253–274.

Wigström, H., McNaughton, B.L. and Barnes, C.A. (1982) Long-term synaptic enhancement in hippocampus is not regulated by postsynaptic membrane potential. *Brain Res.*, 233: 195–199.

Wong, R.K.S. and Prince, D.A. (1978) Participation of calcium spikes during intrinsic burst firing in hippocampal neurons. *Brain Res.*, 159: 385–390.

Yamamoto, C. and McIlwain, H. (1966) Electrical activities in thin sections from the mammalian brain maintained in chemically-defined media in vitro. *J. Neurochem.*, 13: 1333–1343.

Specification of Cortical Neurons
By Visuomotor Experience

MICHEL IMBERT and YVES FREGNAC

Laboratoire de Neurobiologie du Développement, Bâtiment 440, Université de Paris-Sud, 91405 Orsay Cedex
(France)

INTRODUCTION

It is generally accepted that the brain is formed during two successive periods of development of the organism. During the first period, neuroembryological events take place, for example, cellular division and migration, neuronal differentiation and the establishment of interneuronal connections. Both the main cerebral structures and the nerve fiber circuits are established following a very rigorous plan and a precise calender of events. This seems to reflect achievement of intrinsic programs under strict genetic control. However, the network, thus established is neither rigid nor stable. Indeed, this first period is followed by a second one mainly postnatal, during which the neuronal connections become stabilized, giving rise to the adult nervous system organization. This second phase is governed by epigenetic factors including the functioning of the brain itself and processes which are dependent on the experience the organism has of its environment.

Studies of the ontogeny of the functional organization of the visual cortex have given evidence for this two-stage developmental sequence. Combined progress in electrophysiological and neuroanatomical methods, pioneered mainly by Hubel and Wiesel, have clearly demonstrated that the basic features of the adult cortical organization – namely, binocular integration and orientation selectivity – are present before any interaction with visual environment has taken place. However, the extent to which these functional properties are represented in the visual cortex of the neonate animal is the subject of continuing debate. At eye-opening segregation of geniculate afferents from each eye is more prominent in layer IV of monkey cortex than in cat cortex (Rakic, 1977; LeVay et al., 1980; LeVay and Stryker, 1981). Orientation selectivity of visual cortical neurons reaches almost adult standards in neonate primates, whereas experimental evidence is less clear in kittens. Although greater proportions of non-specialized neurons have been found than originally described by Hubel and Wiesel (1963), it is generally agreed that the development of orientation selectivity begins before eye-opening and precedes the extensive growth of the cortical neuropile (Fregnac, 1979; Wolf and Albus, 1981). Oriented cells have been recorded as early as 6 days of age (Wolf and Albus, 1981) at least by the end of the first week (Hubel and Wiesel, 1963; Blakemore and Van Sluyters, 1975; Buisseret and Imbert, 1976; Fregnac and Imbert, 1978). These electrophysiological findings are somewhat surprising, considering the poorness of kitten optical media and the relative paucity of synaptic contacts ($<2\%$ of the final number) found at this age (Cragg, 1972). In this early selectivity state, during which maturation proceeds

428

intrinsically independently of visual experience, a particular relationship is found between ocular dominance and orientation preference (Fregnac and Imbert, 1978). This result seems to hold both for kittens less than 3 weeks of age (Fregnac and Imbert, 1978) and for the neonate monkey (Blakemore and Vital-Durand, 1981). Recent experiments in older kittens support the hypothesis that these monocular, horizontal or vertical detectors which are supposed to be submitted to the strongest endogenous constraints, mature earlier and thus become more functionally stable (Leventhal and Hirsch, 1980; Fregnac et al., 1981; Buisseret et al., 1982). It has also been suggested recently, that such an organization could result from a rigid scheme of afferent connectivity, and be the skeleton of a cortical projection existing earlier in phylogeny (Pettigrew, 1978). This over-representation of horizontal and vertical orientations could reflect an orientation preference which is present at a lower level of integration (Vidyasagar and Urbas, 1982).

The second phase of development, dependent on visual experience, corresponds to the later and major growth of synaptic contacts in kitten visual cortex. During this critical period of postnatal life, the physiology and even the connectivity may be profoundly modified if the visual environment is manipulated. The periods of susceptibility of ocular dominance and orientation selectivity to "visual surgery" start from the beginning of the 3rd week and end around the 12th week (Hubel and Wiesel, 1970; Blakemore et al., 1975; Fregnac, 1979a; Buisseret et al., 1982). While the importance of visual factors in producing cortical functional changes has been extensively stressed, little data has been obtained about the extraretinal factors involved in the sensorimotor experience of the visual world, which might influence the development of cortical function (Berardi et al., 1981).

In this paper we review related results recently obtained in our laboratory showing that:

(1) afferents running through the ophthalmic branch of the trigeminal nerve – among which are found proprioceptive fibers – play an important role in controlling the kinetics of restoration of cortical specificity, following delayed visuomotor experience during the critical period;

(2) specific functional modifications may be recorded from individual cortical neurons, when combining vision and passive eye-movement in a 6-week-old paralyzed and anesthetized kitten.

Taken together, these results stress the importance of ocular motility – and probably of extraocular proprioception – in the development of visual cortical response properties.

ROLE OF EXTRAOCULAR PROPRIOCEPTION IN THE DEVELOPMENT OF CORTICAL SPECIFICITY

Role of extraocular proprioception in the cortical effects of delayed visual experience

In kittens reared in complete darkness during the first 6 weeks of life, the cortical representation of orientation selectivity almost completely disappears (Barlow and Pettigrew, 1971; Imbert and Buisseret, 1975; Buisseret and Imbert, 1976; Fregnac and Imbert, 1978; Fregnac et al., 1981). However, the ocular dominance distribution appears to be normal when compared with normally reared kittens of the same age, i.e. most cells are activated through both eyes (Imbert and Buisseret, 1975).

If 6 hours of visual experience is given following 6 weeks of dark-rearing, the proportion of oriented neurons among visual cortical neurons suddenly reaches a level comparable to that observed in a normally reared kitten of the same age (Imbert and Buisseret, 1975; Buisseret et al., 1978). It has been proposed that such a brief, delayed visual experience leads to the expression at the cortical level of an almost normal process of maturation which had been masked up to this point by the absence of visual experience (Fregnac, 1979b). However, vision is not the only factor involved: if oculomotor activity is prevented during visual experience by using a muscular relaxant, no recovery of orientation selectivity occurs (Buisseret et al., 1978). In contrast, provided that ocular motility is preserved during vision, a striking restoration can be observed. Buisseret and collaborators (1978) conclude that afferents from extraocular muscles, which project to the visual cortex (Buisseret and Maffei, 1977), could play a role in the reappearance of normal orientational properties.

More direct evidence is given by Buisseret and Gary-Bobo (1979) and Trotter et al. (1981a). In the cat, in which a large part of the proprioceptive extraocular afferents and sensory fibers from the eye and the face run through the ophthalmic branch of the trigeminal nerve, these authors have used section of this nerve to suppress such sensory afferents, without affecting the oculomotor innervation. In previously dark reared kittens subjected bilaterally to this lesion, no orientation selectivity is recovered after 6 hours of exposure to light. However, after bilateral

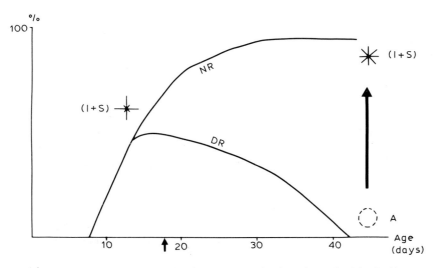

Fig. 1. Effects of visual experience on the development of orientation selectivity in kitten area 17 (adapted from Fregnac, 1979a). The proportion of oriented neurons among visual cells, either broadly tuned (I) or with almost adult specificity (S), is plotted with postnatal age in each rearing condition. The beginning of the period of susceptibility to binocular deprivation begins at around 18 days (black arrow). Six hours of visual experience delayed to after 6 weeks of dark rearing produce a dramatic increase in specificity (I + S) as indicated by a large arrow. All orientation preferences are represented, in contrast to the over-representation of horizontal and vertical orientations found in kittens less than 3 weeks of age. NR, normal rearing; DR, dark rearing.

section of the maxillary branch of the V nerve – which does not contain proprioceptive fibers from eye muscles – a restoration comparable to that in the intact kitten is found. These results indirectly support the hypothesis that it is the proprioceptive message conveyed through the ophthalmic branch of the V nerve which is a necessary cofactor of vision in the re-establishment of orientation selectivity.

Short-term and long-term effects of unilateral section of the ophthalmic branch of the V nerve (V₁)

In order to describe more precisely the role of afferents running through the V_1 nerve during the epigenetic phase of the development of cortical specificity, Trotter, Fregnac and Buisseret have performed unilateral section of V_1 in normally and dark reared kittens of different ages and studied the possible effects at the cortical level a few days to several weeks after the initial surgery. These experiments show an abnormal proportion of monocularly driven neurons when: (1) a sufficient delay exists between surgery and electrophysiology (more than one week) and (2) when section of the maxillary branch of the V nerve – does not contain proprioceptive fibers from eye muscles – a restoration comparable to that in the intact kitten is found. These results indirectly support the hypothesis that it is the proprioceptive message conveyed through the ophthalmic branch of the V nerve which is a necessary cofactor of vision in the re-establishment of orientation selectivity.
period of susceptibility to monocular deprivation of visual information (Hubel and Wiesel, 1970).

In a second series of experiments, Trotter and collaborators made a unilateral section of the V_1 branch a few days before a monocular visual experience of 6 h, in

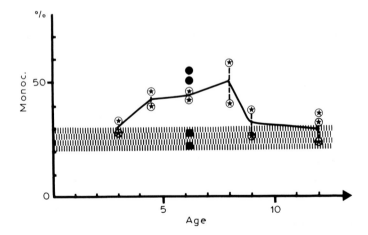

Fig. 2. Period of susceptibility to the unilateral section of the ophthalmic branch of the trigeminal nerve (from Trotter et al., 1981b, with permission). The proportion of monocular cells among visual cells is represented by a continuous line as a function of the age at which the section of the ophthalmic branch was done (expressed in weeks). Each experimental kitten is indicated by a filled symbol (⊛, normally reared; ●, ■, dark-reared). The electrophysiological recordings were done 7 weeks later (●, ⊛) except in two kittens (■) for which the post-operative delay was respectively of 4 and 8 days. The shaded stripe gives the control level of monocularity observed in intact kittens.

6-week-old dark-reared kittens. The short-term effects at the cortical level were studied 12 h after the end of the visual exposure. The results suggest a gating of cortical functional modifications by extraocular proprioception during visuomotor experience: the bilateral suppression of V_1 afferents practically abolishes the effects of 6 h of monocular vision after 6 weeks of dark rearing. In contrast, the unilateral section, whatever its laterality, slightly reduces the breakdown in binocularity and the restoration of orientation selectivity that one observes in control intact monocularly exposed kittens. The cortical capture by the experienced eye is, however, more effective if its proprioceptive afferents are intact. It is concluded that the kinetics of orientation selectivity restoration and of ocular dominance shift are related to the amount of extraocular inflow available during visuomotor experience (Trotter et al., 1981a, c; Trotter, 1981). These observations may give a physiological substrate to the "gate" factor introduced by Fregnac (1979b) in a three-stage description of the maturation of cortical neurons, undergoing successive transformations from unspecified to specified states.

FUNCTIONAL CHANGES INDUCED BY VISION AND PASSIVE EYE-MOVEMENTS, DEMONSTRATED IN SINGLE CORTICAL NEURONS

The electrophysiological approach described in the previous part of this paper relies on comparison of trigger features of visual responses of neurons recorded in the visual cortex of kittens submitted at different ages to various types of visual experience with different nerve sections. This population analysis technique leads to the assessment of a global state of cortical specificity and may be used to describe "critical" periods during which the representation of one functional property depends on visuomotor experience. At this stage, the kinetics of functional development with and without visual experience may be described, and from this one can infer a scheme of development of neuronal selectivity, depending on retinal and extraretinal factors (Fregnac, 1979a, b). However, such analysis gives a limited understanding of how neurons become individually committed to recognize specific attributes of the visual space. All that is known is: (1) from the original state where there are few oriented cells, the *representation* of orientation selectivity becomes generalized in a non-topographic way to the entire visual cortex during ontogeny; and (2) this representation may be altered by visuomotor surgery during a precise phase of postnatal development. Modifications of the statistical distribution of certain properties assessed on limited samples of neurons has been widely assumed to be representative of true modifications of the integrative power of individual neurons. However it has already been mentioned that neither the cortical neuropile nor the population of neurons which may be visually activated can be considered constant or homogeneous during development. It has been shown that certain afferent projections mature more rapidly than others and might show more functional resistance to sensory deprivation (Daniels et al., 1978). Consequently one may observe a reduction in the proportion of Y-type responses by recording in the layers of the thalamic relay innervated by a deprived eye (monocular deprivation: Sherman et al., 1972; binocular deprivation: Kratz et al., 1979). Environmental manipulations could then affect the probability of recording cortical neurons triggered by certain types of afferences, without modifying their own integrative capabilities. This sampling bias reduces the significance of cortical population analysis. In consequence it appears essential to switch from the description of modification of the global properties of the neuronal network to a detailed local analysis of the "evolutive power" (Changeux and Danchin, 1976) of individual neurons.

The first technical question to be answered is to find an experimental situation during which rapid changes of the neuronal function may be observed. We have already described the non-linearity of the susceptibility of cortical neurons to environmental manipulations. It appears that the efficiency of a short delayed visual experience in producing cortical changes is highest when the cortical neuropile reaches its maximum (4–6 weeks of age in the kitten). A necessary condition at this age seems to be the *convergence* of retinal and extraretinal information. We have presented evidence for a gating role exercised by extraocular proprioception. Other workers have shown the possible implication of ascending noradrenergic projections (Kasamatsu and Pettigrew, 1976) or of reticular thalamic nuclei (Singer, 1981) in the mechanisms of cortical plasticity. From these data, it could be hoped that conditioning procedures associating retinal and extraretinal input may result in the modification, in a few hours, of the functional properties of the same neuron recorded in the paralyzed and anesthetized kitten.

Stability of cortical specificity during visual conditioning in the paralyzed kitten

Surprisingly, very few studies concern functional changes of individual neurons in the developing animal. A first attempt was made by Pettigrew and co-workers (Pettigrew et al., 1973), who claimed to have recorded specific shifts in ocular dominance. The iterative presentation of a luminous bar shown to the eye, which initially gave the lesser response, evoked an irregular rise in the level of response, which finally became greater than the response evoked from the other eye. The test stimulus being also the conditioning one, no study of variability was given, which would permit the distinction between spontaneous and stimulus-induced effects. One should note that such modifications in the ocular dominance level are comparable to those observed spontaneously in the adult cat (Hammond, 1981).

Similar experiments, concerning orientation selectivity changes have been carried out in kittens but not reported because of negative results (Maffei, Singer, Stryker, unpublished results). An earlier attempt was undertaken by Imbert and Buisseret using P.S.T.H. techniques. For 6 cells recorded in 6-week-old normally reared kittens, these authors reported an increase in the level of firing following periodic and intermittent binocular presentation of a grating with an orientation orthogonal to the initially preferred one. These unitary modifications observed only in experienced kittens could suggest a modification of orientation selectivity, since the recorded cell seemed to develop a competence for an orientation to which it was not (or poorly) responding at first (Imbert and Buisseret, 1975).

Bienenstock and Fregnac have reproduced these results on a larger sample of neurons but used two types of techniques to characterize the response to the conditioning stimulus (P.S.T.H. synchronized with the onset of a grating or a blank field) and the response to a test stimulus (tuning curve obtained by means of random exploration of the receptive field by a luminous slit). They concluded that the response evoked by the presentation of the conditioning stimulus was not linked either to the orientation or to the contrast content of the figure but that the temporal frequency itself (1/sec) was synchronizing the cortical response with various latencies. In contrast, the orientation tuning assessed with the test stimulus remained stable throughout recording (up to 19 h) (Bienenstock et al., 1979; Fregnac and Bienenstock, 1981).

All these data confirm the stability of the specific visual properties of cortical neurons, even when recorded at the peak of the critical period. It does not seem possible to change the orientation preference of already specified neurons by manipulating solely the visual input. This could explain the success of the paralyzed preparation in developmental studies, when assessing the global state of cortical specificity: in this preparation which abolishes eye-movements, "freezing" of the cortical function is observed and subsequent visual stimulation does not profoundly affect the properties of recorded neurons.

Stimulus-induced modifications following binocular vision associated with passive eye movements

Specific functional modifications have been observed in the paralyzed and anesthetized kitten when binocular vision (typically a vertical grating drifting along the horizontal axis) was associated with unilateral passive eye movement (0.4 Hz, 10–20° of amplitude along the horizontal axis) (Fregnac and Bienenstock, 1981).

Such a conditioning exposure was performed on 12 neurons recorded in 6-week-old, normally reared or deprived kittens. It resulted in: (1) the reversal of ocular dominance or disruption of binocularity (two cells); (2) transitory modifications of orientation preference (six cells) (see Fig. 3).

Although the analysis of the "evolutive power" of a given neuron reflects a particular behavior, a common effect observed at the end of the exposure is the onset of a multicompetence: a gain in the visual response is observed for orientations close to the experienced one, while a loss is found for the initially preferred one. This transitory perturbation is followed either by a relaxation towards the initial state of selectivity in normally reared kittens or by a new unstable competence in deprived animals.

These effects demonstrated in single units were observed in the paralyzed kitten, only when one eye was mechanically moved while the stimulus was presented binocularly. Even variable disparity experiments, in which a discorrelation between retinal images was produced by optical means (instead of by mechanical displacement of the eye) failed to induce any ocular dominance shift or modification in orientation preferences (Fregnac and Bienenstock, 1981).

CONCLUSION

Experimental evidence has been reviewed, which shows the importance of afferent information running through the ophthalmic branch of the trigeminal nerve, during the development of orientation selectivity and binocular integration in kitten visual cortex. It suggests that extraocular inflow during visuomotor experience "gates" the functional modifications induced by specific visual input at the cortical level. In addition, it shows that extraocular proprioception could be needed

434

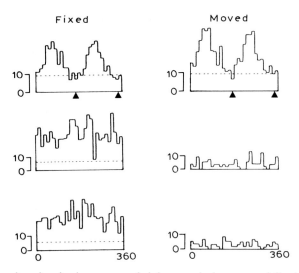

Fig. 3. Modification of ocular dominance recorded from a single neuron, following binocular vision associated with unilateral passive eye movement (from Fregnac and Bienenstock, 1981, with permission). Histograms show orientation tuning curves (number of spikes per sweep as a function of direction of the test stimulus on a 360° scale) at various times. These curves are averaged over 3–5 runs according to the multihistogram technique. Response to stimulation through the eye which is passively moved during the conditioning exposure is given in the right column. Response through the fixed eye is given in the left column. Dotted lines indicate levels of spontaneous activity averaged over 30 acquisition periods. The orientation tuning curves, shown in the upper row, are averaged over a 2 h preliminary observation period and obtained from a cell recorded in a 6-week-old kitten. The conditioning exposure is then given for a 50 min period: passive horizontal movement of one eye is associated with the binocular presentation of a moving grating of vertical bars to which the cell was not initially responding. The corresponding orientation is indicated by filled triangles. The orientation tuning profiles, shown in the middle and lower row, represent respectively the averaged visual responses through each eye during the first and second hour of recording following the end of the conditioning. The cell has lost its initial orientation preference and responds only through the previously fixed eye.

throughout the critical period for the maintenance of binocular integration.

Recordings from individual neurons in the paralyzed animal indicate the temporal stability of the preferred orientation encoded by cortical neurons, even during visual conditioning. However, a direct demonstration of modifications of ocular dominance and orientation selectivity was obtained from a few neurons, when associating vision and passive eye movement.

In the situation where one eye is mechanically moved while the visual stimulus is binocularly presented, the observed behavior of individual neurons is well correlated with evidence inferred from population analysis. Uncorrelated retinal inputs and eye-movements result primarily in a breakdown of binocular interaction for the benefit of either eye. U-shaped ocular dominance histograms seem to be the common initial effect following assymetrical manipulation of visual inputs either in the behaving kitten (Schechter and Murphy, 1976) or in the paralyzed kitten subjected to passive eye movement (Freeman and Bonds, 1979).

Concerning orientation preference, the perturbations described at the single unit level are mainly transitory, although a significant evolution of the neuron's competence towards the experienced orientation is consistently found. These subtle changes in the neuronal evolutive power were not seen by population analysis, i.e.

no significant bias was found in the distribution of orientation preference following the end of the conditioning exposure. This suggests that in such experimental situations, the disruption of the ocular dominance property, depending mainly on direct geniculo-cortical inputs, is more easily observed and that the reorganization of orientation preference in the cortical network, a property depending at least on intracortical connections, needs either more time or some active visuomotor processes, to be permanent.

ACKNOWLEDGEMENTS

The experiments presented in this paper were done in the Laboratory of Neurophysiology, College de France (Paris) with the help of grants from the C.N.R.S. and D.G.R.S.T. We thank Dr. K. Grant for help with the English.

REFERENCES

Barlow, H.B. and Pettigrew, J.D. (1971) Lack of specificity of neurons in the visual cortex of young kittens. *J. Physiol. (Lond.)*, 218: 98P–100P.

Berardi, N., Bisti, S., Fiorentini, A. and Maffei, L. (1981) Section of the ophthalmic branch of the fifth nerve in the cat. *Docum. ophthalmol.*, 30: 109–116.

Bienenstock, E., Fregnac, Y. and Imbert, M. (1979) Stability of orientation selectivity in the visual cortex of curarized kittens. *Neurosci. Lett.*, Suppl. 3: S291.

Blakemore, C. and Van Sluyters, R.C. (1975) Innate and environmental factors in the development of the kitten's visual cortex. *J. Physiol. (Lond.)*, 248: 663–716.

Blakemore, C. and Vital-Durand, F. (1981) Development of spatial resolution and contrast sensitivity in monkey visual cortex. *Neurosci. Abstr.*, 7: 47.1, p. 140.

Blakemore, C., Van Sluyters, R.C. and Movshon, A. (1975) Synaptic competition in kitten's visual cortex. *Cold Spr. Harb. Symp. quant. Biol.*, 40: 601–610.

Buisseret, P. and Gary-Bobo, E. (1979) Development of visual cortical orientation specificity after dark-rearing: role of extraocular proprioception. *Neurosci. Lett.*, 13: 259–263.

Buisseret, P. and Imbert, M. (1976) Visual cortical cells: their developmental properties in normal and dark reared kittens. *J. Physiol. (Lond.)*, 255: 511–525.

Buisseret, P. and Maffei, L. (1977) Extraocular proprioceptive projections to the visual cortex. *Exp. Brain Res.*, 28: 421–425.

Buisseret, P., Gary-Bobo, E. and Imbert, M. (1978) Evidence that ocular motility is involved in the recovery of the orientational properties of visual cortical neurons in dark reared kittens. *Nature (Lond.)*, 272: 816–817.

Buisseret, P., Gary-Bobo, E. and Imbert, M. (1982) Plasticity in the kitten's visual cortex: effects of the suppression of visual experience upon the orientational properties of visual cortical cells. *Develop. Brain Res.*, 4: 417–426.

Changeux, J.P. and Danchin, A. (1976) Selective stabilization of developing synapses as a mechanism for the specification of neuronal networks. *Nature (Lond.)*, 264: 705–712.

Cragg, B.G. (1972) The development of synapses in cat visual cortex. *Invest. Ophthalmol.*, 11: 377–385.

Daniels, D.J., Pettigrew, J.D. and Norman, J.L. (1978) Development of single-neuron responses in kitten's lateral geniculate nucleus. *J. Neurophysiol.*, 41: 1373–1393.

Freeman, R.D. and Bonds, A.B. (1979) Cortical plasticity in monocularly deprived immobilized kittens depends on eye movement. *Science*, 206: 1093–1095.

Fregnac, Y. (1979a) Development of orientation selectivity in the primary visual cortex of normally and dark reared kittens. I. Kinetics. *Biol. Cybernet.*, 34: 187–193.

Fregnac, Y. (1979b) Development of orientation selectivity in the primary visual cortex of normally and dark reared kittens. II. Models. *Biol. Cybernet.*, 34: 195–203.

Fregnac, Y. and Bienenstock, E. (1981) Specific functional modifications of individual cortical neurons, triggered by vision and passive eye movement, in immobilized kittens. *Docum. ophthalmol.*, 30: 100–108.

Fregnac, Y. and Imbert, M. (1978) Early development of visual cortical cells in normal and dark reared kittens: a relationship between orientation selectivity and ocular dominance. *J. Physiol. (Lond.)*, 278: 27–44.

Fregnac, Y., Trotter, Y., Bienenstock, E., Buisseret, P., Gary-Bobo, E. and Imbert, M. (1981) Effect of neonatal unilateral enucleation on the development of orientation selectivity in the primary visual cortex of normally and dark-reared kittens. *Exp. Brain Res.*, 42: 453–466.

Hammond, P. (1981) Non-stationarity of ocular dominance in cat striate cortex. *Exp. Brain Res.*, 42: 189–196.

Hubel, D.H. and Wiesel, T.N. (1963) Receptive fields of cells in striate cortex of very young, visually inexperienced kittens. *J. Neurophysiol.*, 26: 994–1002.

Hubel, D.H. and Wiesel, T.N. (1970) The period of susceptibility to the physiological effects of unilateral eye closure in kittens. *J. Physiol. (Lond.)*, 206: 419–436.

Imbert, M. and Buisseret, P. (1975) Receptive field characteristics and plastic properties of visual cortical cells in kittens reared with or without visual experience. *Exp. Brain Res.*, 22: 25–36.

Kasamatsu, T. and Pettigrew, J.D. (1976) Depletion of brain catecholamines: Failure of ocular dominance shift after monocular occlusion in kittens. *Science*, 194: 206–209.

Kratz, K.E., Sherman, S.M. and Kalil, R. (1979) Lateral geniculate nucleus in dark-reared cats: loss of Y cells without changes in cell size. *Science*, 203: 1353–1355.

LeVay, S. and Stryker, M.P. (1979) The development of ocular dominance in the cats. In J. Ferrendelli (Ed.), *Soc. Neurosc. Symp., 4, Aspects of Developmental Neurobiology*, pp. 83–98.

LeVay, S., Wiesel, T.N. and Hubel, D.H. (1980) The development of ocular dominance columns in normal and visually deprived monkeys. *J. comp. Neurol.*, 191: 1–51.

Leventhal, A.G. and Hirsch, H.V.B. (1980) Receptive-field properties of different classes of neurons in visual cortex of normal and dark-reared cats. *J. Neurophysiol.*, 43: 1111–1132.

Pettigrew, J.D. (1978) The paradox of the critical period for striate cortex. In C.W. Cotman (Ed.), *Neuronal Plasticity*, Raven Press, New York, pp. 311–330.

Pettigrew, J., Olson, C. and Barlow, H.B. (1973) Kitten visual cortex: short-term, stimulus-induced changes in connectivity. *Science*, 180: 1202–1203.

Rakic, P. (1977) Prenatal development of the visual system in rhesus monkey. *Phil. Trans. B*, 278: 245–260.

Schechter, P.B. and Murphy, E.H. (1976) Brief monocular visual experience and kitten cortical binocularity. *Brain Res.*, 109: 165–168.

Sherman, S.M., Hoffmann, K.P. and Stone, J. (1972) Loss of a specific cell type from the dorsal lateral geniculate nucleus in visually deprived cats. *J. Neurophysiol.*, 35: 532–541.

Singer, W. (1981) Diencephalic structures involved in the control of selective attention gate developmental plasticity in kitten striate cortex. *Neurosci. Lett.*, Suppl. 7: S200.

Trotter, Y. (1981) *Role de la Proprioception Extraoculaire dans le Developpement Fonctionnel du Cortex Visual Primaire du Chat*, Doctoral Thesis, Paris VI, 107 pp.

Trotter, Y., Gary-Bobo, E. and Buisseret, P. (1981a) Recovery of orientation selectivity in kitten primary visual cortex is slowed down by bilateral section of ophthalmic trigeminal afferents. *Develop. Brain Res.*, 1: 450–454.

Trotter, Y., Fregnac, Y. and Buisseret, P. (1981b) Periode de sensibilité du cortex visuel primaire du chat à la suppression unilatérale des afférences proprioceptives extraoculaires. *C.R. Acad. Sci. (Paris)*, *Série D*, 293: 245–248.

Trotter, Y., Fregnac, Y. and Buisseret, P. (1981c) Gating control of developmental plasticity by extraocular proprioception in kitten area 17. In *Proc. IVth European Conference on Visual Perception*, Gouvieux.

Vidyasagar, T.R. and Urbas, J.V. (1982) Biases to oriented moving lines in cat LGN and the role of the visual cortical areas 17 and 18. *Exp. Eye Res.*, 46: 157–169.

Wolf, W. and Albus, K. (1981) Postnatal development of receptive field properties in the kitten's visual cortex. *Neurosci. Lett.*, Suppl. 7: S202.

Neurons in Cerebral Cortex Area 4 and Area 5 Increase Their Discharge Frequency During Operant Conditioning

Y. BURNOD, B. MATON and J. CALVET

INSERM U3 CNRS, Hopital Salpêtrière, 47 Bd. Hopital, Paris (France)

INTRODUCTION

Electrical activity of single neurons as waking animals carry out behavioral acts is important to determine time and space constants of the cellular interactions that may be responsible for the organization of behavior. For example, monkeys can learn very precise movement of the arm by a temporal linkage between these movements and a reward. Discharge patterns of the different neuronal systems that are presumably involved in the command and control of this type of movement were studied in naive monkeys and more quantified in overtrained monkeys: in area 4 of the cerebral cortex neurons discharge prior to muscle activity and their discharge frequency is predictive of muscular contraction (Evarts, 1974). Similarly neurons in area 5 discharge prior to arm projection and manipulation (Mountcastle et al., 1975). This led us to focus our attention on two aspects of this system using unit recording in these areas during the first stages of operant conditioning, when repetition of a movement that fit a priori criteria appears: (1) the possible temporal patterns of the frequency of discharge during the behavioral events, i.e. during the conditioned movement itself and the reward-related movement, and (2) a comparison between changes in neuronal discharge frequency and changes in behavior that occur during one conditioning session.

METHODS

Three monkeys were placed in primate chair; the right forearm was attached to a horizontal support which could rotate around a vertical axis corresponding to that of the elbow. The only possible movements of the right arm were flexions around this axis in horizontal plane; therefore this could be described by one parameter, angle of the arm with a starting position A. The flexion had to be performed against a constant load from a fixed position A to an arrival position B; B is any position within a sector determined by the conditioning program, without external signal or cue: a screen prevented the monkey from visually controlling the rotating arm. The EMG of the surface of the biceps and triceps brachii were also recorded. The reward was a piece of fruit given automatically on a tray in front of the free left arm. Movement of the left arm was controlled by photoelectric cells. Two microdrivers

[437]

allowed the parallel but independent penetration of two platinum microelectrodes, one in area 4, the other in area 5. Two well-defined regions of areas 4 and 5 were studied: that of area 4 corresponded to the arm zone and that of area 5 was located in the same laterality. The location of each recorded cell was measured relatively to the four extreme penetrations which were histologically identified and which allowed the reconstruction of the position of each recorded neuron.

CONDITIONING PROGRAM. BEHAVIOR

Movements related to the reward were stereotyped sequences performed by the left arm and did not change during conditioning. Before conditioning the monkey performs few movements of the right arm. Conditioning itself consisted of an increase of the frequency of flexion movements. This increase was observed during several consecutive sessions. During the following sessions the angular zone of arrival was decreased: there was no increase in the frequency of flexion movements but an increase in the frequency of reward due to an increase in the proportion of flexion movements that fit the conditioning criteria. There was at the same time an increase in the temporal regularity of movements.

QUANTIFICATION OF CELLULAR ACTIVITY

The discharge frequency was determined every 20 msec by means of triggers and counters. A mathematical model was proposed to represent patterns of discharge frequency by trapezia (Fig. 1): constant levels separated by linear increases or decreases. The model was computed by the least square method on means triggered by behavioral events (onset of movement, grasping of the reward) and cellular events (levels of discharge frequency, levels of IEMG). Four parameters of the model quantified the cell activity: lower (AB) and higher level (AR + AB), latency of the onset (D1) of the increase and latency of the higher level (D2). These parameters allowed a quantitative comparison of the cell discharge frequency between different events. When events were defined by different thresholds of the same variable, the model allowed us to establish during each period the quantitative relationship between mechanical parameters of the movement (amplitude, velocity, acceleration) and cell discharge frequency.

SETS OF NEURONS

Before examining the time course during one training session, it was necessary to define the sets of cells observed in the explored regions in relation to the behavioral events: flexion movement of the contralateral arm and taking of the reward by the ipsilateral arm. A total of 360 cells discharging in relation to the flexion movement were recorded in each of the two zones: 209 neurons in area 4 and 180 in area 5 (Fig. 1). Fig. 2 shows the distribution of the latencies: many neurons in both areas are active prior to the onset of the movement. The increase of discharge frequency and the latency were more variable for successive movements in area 5 than in area 4.

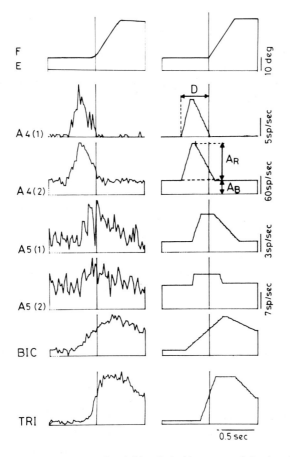

Fig. 1. Quantitative analysis of the neuronal activities. Left: histograms of density of neuronal discharges and of the IEMG synchronized at the onset of successive movements (vertical line). Right: models of activities shown in the same line at left (see text). D measures the latency of the cell activity, A_B the background activity, A_R the increase at the onset of the movement. Upper to lower: F, amplitude of the flexion; A4(1), discharges of one neuron in area 4; A4(2), discharges of a group of neurons in the same place; A5(1), A5(2), same conventions for area 5; BIC, TRI, integrated IEMG of biceps and triceps brachii. Note that this reduction of data preserves most of the information given by histograms.

Another set of neurons contained neurons that were active when the monkey caught the reward with the ipsilateral arm, during one of the three phases: extension of the arm to the tray, grasping of the fruit and flexion to the mouth – 54 neurons in area 4 and 96 in area 5 were in this category.

A third set of neurons was the intersection of the two sets described above. Neurons of this class (46 in area 4, 61 in area 5) were active during the flexion movement with the contralateral arm and during one of the phases of the taking of the reward with the ipsilateral arm (Fig. 3). At the beginning of the training there were two sets of neurons in each area that were active during the conditioned movement and during the taking of the reward. There was a spatial overlap between these two sets and some neurons were thus active two times when a movement was rewarded.

440

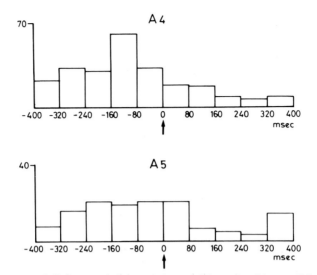

Fig. 2. Latency histogram of all the recorded neurons in area 4 (upper) and in area 5 (lower) active at the onset of the movement (arrow). Latency is the parameter D of the model.

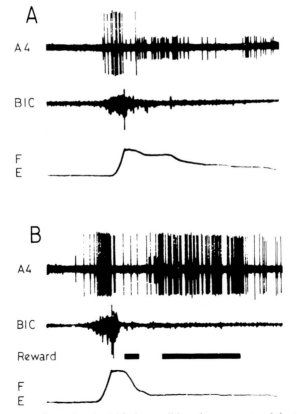

Fig. 3. Activity of a neuron of area 4 active with the conditioned movement and the taking of the reward. A: movement without a reward. B: movement with a reward. Traces show discharges of the neuron of area 4, IEMG of the biceps and amplitude of the flexion. The two signals of reward indicate the rotation of the fruit tray and the catching of the fruit.

NEURONAL ACTIVITY DURING TRAINING SESSION

Throughout each of the training sessions, two neurons, one in area 4 and the other in area 5, were recorded simultaneously and analyzed in relation to the flexion movement. Three monkeys provided a total of ninety such pairs which were studied over periods from 30 min to 2 h.

For neurons in area 4 and area 5 whose maximal discharge frequency occurred in relationship with the flexion movement, changes in cell discharge frequency and changes in behavior (frequency and shape of the flexion movement) were parallel: there was a good correlation between cell discharge frequency and performance: when a movement was rewarded the probability to see a repetition of this movement increased; the probability of firing of these neurons increased in the same way. However, because of some cell variability, the relationship became precise only when the mean value of cell discharge frequency was computed with at least 5 successive movements.

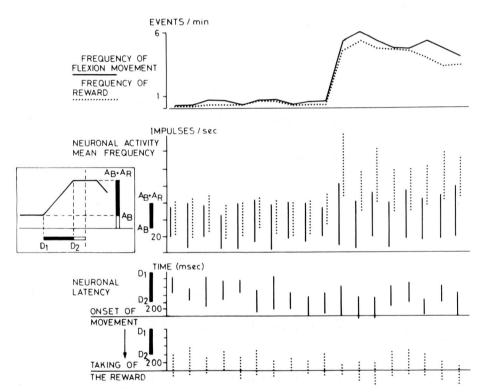

Fig. 4. Changes in the activity of a neuron in area 4 during a session when the frequency of movement increases. Each of the three diagrams represents the results of successive periods of analysis during half an hour of a conditioning session. Upper diagram: frequency of movement and frequency of reward. Middle: each vertical double bar represents the increase of discharge frequency at the onset of the flexion movement (continuous bar) and at the grasping of the fruit (dotted bar); each double bar is the result of one period of analysis of 1 min. Lower and upper limit of each bar represents the two parameters A_R and $A_R + A_B$ computed by the model as shown at left. Lower diagram: latency of the cell activity with respect to the onset of the flexion movement (continuous bar) and to the grasping of the fruit (dotted bar). Each bar represents the two parameters D_1 and D_2 of the model as shown at left. Note the enhancement of discharge frequency that occurs when the frequency of movement increases.

442

(a) Neurons active with movement and reward enhanced their firing rate with reward; this process occurred during the sessions where the frequency of adequate movements increased. Fig. 4 shows such an enhancement: at the beginning of the session, as the movement was still erratic, the cell firing frequency was the same during movement and reward. When the movement became more frequent, there was a strong enhancement of the cell activity with reward.

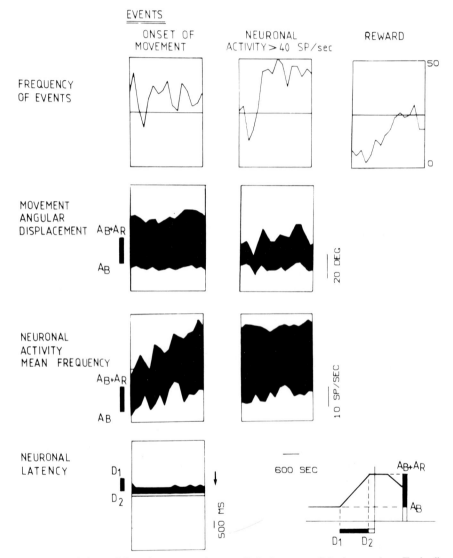

Fig. 5. Changes of the activity of a neuron in area 5 during a conditioning session. Each diagram represents the changes of one parameter during the whole session, with synchronization either by the onsets of flexion (left column) or by the maximal activities of the neuron (middle column). Diagrams use the same convention as in Fig. 4. The bars are jointive and appear in a continuous black surface. Upper to lower row: frequency of events, amplitude of the angular displacement, neuronal activity and neuronal latency. Note the regular increase of discharge frequency at the onset of the flexion (left column, third row) with no correlative change of the mean shape of the flexion (left column, second row) and no change of the maximal frequency of discharge (middle column, third row).

(b) Neurons active with reward discharged until the onset of the next movement; their times of activity overlapped with activity of flexion related neurons. This process appeared during sessions where the temporal regularity of movement became clear.

(c) Neurons active during flexion increased their firing frequency at the onset of the movement during the session where accuracy of flexion became better (Fig. 5). Surprisingly this enhancement did not correspond to parallel changes in amplitude, velocity or IEMG.

DISCUSSION

Since the beginning of training most of the cells recorded in this study could be classified following criteria used by other authors for overtrained animals (see, for example, Evarts, 1974, for area 4; Mountcastle et al., 1975 and Bioulac and Lamarre, 1979, for area 5). Time constants of the cell activities corresponded to the successive derivatives of the behavioral parameters and range from 100 msec to several seconds. Cell activities overlapping in areas 4 and 5 were presumably due to direct connections (Jones et al., 1978). However the activities of the cells recorded in this study present a larger variability than cells studied in overtrained animals even for successive movements that presented similar kinematic characteristics. The histograms of latency were more widely distributed and shifted toward early latencies, mainly for area 5. That may be explained in part by the differences in the paradigm (self initiated movement as opposed to movement triggered by a stimulus).

The enhancement of discharge frequency by reward was not observed on every neuron contingently active before a reward but it was seen for cells which were linked both with the conditioned movement and the reward related movements: this is consistent with the fact that it is easier to obtain operant conditioning by successive differentiation of a natural movement (e.g. taking of the reward): the probability of occurrence of the natural movement is transferred to the conditioned movement; the differentiation from the taking of the reward to the flexion movement of the right elbow can occur via cells which are active in the two situations. This double activity can induce potentiation phenomena with time constants in the range of 1 sec.

During classical conditioning, a number of studies have shown that cells connected to the UR showed an increase of discharge frequency when the CS is given after pairing with the US (e.g. Olds et al., 1972). In area 4 almost all cells connected to a movement of flexion-extension have their discharges modified by the occurrence of the stimulus indicating the direction of the movement to be performed (Evarts, 1974). In this study, the increase of cell activity at the onset of the flexion movement may be interpreted as an anticipation of the maximal activity. This anticipated activity can play a role in the control of the movement; but it is not known if these cells are tuned for afferent inputs that could signal the adequate movement.

SUMMARY

Changes of neuronal activity in areas 4 and 5 of *Macaca speciosa* during learning of a flexion movement were investigated by means of extracellular recordings. A mathematical model was used to quantify neuronal patterns whose changes were compared with the changes in behavior. Before conditioning three categories of neurons were identified: (i) more active with the flexion movement; (ii) more active with the taking of the reward; and (iii) active in the both situations. During the first stage of conditioning, i.e. when the first series of movement appeared, neurons of the first set showed changes parallel with performance; neurons of the third set enhance their discharge frequency with reward. During the sessions where there is an increase of the accuracy of the movement, the cells of the first and third set increased their frequency of discharge at the onset of the flexion movement.

REFERENCES

Bioulac, Y. and Lamarre, Y. (1979) Activity of postcentral cortical neurons of the monkey during conditioned movements of a de-afferented limb. *Brain Res.*, 172: 427.

Evarts, E.V. (1974) Gating of motor cortex reflexes by prior instruction. *Brain Res.*, 74: 479.

Jones, E.G., Coulter, J.D. and Hendry, S.H.C. (1978) Intracortical connectivity of architectonic fields in the somatic sensory, motor and parietal cortex of monkeys. *J. comp. Neurol.*, 181: 291.

Mountcastle, V.B., Lynch, J.C., Georgopoulos, A., Sakata, H. and Acuna, C. (1975) Posterior parietal association cortex of the monkey: command functions for operations within extrapersonal space. *J. Neurophysiol.*, 38: 871.

Olds, J., Disterhoft, J.F., Segal, M., Kornblith, C.L. and Hirsch, R. (1972) Learning centers of rat brain mapped by measuring latencies of conditioned unit responses. *J. Neurophysiol.*, 35: 202.

Excitability Changes in Hippocampal Granule Cells of Senescent Rat

C.A. BARNES and B.L. McNAUGHTON

Institute of Neurophysiology, University of Oslo (Norway) and Department of Anatomy, University College London (U.K.)

INTRODUCTION

Research on senescent nervous systems has tended to emphasize processes of deterioration which, indeed, may be among the most obvious and important kinds of alterations to occur over the lifespan. A number of recent findings, however, suggest that preservation of function, in spite of deteriorative change, occurs at many levels of the nervous system (Adelman et al., 1980; Simpkins et al., 1977; Smith, 1979). One example of a seemingly compensatory change in senescent rat brain function is an increased electrical excitability of hippocampal granule cells in the face of a considerable reduction in the afferent fiber population. One possible mechanism of this change is examined in the present report.

Geinisman and Bondareff (1976) initially reported that the senescent rat fascia dentata showed a significant reduction (27%) in the number of synaptic contacts made onto the middle portion of the granule cell dendritic tree when counts were taken from electron micrographs. Interestingly, although the input to the granule cells changed, there was no change detected in either the number of granule cells or in the depth of the molecular layer which consists primarily of granule cell dendritic arborizations (Bondareff and Geinisman, 1976; Geinisman et al., 1977). From these studies, however, it was not clear whether the reduction of synaptic contacts in the perforant path termination zone was due to a reduction in the number of input fibers, or to a reduction in the number of en passant synapses made by each fiber. It was also not known what the physiological impact of such a massive deafferentation might be. It certainly could result in a substantial change in the integrative properties of these neurons.

Partial answers to these questions were provided by Barnes and McNaughton (1980) in a study of the physiological properties of the granule cells of mature and senescent rats using extracellular recording in chronically prepared animals and both intra- and extracellular recording in the in vitro hippocampal slice preparation. The older animals in this study exhibited a 33% reduction in the amplitude of the extracellular presynaptic fiber potential for a given stimulus intensity. The amplitude of the fiber potential is thought to be an approximately linear measure of the number of fibers activated by the stimulating current (Andersen et al., 1978). Since there was no change in the activation threshold of the afferent fibers between age groups, these physiological data support the anatomical findings and suggest that there is an actual reduction in the number of the perforant path fibers themselves in the old animals. In addition it was found that, for a given presynaptic fiber response, the old animals exhibited larger excitatory postsynaptic potentials (e.p.s.p.s, both intra- and extracellularly), indicating that the remaining synapses were actually about 13% more powerful in this age group.

The intracellular recordings from granule cells revealed a 17% reduction in the voltage threshold for synaptically elicited discharge and a 0.5 msec reduction in the latency of the action potential in the old compared to the young rats. Interestingly, there was no statistically significant change in the discharge threshold when depolarizing current was applied directly to the soma via the recording electrode. Resting potentials, action potential amplitudes, whole neuron time constants, and input impedance were not different between age groups. These data directly confirm earlier extracellular work where senescent granule cells were shown to exhibit a larger population spike for a given magnitude of extracellular e.p.s.p. (Barnes, 1979), which suggested a possible excitability change. In terms of maintenance of input–output characteristics, these data suggest that granule cells could partly compensate for the loss of synapses that occurs during senescence by an increased efficacy of the remaining synapses and by an increase in electrical excitability following synaptic activation.

The possible cause of the increase in electrical excitability was the subject of the experiments to be described here. The particular constellation of results for the intracellular studies discussed above (a reduction in the e.p.s.p. necessary for discharge and a decrease in the latency of the orthodromically elicited action potential) leads to the hypothesis that action potential initiation may occur closer to the site of synaptic input in the dendrites of senescent granule cells. This would explain both the excitability and the latency changes. To examine the electrical excitability of granule cell dendrites in mature and senescent rats, the extent of antidromic invasion of the action potential into the dendritic tree was determined using current source density analysis (Jefferys, 1979; Nicholson, 1973, 1979).

METHODS

Barrier-reared male rats bred by TNO Zeist, The Netherlands, were used in this study: 13 aged 8 months (young) and 13 aged 29 months (old).

Transverse hippocampal slices were prepared as described in detail previously by Barnes and McNaughton (1980a). The brains of one young and one old animal were sliced consecutively on each experimental day (the order counterbalanced for age group) so that the conditions in the chamber were effectively matched between age groups. The slices were cut at a thickness of approximately 525 μm on a Sorvall tissue chopper, and were bathed at 35°C (+1°C) in oxygenated (95% O_2/5% CO_2) Ringer (in mM): NaCl 124; $CaCl_2$ 2; KCl 2; KH_2PO_4 1.25; $MgSO_4$ 2; $NaHCO_3$ 26; glucose 10.

The recording electrode was a Ringer-filled glass pipette with a tip diameter of 10–15 μm. Stimulating electrodes consisted of 114 μm (o.d.) teflon-coated stainless-steel wire. The extracellular signals were amplified (−3 dB filters at 1 Hz and 4 kHz) and sampled on-line by a digital computer at a rate of 10 kHz. Stimulation parameters were kept constant at 140 μA × 150 μS, except when input–output curves were obtained where the current was varied in 10 steps from 140 μA down to 8 μA.

An incubation period of 1.5 h was allowed prior to recording. After this time, a slice was considered acceptable for study if the amplitude of the maximal antidromic population spike recorded in the cell body layer exceeded 10 mV. The recording electrode was first placed in the lower margin of the granule cell body layer (see Fig. 1) and the stimulating electrodes for synaptic (orthodromic) and antidromic activation were positioned in the molecular layer and mossy fiber bundle respectively. The recording electrode was then moved down 40 μm from the bottom of the cell body layer into the hilus and positioned so that the tip of the electrode just touched the surface of the slice, and an average of 10 antidromic responses was collected and stored. Although the surface response was not as large as those recorded deeper within the slice, this method considerably increased the consistency of the results by eliminating the error introduced by attempting to record at a constant depth in a series of penetrations along the dendritic axis. The antidromic population spike potential was recorded in 10 μm steps using this procedure from 40 μm below the cell body layer to the tips of the dendrites at the hippocampal fissure. Input–output curves were recorded both from the cell body layer (to measure the e.p.s.p. and population spike) and from the molecular layer (to measure the presynaptic fiber potential).

Current source densities (CSDs) were computed from the raw antidromic spike potential data by differentiating twice with respect to distance along the dendritic axis. A smoothing algorithm (Nicholson, 1979) was employed which reduced, somewhat, the variance introduced by double differentiation, at the expense of some loss of spatial resolution. Nicholson (1973) and others have shown that such a one dimensional CSD analysis is valid provided that the rate of change of potential with distance is negligible in the other principal axes of the tissue. This occurs when a homogeneous population of neurons is uniformly activated. Jefferys (1979) has shown that these conditions are reasonably well fulfilled in the hippocampal slice preparation.

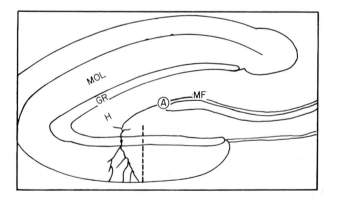

Fig. 1. Schematic diagram of the fascia dentata in the hippocampal slice preparation, illustrating the method used for measuring antidromic invasion of the granule cell dendrites. The stimulating electrode was located within the mossy fiber bundle (at A). The antidromic population spike was measured at 10 μm intervals along the dendritic axis of the granule cells (dashed line). Abbreviations: MOL, molecular layer; GR, granule cell body layer; H, hilus; MF, mossy fiber bundle. In the subsequent figures the zero reference point is taken as the junction between the granule cell body layer and the hilus, which is clearly discernible in the hippocampal slice preparation.

448

RESULTS

The input–output curves for the fascia dentata resembled those found previously when comparing young and old rats (Barnes, 1979; Barnes and McNaughton, 1980a, b). That is, the fiber response was smaller ($P < 0.05$) in the old rats than in the young rats for a given stimulus intensity, with no difference in threshold for fiber activation. The old rats also showed an approximately 35% greater population spike for a given size of field e.p.s.p., a finding that also corroborates earlier work.

The potential waveforms used in the analysis ranged from $40\,\mu m$ below the granule layer–hilus border to $300\,\mu m$ above. This range adequately covered the extent of orthodromic invasion as can be seen from Figs. 2 and 3. Because of the

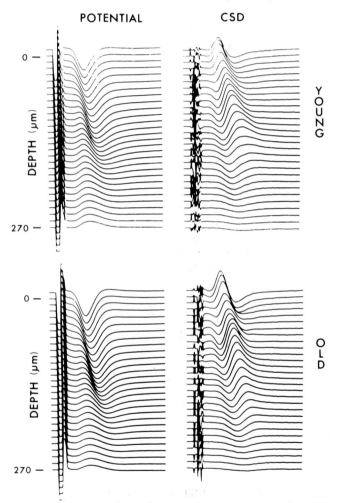

Fig. 2. The average antidromic population spike potentials and corresponding CSDs are shown as functions of depth in the fascia dentata for the two age groups. The zero reference point represents the junction of the granule cell body layer and the hilus. Positive potential and inward current are plotted upwards. The units of current are arbitrary. The average amplitude of the antidromic potentials at the zero reference point were $15.9\,mV + 1.4$ S.E.M. (young) and $16.3\,mV + 4.5$ S.E.M. (old). The prestimulus baseline represents 0.5 msec. The total depth of the molecular plus granule layer was $400\,\mu m$.

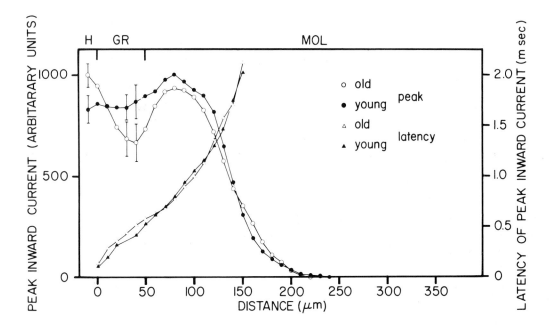

Fig. 3. Plots of peak inward current amplitude (circles) and latency (triangles) versus position along the dendritic axis of the granule cells following antidromic activation. The bottom of the granule cell body layer is taken as the zero reference point. The anatomical boundaries are indicated at the top of the figure: H, hilus; GR, granule cell body layer; MOL, molecular layer. For clarity, standard error bars are shown only for those mean data points for which there was a statistically significant difference between age groups.

smoothing algorithm the 3 waveforms at both ends could not be used, so that the analysis actually extends from 10 μm below the cell body layer to 270 μm into the dendrites above the bottom of the cell body layer. The antidromic field potentials, averaged across animals, and the corresponding CSD profiles are shown in Fig. 2.

In agreement with Jeffery's study, the inward current peak became progressively later and reduced in amplitude with distance from the cell bodies of the granule cells. This can be seen more clearly in Fig. 3, which shows the mean amplitude of the inward current and the latency of the peak as functions of distance from the origin at the bottom of the cell body layer. There was no significant differences between age groups in either the latency profile of the inward current peak (antidromic conduction velocity) or in the distance that this peak propagated into the dendritic tree before declining to zero.

An unexpected complexity in the peak inward current profiles was observed in the granule layer and proximal dendritic tree. Rather than falling monotonically with distance, the inward current showed a maximum at about 100 μm into the dendritic zone. This was characteristic of each of the individual CSDs, and was not due to several odd cases. At present we can offer no explanation for this observation, nor for the apparent between-group differences in current amplitude within the granular layer itself.

DISCUSSION

The present results confirm earlier extracellular work and are in agreement with intracellular studies showing an increased excitability of hippocampal granule cells in senescent rats. Since it previously has been shown that the excitability change is not due to tonic resting membrane potential differences or differences in the passive electrical characteristics of senescent granule cells (Barnes and McNaughton, 1980a), we proposed that active currents should be detected further out into the dendrites of senescent granule cells. This could occur, for instance, by an increased distribution of sodium channels in the proximal dendrites. There was not, however, a detectable difference (within our approximately 50 μm resolution capacity) in the distance travelled by the peak inward current or in the conduction velocity between age groups.

It is clear from these results that these classically mediated active currents can play no major role in dendritic integration beyond the most proximal portion of the dendritic tree. These results also tend to rule out an age-associated change in ordinary sodium-channel mediated mechanisms for electrical excitability in the granule cell dendrites. The possibility remains, however, that some other type of voltage-dependent conductance may be present in granule cell dendrites which is activated only by more slowly changing potentials such as during synaptic input. A change in such a slowly activated conductance system appears at present to be the most likely explanation for the fact that excitability increases appear only following synaptic activation, and not following either antidromic activation or direct activation via intracellular current pulses. This possibility is under investigation.

ACKNOWLEDGEMENTS

We would like to thank Prof. P. Andersen for the use of his laboratory facilities and Dr. H. Rigter and Organon International B. V., Oss, The Netherlands, for the gift of the animals. This work was supported by postdoctoral fellowships from the National Institute on Aging (U.S.A.) to C.A.B. and from the NSERC (Canada) to B.L.M.

REFERENCES

Adelman, R.C., Roberts, J., Baker, G.T., Baskin, S.I. and Cristofalo, V.J. (Eds.) (1980) *Neural Regulatory Mechanisms During Aging*, Alan R. Liss, Inc., New York.

Andersen, P., Silfvenius, H., Sundberg, S.H., Sveen, O. and Wigstrom, H. (1978) Functional characteristics of unmyelinated fibers in the hippocampal cortex. *Brain Res.*, 144: 11–18.

Barnes, C.A. (1979) Memory deficits associated with senescence: a neurophysiological and behavioral study in the rat. *J. comp. physiol. Psychol.*, 93: 74–104.

Barnes, C.A. and McNaughton, B.L. (1980a) Physiological compensation for loss of afferent synapses in rat hippocampal granule cells during senescence. *J. Physiol. (Lond.)*, 309: 473–485.

Barnes, C.A. and McNaughton, B.L. (1980b) Spatial memory and hippocampal synaptic plasticity in senescent and middle-aged rats. In D. Stein (Ed.), *The Psychobiology of Aging: Problems and Perspectives*, Elsevier/North-Holland, New York, pp. 253–272.

Bondareff, W. and Geinisman, Y. (1976) Loss of synapses in the dentate gyrus of the senescent rat. *Amer. J. Anat.*, 145: 129–136.

Geinisman, Y. and Bondareff, W. (1976) Decrease in the number of synapses in the senescent brain: a quantitative electron microscopic analysis of the dentate gyrus molecular layer in the rat. *Mech. Age. Develop.*, 5: 11–23.

Geinisman, Y., Bondareff, W. and Dodge, J.T. (1977) Partial deafferentation of neurons in the dentate gyrus of the senescent rat. *Amer. J. Anat.*, 152: 321–330.

Jefferys, J.G.R. (1979) Initiation and spread of action potentials in granule cells maintained in vitro in slices of guinea-pig hippocampus. *J. Physiol. (Lond.)*, 289: 375–388.

Nicholson, C. (1973) Theoretical analysis of field potentials in anisotropic emsembles of neuronal elements. *IEE Trans. Biomed. Engng*, 20: 278–288.

Nicholson, C. (1979) Generation and analysis of extracellular field potentials. In *Society for Neuroscience Short Course, Electrophysiological Techniques*, Atlanta, Georgia.

Simpkins, J.W., Mueller, G.P., Huang, H.H. and Meites, J. (1977) Evidence for depressed catecholamine and enhanced serotonin metabolism in aging male rats: possible relation to gonadotropin secretion. *Endocrinology*, 100: 1672–1678.

Smith, D.O. (1979) Reduced capabilities of synaptic transmission in aged rats. *Exp. Neurol.*, 66: 650–666.

Two Spatial Systems in the Rat Brain – Implications for the Neural Basis of Learning and Memory

JOHN O'KEEFE

Cerebral Functions Group, Department of Anatomy, University College London, Gower Street, London WC1E 6BT (U.K.)

INTRODUCTION

One of the most powerful approaches to a scientific problem is to find a simple "model" system which exemplifies the interesting features of the problem. Principles which have been worked out on the simple "model" system can subsequently be checked to insure their validity on more complex systems. This approach has yielded results in biology in general (e.g. *E. coli* or tobacco mosaic virus) and in neurobiology in particular (e.g. the squid axon and the cholinergic synapse of *Torpedo*).

There are two ways which this model approach can be used in the study of the neural basis of learning and memory. The first involves the study of learning in relatively simple organisms such as invertebrates (e.g. Kandel, 1976); the second involves the study of apparently simple types of learning in higher organisms such as habituation of spinal reflexes (e.g. Thompson and Spencer, 1966) or classical conditioning of the nictitating membrane (e.g. Thompson, 1976). The hope is that the properties of learning derived from the study of these preparations can be generalized to cover more complex types of learning.

My primary reservation about this approach concerns the generality of the results drawn from any particular model system. I will argue in this paper that there are at least two markedly different neural systems which a vertebrate such as the rat uses to find its way around an environment and that changes within these systems during learning are probably based on different principles. The two systems are the hippocampal cognitive mapping system and the ego-centric orientation system. They are part of a more general theory put forward by Nadel and myself (O'Keefe and Nadel, 1978) which I will outline before discussing the two spatial systems.

THE THREE-FOLD WAY: A GENERAL APPROACH TO HYPOTHESIS LEARNING

Krechevsky (1932) originally suggested that when an animal such as the rat is faced with a problem it does not act randomly but generates and tests a series of "hypotheses" about the solution to the problem. In one of his experiments, rats were trained to run in a linear maze in which they had to make four successive choices between pairs of doors to get to the goal. There was no "correct" solution to the

[453]

problem since the "correct" door of each pair was changed in a random fashion from trial-to-trial. In spite of this many rats behaved consistently, trying a particular hypothesis for several trials before changing to a different one. For example, an animal might consistently choose the left doors for several trials and then switch to the right doors for a further series of trials.

Nadel and I have elaborated on this theory and suggested that there are three different types of hypothesis and that these hypotheses are dependent on different brain structures (O'Keefe and Nadel, 1978, pp. 89–101). The three hypotheses we suggested are: (1) place, (2) orientation and (3) guidance. In this paper I will not touch on guidance hypotheses but will restrict myself to a comparison of place and orientation hypotheses and in particular the properties of learning and memory based on them. One of my conclusions will be that place learning can support large shifts in behavior as the result of a single experience whereas orientation hypotheses only support small changes in behavior with each experience and that the neural changes within this system are incremental and cumulative.

PLACE LEARNING AND THE HIPPOCAMPUS

One of the ways an animal can solve a problem is to approach or avoid a particular place in the environment. We have suggested that the ability to do this depends on a neural structure which, following Tolman (1932), we have called a cognitive map. The cognitive map consists of a set of place representations and a subsystem for relating these representations to each other in terms of their relative spatial location. Each place representation consists of a set of place cells in the hippocampus and related areas of the brain such as the entorhinal cortex. As far as can be ascertained, there is no structure to the set of place cells representing a location in an environment nor is there any obvious topographic relationship between place representations in the hippocampus and the parts of the environment which they represent (O'Keefe, 1979). The same cells in the hippocampus represent different places in different environments (Kubie and Ranck, 1981).

Damage to the hippocampal system leads to a loss of place learning and exploration. The evidence for this is extensive and is summarized in Black et al. (1977) and O'Keefe and Nadel (1978, pp. 231–379). The most striking evidence for this claim is the recent demonstration that animals with hippocampal lesions have a total deficit in the place learning version of the Morris (1981) swimming pool maze. In this task, rats are placed into a large swimming pool and required to find a small platform in order to escape from the water.

Two different platforms are used: one is tall enough to protrude above the surface of the water and acts as a guidance cue which can be directly approached by the rat; the other sits below the surface of the water and cannot be perceived until the rat touches it. If the hidden platform remains in the same location in the pool from trial-to-trial the rat should be able to find it using the place system. Animals with hippocampal lesions never learn the location of the hidden platform (Fig. 1) but have no difficulty in learning to escape to the visible platform (Morris et al., 1982). The fact that the brain-damaged rats can learn the guidance version of the task rules out an explanation of the deficit in terms of changes in motivation or motor ability.

The most likely explanation for the deficit is that the animals lack place learning

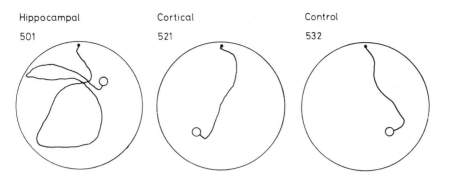

Fig. 1. The actual navigated path of the median rat from the hippocampal-lesioned (left), the cortical-lesioned (middle), and the control (right) groups on the 28th trial of place learning in the Morris swimming pool maze. As a group the hippocampal lesioned rats took 4.66 ± 0.86 m to reach the hidden platform while the cortical and control rats took 2.35 ± 0.98 m and 1.20 ± 0.34 m, respectively.

and must attempt to solve the problem using either orientation or guidance hypotheses. An alternative explanation is that the brain damaged rats have a selective deficit in the perception of the distal cues outside of the swimming pool and that the solution of the place task, but not the guidance task, is dependent on these cues. Another recent experiment from our laboratory controlled for such a difference and also examined the question as to whether the place system could support memory as well as learning.

Conway, Schenk and I wanted to train rats on a place task where the cues were identified and under control. The environment consisted of a set of curtains within which there were a set of cues which the animal could use to locate itself. The cues were spread around the environment and always maintained a constant spatial relationship to each other but the constellation of cues changed from one trial to the next (Fig. 2). The animal's were trained on an elevated +-shaped maze in which one arm always contained food. The problem was to find this goal arm when started from any of the other three arms. The goal arm was defined by its constant relationship to the controlled cues and therefore changed with them from trial to trial in terms of its spatial relation to the external environment. The general idea was to fool the rats into accepting the environment as stable and to disregard the external environment.

Several conclusions can be derived from a series of studies we have done in this type of environment.

(1) With the cues shown in Fig. 2, most normal rats find the task relatively easy to learn. Under the specific training conditions that we used, the median trials to criterion for a typical group of 4 rats would be between 10 and 20 trials.

(2) Some hippocampal cells have place fields inside the cue-controlled environment. The fields maintain their spatial relation to the goal as the cues are rotated from trial to trial. Fig. 3 shows an example of such a result.

(3) Some of these cells maintain their place fields on trials when some of the controlled-cues are removed. For some cells any subset can be removed without serious alteration of the field. The unit shown in Figs. 3 and 4 displayed this behavior. It was somewhat atypical, however, in that part of the sensory control was exerted by intra-maze cues. This was clearly shown when the goal was located in the south east. On such trials the cell refused to fire in the place field. When the

456

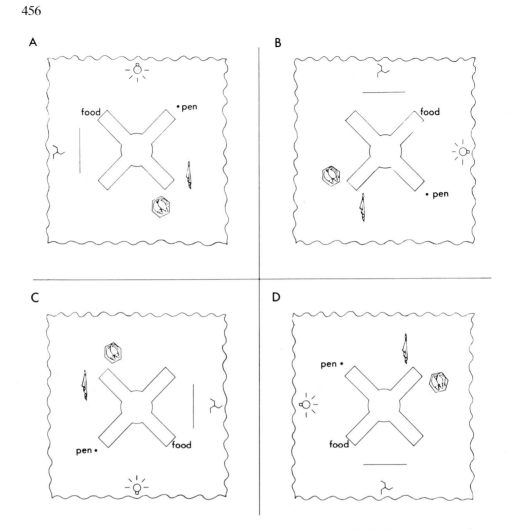

Fig. 2. Four possible configurations of controlled cues and the goal in the distributed-cue task.

south east and north east corners were interchanged, the place field response returned (Fig. 3F).

(4) The problem to be solved within the cue-controlled environment could be altered from a perceptual task to a memory task. This was done by forcing the rats to attend to the controlled cues at the beginning of the trial and then removing the cues before the animal was allowed to run to the goal (see O'Keefe and Conway, 1980). This meant that on each trial the rat had to remember the location of the goal and that this information changed from trial-to-trial.

(5) To our surprise many of the rats learned this memory task relatively quickly. I say surprise because the cued version of the delayed reaction task has proven very difficult for rats (Hunter, 1913; Miles, 1971). When we tested how long the rats could remember the location of the goal on each trial by increasing the time between the offset of the cues and the animal's choice we found no deterioration with delays up to 30 min. This suggests that once established the memory trace held within the place system persists for a long time.

GROUND TRIALS 11/3/1

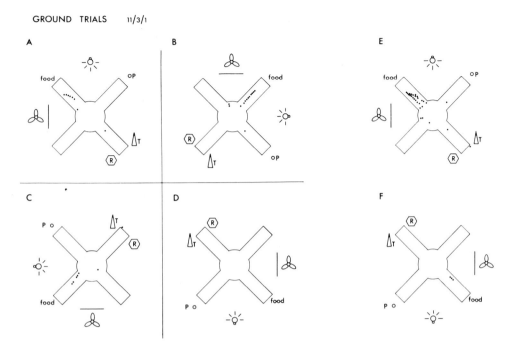

Fig. 3. Place cell. The cell fired when the rat ran to the goal (A, B, C) except when the goal was located in the southeast arm (D). Substitution of the northeast arm for the southeast arm showed that the cell would fire in the southeast but that there must have been an intra-maze cue in that arm which prevented it from doing so (F). E shows the superimposition of A–D after they have been realigned relative to the controlled cues.

(6) Lesions of the fornix, one of the major fiber tracts associated with the hippocampal system, have a marked effect on both the perceptual and memory aspects of the task (O'Keefe, Conway and Schenk, 1983). The animals can relearn the perceptual task but most cannot relearn the memory task in spite of extensive retesting. In order to control for motivational and motor changes following the lesions, we trained another group of rats on a task which was identical except for the configuration of the cues. Instead of having the cues distributed around the maze as in the place task the same cues were clustered behind the goal. We assumed that this would make it more difficult to adopt a place hypothesis and more likely that they would learn on the basis of a guidance hypothesis such as "approach one of the cues". On average the animals in this group took twice as long to learn as the animals in the distributed group. Furthermore none of the animals reached criterion in the memory task and only two scored significantly above chance. Finally, fornix lesions had virtually no effect on the animals performance on the perceptual task suggesting that whatever hypothesis they had used was not based on the hippocampal system.

THE ORIENTATION SYSTEM

The second spatial system consists of a space (or spaces) which emanates from the body (or parts of the body) and is carried around with the body as it moves. In this

458

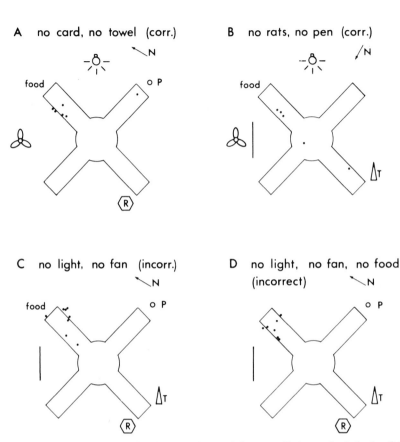

A   no card, no towel (corr.)

B   no rats, no pen (corr.)

C   no light, no fan (incorr.)

D   no light, no fan, no food
(incorrect)

Fig. 4. The results of 4 trials on which different subsets of the controlled cues (and the food) had been removed. The cell continues to identify the goal arm even on trials where the animal chooses incorrectly (C and D). Note that the trials have been displayed so that the goal is in the northeast corner. The actual direction of North is shown by the arrow. On these trials we deliberately tried to avoid using the southeast arm as the goal arm.

section I will only concern myself with the major orientation system which is centered on the body midline axis but it is clear that other spaces with axes centered on individual limbs, the head, or the eye, may also exist.

The simplest way to conceptualize the orientation system is in terms of a polar coordinate system with the origin centered on the animal's head. Directions are specified within this system by an orientation vector which determines the amount of turn around its body axis the animal makes in response to a cue. Fig. 5 shows the polar coordinate system we used to represent the orientation vector. Straight ahead is called 0° while an about face is 180°. Turns to the left are denoted by angles running from L1° to L179°: those to the right by angles R1 to R179°. This system makes mathematic computations more difficult than the standard notation in which 0° denotes the X axis and the angle of the vector increases in an anti-clockwise direction but it has a certain intuitive appeal and is much easier to use while running experiments.

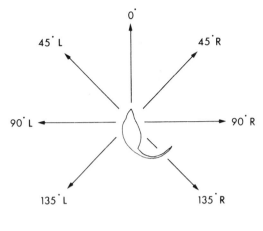

Fig. 5. Schematic diagram showing the representation of body turns within the egocentric orientation system. Any particular turn is represented by a swing of the orientation vector from 0° straight ahead to the angle corresponding to the deviation of the turn from straight ahead.

Our understanding of the orientation system is still at a rudimentary level but some of its properties are becoming clear. The first is that the direction of the orientation vector cannot be read off the animal's behavior in any simple way. Let us consider, for example, an animal which has been trained to make a right turn in a T-shaped maze and which learns to do so on the basis of an orientation hypothesis. On the basis of its surface choice behavior it might be assumed that it is operating on the hypothesis "go straight to the choice point, rotate the orientation vector R90°, go straight to goal". However, when we tested this assumption (O'Keefe, 1983), we found that it was not valid. Rats were trained to make a 90° turn in a T-maze under circumstances which forced them to use an orientation hypothesis: the intra-maze and extra-maze cues were changed sufficiently often during the experiment so that they could not provide consistent cues for solution. One group consisted of 6 control rats and another group consisted of 6 rats with lesions of the fornix. After they had learned, probe experiments were given during which the animals were tested on an 8-arm radial maze and could choose amongst 7 directions instead of the usual 2 of the T-maze (Fig. 6). Eleven of the 12 animals chose arms on the same side of the 7-arm maze as they had on the T-maze but many of them choose directions other than the 90° one on which they had been trained. Some of the animals preferred angles which were closer to 45° while others preferred more acute angles towards the 135° extreme.

Another aspect of this experiment addressed itself to the question of neural plasticity within the orientation system. I looked at the way in which an animal which has learned to choose one of the two arms of a T-maze on the basis of an orientation hypothesis learns to alter its behavior. After the animals had learned to choose one arm I reversed the reward from this arm to the previously incorrect arm. An animal which had been trained to go right, now found no food in the right arm and had to learn to go to the left arm. The changes in the orientation vector during reversal were monitored by giving the animals a probe trial on the 8-arm maze on every third trial. There was no food in any arm on these trials. The results strongly

460

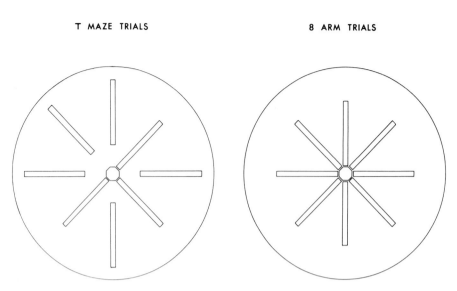

Fig. 6. Plan of the T-maze (left) and the 8-arm probe maze (right).

support the notation that changes within the orientation system take place in an incremental fashion. The animals with damage to the hippocampal system showed this very clearly. The lesioned animal whose data are shown in Fig. 7, gave the clearest evidence for this incremental shift. The animal was originally trained with the left goal correct. It learned the task in 18 trials which was considerably faster than the average.

During reversal, this animal continued to choose the now incorrect left arm for nine trials before abruptly switching to the correct right arm which it continued to choose thereafter. During this period there was no significant change in its latency as shown on the top panel of Fig. 7. In contrast, the bottom panel of Fig. 7 shows that the orientation vector was steadily shifting from the left direction towards which it pointed before reversal to a position on the right side after reversal on the T-maze was completed. Two aspects of this change in the direction of the orientation vector are noteworthy. First, the shift is incremental. The vector shifts by a small amount from trial-to-trial and these increments are cumulative. Second, the change in the animal's choice on the T-maze from left to right roughly coincides with the point that the orientation vector curve crosses the midline (0°). This strongly suggests that the apparent abrupt all-or-none shift in the T-maze performance is a product of the incremental continuous shift in the underlying orientation vector and the dichotomous choice offered by the T-maze. The group data for the lesioned rats show a similar pattern (Fig. 8) but the results of the control animals differ in several important respects (Fig. 9). The clearest difference can be seen in the latency curves. While the lesioned rats showed almost no change in latency, the normal animals showed an increase in latency which began very early during the reversal training. I believe this increase is due to the operation of the hippocampal cognitive map system which must still be operating in this environment despite our attempts to produce an "environmental lesion".

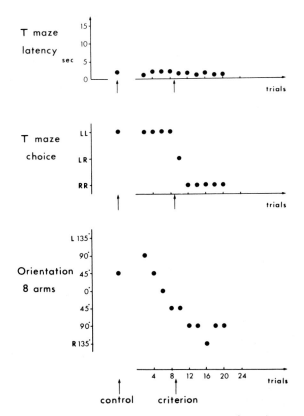

Fig. 7. Three graphs representing the behavior of a fornix-lesioned rat during reversal of an orientation habit on a T-maze. The top graph shows the median latencies for each two trials of a block; the middle graph shows the animals choices on the T maze on these two trials; and the bottom graph shows the choices made by the animal on the 8-arm maze on the probe trial immediately after the two trials on the T maze. The animal switches from the non-rewarded to the rewarded side of the T maze at approximately the point that its orientation vector crosses from the left quadrant to the right quadrant.

IMPLICATIONS FOR THE NEURAL BASIS OF LEARNING AND MEMORY

The data that we have thus far suggest that changes in the two spatial systems occur in markedly different ways. In the place system, information about the spatial cues in an environment can be incorporated into the map in a single exposure and the neural changes are large enough to produce large behavioral changes, e.g. the shift from one goal arm to another on a T-maze. In contrast, the change which occur within the orientation system after a single experience are incremental and, in many behavioral situations, will not be large enough to result in overt changes in an animal's behavior.

462

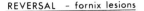

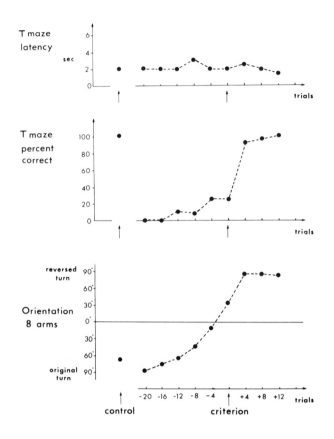

Fig. 8. The graphs for the fornix-lesioned rats plotted in a manner similar to the individual animal shown in Fig. 7. The data are plotted backward and forward from the trial on which the animal began its criterion run. Each point for the latency (top) is the median of 4 trials. The percentage correct on the T maze (middle) is also based on 4 trials. The orientation vector (bottom) is based on two probe trials on the 8-arm maze. Notice that the group shifts from the incorrect to the correct arm at approximately the point when the orientation vector swings from the non-rewarded side to the reversal side.

It seems unlikely, but not impossible, that the synaptic events underlying these two very different types of behavior change would be similar. From this it follows that an understanding of the neurophysiology of one type of learning may tell us little or nothing about the neural processes underlying the other. If this is accepted it places limitations on the generality of the conclusions which can be drawn from either the invertebrate "model system" of Kandel or the nictitating membrane "model system" of Thompson, discussed in the Introduction. In particular it seems to me not unreasonable to suppose that the cognitive mapping system is a recent development in evolution and may be restricted to the vertebrates or to a subsection of them. We will need a whole series of "model systems" on which to base our theories of vertebrate learning and memory.

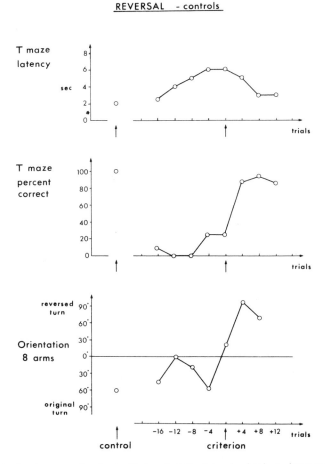

Fig. 9. The graphs for the control animals. Notice that the latencies begin to increase almost from the beginning of reversal training. Furthermore, although the graph of the group data suggests an incremental shift in the orientation vector, none of the individual control rats showed as striking a pattern as seen in the fornix-lesioned rat of Fig. 7.

ACKNOWLEDGEMENTS

I would like to thank Dulcie Conway and Francoise Schenk who participated in some of the experiments described in this paper and the Medical Research Council (U.K.) for their continued support.

REFERENCES

Black, A.H., Nadel, L. and O'Keefe, J. (1977) Hippocampal function in avoidance learning and punishment. *Psychol. Bull.*, 84: 1107–1129.

Hunter, W.S. (1913) The delayed reaction in animals and children. *Behav. Monogr.*, 2: 1–86.

Kandel, E.R. (1976) *Cellular Basis of Behavior*, W.H. Freeman, San Francisco, CA.

Krechevsky, I. (1932) "Hypotheses" in rats. *Phychol. Rev.*, 39: 516–533.

Kubie, J.L. and Ranck, J.B. (1981) Sensory-behavioral correlates in individual hippocampal neurons of the rat across four situations. *Neurosci. Abstr.*, 7: 119.2.

Miles, R.C. (1971) Species differences in "transmitting" spatial location information. In L.E. Jarrard (Ed.), *Cognitive Processes of Non-Human Primates*, Academic Press, New York, pp. 165–179.

Miller, V.M. and Best, P.J. (1980) Spatial correlates of hippocampal unit activity are altered by lesions of the fornix and entorhinal cortex. *Brain Res.*, 194: 311–323.

Morris, R.G.M. (1981) Spatial localization does not require the presence of local cues. *Learn. Motiv.*, 12: 239–260.

Morris, R.G.M., Garrud, P., Rawlins, J.N.P. and O'Keefe, J. (1982) Place navigation impaired in rats with hippocampal lesions. *Nature (Lond.)*, 297: 681–683.

O'Keefe, J. (1979) A review of the hippocampal place cells. *Progr. Neurobiol.*, 13: 419–439.

O'Keefe, J. (1983) The behavioral orientation system: effects of fornix lesions, prior turns, and reversal training. Submitted.

O'Keefe, J. and Conway, D.H. (1980) On the trail of the hippocampal engram. *Physiol. Psychol.*, 8: 229–238.

O'Keefe, J. and Nadel, L. (1978) *The Hippocampus as a Cognitive Map*, Clarendon Press, Oxford.

O'Keefe, J., Conway, D.C. and Schenk, F. (1983) Learning and memory in a cue-controlled environment: the effects of spatial configuration of the cues, delay interval and damage to the hippocampal system. Submitted.

Thompson, R.F. and Spencer, W.A. (1966) Habituation: a model phenomenon for the study of neuronal substrates of behavior. *Psychol. Rev.*, 73: 16–43.

Thompson, R.F., Berger, T.W., Cegavske, C.F., Patterson, M.M., Roemer, R.A., Teyler, T.J. and Young, R.A. (1976) The search for the engram. *Amer. Psychol.*, 31: 209–227.

Tolman, E.C. (1932) *Purposive Behavior in Animals and Man*, Century Co., New York.

Concluding Remarks: On
the "Singularity" of Nerve Cells
and its Ontogenesis

JEAN-PIERRE CHANGEUX

Collège de France and Neurobiologie Moléculaire, Laboratoire associé au Centre National de la Recherche Scientifique, Interactions Moléculaires et Cellulaires, Institut Pasteur, 25, rue du Docteur Roux, 75015 Paris (France)

INTRODUCTION

Those who attended the Meeting under the Cistertian vaults of the Abbaye de Fontevraud and those who have read the impressive group of papers written by its participants, will agree that its title "Molecular and Cellular Interactions Underlying Higher Brain Functions" is still quite ambitious. However, they will agree also, I hope, that, even ambitious, the topic is up to date. During the past ten years, the neurosciences have evolved in a rapid and progressive manner which can be compared to the development of molecular biology in the 1950s. Molecular biology arose from the convergence of biochemistry and genetics. Neurosciences acquired recently a new identity through the convergence of electrophysiology and biochemistry, anatomy and immunology, genetic engineering and phamacology, physics and behavioral sciences. The 20th century began with a revolution in our understanding of matter, it will end, hopefully, with a comparable revolution in our understanding of the brain through that of the functional properties of the neuron and of the neuronal networks.

THE COMPLEXITY OF THE FUNCTIONAL ORGANIZATION OF THE NERVOUS SYSTEM

Understanding the brain stumbles on its "complexity". The word, complexity, often used as a deterrent against simple-minded biochemists or molecular biologists, in fact covers a dramatic ignorance of the anatomical and functional organization of the nervous system at the level where its main originality lies, i.e. the cellular level.

The description of the nerve cells and of their mutual relationships has been investigated in the past by two distinct although complementary approaches. "Histological" techniques led to the description of neuronal morphology and of the local distribution of some biochemical and antigenic markers. "Microphysiological" techniques, thanks to the use of juxta- or intracellular electrodes, have defined the functional modalities of individually recorded cells.

The nervous system of vertebrates contains an ensemble of cells which show the same general shape (soma, axonal and dendritic arborizations), synthetize and release the same neurotransmitter, contain the same receptors for neurotransmitters, and display the same surface antigens. This is, for instance, the case for the Purkinje cells of the cerebellar cortex. Even if in the near future subgroups might be defined within the Purkinje cells (see Chan-Palay et al., 1981), the number of these subgroups is expected to be small compared to the actual total number of Purkinje cells (which may reach $1-2 \times 10^7$ in man) (Palay and Chan-Palay, 1974). The recent subdivision of the amacrine cells in the retina (Morgan, this volume, p. 191; Karten and Brecha, 1980) according to the neurotransmitter they produce, which actually fits with subtle differences in morphology, is not expected to lead to a diversity as large as the number of amacrine cells themselves. Thus it appears legitimate to group, within the same *category*, the smallest ensemble of cells with the same morphological characters (including rules of connectivity) and the same biochemical (and immunological) properties. At least in principle, the category could be defined by a *common repertoire of "open" genes* (able to be transcribed and translated into proteins), in other words, by its *differentiated state*.

On the other hand, microphysiological recordings of single cells within a category disclose clearcut differences. For instance, in the area of projection of eye muscles on the cerebellar vermis, a given Purkinje cell will respond by a *decreased* firing rate when the right lateral rectus muscle is stretched, yet another one will respond by an increased firing rate when the right median rectus muscle now is stretched (see Schwarz and Tomlinson, 1977). In some areas of the cerebellum, Purkinje cells will be characterized by several sensory modalities, in other areas by single ones. Therefore, within a given cell category, a remarkable functional diversity exists. The word *singularity* (Changeux, 1980) can be proposed to qualify this diversity. In principle, the singularity of any cell within a given category can be described by the *repertoire* of *its afferent and efferent synapses*, in other words by its precise *connectivity*. At this level of resolution, little true redundancy exists within a cell category.

Comparative anatomy of the nervous system of vertebrates and invertebrates discloses two different evolutionary trends. Starting from a diffuse (coelenterates), highly redundant, metamerized (worms) organization, one trend is an increase of the number of categories without changing the number of cells; the number of categories therefore approximates the number of cells. This is the case of the nervous system of *Aplysia* (Segal, this volume, p. 157; Kandel, 1976), of the leech (Stent, this volume, p. 147) or of nematodes (Sulston and Horvitz, 1977). Another trend, which manifested itself at least twice in the course of evolution, in cephalopods (Young, 1971) and in vertebrates, results in an increase of the number of cells within a category rather than in the number of categories. Then, a diversification by "singularization" takes place. Interestingly, this diversification often conserves some common functional features or discloses some regularities in the distribution of properties among cells from a given area which may thus form a *map* (of a sensory or motor organ or of another nerve center) (Martin and Perry, this volume, p. 321; Van der Loos and Woolsey, 1973). The first evolutive trend could be referred to as "evolution by categorization", the second one as "evolution by singularization". The complexity of the first group of nervous systems would be directly linked to the repertoire of active genes in any given cell, but this would not be necessarily the case in the second.

If this is true for the cerebral cortex in mammals, then it might be rewarding to look for simple rules of organization common to a cell category or to an ensemble of cell categories, whatever the precise singularity of each individual neuron within a given category. An organization into repetitive vertical "modules" has been emphasized in the past. The recent analysis of simple systems such as the retina (Wässle et al., this volume, p. 183) offers new perspectives. The remarkable regularities noticed in the disposition of cells within the plane of the retina which lead to some kind of "crystalline organization" might not be limited to this system. Indeed, such an organization was already suggested and documented in the case of the cerebellar cortex (Eccles et al., 1967) but for unknown reasons, not considered in the case of the cerebral cortex. It is thus tempting to view the cerebral cortex as a superposition of "*cellular crystals*", analogous (though different) to retina and/or cerebellar cortex. Of course, diversity between areas would then result from differences in the nature and densities of the afferent and efferent fibers. In addition, their orientation and mutual organization might create the well-recognized regularities in vertical organization. Extension to the cerebral cortex of the immunoanatomical methods used with the retina might reveal, in the future, such tangential "crystalline" organizations.

THE ONTOGENESIS OF THE COMPLEXITY OF THE NERVOUS SYSTEM

The differentiation of the neural ectoderm and of the different cell categories, the morphogenesis of the ganglia and/or neural tube are processes of embryonic development which might follow rules similar to those of any other organ of the body. They are thus excluded from this discussion limited to the complexity linked to connectivity.

(a) *Complexity of the genome and complexity of the nervous system compared*

A rather crude and naive manner to relate the organization of the genome with that of the nervous system is to compare the weight of DNA in the fertilized egg and the total number of cells in the adult nervous system. *Drosophila* diploid genome consists of 0.24×10^{-6} µg DNA and there are about 100,000 neurons. In the mouse, the fertilized egg contains 27 times more DNA than in *Drosophila* but the nerve cells are, at least, 60 times more abundant. Man possesses 2–16.5 billion nerve cells in its brain and nearly the same amount of DNA as the mouse per diploid genome. Hybridization experiments between total DNA of chimpanzee and man reveal not more than a 1.1% difference of nucleotide sequences (King and Wilson, 1975). Finally, the estimation of the *absolute* number of different structural genes (of average size) give astonishingly small numbers of 5–6000 in *Drosophila* and 20–100,000 in mammals.

A first answer to this paradox consists in the striking economy of genetic information uncovered recently, within the organism and within the nervous system, at the molecular level. Peptides identified as peripheral hormones, such as VIP or LH-RH, have been recognized as authentic neurotransmitters in the nervous system (see Jan and Jan, this volume, p. 49). The storage and release of different neurotransmitters, such as norepinephrine and acetylcholine, might involve several membrane proteins in common (see Winkler et al., p. 11; Bader et al., p. 21; Morel, p. 31 this volume). Receptor mechanisms might also present striking analogies at the periphery and in the central nervous system. Even though a reluctance has been noticed in the past (perhaps for ideological reasons) to accept that "what is true for the periphery is true for the center", this statement appears largely correct. In a general manner, the *sharing of genetic information* within the organism, leads to an economy of structural genes.

The complex organization of the nervous system thus develops during the course of evolution starting from a small set of genes. Moreover, at least in vertebrates and particularly in mammals, a remarkable *non-linear* relationship is noticed between the evolution of the complexity of the genome and that of the fine anatomy of the nervous system. The complexity of the anatomy increases much faster than that of the genome.

A first formal solution to this paradox is that since no simple relationship exists between genes and neuronal morphology, *combinations* of genes might be used to label each cell and each synapse of a given cell. The number of genes would be, in any instance, sufficient to create a large repertoire of labels. However, this reasoning does not explicitly deal with the non-linearity mentioned above.

Another plausible solution is that a *combinatory* mechanism of another nature accounts for the diversification of nerve cells and requires only a small number of genes which would be "regulatory" in nature.

(b) *Limits of the genetic determinism*

Evidence for such a combinatory mechanism might come from the analysis of the limits occurring in the genetic determinism of the functional organization of the nervous system. It is difficult to define the minimal effect of a gene mutation since it is a priori determined by the sensitivity of the method of mutants selection. For example, some known lesions, caused by point mutations, affect: (1) Purkinje cells (PCD) or granular cells in the mouse (weaver) (Sotelo and Privat, 1978; Caviness and Rakic, 1978); (2) a given photoreceptor cell (e.g. R7) common to all the ommatidia of *Drosophila* eye (Harris et al., 1976), and (3) probably one class of synapses between parallel fibers and Purkinje cell dendrites in the staggerer mouse (Landis and Sidman, 1978; Mariani and Changeux, 1980). The minimal known effect of gene mutations seems to affect all cells (or all synapses) which belong to a given *category*.

Limits in the genetic determinism are also expressed by the phenotypic variance of the fine neuroanatomy of isogenic animals (Levinthal et al., 1976). This variance is significant in small invertebrates like *Daphnia* (Macagno et al., 1973) where it affects the number of morphological synapses within a given category. It may be more important, though difficult to estimate, in mammals where the number of neurons is large (Wimer et al., 1976).

The existence of such limits justifies the concept of a "genetic envelope" which contains the invariant characters of the adult nervous system but also allows significant phenotypic variance.

(c) *Transient structural redundancy: an ontogenetic mechanism of amplification with a low gene cost*

The setting out of neuronal *somas* in highly "categorized" nervous systems such as that of *C. elegans*, of the leech and of the grasshopper (and presumably all the nervous systems with a fixed number of cells), takes place through a sequence of cell divisions and differentiation (including cell death) which follow invariant patterns (Weisblat, this volume, p. 277; Goodman et al., this volume, p. 283).

This is not the case in the nervous systems of high vertebrates. For instance, the lineage of Purkinje cells in the cerebellum of allophenic mice (Mullen, 1978) does not suggest any simple relationship between the adult distribution of these cells and the pattern of division of their immature precursors. After their last division, the precursors of the Purkinje cells migrate to their final location in a quasi-random manner. When they reach the cerebellar cortex they likely are all equivalent. At this stage, before neurite growth, the structural redundancy is maximal. A similar situation might occur during the development of the cerebral cortex, in particular, if its cellular organization appears to be "crystalline", as in the case of the cerebellar cortex.

A redundancy has also been noticed later in development when functional synapses become established. For instance, in the newborn rat, up to five climbing fibers make functional contacts with each Purkinje cell (Crepel et al., 1976; Mariani and Changeux, 1980, 1981) but, in the adult, only a single one persists (Eccles et al., 1966). A similar situation has been reported in the case of sympathetic and parasympathetic (Lichtman, 1977; Lichtman and Purves, 1980) ganglia and in the well known case of the motor endplate (Redfern, 1970; rev. Changeux, 1979). It may simply result from the fact that the elements of structure which determine the formation of the early contacts are not unique to each individual contact but common to the *category* of contacts (for instance the climbing fiber–Purkinje cell synapses). Again, the setting out of this redundant synaptic organization may not require a large number of genes.

A common feature of this redundancy is its *transient* character. During development, significant cell death (up to 40%) occurs and, at later stages, many of the synaptic contacts regress (Mariani, this volume, p. 383; Cowan, 1979) (up to 80%). These regressive phenomena accompany the "singularization" of the nerve cells.

(d) *The activity of the developing neuronal network: its contribution to epigenesis*

Classical cybernetics considers nerve activity mainly as an intermediate component of the input–output relationship of the adult organism in its environment. The activity of the developing neuronal network might also be viewed as an *internal* signalling mechanism which plays a morphogenic role during embryogenesis and postnatal development. The word activity will describe any process, which, directly or indirectly, results in a change of electrical properties of the neuronal membrane including the propagation of action potentials, electrical coupling, chemical transmission and modulation and, eventually, the evoked release of so-called "trophic" factors.

Various electrical phenomena have been recorded during early stages of development, even in the egg (review in Harris, 1981). For instance, *Xenopus* oocytes respond to acetylcholine by a depolarization and to dopamine (or serotonin) by a hyperpolarization (Kusano et al., 1977). In *Amblystoma*, at the early stages of neural tube formation, a difference of membrane potential appears between the ectodermic (about −30 mV) and embryonic neural cells (−44 mV) (Warner, 1973). At later stages regenerative phenomena develop only in this last class of cells.

Spontaneous movements are observed in chick embryos as early as 3–5 days in ovo. These movements last throughout embryogenesis and are neurogenic of origin (Hamburger, 1970). Even growth cones may release significant amounts of neurotransmitter (Cohen, 1980). Such spontaneous neural activity has been recorded in embryos of all groups of vertebrates including man (Bergstrøm, 1969). Most often the spontaneous firing of the neurons occurs as bursts of action potentials. Similar oscillatory behavior of membrane properties has been recorded in many different categories of cells (*Aplysia* neurons, Purkinje fibers of the heart, pancreatic islets (see Berridge and Rapp, 1979)). In all instances the ionic mechanism for generation of these oscillations appears rather simple: two"rapid" Na^+ and K^+ ionic channels for the action potential, and two "slow" K^+ and Ca^{2+} channels for the pacemaker. Genesis of spontaneous activity probably requires only a few structural genes and, in addition, the same gene products can be utilized in different cells and organs.

Sense organs also generate spontaneous activity even before they begin to respond to physical stimuli from the outside world. This is the case for retina ganglion cells (Cavaggioni, 1968) and for vertibular receptors (Wilson and Melvill-Jones, 1979). In a general manner, embryonic sensory receptors may behave as *peripheral* oscillators which contribute to the spontaneous activity recorded in the centers.

Of course, as soon as the sense organs become functional, the contribution of the evoked activity circulating in the developing nervous system becomes more and more significant. It is worth noting that the nervous system where the most striking non-linearity exists between genomic vs neural complexity are precisely those where the period of post natal synaptogenesis lasts longer. This is, of course, highly suggestive of a plausible role of evoked activity, in addition to the spontaneous one, in the regulation of synapse formation.

The working hypothesis that spontaneous and evoked activity plays a morphogenic role during development of the nervous system offers a significant number of possibilities. The activity propagated in the developing network is a long distance mechanism of interaction between cells and even organs. The "convergence" and "divergence" properties of neurons make possible the integration of many signals at the neuronal level. A *combinatory mechanism* can thus be generated by the propagated activity.

THE SELECTIVE STABILIZATION OF DEVELOPING SYNAPSES: A PLAUSIBLE MECHANISM FOR THE SINGULARIZATION OF NERVE CELLS

The theory of epigenesis by selective stabilization (Changeux, 1972; Changeux et al., 1973, 1981; Changeux and Danchin, 1974, 1976) deals with the main issues presented in the previous section. The mechanism proposed is a combinatory mechanism able to generate a considerable diversification of nerve cells on the basis of a small number of genetic determinants. It primarily concerns the highly singularized nervous system of vertebrates (particularly mammals and primates).

The stage of development that was referred to as structural redundancy is taken as the initial state. The theory was originally designed for developing synapses but can be extended to the neuronal somas. At this stage, excitatory (or inhibitory) synapses of the considered category, may exist under at least three states, labile (L), stable (S) and degenerate (D). Only the L and S states transmit nerve inpulses and the acceptable transitions between states are L→S, L→D and S→L. The evolution of the connective state of a given synapse δ is governed by the total message of activity, U(t), afferent to the post-synaptic soma during a prior time interval. This regulatory function of the neuronal soma is referred to as its "evolutive power" Δ. The maximal connectivity, at the peak of transient redundancy, the main stages of development of the network of synaptic connections, the evolutive power of the soma and its integrative properties Φ, in other words the rules of growth and stabilization by activity of the redundant and labile synaptic contacts, is a determinate expression of the genome (the genetic "envelope" of the network).

Neuronal graphs (C, Σ) provide a model of the connective organization of the network where the synapses are labeled by the elements of Σ. If Φ and η respectively represent the rules of propagation and "memorization" by the soma of the afferent multi-messages, then one may consider a mathematical structure R = (C, Σ, θ, η, Φ, Δ) or "neuronal program". The "actualization" of R for a given afferent multimessage during the "critical period" of synaptic plasticity results in the stabilization of a particular set of synapses from the graph (C, Σ) while the other ones regress.

A first consequence of the theory offers a plausible mechanism for the recording of a temporal sequence of nerve impulses as a stable trace which can be described in terms of network growth (and not solely in terms of synapse efficacy – see Kandel, 1976). This trace is printed as a particular pattern of connective organization which exists *before* the critical period of stabilization. It differs from instructive mechanisms which assume, for instance, that a particular message directs the growth of nerve endings towards suitable targets or causes the appearance of new molecular species. The proposed mechanism is a strictly *selective* one.

A second consequence, which can be demonstrated rigorously, is that the same afferent multimessage may stabilize different connective organizations that nevertheless result in the same input–output relationships. What we referred to as "variability" (Changeux et al., 1973) may account for the phenotypic variance noticed in isogenic individuals. It, of course, accounts for the *singularization* of nerve cells within a given *category* at the stage of transient synaptic redundancy. According to these views several different connective combinations may result in the *same* behavior. The code for behavior would thus be "degenerate".

Finally, the genes which compose the genetic envelope, in particular those which determine the rules of growth and stabilization of synaptic contacts might be "open" in the highly singularized nervous systems, in all the nerve cells which belong to the *same category*. Thus the cost in genes might be rather low. The development of an amplification device by transient structural redundancy associated with a combinatory epigenetic mechanism may account at least in part for the paradoxical non-linearity noticed between the complexity of the genome and that of the connective organization of the mammalian nervous system.

EXPERIMENTAL TEST OF THE THEORY

Only fragmentary data are yet available. The central issue of the theory, (that synapse stabilization and elimination is the mechanism for nerve cells' singularization and thus for the development of their specific functional modalities), still requires an unambiguous demonstration. The experimental observations reported here concern only two systems: (1) the neuromuscular junction from chick embryo and newborn rat, and (2) the cerebellar cortex from rat and mouse. Moreover, *only data from our laboratory shall be mentioned* (for a general recent review see Harris, 1981)

(a) *Consequences of the chronic paralysis of chick embryos on the development of the neuromuscular junction*

When nicotinic antagonists such as curare, flaxedil or snake α-toxins are chronically injected into yolk sacs of chick embryos, spontaneous movements of the embryos are blocked without systematically causing their death. (In adults, death results from the paralysis of the respiratory muscles.) This essentially post-synaptic (the antagonists bind to the acetylcholine receptor) and peripheral (the pharmacological agents do not cross the blood–brain barrier) blocking has consequences both on the pre- and post-synaptic sides of the motor endplates.

A significant decrease of the total content of the *pre-synaptic* enzyme choline acetyltransferase (responsible for acetylcholine synthesis) in the muscle and sciatic nerve takes place after paralysis by α-bungarotoxin from the 3rd to 12th day of incubation (Giacobini et al., 1973, 1975; Betz et al., 1980). The total number of motor neurons which persist in the spinal cord also decreases below the normal level under the same conditions. However, different conditions of paralysis (such as by curare instead of α-bungarotoxin from the 6th to 9th day in ovo) have the opposite effect (refs. in Pittman and Oppenheim, 1978). Many more motor neurons persist in the paralyzed compared to control embryos. Under these conditions, paralysis prevents cell death. In any case, and in agreement with the selective stabilization hypothesis, cell death, and therefore the survival of the adult neurons, appears regulated by the activity of the neuromuscular junction.

At the *post-synaptic* level, chronic paralysis does not interfere with the subsynaptic accumulation of the acetylcholine receptor but interferes with the disappearance of the extrajunctional receptor (refs. in Betz et al., 1980). More extrasynaptic receptors persist in the paralyzed embryo. Since the half life of the receptor molecule does not change under these conditions, the regulation must take place at the level of the receptor protein synthetic machinery. In the course of normal development, the neurally evoked electrical activity of the muscle thus represses the synthesis of acetylcholine receptor. An involvement of Ca^{2+} and/or cyclic nucleotides as "second messengers" in this regulation appears plausible (Betz and Changeux, 1979).

Chronic post-synaptic block prevents the localization of the degradative enzyme acetylcholinesterase. Activity of the muscle is *required* for the local accumulation of the enzyme in the basal lamina which covers the subsynaptic membrane (Giacobini et al., 1973; Gordon et al., 1974; Oppenheim et al., 1978; Rubin et al., 1980). Since the transmission efficiency of the endplate depends on the synaptic content of acetylcholinesterase, this regulation can be taken as a model for the effect of "disuse" or "experience" on the functional (and biochemical) properties of a synapse.

(b) *Effect of chronic stimulation of chick embryo spinal cord on the pattern of motor endplates*

In the chick, the wing muscles, latissimus dorsi, receive two distinct types of innervation. The slow *anterior* muscle (ALD) shows several endplates distributed at approximately equal distances along the muscle fiber, while the fast *posterior* muscle (PLD) receives a single focal endplate in the middle of the fiber.

Cross-innervation experiments in the embryo have shown that the nerve, not the muscle, determines the pattern of endplates (Hnik et al., 1967; Zelena et al., 1967). Moreover, during development, the programs of neurally evoked spontaneous activity differ in the two muscles: in 15-day-old embryos, the ALD shows a sustained low activity of around 0.2–1 Hz, whereas the PLD shows high frequency bursts of activity around 8 Hz interrupted by periods of silence (Gordon et al., 1977).

To test the hypothesis that the activity of the nerve regulates or even determines the pattern of endplates, electrodes were chronically implanted around the brachial spinal cord in 7-day embryos in ovo by the method developed by Renaud et al. (1978) and electric pulses delivered at 0.5 Hz frequency from the 10th to 15th day of incubation. Quantitative analysis of the number and distribution of clusters of acetylcholine receptor (Toutant et al., 1980) and of patches of acetylcholinesterase activity (Toutant et al., 1981) discloses a significant increase of their number per individual PLD muscle fiber and per total PLD muscle (by a factor of 1.8–2.0). However, the distribution of the multiple clusters of acetylcholine receptor which appear in the normally focally innervated PLD is not as regular as in ALD. The parallel evolution of the clusters of acetylcholine receptor and esterase supports the conclusion that the chronic stimulation of the PLD muscle with a program close to that of ALD, results in a distributed pattern of endplates over the fiber. An electrophysiological demonstration of this point is, as yet, lacking.

A still theoretical, and thus speculative, biochemical mechanism (Changeux et al., 1981) has been proposed to account for the epigenetic dependence of the ALD and PLD synaptic topologies upon the afferent multimessage resulting from the spontaneous activity of the spinal cord during development. In its initial state the muscle fiber receives exploratory motor nerve endings (originating from the same neuron) at multiple points randomly distributed along the fiber. At each of these points the nerve endings release acetylcholine and, as a consequence, the neurally evoked activity of the muscle fiber stops the synthesis of receptor. The biochemical postulates of the model are restricted to: (1) the interconversion of the receptor protein from a labile L form to an A form, which may aggregate under a nerve terminal (while the L does not) but still diffuses laterally in the muscle membrane; (2) the release by the nerve endings of an "anterograde factor" with a finite half-life, the amount of factor liberated being directly linked to the afferent multimessage $U(t)$; once liberated the factor triggers the transformation of L to A; (3) the aggregation of the receptor begins and continues with a faster rate when the local concentration of A reaches a threshold value. The computer simulation of the mathematical model confirms that the biochemical hypotheses made are sufficient to obtain a distributed pattern of acetylcholine receptor clusters (nevertheless in numbers smaller than the initial number of contacts) when the afferent multimessage is continuous and a focal pattern when it is in bursts. Even though plausible, none of the biochemical hypotheses made have yet been demonstrated experimentally.

(c) *Experimental analysis of the regression of polyneuronal innervation of skeletal muscle in newborn rats*

At birth, in the rat, acetylcholine receptor and esterase are localized at the motor endplate which receives several functional nerve terminals originating from different motor neurons. Twenty days after birth, a single nerve ending persists per endplate. This regression coincides with the segregation of the motor units. In the simplest situation, each motor neuron innervates the same number of muscle fibers (motor unit) but no regularity exists in the relative distribution of the muscle fibers in any given motor unit. In other words, the muscle fibers from different motor units are randomly mixed (review in Brown et al., 1976). In a first attempt to demonstrate an effect of activity on the regression of multiple innervation, one tendon of the sartorius muscle was sectioned in newborn rats. As a consequence, the mechanical activity of the muscle becomes negligible and an important delay in the regression of the multi-innervation takes place (Benoit and Changeux, 1975). The paralysis of the motor nerve by a cuff of local anesthetic has the same effect (Benoit and Changeux, 1978). Finally, chronic electrical stimulation accelerates the regression of the multiple innervation. In conclusion, the stabilization of one motor nerve ending per muscle fiber is an "active" process that nerve activity regulates.

A theoretical model (Gouzé et al., 1983) accounts for this evolution, if one assumes that: (1) a *retrograde* post-synaptic factor, produced in limiting amounts by the muscle fibers, is required for the stabilization of the motor nerve ending; (2) an uptake of the retrograde factor by the nerve terminal takes place; (3) when an impulse reaches the nerve terminal the retrograde factor combines with an *internal* presynaptic factor to yield an active complex which triggers the stabilization of the nerve endings.

(d) *Post-natal evolution of the olivo-cerebellar relationships in rat and mouse*

If the occurrence of transient polyneuronal innervation were unique to the neuromuscular junction, this phenomenon could not be taken as a model for a general mechanism of neurogenesis. It was thus essential to examine, in this respect, another system. The innervation of the Purkinje cells from cerebellar cortex by the climbing fibers (which originate from olivary neurons) appears adequate since, in the adult, only one climbing fiber innervates each Purkinje cell (Eccles et al., 1966). Interestingly, in newborn rat, *several* functional climbing fibers (up to 5) end on each Purkinje cell (Crépel et al., 1976) but all of them, except one, are eliminated later during development (Mariani and Changeux, 1980b). An important spontaneous activity is recorded in the system (Mariani and Changeux, 1981) but its contribution to the stabilization of the adult synapses is not demonstrated. On the other hand, the elimination of granular cells in the newborn by X-ray irradiation or mutation is followed by the maintenance, in the adult, of the multi-innervation of the Purkinje cell by several climbing fibers (Crépel and Mariani, 1976; Mariani et al., 1977; Mariani and Changeux, 1980a, 1981; Mariani, this volume, p. 383).

CONCLUSION

The selective stabilization as a theory of developing synapses brings one, but
— necessarily limited, answer to the questions raised by the ontogenesis of complexity

at a low gene cost. It offers a plausible mechanism for nerve cell "singularization" based on the combination of elementary activities working on a redundant and labile framework of developing synapses. It is neither unique nor exclusive of other mechanisms of diversification, for instance associated with an ordered growth of axons (Martin and Perry, this volume, p. 321) leading to the formation of topographical representations (or "maps") of the periphery into the centers and of one center into another. Its extension to complex systems such as the cerebral cortex (see Rakic, this volume, p. 393; Goldman-Rakic, this volume, p. 405; and Imbert and Frégnac, this volume, p. 427) appears worth trying.

ACKNOWLEDGEMENTS

We thank B. Holton for her criticisms of the manuscript and M. Spear for typing it. This work was supported by grants from the Muscular Dystrophy Association of America, the Fondation de France, the Fondation pour la Recherche Médicale, the Collège de France, the Délégation Générale à Recherche Scientifique et Technique, the Centre National de la Recherche Scientifique, the Institut National de la Santé at de la Recherche Médicale and the Commissariat à l'Energie Atomique.

REFERENCES

Benoit, P. and Changeux, J.P. (1975) Consequences of tenotomy on the evolution of multi-innervation in developing rat soleus muscle. *Brain Res.*, 99: 354–358.

Benoit, P. and Changeux, J.P. (1978) Consequences of tenotomy on the evolution of multi-innervation at the regenerating neuromuscular junction of the rat. *Brain Res.*, 149: 89–96.

Bergstrøm, R. (1969) Electrical parameters of the brain during ontogeny. In R.J. Robinson (Ed.), *Brain and Early Behavior*, Academic Press, New York, p. 15.

Berridge, M.J. and Rapp, P.E. (1979) A comparative survey of the function, mechanism and control of cellular oscillators. *J. exp. Biol.*, 81: 217–279.

Betz, H. and Changeux, J.P. (1979) Regulation of muscle acetylcholine receptor synthesis in vitro by derivatives of cyclic nucleotides. *Nature (Lond.)*, 278: 749–752.

Betz, H., Bourgeois, J.P. and Changeux, J.P. (1980) Evolution of cholinergic proteins in developing slow and fast skeletal muscles in chick embryo. *J. Physiol. (Lond.)*, 302: 197–218.

Brown, M.C., Jansen, J.K.S. and Van Essen, D. (1976) Polyneural innervation of skeletal muscle in new-born rats and its elimination during maturation. *J. Physiol. (Lond.)*, 261: 387–422.

Cartaud, J., Sobel, A., Rousselet, A., Devaux, P.F. and Changeux, J.P. (1981) Consequences of alkaline treatment for the ultrastructure of the acetylcholine receptor-rich membranes from *Torpedo marmorata* electric organ. *J. Cell. Biol.*, 90: 418–426.

Cavaggioni, A. (1968) The dark discharge of the eye in the unrestrained cat. *Pflüger's Arch.*, 304: 75–80.

Caviness, V. and Rakič, P. (1978) Mechanisms of cortical development: a view from mutation in mice. *Ann. Rev. Neurosci.*, 1: 297–326.

Chan-Palay, V., Nivaler, G., Palay, S.L., Beinfeld, M., Zimmerman, E.A., Jang-Yen Wu and O'Donohue, T.L. (1981) Chemical heterogeneity and cerebellar Purkinje cells: existence and co-existence of glutamic acid decarboxylase-like and motiline-like immunoreactivity. *Proc. nat. Acad. Sci. U.S.A.*, 78: 7787–7791.

Changeux, J.P. (1972) Le cerveau et l'évènement. *Communications*, 18: 37–47.

Changeux, J.P., Courrège, Ph. and Danchin, A. (1973) A theory of the epigenesis of neural networks by selective stabilization of synapses. *Proc. nat. Acad. Sci. U.S.A.*, 70: 2974–2978.

Changeux, J.P. and Danchin, A. (1974) "Apprendre par stabilisation sélective de synapses en cours de développement". In E. Morin and M. Piatteli (Eds.), *L'Unité de l'Homme*, Le Seuil, Paris, pp. 320–357.

Changeux, J.P. and Danchin, A. (1976) Selective stabilization of developing synapses as a mechanism for the specification of neuronal networks. *Nature (Lond.)*, 264: 705–712.

Changeux, J.P. (1979) Molecular interactions in adult and developing neuromuscular junction. In F.O. Schmitt and F.G. Worden (Eds.), *The Neurosciences. Fourth Study Program*, The MIT Press, Cambridge, MA, pp. 749–778.

Changeux, J.P. (1980) *Ann. Collège de France*, 80: 309–343.

Changeux, J.P., Courrège, Ph., Danchin, A. and Lasry, J.M. (1981) Un mécanisme biochimique pour l'épigénèse de la jonction neuromusculaire. *C.R. Acad. Sci. (Paris)*, 292: 449–453.

Cohen, S.A. (1980) Early nerve–muscle synapses in vitro release transmitter over synaptic membrane having low acetylcholine sensitivity. *Proc. nat. Acad. Sci. U.S.A.*, 77: 644–648.

Cowan, W.M. (1979) Selection and control in neurogenesis. In F.O. Schmitt and F.G. Worden (Eds.), *The Neurosciences. Fourth Study Program*, The MIT Press, Cambridge, MA, pp. 59–81.

Crepel, F. and Mariani, J. (1976) Multiple innervation of Purkinje climbing fibers in the cerebellum of the weaver mutant mouse. *J. Neurobiol.*, 7: 579–582.

Crepel, F., Mariani, J. and Delhaye-Bouchaud, N. (1976) Evidence for a multiple innervation of Purkinje cells by climbing fibers in the immature rat cerebellum. *J. Neurobiol.*, 7: 567–578.

Eccles, J.C., Llinas, R. and Sasaki, K. (1966) The excitatory synaptic action of climbing fibers on the Purkinje cells of the cerebellum. *J. Physiol. (Lond.)*, 182: 268–296.

Eccles, J., Ito, M. and Szentagothai, J. (1967) *The Cerebellum as a Neuronal Machine*, Springer-Verlag, Berlin.

Giacobini, G., Filogamo, G., Weber, M., Boquet, P. and Changeux, J.P. (1973) Effects of a snake α-neurotoxin on the development of innervated motor muscles in chick embryo. *Proc. nat. Acad. Sci. U.S.A.*, 70: 1708–1712.

Giacobini-Robecchi, M.G., Giacobini, G., Filogamo, G. and Changeux, J.P. (1975) Effect of the type A-toxin from *C. botulinum* on the development of skeletal muscles and of their innervation in chick embryo. *Brain Res.*, 83: 107–121.

Gordon, T., Perry, R., Tuffery, A.R. and Vrbova, G. (1974) Possible mechanisms determining synapse formation in developing skeletal muscles of the chick. *Cell Tiss. Res.*, 115: 13–25.

Gordon, T., Purves, R. and Vrbova, G. (1977). Differentiation of electrical and contractile properties of slow and fast muscle fibers. *J. Physiol. (Lond.)*, 269: 535–547.

Gouzé, J.L., Lasry, J.M. and Changeux, J.P. (1983) The selective stabilization of motor units during development of muscle innervation: a mathematical model. *Biol. Cybernet.*, in press.

Hamburger, V. (1970) Embryonic mobility in vertebrates. In F.O. Schmitt (Ed.), *The Neurosciences. Second Study Program*. The Rockefeller University Press, New York, pp. 141–151.

Harris, W.A., Stark, W.S. and Walker, J.A. (1976) Genetic dissection of the photoreceptor system in the compound eye of *Drosophila melanogaster*. *J. Physiol. (Lond.)*, 256: 415–439.

Harris, W.A. (1981) Neural activity and development. *Ann. Rev. Physiol.*, 43: 689–710.

Henderson, C.E., Huchet, M. and Changeux, J.P. (1981) Neurite outgrowth from embryonic chicken spinal neurons is promoted by media conditioned by muscle cells. *Proc. nat. Acad. Sci. U.S.A.*, 78: 2625–2629.

Hnik, P., Jirmanova, I., Vyklicky, L. and Zelena, J. (1967) Fast and slow muscles of the chick after nerve cross-union. *J. Physiol. (Lond.)*, 193: 309–325.

Kandel, E. (1976) *Cellular Basis of Behavior*, W.H. Freeman, San Francisco, CA, 727 pp.

Karten, J.J. and Brecha, N. (1980) Localization of substance P immunoreactivity in amacrine cells of the retina. *Nature (Lond.)*, 283: 87–88.

King, M.C. and Wilson, A.C. (1975) Evolution at two levels in humans and chimpanzees. *Science*, 188: 107–116.

Kusano, K., Miledi, R. and Stinnakre, J. (1977) Acetylcholine receptors in the oocyte membrane. *Nature (Lond.)*, 270: 739–741.

Labat-Robert, J., Saitoh, T., Godeau, G., Robert, L. and Changeux, J.P. (1980) Distribution of macromolecules from the intercellular matrix in the electroplaque of *Electrophorus electricus*. *FEBS Lett.*, 120: 259–263.

Landis, D.M. and Sidman, R.L. (1978) Electron microscopic analysis of postnatal histogenesis in the cerebellar cortex of staggerer mutant mice. *J. comp. Neurol.*, 179: 831–863.

Levinthal, F., Macagno, E. and Levinthal, C. (1976) Anatomy and development of identified cells in isogenic organisms. *Cold Spr. Harb. Symp. quant. Biol.*, 40: 321–332.

Lichtman, J.W. (1977) The reorganization of synaptic connexions in the rat submandibular ganglion during postnatal development. *J. Physiol. (Lond.)*, 273: 155–177.

Lichtman, J.W. and Purves, D. (1980) The elimination of redundant preganglionic innervation to hamster sympathetic ganglion cells in early postnatal life. *J. Physiol. (Lond.)*, 301: 213–228.

Macagno, E., Lopresti, V. and Levinthal, C. (1973) Structure and development of neuronal connexions in isogenic organisms: variations and similarities in the optic system of *Daphnia magna. Proc. nat. Acad. Sci. U.S.A.*, 70: 57–61.

Mariani, J. and Changeux, J.P. (1980a) Multiple innervation of Purkinje cells by climbing fibers in the cerebellum of the adult *staggerer* mutant mouse. *J. Neurobiol.* 11: 41–50.

Mariani, J. and Changeux, J.P. (1980b) Etude par enregistrements intracellulaires de l'innervation multiple des cellules de Purkinje par les fibres grimpantes dans le cervelet de rat en développement. *C.R. Acad. Sci. (Paris)*, 291: 97–100.

Mariani, J. and Changeux, J.P. (1981) Ontogenesis of olivocerebellar relationships: I – Studies by intracellular recordings of the multi-innervation of Purkinje cells by climbing fibers in the developing rat cerebellum. *J. Neurosci.*, 1: 696–702. idem. II – Spontaneous activity of inferior olivary neurons and climbing fiber-mediated activity of cerebellar Purkinje cells in developing rats and in adult cerebellar mutant mice. *J. Neurosci.*, 1: 703–709.

Mariani, J., Crépel, F., Mikoshiba, K., Changeux, J.P. and Sotelo, C. (1977) Anatomical, physiological and biochemical studies of the cerebellum from *reeler* mutant mouse. *Phil. Trans. B*, 281: 1–28.

Monod, J. (1980) In M. Piattelli-Palmarini (Ed.), *Language and Learning*, Harvard University Press, p. 199.

Mullen, R.J. (1978) Mosaicism in the central nervous system of mouse chimeras. In S. Bubtelny and I.M. Sussex (Eds.), *The Clonal Basis of Development*, Academic Press, New York.

Oppenheim, R.W., Pittman, R., Gray, M. and Madredrut, J.L. (1978) Embryonic behavior, hatching and neuromuscular development in the chick following a transient reduction of spontaneous mobility and sensory input by neuromuscular blocking agents. *J. comp. Neurol.*, 179: 619–640.

Palay, S. and Chan-Palay, V. (1974) *Cerebellar Cortex*, Springer-Verlag, Berlin.

Pittmann, R. and Oppenheim, R.W. (1979) Cell death of motoneurons in the chick embryo spinal cord. *J. comp. Neurol.*, 187: 425–446.

Redfern, P.A. (1970) Neuromuscular transmission in new-born rats. *J. Physiol. (Lond.)*, 209: 509–534.

Renaud, D., Le Douarin, G. and Khaskiye, A. (1978) Spinal cord stimulation in chick embryo: effects on development of the posterior latissimus dorsi muscle and neuromuscular junction. *Exp. Neurol.*, 60: 189–200.

Rousselet, A., Cartaud, J. and Devaux, P.F. (1979) Importance des interactions protéine-protéine dans le maintien de la structure des fragments excitables de l'organe électrique de *Torpedo marmorata. C.R. Acad. Sci. (Paris) D*, 289: 461–463.

Rubin, L.L., Schuetze, S.M., Weill, C.L. and Fischbach, G.D. (1980) Regulation of acetylcholinesterase appearance at neuromuscular junction in vitro. *Nature (Lond.)*, 283: 264–267.

Saitoh, T., Wennogle, L. and Changeux, J.P. (1979) Factors regulating the susceptibility of the acetyl-choline receptor protein to heat inactivation. *FEBS Lett.*, 108: 489–494.

Saitoh, T. and Changeux, J.P. (1981) Change in the state of phosphorylation of the acetylcholine receptor during maturation of the electromotor synapse in *Torpedo marmorata* electric organ. *Proc. nat. Acad. Sci. U.S.A.*, 78: 4430–4434.

Schwarz, D.W. and Tomlinson, R.D. (1977) Neuronal responses to eye-muscle stretch in cerebellar lobule VI of the cat. *Exp. Brain Res.*, 27: 101–111.

Sotelo, C. and Privat, A. (1978) Synaptic remodeling of the cerebellar circuitry in mutant mice and experimental cerebellar malformations. *Acta neuropath.*, 43: 19–34.

Sulston, J.E. and Horvitz, H.R. (1977) Postembryonic cell lineage of the nematode *Caenorhabditis elegans. Develop. Biol.*, 56: 110–246.

Toutant, M., Bourgeois, J.P., Toutant, J.P., Renaud, D., Le Douarin, G. and Changeux J.P. (1980) Chronic stimulation of the spinal cord in developing chick embryo causes the differentiation of multiple clusters of acetylcholine receptor in the posterior latissimus dorsi muscle. *Develop. Biol.*, 76: 384–395.

Toutant, M., Toutant, J.P., Renaud, D., Le Douarin, G. and Changeux, J.P. (1981) Effet de la stimulation médullaire chronique sur le nombre total de sites d'activité acétylcholinérasique du muscle posterior latissimus dorsi de l'embryon de poulet. *C.R. Acad. Sci. (Paris)*, 292: 771–775.

478

Van der Loos, H. and Woolsey, T. (1973) Somatosensory cortex: structural alterations following early injury to sense organs. *Science*, 179: 395–398.

Warner, A.E. (1973) The electrical properties of the ectoderm in the amphibian embryo during induction and early development of the nervous system. *J. Physiol. (Lond.)*, 235: 267–286.

Wilson, V.J. and Melvill-Jones, G. (1979) *Mammalian Vestibular Physiology*, Plenum Press, New York.

Wimer, R.E., Wimer, C.C., Vaughn, J.E., Barber, R.P., Balvanz, B.A. and Chernow, C.R. (1976) The genetic organization of neuron number of Ammon's horns of house mice. *Brain Res.*, 118: 219–243.

Young, J.Z. (1971) *The Anatomy of the Nervous System of Octopus vulgaris*, Clarendon Press, Oxford, 690 pp.

Zelena, J. and Jirmanova, I. (1973) Ultrastructure of chicken slow muscle after nerve cross union. *Exp. Neurol.*, 38: 272–285.

Subject Index